Functional MRI

An Introduction to Methods

Edited by

PETER JEZZARD, PAUL M. MATTHEWS, and
STEPHEN M. SMITH

Centre for Functional Magnetic Resonance Imaging of the Brain,
Department of Clinical Neurology, University of Oxford, UK

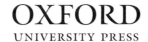

OXFORD

UNIVERSITY PRESS

Great Clarendon Street, Oxford OX2 6DP

Oxford University Press is a department of the University of Oxford.
It furthers the University's objective of excellence in research, scholarship,
and education by publishing worldwide in

Oxford New York

Athens Auckland Bangkok Bogotá Bombay Buenos Aires Kolkata
Cape Town Dar es Salaam Delhi Florence Hong Kong Istanbul Karachi
Kuala Lumpur Madrid Melbourne Mexico City Mumbai Nairobi Paris
São Paulo Shanghai Singapore Taipei Tokyo Toronto Warsaw

and associated companies in Berlin Ibadan

Oxford is a registered trade mark of Oxford University Press
in the UK and in certain other countries

Published in the United States
by Oxford University Press Inc., New York

A catalogue record for this title is available from the British Library

Library of Congress Cataloging in Publication Data
Functional MRI : an introduction to methods / edited by Peter Jezzard,
P.M. Matthews, and Stephen M. Smith.
Includes bibliographical references and index.
1. Brain–Magnetic resonance imaging   I. Jezzard, Peter
II. Matthews, Paul M.   III. Smith, Stephen M.
RC386.6.M34 F863 2001   616.8′047548–dc21   2001035793

ISBN 0 19 263071 7

2 4 6 8 9 7 5 3 1

Typeset by Florence Production Ltd,
Stoodleigh, Devon
Printed in Great Britain on acid-free paper by
Bookcraft Ltd, Midsomer Norton, Avon

OXFORD MEDICAL PUBLICATIONS

Functional MRI

Preface

The growth of magnetic resonance imaging (MRI) as a tool for studying brain function, as opposed to its more traditional role as a tool for studying brain anatomy and pathology, has been quite remarkable over the past decade. This has been driven in large measure by an appreciation of the considerable potential for functional magnetic resonance imaging (fMRI) to increase our understanding of how the human brain works, both in the normal and diseased states. FMRI-based research has drawn together a multi-disciplinary community of neuroscientists, clinicians, engineers, physicists, and image analysis specialists focusing on common problems. However, as fMRI and related methods mature, there is an increasing tendency for studies employing them to be performed in smaller hospitals and research institutions, often without the benefit of large teams for research support, but with important questions ripe for exploration. To those newcomers who wish to exploit fMRI and related methods in solving neurobiological problems, it can seem as though there is a bewildering range of information that must be absorbed.

The motivation for compiling this book was to provide a rigorous yet accessible introduction to the burgeoning field of fMRI and, in particular, the method of blood oxygenation level dependent (BOLD) contrast. Although other books, chapters, and review articles which deal with fMRI have appeared, there is a conscious effort in this book to cater more for the needs of the novice fMRI researcher, than for the expert fMRI scientist. In this respect, we have tried to keep the needs of the neuropsychologist, the experimental cognitive neuroscientist, or the research-oriented physician in mind in tailoring the chapters. In each chapter in this book, little or no previous knowledge of the principles or practice of fMRI is assumed. At the same time, a high level of rigour is also sought.

The target audience is a wide group of individuals who participate in this multi-disciplinary endeavour. In particular we hope to provide a useful text book to those who are new to fMRI, but want to use it as a tool for study of the brain. Our own experience with graduate students and postdocs is that the best fMRI experiments are performed by those who appreciate the underlying brain physiology, and seek to understand the 'black box' beneath the MRI scanner and the analysis computer. By doing so, the complexity of question that can be asked, and the level of interpretation that can be made, are vastly improved. This book is aimed at those inquiring individuals.

The book is divided into six main parts. In Part I a broad overview of the field is provided, which also serves to set the remainder of the book in context. In Part II the physiological and physical background to fMRI is given. This includes a consideration of the necessary hardware and pulse sequence selection. Practical issues involving experimental design of the paradigms and also psychophysical stimulus delivery and subject response are provided in Part III, followed by a comprehensive treatment of data analysis in Part IV. General issues underlying applications, both to questions in neuroscience and to questions in clinical science, are given in Part V. The book concludes in Part VI with a discussion of how fMRI can be integrated with other neuro-electro-magnetic functional mapping techniques.

The scope of expertise required to write a book with authority on this range of topics demanded that it became a multi-authored work. We have been remarkably fortunate to have secured chapters and input from colleagues of the highest calibre. As such, our primary duty is to thank them all sincerely for their scholarly didactic contributions. We also thank a number of individuals who have read parts of this book in an attempt to provide feedback which should ensure that the book remains accessible to its target audience. We also thank Oxford University Press for their patience and help.

Oxford
February 2001

P.J.
P.M.M.
S.M.S.

Basic . 1, 9 - 16
Intro°

Contents

Contributors

P.A. Bandettini   Unit on Functional Imaging Methods, Laboratory of Brain and Cognition, National Institute of Mental Health, Bethesda, MD, USA.

M.J. Brammer   Brain Image Analysis Unit, Institute of Psychiatry, London, UK.

J.A. Brookes   Resonance Magnetiques des Systemes Biologiques, UMR 5536, CNRS/University Victor Segalen Bordeaux2, Bordeaux, France.

C. Büchel   Department of Neurology, University of Hamburg, Germany.

R.L. Buckner   Department of Radiology, Department of Anatomy and Neurobiology, Washington University, St Louis, MO, USA.

S. Clare   Centre for Functional Magnetic Resonance Imaging of the Brain, Department of Clinical Neurology, University of Oxford, UK.

D.I. Donaldson   Department of Psychology, Department of Anatomy and Neurobiology, Washington University, St Louis, MO, USA.

R. Epstein   MRC Cognition and Brain Sciences Unit, Cambridge, UK.

K. Friston   Wellcome Department of Cognitive Neurology, University College London, UK.

J.S. George   Biophysics Group, Los Alamos National Laboratory, Los Alamos, NM, USA.

A. Gisbert   MR Research Programmme, Univerisity of Illinois, Chicago, USA.

A. Gjedde   Pathophysiological and Experimental Tomography Centre, Aarhus General Hospital, Aarhus, Denmark.

G.H. Glover   Department of Radiology, Lucas MR Building, Stanford University, USA.

B.G. Goodyear   Department of Clinical Neurosciences and Radiology, Seaman Family Magnetic Resonance Research Centre, University of Calgary, Alberta, Canada.

R.D. Hoge   Nuclear Magnetic Resonance Centre, Massachusetts General Hospital, Department of Radiology, Harvard Medical School, Charlestown, MA, USA.

M. Jenkinson   Centre for Functional Magnetic Resonance Imaging of the Brain, Department of Clinical Neurology, University of Oxford, UK.

P. Jezzard   Centre for Functional Magnetic Resonance Imaging of the Brain, Department of Clinical Neurology, University of Oxford, UK.

I.S. Johnsrude MRC Cognition and Brain Sciences Unit, Cambridge, UK.*R.A. Jones* Resonance Magnetiques des Systemes Biologiques, UMR 5536, CNRS/University Victor Segalen Bordeaux2, Bordeaux, France.

R.A. Jones Resonance Magnetiques des Systems Biologiques, UMR 5536, CNRS/University Victor Segalen Bordeaux2, Bordeaux, France.

P.M. Matthews Centre for Functional Magnetic Resonance Imaging of the Brain, Department of Clinical Neurology, University of Oxford, UK.

R.S. Menon Laboratory for Functional Magnetic Resonance Research, The John P. Robarts Research Institute, London, Ontario, Canada.

C.T.W. Moonen Resonance Magnetiques des Systemes Biologiques, UMR 5536, CNRS/University Victor Segalen Bordeaux2, Bordeaux, France.

A.M. Owen MRC Cognition and Brain Sciences Unit, Cambridge, UK.

G.B. Pike McConnell Brain Imaging Centre, Montreal Neurological Institute, McGill University, Montreal, Quebec, Canada.

D.M. Rector Biophysics Group, Los Alamos National Laboratory, Los Alamos, NM, USA.

R. Savoy The Rowland Institute for Science, Cambridge, MA, USA.

D.M. Schmidt Biophysics Group, Los Alamos National Laboratory, Los Alamos, NM, USA.

S.M. Smith Centre for Functional Magnetic Resonance Imaging of the Brain, Department of Clinical Neurology, University of Oxford, UK.

K.R. Thulborn MR Research Programmme, Univerisity of Illinois, Chicago, USA.

C. Wood Biophysics Group, Los Alamos National Laboratory, Los Alamos, NM, USA.

K.J. Worsley Department of Mathematical Statistics, McGill University, Montreal, Quebec, Canada.

Abbreviations

AFNI	analysis of functional neuroimages
AIR	automated image registration
ASL	arterial spin labelling
ADP	adenosine diphosphate
ATP	adenosine triphosphate
ATPase	enzyme catalysing the hydrolysis or synthesis of ATP
BEM	boundary element method
B_0	static magnetic field applied for MRI
BOLD	blood oxygenation level dependent
CBF	cerebral blood flow
CBV	cerebral blood volume
CCD	charge-coupled device
Cho	choline
CK	creatine phosphokinase
$CMRO_2$	cerebral metabolic rate of oxygen consumption
CNR	contrast-to-noise ratio
Cr	creatine
CRT	cathode ray tube
CSF	cerebro-spinal fluid
CT	computed tomography (X-ray imaging method)
dHb	deoxyhaemoglobin
DLP	digital light processing
DOF	degrees of freedom
DTI	diffusion tensor imaging
DWI	diffusion weighted imaging
ECD	equivalent current dipole
EDRF	endothelium-derived relaxation factor
EAAT	excitatory amino acid transporter
EEG	electroencephalography
EIT	electrical impedance tomography
EMG	electromyography
ENOS	endothelial nitrous oxide synthases
EPI	echo planar imaging
EPISTAR	echo planar imaging with signal targeting and alternating RF
EROS	event related optical signals
ERP	event-related potential
FAIR	flow-sensitive alternating inversion recovery (perfusion pulse sequence)
FDA	Food and Drug Administration
FEAT	fMRI expert analysis tool
FFA	fusiform face area

FFT	fast Fourier transform
FID	free induction decay
FLASH	fast low angle shot. (Also known as SPGR and T1FFE)
FLIRT	FMRIB's linear image registration tool
fMRI	functional magnetic resonance imaging
FOV	field of view
FSE	fast spin echo
FWHM	full-width-half-maximum
g	gram
G	Gauss
GE	gradient echo (also known as gradient recalled echo, GRE)
GRF	Gaussian random field
GSR	galvanic skin response
HK	hexokinase
HRF	haemodynamic response function
ICA	independent components analysis
IEI	inter echo interval
INOS	inducible nitrous oxide synthases
J_{O2}	net oxygen consumption
K_t	Michaelis constants
LDH	lactate dehydrogenase (enzyme)
MCMC	Markov chain Monte Carlo
MCT	monocarboxylate transporter
MFT	magnetic field tomography
MMCT	mitochondrial-specific monocarboxylate transporter
MEG	magnetoencephalography
MI	myoinositol
MION	monocrystalline iron oxide nanocolloid
Mol, mole	an Avagadro's number of atoms or molecules
μmol	micromole (10^{-6} mole)
MR	magnetic resonance
MRI	magnetic resonance imaging
mRNA	messenger ribonucleic acid
MRS	magnetic resonance spectroscopy
MRSI	magnetic resonance spectroscopic imaging
ms	millisecond (10^{-3} second)
NAA	N-acetylaspartate
NADH/NAD	nicotinamide adenine dinucleotide (reduced form/oxidized form)
NEM	neural electromagnetic techniques
NIRS	near infrared spectroscopy
NMR	nuclear magnetic resonance
NNOS	neuronal nitrous oxide synthases
NO	nitric oxide
NOS	nitric oxide synthase
PCr	phosphocreatine
PCA	principle components analysis
PDH	pyruvate dehydrogenase
PET	positron emission tomography

PFK	phosphofructokinase
pH	logarithm of the reciprocal of the hydrogen ion concentration
Pi	inorganic phosphate
PPA	parahippocampal place area
Pixel	single picture element in a 2D slice
P_{O2}	partial pressure of dissolved oxygen
PR	projection reconstruction
QC	quality control
QUIPSS	quantitative imaging of perfusion using a single subtraction
RARE	fast spin echo (pulse sequence) (see FSE)
Resel	resolution element
RF	radio-frequency
RT	room temperature
ROI	region of interest
s	second
SAR	specific absorption rate
SE	spin echo
SEM	structural equation modelling
SENSE	sensitivity encoding
SMA	supplementary motor area
SMASH	simultaneous acquisition of spatial harmonics
SNR	signal-to-noise ratio
SOR	successive over relaxation
SPL	superior parietal lobule
SPECT	single photon emission computed tomography (also known as SPET)
SPM	(1) statistical parametric map
	(2) Statistical Parametric Mapping (a popular software package for the analysis of functional and structural imaging data)
SVD	singular value decomposition
T1	longitudinal (z-direction) magnetization recovery time constant
T2	transverse (xy-direction) magnetization decay time constant
T2*	transverse decay time constant including magnetic field inhomogeneity effects
T	Tesla
TCA	tricarboxylic acid (or Krebs) cycle
TE	time to echo (from the radio-frequency excitation pulse)
TG	transmitter gain
TI	inversion time (time following inversion of the spins with a 180° inversion pulse)
TMS	trans-cranial magnetic stimulation
T_{max}	maximal transport capacity of a transporter (influx or efflux)
TR	time for repetition
TSP	tri-methylsilyl propionic acid
UNFOLD	Unaliasing by Fourier-encoding Overlaps using the temporal Dimension
V_{max}	maximal reaction rate
Voxel	single volume element in a 3D volume (see also pixel)
VPR	variable parameter regression

I | Introduction

1 | An introduction to functional magnetic resonance imaging of the brain

Paul M. Matthews

1.1 Introduction: What is functional imaging of the brain?

This chapter is intended to provide an overview of fMRI methods and applications. Like the rest of the book, it is intended to highlight key concepts or strategies rather than to provide a review of the literature. It also should provide a guide to the chapters that follow. We hope that it will help to place them in context. In doing so, this chapter makes later repetition inevitable, but we have embraced this in the belief that learning can be made easier by having ideas presented more than one time and in more than one way.

1.1.1 The physiology of brain activation

Functional brain imaging can be strictly or more broadly defined. We consider it broadly to include the full range of techniques by which physiological changes accompanying brain activity are defined. Different techniques are sensitive to different types of changes. As outlined in the chapters of Part II, the focus on magnetic resonance-based techniques in this book arises from the extraordinary flexibility and range of potential applications for magnetic resonance methods, as well as the safety and widespread availability of MRI scanners.

In contrast to many of the *in vitro* methods used to define brain function, methods used *in vivo* generally are concerned not with the behaviours of single neurones but with the activities of large populations of neurones. This nonetheless is highly informative, as single neurones do not work independently, but function in large aggregates (consider, for example, the vertical integration of neurones in columns in primary sensory cortex). Despite the small sizes of individual neurones, useful information concerning brain function therefore can be obtained using methods that have an in-plane spatial resolution of 3 mm or greater.

Information transfer in the brain along axons occurs by electrical conduction. Information is transferred between neurones by the release of neurotransmitter molecules at synapses and their subsequent interactions with specific receptors on target neurones. These neurotransmitter–receptor interactions then lead to changes in membrane current flow which change the post-synaptic neuronal membrane potential (and the accompanying extracellular electrical field) and alter depolarization frequency.

As discussed in some detail in Chapter 2, the metabolic changes in neurones and glia that accompany neurotransmitter release are energy-requiring. Most of this energy is used at or around synapses. As normal brain energy production depends ultimately on oxidative metabolism, there thus is greater local demand for delivery of oxygen with increased synaptic activity. To meet this increased metabolic demand, neuronal activation is accompanied by increased local blood flow.

In, 1890, the physiologist Arthur Sherrington demonstrated that stimulation of the brain caused a local increase in blood flow. However, he also observed that the relative proportion of oxygen extracted from this blood was reduced: the increase in total oxygen delivery exceeded the increase in oxygen utilization. Evidence cited in Chapter 2 highlights the potential physiological significance of an increased rate of oxygen delivery to the working brain and shows that rates of oxygen diffusion from capillaries may limit its utilization rate (Kuwabara *et al.* 1992; Buxton and Frank 1997). By increasing the relative proportion of oxygenated haemoglobin in blood, the oxygen gradient between capillaries and cell mitochondria is increased, helping to match diffusion-limited transport to the rate of utilization. Accompanying the increase in blood flow is a small increase in local blood volume.

These elements of the physiology of information transfer in the brain–generation of an extracellular electrical potential, increased oxidative metabolism (and glucose substrate utilization), and enhanced local blood flow and relative oxygenation – provide the basis for a number of functional imaging methods. Changes in blood oxygenation and flow have been used for the functional magnetic resonance imaging methods that are the primary focus of this book (see Chapters 6 and 8), but advances in spectroscopic imaging suggest some potential for using magnetic resonance metabolic imaging in similar ways (Hyder *et al.* 1996; Hyder *et al.* 1997).

1.1.2 Techniques for functional brain mapping

Functional imaging methods define dynamic brain changes having a time course similar to that of brain sensory, motor or cognitive activities. Specific interpre-

tations demand methods that also can define the neuro-anatomical localizations for these dynamic changes.

Different functional brain imaging methods, therefore, are usefully compared and contrasted in terms of both their temporal and spatial resolution (Fig. 1.1). In general, electrophysiological methods based on direct mapping of transient brain electrical dipoles generated by neuronal depolarization (e.g. electroencephalography or EEG) or the associated magnetic dipoles (magnetoencephalography or MEG) define the underlying cortical neuronal events in real time (10–100 msec), but provide relatively poor spatial resolution (many mm–cm). In contrast, functional magnetic resonance imaging (fMRI) and positron emission tomography (PET) provide information on the increases in blood flow accompanying neuronal activation with relatively high spatial resolution (approximately, 1–10 mm), but have a temporal resolution limited (at best) by the rate of the much slower haemodynamic changes that accompany neuronal depolarization. Factors determining the potential spatial and temporal resolution of fMRI are discussed in Chapter 7.

Optical imaging methods (e.g. near infrared spectro-

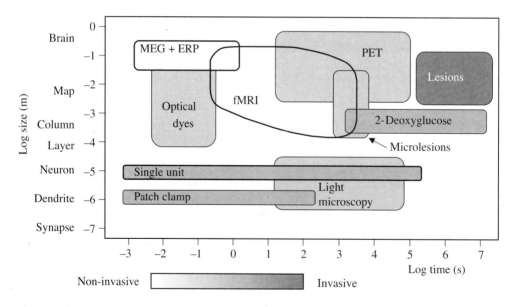

Fig. 1.1 FMRI occupies a unique niche among the functional brain mapping techniques available. This is an adapted version of a popular illustration of the relative spatial and temporal sensitivities of different functional brain mapping methods that can be used in animals, man, or isolated tissue preparations. FMRI has the potential to link high spatial and temporal resolution studies to an understanding of systems organization across the brain. This integration of brain mapping techniques constitute use of the most important area in current research (adapted from Cohen and Bookheimer 1994).

scopy or NIRS) also measure changes in cortical blood flow, but, because of light scattering particularly by the skull, have poor spatial resolution unless the cortical surface is exposed. Optical imaging methods also are restricted to study of the cortical surface. An important relative advantage of PET or fMRI methods is that they allow mapping of neuronal activation deep in the brain. Metabolic imaging by magnetic resonance spectroscopic imaging (MRSI) or PET is also possible, but these methods have a more variable and generally lower spatial resolution (depending on the nature of the chemical species being imaged) and rather poor temporal resolution (on the order of 30 s to min). However, the specificity of the information that they can provide is high and complements that available from fMRI.

This book will focus primarily on blood oxygenation level dependent (BOLD) fMRI, in which the imaging contrast arises as a consequence of the higher ratio of oxy- to deoxyhaemoglobin in local draining venules and veins that accompanies neuronal activation (Ogawa *et al.* 1993). Direct imaging of the blood flow response using perfusion MRI is also discussed in Chapters 6 and 8, but has been used less widely because of its much lower sensitivity. Similar analysis problems and methods would be used for both BOLD and perfusion fMRI. These are discussed in the context of BOLD fMRI in the chapters of Part IV. Ways in which BOLD fMRI can be integrated with electrophysiological methods (e.g. direct linking of transcranial magnetic stimulation (TMS) and fMRI (Roberts *et al.* 1997) or event-related potential (ERP) and fMRI (McCarthy 1999)) are becoming increasingly important (see Chapter, 19).

The singular focus on MRI-based techniques in this book is a response to the explosion of interest in this specific modality. The widespread availability of the technology, its relatively low cost per examination, and the lack of recognized risks to repeated applications have already ensured that fMRI will have a major role in both basic and clinical neuroscience for some time to come.

1.2 Principles of magnetic resonance imaging

The nuclear magnetic resonance phenomenon is introduced more fully in Chapter 3. Very briefly, magnetic resonance arises from the interaction of nuclei which have a magnetic moment with an applied magnetic field. (For more detail, see Hashemi and Bradley 1997.) Nuclei of many atoms with a nuclear 'spin' (e.g., 1H, 1^3C, ^{31}P) (Table 3.1) can behave as simple magnetic dipoles and (notionally) can assume either a high-energy state (behaving as if oriented against the applied field) or a low-energy state (as if aligned with the applied magnetic field). Transitions between the two energy states accompany absorption or emission of energy in the radiofrequency range.

The frequency of the energy emitted by an excited nucleus is proportional to the magnetic field experienced. The magnetic field at the nucleus is determined primarily by the strong magnetic field that is applied to the sample in the imaging experiment. As the precise relation between the resonance frequency and the applied magnetic field is different for different nuclei, magnetic resonance imaging systems can be 'tuned' to detect specific types of nuclei independently. However, the magnetic field at the nucleus is also modulated by small 'shielding' effects of electrons around the nucleus. These 'shielding' effects cause changes on the order of only ppm in the precise resonance frequencies of nuclei that are observed. These small differences between resonance frequencies of protons in different molecules are ignored in conventional MRI or fMRI applications, but they provide the basis for MR spectroscopic methods.

1.2.1 Spatial localization in MRI

Hardware for magnetic resonance imaging is discussed in Chapter 5. Magnetic field strengths are measured in units of Tesla (T) or Gauss (G). Imaging the location of resonating nuclei in a sample (e.g. protons in water molecules of the human brain) is made possible with the use of small magnetic field gradients (e.g. 2.5–4.0 G/cm or 25–40 mT/m) that are superimposed on the larger homogenous static magnetic field of the imaging magnet (typically of, 1.5 T or greater, which is more than 25 000-times the Earth's magnetic field). The relative positions of molecules along the smaller gradient field are measured (or encoded) simply from differences in resonance frequency, as the resonance frequency for a nucleus (e.g., 1H) in a compound (e.g. water) is proportional to the applied field strength (the sum of the large static field of the magnet and the smaller field of the gradient coil). Elegant methods have been developed that allow an extension of this simple concept for one-dimensional imaging into methods for multi-slice two-dimensional (with application of gradients along two directions) or three-dimensional (with application of gradients along three dimensions) imaging. These are introduced in Chapters 3 and 4.

Switching the small gradient magnetic fields on and off takes time. FMRI really became robust and practical with the availability of fast gradients integrated with imaging techniques that allow several brain images to be acquired over the time course of the haemodynamic response (which lasts several s). As discussed in Chapter 4, several strategies are available, although echo-planar imaging (EPI) has been the most popular.

1.2.2 Generation of contrast in MRI

Second only to spatial localization, generating contrast between tissues is a major goal in imaging. Once nuclear spins are excited from a low- to a high-energy state, they can return (or 'relax') to the low-energy state by emission of the radiofrequency energy that is detected in MRI. The efficiency with which this spin relaxation occurs is determined by the nature of interaction of the spins with their surrounding environment

(referred to as the 'lattice' in the literature of physics). This is governed by a 'spin-lattice' relaxation process that has a rate constant, $1/T1$, where T1 is the so-called 'spin-lattice relaxation time'. This is an exponential process. Excited spins regain 66 per cent of their equilibrium magnetization over one T1 period and regain 95 per cent of the equilibrium magnetization (or 'relax') over three T1 periods. If excitation pulses are applied more rapidly than allows for full relaxation, then the proportion of spins that can be excited is lower and the resonance signal decreases. This provides a source of image contrast, as the T1 for a water molecule will depend on the local chemical environment, which varies between different parts of the brain, e.g. it is longer for water in the cerebrospinal fluid (CSF) than for water in tissue. As the rate at which radiofrequency pulses are applied to the sample rises (by shortening the inter pulse delay or 'TR' in a pulse sequence), signal from parts of the brain with a shorter T1 (e.g. tissue) will increase relative to that in parts of the brain with a longer T1 relaxation time (e.g. cerebrospinal fluid) (Fig. 1.2).

In principle, if one could observe the signal from an isolated single resonating nucleus, it would decay with a time constant equal to T1. This simply reflects the fact that emission of energy can occur as long as the nucleus is in an excited state. However, in a real

(a) (b)

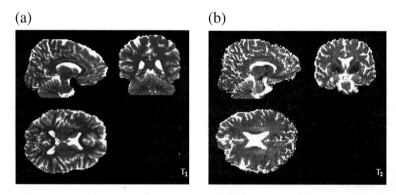

Fig. 1.2 (a) MRI contrast in the brain is determined not only by differences in the distribution of protons in water and fat, but also by differences in their relaxation times. The images on the *left* demonstrate the differences in T1 or 'spin lattice' relaxation times across the brain. Longer T1 values are indicated by lighter colours. Water in cerebrospinal fluid has the longest T1 value of water in any of the brain compartments. (b) The image on the *right* shows the distribution of T2 or 'spin-spin' relaxation times across the brain. Tissue differences in T2 values are not identical to those of T1 values, although both the longest water T2 and T1 relaxation times in the brain are found for the cerebrospinal fluid. Relative differences in T1 and T2 between different tissue types generate contrast with variation of parameters in pulse sequences. A variation of the TR or inter-pulse interval alters the relative amount of T1 contrast. Variations in the TE or the 'time to echo' alter the relative T2 relaxation time weighting of contrast. (Images acquired at 3T by Dr S. Clare, FMRIB Centre, University of Oxford.)

(a) 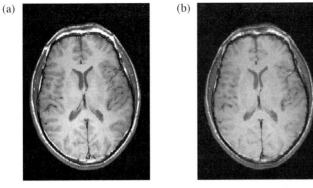 (b)

(c) 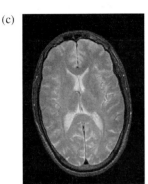 (d)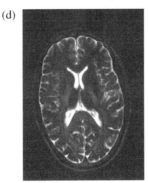

Fig. 1.3 Differences in T1 and T2 relaxation times for water indifferent brain compartments generates contrast. The relative contrast can be varied by changes in radiofrequency excitation pulse seqeunce parameters. Changes in contrast from differences in T1 can be generated by varying the TR or interpulse interval (a) TR = 500 ms; (b) TR = 1000 ms [spin-echo sequence, TE 18 ms]. Changes in contrast from differences in T2 can be generated by varying the TE or time to echo (c) TE = 60 ms; (d) TE = 180 ms [spin-echo sequence, TR = 2000 ms]. (All images were acquired at 3T and provided courtesy of Mr Peter Hobden, FMRIB Centre, University of Oxford.)

sample one is observing emissions from huge numbers of spins simultaneously (in the brain, for example, there are more than 4×10^{19} water protons/mm^3!). On a molecular scale these nuclei are each experiencing continuous very small local changes in magnetic field. These shifting fields allow an exchange of energy between the nuclei which leads to a loss of coherence in the phases of their resonance emissions. This loss of coherence leads to an exponential loss of intensity for the summed resonance signal from all of the nuclei together, which is described by the so-called 'spin-spin' or T2 relaxation time. The T2 is an intrinsic property of nuclei in a particular chemical environment. By increasing the delay before signal detection in a pulse sequence (i.e. lengthening the 'TE'), signal from tissues with a longer T2 (e.g. brain grey matter) will be increased relative to those from tissues with a shorter T2 (e.g. brain white matter) (Figs. 1.2, 1.3) (see Chapter 3).

In both conventional MRI and BOLD fMRI, the distribution of protons in tissue water is imaged (in most brain studies the strong signal from protons in fat is ignored or even 'edited' out of the image). Variations in the relative concentrations of water protons provide contrast between some structures, allowing clear discrimination between bone (little water, low MR signal) and brain (approximately 70 per cent water, high signal), for example. Further contrast arises from differences in the relaxation times of the excited proton nuclei of water molecules in different local environments.

Contrast differences arising from differences in relaxation times are realized by changing the way in which the spins are excited and observed using different 'pulse sequences' (e.g. a 'T2-weighted spin-echo pulse' sequence). The principles of MRI pulse sequence design are discussed more fully in Chapters 3 and 6. Here we will note only that there are three principal parameters of pulse sequences that can be varied to generate contrast. First is the energy per pulse of radiofrequency excitation energy, which is expressed as the 'flip angle' (a measure in notional degrees of the extent to which the net magnetization vector of the nuclear 'spins'—that one can classically visualize as a spinning gyroscope—is 'tipped' away from the equilibrium alignment with the applied magnetic field). The more energy that is put into the sample, the greater the amount of time needed for full relaxation, all other factors being constant. Second is the rate at which these pulses are applied. This increases as the 'TR' interval (measured in s) between each pulse become shorter. The shorter the 'TR', the less time is allowed for T1 relaxation. Finally, the time that is waited before the resonance is detected after excitation ('TE', measured in milliseconds) can be varied. Nuclei that have a shorter T2 will contribute relatively less signal, the longer the 'TE' value used.

The rate of decay of signal is faster if there are local field gradients that the molecules can diffuse through over the time course of a single TE. As molecules move into regions of different local fields, their resonance frequencies change slightly, lowering the coherence of the nuclear spins. This leads to more rapid decay of the net signal. In the presence of local magnetic field inhomogeneities the rate of signal decay is expressed by the T2* relaxation time. In regions of rapidly changing local magnetic fields (e.g. in tissue adjacent to a blood vessel filled predominantly with paramagnetic deoxyhaemoglobin), the T2* can be substantially shorter than the T2. This provides yet another mechanism for generating contrast that has proven particularly important for functional MRI, as will be further discussed below.

1.2.3 Magnetic resonance spectroscopic imaging

Magnetic resonance spectroscopic imaging (MRSI) can be used to provide information on the relative concentrations and distribution of compounds or ions with nuclei that have a magnetic moment (including, ^1H, ^{13}C, ^{31}P, ^{23}Na). There are large differences between resonance frequencies for different nuclei in an applied magnetic field. Even the same nuclei will resonate at slightly different frequencies (varying over a few to tens of ppm) in different molecules or at different positions in a molecule because of differences in the magnetic 'shielding' afforded by the different electronic environments. A 'fingerprint' of the biochemicals present at high concentrations in the tissue is provided by the relative signal intensities and frequencies of resonance of the constituent 'MR visible' nuclei (Fig. 1.4). The overall intensity of each resonance is proportional to the concentration (all other parameters being constant) of the molecular species being observed. Because the frequency of the signals provides the chemical information of interest, spatial localization does not rely on frequency encoding in the same way as for MRI.

1.3 The physiological basis for blood oxygenation level dependent fMRI

1.3.1 Mechanisms of haemodynamic change

The locally increased blood flow in regions of the brain that become active appears to be a consequence of increased energy utilization at the synapse (Duncan *et al.* 1987; Duncan and Stumpf 1991). Precisely which processes account for the metabolic changes is unclear. A major contribution to increased energy utilization may arise from metabolic changes in adjacent astrocytes with the uptake of the excitatory neurotransmitter, glutamate (Magistretti and Pellerin 1996). Astrocytes are abundant in the brain and are found in close proximity to the neurones. Elegant, ^{13}C MRS experiments have suggested a 1:1 coupling stoichiometry of oxidative glucose metabolism with glutamate neurotransmitter cycling between neurones and astrocytes (Sibson *et al.* 1998). However, as discussed in Chapter 2, it does not appear as though there is necessarily a simple relationship between increased energy utilization and increased blood flow. This complexity is obvious particularly with consideration of inhibitory synaptic activity. Theoretical arguments suggest that inhibitory neurotransmitter release may not lead directly to substantially increased energy utilization (Gjedde 1997). Consistent with the most obvious prediction of this, there is no detectable activation in the motor cortex during the 'no go' phase of a 'go/no go' paradigm when there is electrophysiologically demonstrable motor cortex inhibition (Rees *et al.* 2000). However, other evidence challenges this as a general notion. Ipsilateral afferents to the lateral superior olive are excitatory, while those from the contralateral ear are inhibitory. Stimulation of *either* pathway leads to increased deoxy-glucose uptake (a measure of energy utilization) (Glendenning *et al.*

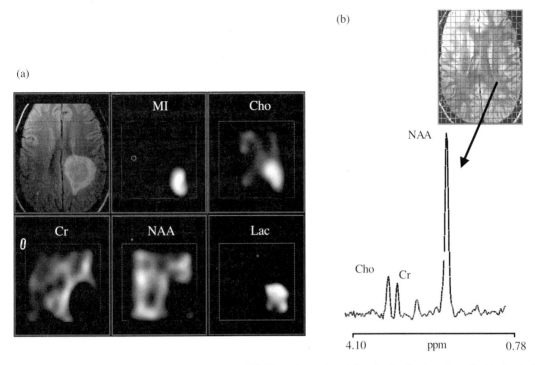

Fig. 1.4 (a) Magnetic resonance spectroscopic imaging (MRSI) can be used to define the distribution of specific biochemicals in the brain. The upper left panel shows conventional T2-weighted MRI image from a patient with a large, acute demyelinating lesion. The other panels show the distributions of specific proton- containing biochemicals in a central large region of this axial slice from left to right: MI, myoinositol; Cho, choline; Cr, creatine; NAA, N-acetylaspartate; Lac, lactate. These images were generated by thresholding at defined relative concentration levels for each of the metabolites. They show, for example, increased concentrations of lactate and myo-inositol in the core of the demyelinating lesion.

Quantitative information concerning the distribution of biochemcials also can be provided by MRSI. From a single voxel (approximately $1 \times 1 \times 1$ cm^3) in the area of the conventional imaging shown a proton magnetic resonance spectrum can be obtained as shown on the bottom of the image. The spectrum is a plot of frequency (along the abscissa) expressed as 'ppm' or ppm from a reference frequency as a function of signal intensity (ordinate). The frequencies are distinct for protons in different chemical environments of different molecules (NAA, N-acetylaspartate; Cr, creatine; Cho, choline). In fully-relaxed spectra the signal intensities are proportional to concentrations. These proton magnetic resonance spectroscopic images in the spectra were acquired at 1.5 T. (Images courtesy of Drs D.L. Arnold and N. de Stefano, Montreal Neurological Institute).

1985). Similarily, stimulation of both the disynaptic, inhibitory parallel fibre system and monosynaptic, excitatory climbing fibres causes increased local blood flow in the rat cerebellum (Mathiesen *et al.* 1998). In this system blood flow changes were correlated directly with the product of the stimulation frequencies and the magnitude of the field potentials, implying a contribution from both pre- and post-synaptic metabolic factors to control. More work needs to be done to clarify the interpretation and mechanisms of coupling the haemodynamic response to neuronal activity.

These observations highlight fundamental charac-

teristics of the BOLD fMRI response. First, it should be useful for identifying activation-related changes in grey matter (where the synapses are found) and not in the white matter. Second, the changes measured reflect synaptic activity or a combination of synaptic and dendritic electrical changes, but not neuronal activity directly. Third, as cortical signal changes are triggered by excitatory synaptic activity, at least under some conditions there should be a direct relationship between neuronal discharge rate and the magnitude of the BOLD response (Rees *et al.* 2000). However, the relationship should be modulated by the relative inhibitory input. Under some conditions at least, increases in inhibitory synaptic input may also contribute independently to increases in the fMRI BOLD signal.

1.3.2 Coupling of haemodynamic changes to neuronal activation

Understanding of this phenomenon is still limited by an incomplete appreciation for the fundamental mechanisms responsible for regulation of local cerebral blood flow.

Multiple mechanisms interact in the control of blood flow to the brain. Global brain perfusion is regulated by sympathetic, hormonal (e.g. the renin-angiotensin system), and myogenic mechanisms. Local tissue perfusion demands additional, more specific regulation to meet changes in energy demands with neuronal activation. There is a variety of factors likely to contribute to this local response, including K^+ release with neuronal depolarization and H^+ and adenosine release when there is a mismatch between oxygen delivery and utilization. However, nitric oxide (primarily from neuronal nitric oxide synthase) is likely to be the most important chemical signal responsible for local increases in perfusion with neuronal activation and also cerebral vasodilatory response to hypercapnia. Locally generated eicosanoids (e.g. prostacyclin) (Kuschinsky 1991) and circulating factors (e.g. norepinephrine, serotonin) can modulate blood flow regulation, as can some drugs in common use (e.g. theophylline or scopolamine inhibit the haemodynamic response to neuronal activation) (Ogawa *et al.* 1993; Dirnagl *et al.* 1994).

There may be age-dependent changes in the coupling between neuronal activation and increased blood flow. For example, in neonates the relative local concentration of deoxyhaemoglobin may increase (rather than decrease) with neuronal activation (Meek *et al.* 1998). In ageing adults there may be some attenuation of blood flow increases accompanying neuronal activation (Hock *et al.* 1995).

1.4 Perfusion fMRI

1.4.1 Use of contrast agents

Conceptually the most direct approach to measuring functional activation with MRI would be to define directly the changes in perfusion or the related local increase in blood volume. The first functional MRI studies were based on defining changes in local blood volume with increased activation (Belliveau *et al.* 1991). Paramagnetic MRI contrast agents alter the relaxation properties of blood water and of the tissue water which surrounds blood vessels. In the study by Belliveau *et al.*, subjects were given an intravenous bolus of one such agent (gadolinium-DTPA) before and then during photic stimulation (Belliveau *et al.* 1991). By application of tracer kinetic principles to analysis of the time course of signal changes induced by the bolus of contrast agent passing through the brain, maps of relative blood volume for the resting and the activation states with photic stimulation were calculated. Direct contrast of these two maps then functionally defined the visual cortex as the region of brain in which blood volume increased with visual stimulation. In principle, this method (or similar methods measuring changes in perfusion based on signal changes with transit of a bolus of exogenous contrast (Ostergaard *et al.* 1998)) is quite generally applicable. An advantage is that an agent such as gadolinium-DTPA provides a relatively large contrast change. However, the method demands injection of a contrast agent and only a very limited number of doses can be given safely in a single imaging session. Possible future availability of long-lived circulating contrast agents such as MION particles (Palmer *et al.* 1999) could make measurements of activation-induced changes in local brain blood volume using exogenous contrast agents feasible, even when multiple observations need to be made.

1.4.2 Arterial spin-tagging methods

For the present, because activation studies demand repeated (due to the generally low signal changes) measurements in multiple (due to the typical need to test several potential variables) cognitive states, the most practical approach to measuring functional activation changes from direct perfusion measurements may be to use non-invasive arterial spin-tagging (Detre *et al.* 1994; Wong *et al.* 1995,1997; Kim *et al.* 1997). Arterial spin-tagging methods use radiofrequency pulses from the MRI system itself to transiently 'label' flowing blood without the need for an exogenous contrast agent. A variety of techniques are available (see Chapter 6). Even so, these methods are not yet in widespread use for functional imaging because they provide lower (perhaps half or less) signal-to-noise than BOLD-based fMRI.

Considerable interest remains focused on arterial spin-tagging perfusion methods for functional imaging, however. Theoretically, perfusion changes should be better localized to active volumes of brain tissue than are BOLD-contrast changes. Perfusion fMRI also measures a single physiological parameter, while (as will be described below) BOLD-contrast changes depend on several (although determined primarily by changes in blood oxygenation). This may account in part for the reportedly rather poor correlation between the magnitudes of BOLD and perfusion functional activation changes (Kim *et al.* 1997).

An exciting development described in detail in Chapter 8 has been the combined use of perfusion and BOLD fMRI to allow estimation of activity-dependent changes in local tissue oxygen consumption (Hoge *et al.* 1999). This is possible because BOLD fMRI is sensitive to changes in local oxygen content with activation, while perfusion fMRI measures associated changes in local blood delivery. To determine oxygen consumption, the component of the BOLD response due to increases in oxygen content alone (independent of the flow component) needs to be calibrated for individual subjects. Kastrup *et al.* (1998) have described how this can be performed even just using a simple breath holding period (which transiently increases blood flow during the consequent period of hypercapnia without increasing brain oxygen consumption).

1.5 Blood oxygenation level dependent (BOLD) fMRI

1.5.1 How is blood oxygenation level dependent contrast generated?

Understanding the BOLD response is important for appreciating aspects of fMRI, including the spatial and temporal limitations to activation mapping, optimization of those responses and their potential changes with pathology. The basis of the BOLD response is therefore described in different ways in several chapters, including particularly Chapters 2, 6 and 8. ·

BOLD fMRI images signal contrast arising from changes in the local 'magnetic susceptibility', an index of the extent to which an applied magnetic field is distorted as it interacts with a material. Normal blood can be considered simply as a concentrated solution of haemoglobin (10–15 gm haemoglobin/100 cm³). When bound to oxygen, haemoglobin is diamagnetic, while deoxygenated haemoglobin is paramagnetic (Pauling and Coryell 1936). Magnetic flux is reduced in diamagnetic materials, i.e. the applied magnetic field is repelled. Paramagnetic materials, in contrast, have an increased magnetic flux, i.e. the applied magnetic field is attracted into the material. A change in haemoglobin oxygenation therefore leads to changes in the local distortions of a magnetic field applied to it.

Thulborn *et al.* demonstrated that the T2-relaxation rate of blood varies exponentially with the proportion of deoxygenated haemoglobin in a fashion precise enough to allow determination of blood oxygenation directly from the line width (which is proportional to, 1/T2) of the water proton MR resonance signal of blood (Thulborn *et al.* 1982). The effect was shown to increase with applied magnetic field strength, as predicted for a phenomenon based on differences in magnetic susceptibility between blood cells and the surrounding medium (or tissue).

However, it was Ogawa who described the first true blood oxygenation level dependent (BOLD) contrast imaging experiment with a report that gradient echo MR images of a cat brain showed signal loss around blood vessels when the animal was made hypoxic (Ogawa *et al.* 1990). This effect was reversed with normoxia. Blood deoxygenation increased the magnetic susceptibility of blood vessels relative to the surrounding brain tissue, which generated local field gradients and locally decreased tissue T2* in tissue water around the blood vessels. Ogawa then had the insight to suggest that the effect could be used to image the smaller changes in the relative blood oxygenation that accompany neuronal activation in the brain.

In fact, the experiments of Thulborn (characterizing T2 changes) and Ogawa (characterizing T2* changes) define distinct phenomena, although they are related.

Increased oxygenation of blood gives rise to increased signal from water both in blood vessels and from the surrounding brain tissue, but the mechanisms are somewhat different. The distinction is in the basis of methods described in Chapters 6, 7 and 8 to image activation-related changes selectively in tissue as opposed to the draining blood vessels. Both T2 and T2* changes contribute to BOLD contrast.

What is happening to the signal inside a vessel? This is effectively a single compartment. Water diffuses freely between red blood cells and serum, but cannot exchange across the vessel wall to a significant extent in the time course of a single TE (typically approximately 50 msec or less). However, during this time, a water molecule can diffuse in or out of a red blood cell or encounter several red blood cells in the surrounding medium. In consequence, its precise resonance frequency shifts because of the rapidly changing magnetic fields immediately around each red blood cell and with the change in magnetic flux inside red blood cells relative to the surrounding serum. As the blood oxygen content decreases, the magnitude of these local magnetic field differences increases with the proportion of haemoglobin that changes from a diamagnetic to paramagnetic state. This gives rise to apparent water MRI signal decreases from a T2 effect.

What is happening to signal in the tissue immediately surrounding a vessel? With blood deoxygenation, extravascular water within a voxel located close to the vessel experiences a significant local field gradient across the voxel, the magnitude of which depends on the proximity and relative orientation of the vessel and the extent of the change in haemoglobin oxygenation (which changes the magnetic susceptibility of the vessel). The variation in magnetic field across the voxel leads to signal dephasing and hence to a T2* signal loss. Additional T2-like signal loss occurs if the nuclei diffuse significantly through the field gradient.

Changes in both T2 and T2* relaxation times for intra- and extravascular water (respectively) become greater with higher imaging magnetic field strength, but for intra-vascular water the increase is linear and for extravascular water the increase is exponential (Ogawa *et al.* 1993). Thus, at higher magnetic fields the contribution of contrast change in the brain tissue should increase relative to that from blood in vessels (Gati *et al.* 1997). At usual clinical (1.5 T) field strengths there is a major intravascular component which can limit the accuracy with which an activation volume in the brain parenchyma can be mapped.

1.5.2 Temporal resolution of the BOLD response

The temporal resolution of fMRI and its relationship to the time course of underlying neuronal events is discussed in Chapter 7. Here we wish to introduce the important idea that the time course of the BOLD

(a) 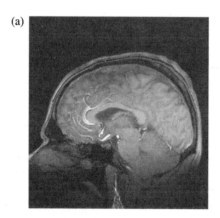 (b)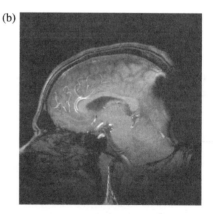

Fig. 1.5 Gradient echo sequences are very sensitive to magnetic susceptibility effects (which is, in fact, one reason why it has been so useful for BOLD fMRI). In panel (a) is a typical sagittal brain image (TE = 30 ms at 3 T). In panel (b) is the same brain imaged again with an approximately 5 mm ferromagnetic washer placed behind the occiput. Note the widespread loss of signal arising from the magnetic field inhomogeneities introduced by the washer. It is striking how far beyond the immediate region of the washer the imaging artefact extends.

response in a region of activation is complex, and that different parts of the time course may provide distinct information. It has been defined best for the primary visual cortex, where the timing of the stimulus can be controlled precisely (Ernst and Hennig 1994). In the primary visual cortex there is an initial small decrease in signal intensity (the early 'dip') that evolves over the first second following a stimulus. There is a progressive increase in signal intensity over the next 2–4 s. For a simple stimulus that does not cause physiological habituation, the signal change is maintained at a relatively constant level for the period of stimulation (Bandettini *et al.* 1997). After the stimulus stops, the BOLD signal decreases over a few s to a level below the initial baseline (the 'undershoot'), from which it recovers slowly over a further few s. Overall, even for a brief stimulus, the time from onset to final return of the signal intensity to baseline may be, 12–18 s.

Optical imaging techniques allow more direct measurement of changes in blood volume and in the relative proportions of oxy- to deoxyhaemoglobin from the absorption spectra of the haemoglobin. The time course of changes following cortical stimulation in the cat brain is remarkably similar to that of the fMRI response in humans (Malonek *et al.* 1997), suggesting a specific physiological interpretation of the time course of the BOLD response. In this interpretation, the initial signal 'dip' is hypothesized to arise from the rapid deoxygenation of capillary blood accompanying the greater oxygen utilization associated with increased synaptic activity. There then is an increase of blood volume in draining veins (which also contributes to the 'dip', as this increases the partial volume of blood in the voxel and the resonance intensity of blood water is lower than that of tissues). Over the 2–5 s after stimulation there is an increase in blood flow (typically on the order of 50–70 per cent). As this is proportionally greater than the increase in local oxygen utilization (which increases by only 5–20 per cent), the oxyhaemoglobin/deoxyhaemoglobin ratio increases, causing an increased signal intensity in the gradient echo image. After the stimulus stops, synaptic activity decreases and both blood flow and the oxyhaemoglobin/deoxyhaemoglobin ratio decay back towards baseline. There is a brief 'undershoot' of signal below that initial baseline that is thought to be due to the effects of a more slowly resolving increase in cerebral blood volume.

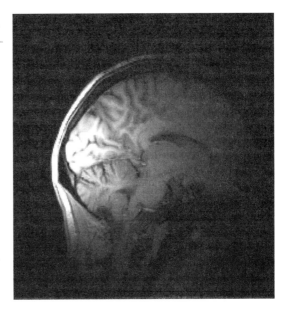

Fig. 1.6 Improved signal-to-noise from any region of the brain can be obtained with improved coupling of the radiofrequency coil to the sample, which is in this case the brain. One of the most straightforward ways of doing this is to move the coil as close as possible to the region-of-interest and to limit the size of the coil to that needed. This approach is embodied in the design of a 'surface coil' which, in its simplest form, is a radiofrequency antennae shaped like a simple coil of wire. A surface coil is sensitive to signals from an approximately disk-shape region below the coil. To generate this image a surface coil was placed over the occipital cortex, which gives the very strong signal shown as the very bright areas on the image. The farther tissue is from the sensitive volume of the coil the lower the signal. Thus, there is a rapid fall-off in signal intensity in parts of the brain away from the occiput, against which the coil was placed. This is an extreme example of B1 in-homogeneity or 'bias field' effects.

The total intravascular blood volume in a voxel including only brain tissue is about 4 per cent. Venules and capillaries contribute similar volumes of blood per voxel, but the venules make a greater relative contribution to the BOLD effects as they carry the less oxygenated blood. BOLD fMRI signal changes in typical tissue voxels (on the order of $3 \times 3 \times 3$ mm^3) with usual sorts of stimuli are no more than 0.5–3 per cent at 1.5 T (larger changes can of course be found in voxels localized to draining veins).

1.5.3 Spatial resolution of the BOLD response

Chapter 7 more fully describes factors determining spatial localization using BOLD fMRI, but here a few basic notions will be noted. The spatial resolution of the BOLD effect depends first on the intrinsic resolution of the imaging experiment. But, more important is that the haemodynamic response is not spatially very specific to areas of neocortical activation (provoking the metaphor that the brain 'waters the whole garden for the sake of one thirsty flower'). Signal changes from draining veins (e.g. more particularly at, 1.5 T or lower fields) spatially 'blur' the activation response. As they drain relatively large cortical regions, signal intensity changes in veins may also be displaced from the relevant activation volume. Even so, activation in two very closely adjacent cortical volumes (e.g. adjacent cortical columns) may be resolved in a difference image made by subtraction of the activation image generated with separate stimulation of the two individual volumes (Menon and Goodyear 1999) (Fig. 1.7). If two adjacent cortical areas drain into common veins, activation of the areas individually should give nearly identical venous signal changes. However, this common venous activation can be nulled in the difference image generated from separate activations for the two adjacent cortical areas, while the *unique* areas of signal change associated with the individual activations are highlighted as regions of positive or negative signal change (depending on the relative order of the subtraction).

An alternative approach to direct high-resolution BOLD mapping is possible at very high fields by defining volumes that show an 'early dip' in signal intensity after the onset of the stimulus (Fig. 1.8) (Grinvald *et al.* 2000; Kim *et al.* 2000). Whether the 'early dip' results from initial capillary deoxygenation or an increase in blood volume (Buxton and Frank 1997), it is an effect that appears to occur local to the volume of activation. This approach therefore may define the volume of activation more directly than do those based on the signal intensity increase, for which resolution is determined by the volume over which haemodynamic regulation occurs.

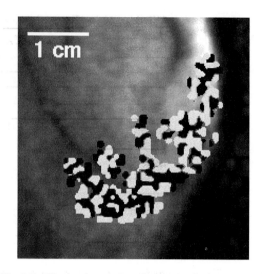

Fig. 1.7 The local perfusion changes in the brain extend beyond the aggregate of neurones activated, prompting the metaphor that the brain 'waters the entire garden for the sake of one flower'. Spatial resolution for defining activation changes on the basis of a haemodynamic response can be maximized by contrasting the haemodynamic responses from adjacent aggregates of neurones with a subtraction procedure. Common areas of activation that are non-specifically perfused by the haemodynamic response in adjacent territories are nulled, highlighting activations very local to the areas recruited. This is nicely demonstrated by results from this study in which the visual cortical activation with stimulation of alternate eyes was subtracted, yielding high spatial resolution maps of the ocular dominance columns. (Image courtesy of Dr Ravi Menon, University of Western Ontario). (See also colour plate section.)

1.6 Hardware for MRI

There are four key components in an MRI system: the magnet, the gradient coil, the radiofrequency transmitter and receiver coil, and the associated electronics and computer hardware for control of the experiment and data acquisition. Along with some elements of the underlying theory, these are described in Chapter 5.

1.6.1 What is the best magnetic field strength?

The magnet provides the strong, homogeneous static magnetic field necessary to observe the magnetic resonance phenomenon. Experimenters new to fMRI are generally interested in understanding what determines

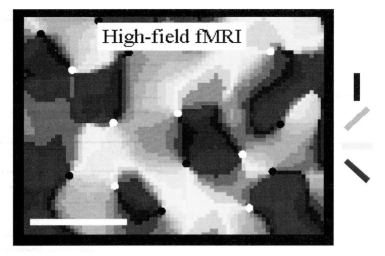

Fig. 1.8 The time course for the haemodynamic response in the visual cortex begins with a decrease in signal over approximately the first second after stimulation. By comparison of the time course of a gradient echo MRI sequence with that from optical imaging studies in animals, it has been suggested that this early decrease in signal is related to a transient increase in oxygen extraction fraction from blood in capillaries local to the area of neuronal activation occurring as a direct result of the increase in oxidative metabolism. It is argued that because such an increase in oxygen extraction can occur only within oxygen diffusion distance of activated cells, mapping of the cortical volume that shows this decreased signal provides a more localized measure of the region of cortical activation than does the later increase signal resulting from the subsequent hyperaemia. This image shows cortical columns in the cat visual cortex mapped out on the basis of the early negative response in BOLD fMRI using a 4.7 Tesla imaging system. Cats were exposed to moving grating stimuli with different orientations, as illustrated in the colour boxes to the *right*. The composite angle map was attained through pixel-by-pixel vector addition of the four single orientation maps to display the resulting orientation preference at each cortical location. There is an interruption of the smooth changes in preferred orientations along the cortical surface at so-called 'orientation pinwheels', where cortical columns for different orientations are arranged in a circular manner. These generate two types of topological singularities based on their rotational symmetries. White and black circles represent clockwise and counter-clockwise pinwheels, respectively. The scale bar shown represents 1 mm. (Image courtesy of Dr D.S. Kim, T.Q. Duong and S-G. Kim of the University of Minnesota.) (See also colour plate section.)

(a) (b)

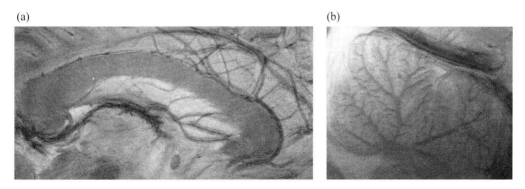

Fig. 1.9 Ultra-high field magnetic resonance imaging offers the potential for increased spatial resolution and some forms of improved contrast, particularly between blood vessels and tissue. Another advantage of ultra-high field MRI may be the enhanced signal-to-noise, which allows extremely small voxel dimensions for ultra-high resolution mapping. (a) This 8 Tesla image from a sagittal section through the human corpus callosum demonstrates the delicate tracery of the draining venous system in fine detail. (b) The folia of the cerebellum are displayed with very high resolution in this image. (Images courtesy of Dr Pierre Robitaille, Ohio State University.)

the ideal imaging system for their work. There is no simple answer to the question of what the optimal field strength is for functional imaging. From the theory outlined in Chapter 3, it is clear that the intrinsic signal-to-noise in MRI increases with the strength of the applied static magnetic field. Descriptions of the BOLD effect above and in later chapters describe how the contrast-to-noise in BOLD imaging and the relative proportion of BOLD signal arising from tissue rather than draining veins increase with the applied static magnetic field strength (Gati *et al.* 1997a). However, radiofrequency coil design becomes more difficult at higher fields and large-scale magnetic susceptibility artefacts (leading to geometric distortion and signal loss) rise, particularly near the air-filled sinuses (Fig. 1.5). In addition, energy deposition in tissue by the radiofrequency pulses increases at higher frequencies (and thus at greater magnetic field strengths) to the extent that some pulse sequences commonly used at lower fields (e.g. fast spin echo) may lead to undesirable levels of tissue heating at very high fields. Nonetheless, it is clear that structural and functional imaging of humans even at extremely high fields (7–9 T) is possible (Fig. 1.9) (Robitaille *et al.* 2000). Thus the optimal field strength for any institution is determined by several factors, including the imaging goals and the extent of the local expertise for support of imaging – as well as the funding available!

1.6.2 Defining characteristics of the ideal gradient coil

Gradient coils are used to provide the smaller, rapidly changing magnetic fields necessary for spatial encoding of spins in the volume being imaged. Gradient coils are maintained at room temperature and are placed inside the bore of the superconducting magnet. Gradient coil performance is a central concern for ultra-fast imaging techniques (see Chapter 4).

Important issues in gradient coil design are described in Chapter 5. Two major characteristics of gradient coils that compete for optimization will be highlighted here. The first is the need to achieve high magnetic field gradients. Higher magnetic field gradients allow higher resolution spatial encoding and are also essential for particular forms of MRI such as diffusion imaging. The second major requirement is for fast gradient switching. Ultra-fast imaging (e.g.

with EPI) requires that gradients can be switched rapidly. But there is a trade-off: as gradients become more powerful, the inductance of their coils rises, reducing the maximum rate at which they can be switched (inductance can be considered as a measure of resistance to change of the electrical current in a circuit).

For brain imaging, one approach to balancing these competing needs is to use the smallest possible 'head-only' gradient coil design. By reducing the size of the region that can be imaged as much as possible, higher gradient strengths can be achieved with relatively lower inductance to realize higher switching speeds. In practice, gradient coil design is already constrained more by the physiological limits to gradient switching than by the technology itself. A changing magnetic field (dB/dt) induces an electric current in a conducting medium such as a human body. As the gradient changes become faster (i.e. as dB/dt rises) the induced current in the body rises. Thus very rapid gradient switching can generate currents that can cause unpleasant muscle twitching. The magnitude of this induced current increases with the cross-sectional area of the body region across which the gradient is applied, so it should be greatest across the shoulders (described by convention as in the gradient y-axis).

1.6.3 The importance of the radiofrequency coil

A radiofrequency pulse is used for excitation of nuclei and the resulting resonance is also a radiofrequency signal. To maximize detection sensitivity the volume being imaged (e.g. the head) must be placed in close proximity to the radiofrequency transmit and receive coil, which therefore must be positioned inside the gradient coils. Typically, the radiofrequency coil slides in and out of the bore of the magnet with the subject.

The importance of radiofrequency coil design and sensitivity to the MR experiment cannot be overstated. The benefits of higher field strengths for signal-to-noise simply are not realized if the relative coil sensitivity is not maintained at higher frequencies (although this will not affect directly the improvements in BOLD contrast-to-noise at higher field strengths). Less optimal volume coil designs can also lead to greater inhomogeneities of the radiofrequency field across the coil, giving rise to undesirably large signal intensity variations across the imaged volume. These can complicate precise determinations of the stimulus-induced time course of signal changes in the functional imaging experiment.

In general there is a trade-off between the flexibility of the coil for examination of the whole brain and sensitivity of the coil for examination of a specific region of the brain. There are two general types of coil. So-called 'volume' coils are placed completely around the head and can be used to image any part of the brain. However, the cost of this flexibility is that the size and position of the coil are not optimized for examination of any one brain region. Higher signal-to-noise for a specific region can be achieved with a 'surface' coil, a flat or curved coil that is positioned immediately next to the part of the head being imaged (Fig. 1.6). Surface coils provide good images from the volume immediately beneath the coil, but suffer from considerable image intensity distortions (from radio-frequency inhomogeneities or 'bias field') as the edges of the sensitive region are approached (Fig. 1.6) and are not sensitive to volumes farther from the coil. In some applications (e.g. spine imaging) a series of surface coils is used together as a 'phased array'. This approach combines the advantages of a small coil positioned close to the volume to be imaged with the need to image a larger volume. It could provide a useful strategy for future higher sensitivity brain imaging.

1.6.4 Practical constraints in functional imaging

Optimization of the fMRI experiment is particularly challenging because it demands simultaneous optimization of the imaging experiment (see Chapter 6), the stimulus presentation, response measurement and subject management (see Chapter 9), and the design of the psychophysical experiment (see Chapter 10). Because of the need to wait for some seconds between delivery of stimuli to allow full scanning coverage of the brain and recovery of the haemodynamic response, fMRI experiments can be of relatively long duration, so subject fatigue and boredom (during 'rest' periods) may become a particular concern. It is also important not to minimize the importance of considering the potential impact of the peculiar physical environment that the scanning magnet poses for any experiment. For example, visual fields may be limited to, 15–20°

for stimulus presentations. This limited field-of-view and the small space in a typical magnet bore may create a sense of claustrophobia in many subjects, the extent of which can depend very much on how well the subject is prepared for the experience.

Above all in the experiment, the safety of the subject must be assured. The problems of delivery or recording of stimuli from subjects can be among the most challenging because the high magnetic field makes the use of any ferromagnetic materials in stimulus presentation or response recording hazardous. Any metal in the subject (e.g. braces on teeth) can reduce image quality or put the subject at risk of injury. Cardiac pacemakers, particularly, use an externally applied magnetic field to switch operating mode and therefore should never be allowed even near an imaging magnet. Every subject should be questioned carefully regarding past surgeries and related matters prior to an examination. Materials having significantly different magnetic susceptibility than tissues generally should be kept away from the imaging volume as they can induce substantial imaging artefacts. In addition, the physical space is very limited and the subject must lie supine (at least with current magnet designs).

To minimize radiofrequency noise that degrades image quality, the imaging room must be insulated against external radiofrequency interference. This means that all equipment that could act as radio-frequency antennae (e.g. leads for electromyography (EMG) or electroencephalography (EEG)) must be shielded from environmental radiofrequency noise (which comes from such things as electric motors or local radio stations) or be entirely contained within the radiofrequency-shielded magnet room. As the rapidly switching gradient fields can induce currents substantial enough to cause severe burns, the subject must be electrically insulated from any potential conducting loops (e.g. arising from moisture or wires). Many types of electrical devices (e.g. many computer screens, electrical motors) simply may not function near the magnet, aside from any safety concerns.

The imaging system also generates considerable acoustic noise with gradient switching. In 3–4 T imaging systems, for example, the noise level may rise to 120 dB with some EPI sequences. Subjects need to be protected from the effects of noise using earplugs or headphones. Acoustic noise can cause more specific problems for experiments in which an auditory stimulus must be delivered. Finally, because the subject is positioned at some distance from the experimenter, interactions between the patient and the experimenter are limited and appropriate monitoring of behavioural responses is made more difficult.

1.7   Experimental design for fMRI

1.7.1   Design of the fMRI experiment

A fundamental limitation to experimental design with fMRI arises from the fact that the signal changes being measured are so small. The magnitudes of signal differences between different cognitive or stimulus-induced states can be substantially lower than the reproducibility of signal intensities in independent serial examinations even of the same subject using MRI! Thus, fMRI can be used only for determining *relative signal intensity changes within a single imaging session.* Even so, as Chapter 9 describes, one of the most important ways in which fMRI has advanced functional imaging has been in the experimental flexibility that it allows. This theme is taken up further in Chapter 19.

General strategies for fMRI experimental design

Once a set of specific hypotheses are generated that have functional neuroanatomical predictions, there are two general strategies that can be used in experimental design. The first involves *isolation of variables.* With this strategy, experiments are designed that notionally differ in the contribution of a defined cognitive process. Parts of such experiments then are contrasted serially to determine the independent effects of the factors of primary interest. The simplest way to do this is to effectively subtract the rest from the activation signals and test for significant changes. This assumes that the effects of activation of individual cognitive processing elements are linearly additive in a complex cognitive task. All of the methods for *isolation of variables* rely on an underlying model for the cognitive processing task. The validity of interpretation of the results therefore depends on the accuracy of this model.

An alternative strategy involves analysis by *conjunction.* Here, multiple tasks are chosen that are assumed to share a common processing element. Regions of the brain that are commonly activated by all of the tasks then reasonably can be inferred to be concerned with the common processing element. However, in using conjunction approaches (and more generally in the interpretation of functional imaging, in fact) it is also important to consider that any given anatomical region (particularly if not defined to very high spatial resolution) may have multiple processing functions that can be engaged, depending on the task involved.

Alternative stimulus presentation designs

The most time-efficient approach for comparing brain responses to different tasks during the imaging experiment is the 'block' design (Friston *et al.* 1999). This design uses relatively long alternating periods (e.g. 30 s), during each of which a discrete cognitive state is maintained. In the simplest form, there may only be two such states, a 'rest' and an 'active' state (although 'rest' is defined only with respect to the specific activity being considered). These are alternated through the experiment in order to ensure that signal variations from small changes in scanner sensitivity, patient movement, or changes in attention have a similar impact on the signal responses associated with each of the different states.

The block design is relatively straightforward to analyse, as the shape of the response function can be assumed to be simple. It remains an ideal design for many types of experiment, particularly in an early, exploratory stage. However, it creates a highly artificial psychological constraint. The task switching itself may also pose specific psychological demands. Finally, it can become difficult to control a cognitive state precisely for the relatively long periods of each block. A 'rest' state is rarely a true rest, as the mind 'wanders' in a subject who is not engaged in a specific task. Many types of stimuli (particularly sensory stimuli) may show rapid habituation (a particular problem in studies of olfaction (Sobel *et al.* 1998)). More complex cognitive tasks simply may not be amenable to a block design. For example, an 'oddball' paradigm (in which the reaction to an unexpected stimulus is probed) cannot be adapted to a classical 'block' design directly. Finally, information regarding the time-course of an individual response is lost within a block.

An interesting interpretative problem can arise as a

consequence of the lack of information on activation response time courses in the block design. When comparing activations between more complex cognitive tasks performed as 'blocks', differences in the relative length of activation after a stimulus can give rise to differences in the average magnitude of activation over the period of the block. Thus, a more long-lived activation that gives rise to a lower signal intensity change *per stimulus* delivered can lead to a greater intensity change *over the block* than does a shorter-lived activation that gives a higher signal change *per stimulus* (Carpenter *et al.* 1999).

A major focus of Chapter 9 is the description of so-called single-event fMRI (Buckner *et al.* 1996). In this design activation data are acquired serially after discrete stimuli or responses. By averaging data acquired after many such discrete events, the time course of the haemodynamic response can be defined. This is a potentially powerful approach, as it allows considerable flexibility for determining, e.g. responses to novel or aperiodically presented stimuli.

A related approach is to present stimuli in an entirely periodic fashion and then to map responses in terms of their phase relative to that of the stimulus presentation. This was used first for study of the visual cortex, which is organized functionally in multiple retinotopic maps arranged according to increasing eccentricity and polar angle. 'Edges' of functionally distinct areas within the visual cortex are defined by reversing patterns of map organization, e.g. the primary visual cortex, V1, represents a mirror image of the visual field, whereas adjacent secondary visual cortex represents the field directly. These differences allow adjacent functionally distinct regions of the visual cortex to be defined based on reversal of the patterns of response to a stimulus with periodically varying eccentricity and polar angle where phase-reversals mark the edges of distinct cortical areas (Sereno *et al.* 1995). Because it is effectively a difference mapping procedure (Grinvald *et al.* 2000), the edge contrast between adjacent regions is emphasized. Tonotopy in the auditory system and somatotopy of the arm have been mapped using a similar strategy (Servos *et al.* 1998).

Behavioural monitoring

A critical issue in fMRI is to ensure that the subject is performing the required task. This can be important particularly in clinical studies (see Chapter 18), in which full subject cooperation may be less certain.

Motor responses can be measured using a variety of devices. A button press can be used to indicate alternate choices (e.g. with multiple choice tasks) and to measure reaction times. More complex motor response devices (e.g. joystick movement) can also be used. Sensors for measuring kinematics (e.g. surface EMG coupled with goniometers) in principle could be used to provide an even more refined description of motor output. The primary issues in the design of such devices are that they should be safe for use in the magnet, do not introduce radiofrequency noise, and do not lead to head or proximal body movement sufficient to generate artefacts in the images.

Head movements invariably occur with speaking. Speaking also variably induces magnetic susceptibility artefacts in caudal brain regions arising from the changes in sizes of air cavities in the oropharynx and lungs. However, as the time course of these changes is brief relative to the haemodynamic response, their effects can be edited out of an image time series without diminishing sensitivity to the later haemodynamic response associated with vocalization (Birn *et al.* 1999). Assessment of cognitive activation using some forms of time series analysis (e.g. using a model-free method such as independent components analysis) also may be less sensitive to these artefacts. Most experimenters have thus far relied on non-verbal responses, however.

Eye movements may need to be controlled or monitored for a variety of types of experiments (e.g. in visual attention tasks). This now is possible with commercially supplied infrared optical fibre camera systems or high intensity light sources that can be reflected off the eye to provide an index of eye movement.

1.8 *Analysis of fMRI experiments*

Methods for the analysis of fMRI data are described in some detail in Part IV of this book. The basic problem in analysis of functional imaging experiments is to identify voxels that show signal changes varying with the changing brain states of interest across the serially acquired images. This becomes a challenging problem for fMRI data because the signal changes are small (giving potential false negatives or Type II error) and the number of voxels simultaneously interrogated across the imaged volume is very large (giving potential false positives or Type I error).

The major issues in statistical analysis for fMRI are outlined in Chapters 11 and 14, whilst Chapters 12 and 13 address ways in which the data can be prepared for analysis to minimize artefacts and maximize sensitivity for the detection of activation changes. One of the potentially most significant artefacts for fMRI that distinguishes it from other functional imaging techniques is its extreme susceptibility to *motion* from movements, either of the head or brain (e.g. with the respiratory or cardiac cycles) (Liepert *et al.* 1995) (see Chapter 13). Additional challenges can arise from EPI imaging artefacts, e.g. image 'ghosting' and reduced sensitivity or image 'holes' near regions of magnetic susceptibility changes (e.g. the sinuses) (Devlin *et al.* 2000).

After artifact removal two general approaches to maximising the signal-to-noise ratio for the time course data then are applied typically: *spatial and temporal filtering*. fMRI is being used to detect a signal change that lasts for only a limited period of time and covers just a small region of the brain. A general result of signal detection theory is that blurring of a signal (in this case both the dimensions of space and time need to be considered) can enhance the signal-to-noise. This important conclusion can be rationalised if one considers that any noise changing faster in space or time than the signal of interest is 'flattened' to a greater extent than is the signal of interest after such blurring.

After optimization of the signal-to-noise by filtering, analysis of the time course by comparison of signals in the 'baseline' and 'active' states must be made. Statistical inference from fMRI data is discussed in Chapter 14. There are many valid ways of performing statistical comparisons between signals in images associated with different brain states and their time courses of change. A common approach is to generate a map of t statistics (the ratio of the mean signal intensity to its standard error) on a voxel-by-voxel basis and use this to identify voxels with significance levels exceeding a chosen threshold (e.g. $t > 3$, which might correspond in a particular case to $p < 0.01$). A natural extension of the creation of the t map in this simple way is to correlate the time course with a more general model of expected response, again resulting in a t map,

which can then be tested for significant activation. However, it has been argued that non-parametric approaches may be more valid, as they make fewer assumptions about the behaviour of the data. One strategy is to set the threshold on the basis of voxel-by-voxel comparisons with changes seen in data sets after randomisation of the serially acquired images (Brammer *et al.* 1997). Other approaches are now being developed which are even less dependent on setting up a prior activation model. For example, independent component analysis (ICA) identifies regions of activation on the basis of finding independent modes of signal variation through space or time (McKeown *et al.* 1998).

A crucial point made in Chapter 14 is that valid statistical inference from the image time course data is complicated by the fact that large numbers of voxels are being assessed simultaneously for changes. The significance level must be corrected for the number of truly independent comparisons that are being made. For example, if 10 000 independent voxels are being tested and a threshold for significance of change in each of the individual voxels of $p = 0.05$ is chosen, then 500 (= $0.05 \times 10\,000$) would be 'active' by chance alone! The significance threshold therefore must be made more stringent in proportion to the number of independent comparisons. A related problem is to define the extent of independence of signal change between image volume elements across the brain.

A sometimes troubling early lesson in analysis is that the apparent pattern of brain activation changes with the statistical significance threshold chosen. In fact, the notion that a single statistical map could fully represent the complex, highly distributed and dynamic patterns of neuronal activation during a task is certainly over simplistic! Direct recordings make clear that neurones differ in firing rates over a continuum. The discrimination of activities that are relatively uniquely associated with a cognitive task is therefore only relative. Thus, to be as inclusive as possible in identifying regions involved in a cognitive task, a low significance level for activation would be needed. In contrast, to identify only those areas that show the greatest changes in activity during a cognitive task, a higher significance level may be ideal. The optimal choice will ultimately depend on the data set and the goals of the experiment.

1.8.1 Quantitative fMRI

Many applications (see Part IV) demand quantitation of results from studies performed before and after interventions or when comparisons are desired between studies performed over multiple occasions, e.g. in correlations of fMRI and behavioural responses (Wagner *et al.* 1999) or in studies of drug effects (Levin *et al.* 1998). In applications of BOLD fMRI different measures can be used to express activation in a region-of-interest, including the absolute or relative numbers of activated voxels, the mean percent signal change in significantly activated voxels, or the maximum signal change. Interpretations of changes in the different measures will be different. There is a high variance in counts of numbers of voxels that exceed a given threshold, as this index of change is very dependent on measuring the 'tails' of the activation distribution, where contrast-to-noise (i.e. the magnitude of signal change) is lowest (Cohen and DuBois 1999). However, caution should be exercised in selecting a single strategy for quantitative activation analysis. It should not be assumed that there is a fixed relationship between measures of the *magnitude* of signal intensity change and the *extent* of activation in a region-of-interest, particularly in studies of pathology. Alternative strategies may use different measures of activation response, e.g. perfusion or oxygen consumption changes. It is possible that such measures may show less intersession or inter-individual variation that does BOLD fMRI.

1.8.2 Real-time fMRI

A specialized area of research has been the development of fMRI as a technique for *real-time* physiological analysis of the brain. This could allow improved quality control by allowing determination whether a study had been technically successful even before the subject has left the scanner. More exciting, it would allow subjects to monitor their own performance directly, potentially allowing modification of cognitive state (e.g. in studies of meditation or imagery) using the neurophysiological feedback of fMRI (Voyvodic 1999).

1.9 Neuroanatomical interpretation of functional data

1.9.1 A common brain space

Generally, the primary goal of functional imaging experiments is to interpret functional changes in terms of the underlying neuroanatomy. The most important step in doing this is the registration of regions of significant change in the functional image with the structural image of an individual brain. This is a challenging problem because the image resolution, contrast, and distortions in the high resolution conventionally acquired structural image usually are different from those in the lower resolution (typically EPI) functional image. Problems of registration are outlined in Chapter 15. With BOLD EPI fMRI difficulties can be minimized by using a high resolution EPI image (e.g. a 'multi-shot' EPI image) for defining brain structure, as this has similar geometric distortions as the individual single-shot EPI images used for generation of the functional image.

Averaging results from studies of many subjects often is useful for identifying areas of activation common to many members of the group or for increasing sensitivity to low level activation effects. This is possible with use of a common brain space. The most well-known common brain space was developed by Talairach and Tournoux as a simple geometric parcellation of the brain according to major anatomical landmarks. The concept behind this development was to develop a common coordinate framework for expressing relative neuroanatomical positions in any brain. It is important to recognize that different common brain spaces (e.g, the Montreal Neurological Institute average brain vs. that of the Talairach atlas (Talairach and Tournoux 1988)) may have different shapes, so that there are different relations between specific structures and coordinate positions.

In order to represent individually variable brain shapes in a standard coordinate framework computational methods for 'warping' one brain geometry into that of another have been developed (Collins *et al.* 1994). Such methods fit one brain shape to another by optimising the alignment of neuroanatomically similar features of the two brains.

However, even when both linear and non-linear 'warping' is allowed such procedures do not lead to brains that are perfectly co-registered everywhere. There are substantial anatomical differences between brains (and even greater variations in the underlying cytoarchitectonic structures (Amunts *et al.* 1999, 2000; Geyer *et al.* 2000)) affecting the relative sizes and shapes of subcortical grey matter and the sizes, orientations, and even the number of gyri. To allow accurate structural inferences in group data analysis, it is important to be able to express the range of this variation in brain anatomy across a population quantitatively. One powerful approach has been to combine maps of individual brains in a common brain space in order to generate a probabilistic map of brain structure. Within such a probabilistic brain space, the *likelihood* of finding a specific neuroanatomical feature in a given voxel can be expressed with precision even if mappings between structures in individual brains are not exact. When applied to a functional activation map, the relative likelihood of finding activation in a probabilistic brain structural space is expressed.

It is therefore important to appreciate that brain atlases do not provide a neuroanatomical 'Bible' for understanding functional activation. Brain atlases do not directly address the problem of what the neuroanatomical position of activation is in any individual brain, they simply are not reliable for determining anatomical positions in structurally abnormal brains. However, a probabilistic brain atlas provides an important tool for interpretation of activation data from the normal groups for which it was derived.

1.9.2 Cortical 'flat map' representations

Chapter 15 also addresses a potentially highly informative strategy for reducing confounds to understanding the functional interrelations between brain regions that are introduced by the convoluted surface of the cortex. As the relative localization of different function regions sometimes can be defined better using flattened representations, a number of strategies have been presented for computationally unfolding the cortex based on structural MRI data (e.g. Van and Drury 1997; Van *et al.* 1998; Dale *et al.* 1999; Fischl *et al.* 1999). 'Inflating' the brain to provide a continuous closed surface can cause distortions of relative distances (depending on the geometry of inflation). Unfolding such a surface into a flat map demands introducing 'cuts' into the surface to minimize intro-

duction of further distortions (consider the problem of flattening an orange peel). However, these need not affect quantitative measurements of relative positions substantially, particularly for closely adjacent areas. Other representations using standard geometric shapes for which coordinate systems are derived readily and that demand less distortion (e.g. a sphere) also are possible (Fischl *et al.* 1999). These methods all share the theoretical advantage that the relative coordinates in the new frame of reference more accurately reflect relative distances along the cortex between regions than do apparent distances across the surface of the normally-folded brain.

1.10 Applications of fMRI

1.10.1 Cognitive neuroscience

The range of applications of fMRI to neuroscience is growing rapidly. It is impossible to provide a textbook review that could be up-to-date. Chapter 17 describes the potential for fMRI applications from the standpoint of the cognitive neuroscientist. Here a more limited range of examples is offered to illustrate major research areas in which fMRI is proving to be an important tool:

(1) Defining neurophysiological correlates of behaviour;
(2) Defining ways in which brain functions can be modulated;
(3) Establishing a 'systems-level' description for the brain basis of learning;
(4) Defining 'networks' for cognitive processing.

Neurophysiological correlates of behaviour

One goal of neurophysiological studies of the brain is to localize cerebral functions. Ultimately this description contributes to an understanding of mechanisms for cognitive processing.

The first major application of fMRI was for the localization of cerebral functions. fMRI is established now as a powerful, relatively general technique for doing this. Activation maps can be generated with linear dimensions on the order of millimeters. In specialized applications (e.g. the primary visual cortex) it has been possible to refine spatial localization to the level of cortical columns (tens of microns) (Kim *et al.* 2000). The range of processes that can be studied and the precision of assignment of functions to the areas mapped depend largely on the imagination of the experimenters in designing the paradigm. Applications to understanding sensation, motor control, and cognitive processes such as language and memory have all been explored widely. A limitation to be borne in mind is that sensitivity to neuronal activity varies across the brain (Devlin *et al.* 2000).

Initial applications used tasks that could be constrained to periodic designs with repeated blocks stimuli. They also were confined to simple contrasts. With the availability of more sophisticated methods of analysis and the increased contrast-to-noise afforded by higher field systems, the requirement for stimulus repetition has become less limiting. In addition, application of single event designs have allowed a brief stimulus to be delivered even aperiodically, reducing the confounds of habituation and anticipation. This has allowed an extension of applications to include mapping for brain activation associated with such classic neuropsychological phenomena as 'oddball' detection (Linden *et al.* 1999).

Modulation of brain function

An intermediate goal in trying to define ways in which different areas of the networks for cognitive processing interact has been to study the modulation of brain responses. One area of applications has been to understand the way in which the sensory cortex integrates information from multiple modalities. Here, for example, it has been shown how the cortical response to touch is modulated by a visual stimulus (Macaluso *et al.* 2000). Such approaches have demanded improved methods for quantitative fMRI. These rely primarily on detection of changes in signal intensity, a characteristically more robust measure of activation than numbers of significantly activated pixels.

A particular class of such experiments have been those focused on understanding the phenomenon of 'attention'. These studies probe the nature of cognitive set changes and their influences on cortical activations. Such work has emphasized primarily that mechanisms of attention involve highly distributed changes in activation throughout the cortex in networks specific for a particular cognitive task (Johansen-Berg *et al.* 2000; O'Craven *et al.* 1997).

Understanding mechanisms of learning

Another early application of fMRI was to define changes in brain activation with motor learning. A complex finger movement paradigm was presented to subjects, who were asked to practice it over days (Karni *et al.* 1995). With improved rates of performance there was increased activation in the primary sensorimotor cortex contralateral the hand moved. This suggested that one aspect of motor learning involves expanding the cortical representation for the movement.

Shorter-term changes in activation with learning later were studied for a more complex puzzle-solving task (Toni *et al.* 1998). Subjects had to learn the correct order of button presses and then serially execute them. This could be done within the time-scale of a single imaging session. Shifts in the relative magnitude of activations between cortical and sub-cortical structures could be defined.

Learning of other types also has begun to be explored. Better methods of analysis and improved sensitivity of detection have been developed, allowing short-term modulation of responses to be detected. This has allowed, for example, mapping of areas of the brain that respond both to learning a noxious stimulus and to 'reverse learning' (i.e. having an expectation disappointed) (Ploghaus *et al.* 1999; Ploghaus *et al.* 2000).

Defining networks for cognitive processing

A longer-term goal of mapping and activity modulation studies is to define the ways in which brain regions interact to create a full processing network used by the brain for cognitive tasks. Defining networks begins with identification of at least a subset of its constituent nodes by mapping methods as described above. Analytical techniques can then be applied to define the functional interrelations between activated cortical areas, e.g. using methods such as path or independent components analysis (McKeown 2000; Bullmore *et al.* 2000). Both of these techniques provide measures of the strengths of the correlations between activation changes in different areas of the brain. Diffusion MRI promises to add an additional dimension to this work by defining at least the larger white matter axonal tracts that provide the physical basis for the functional connectivities underlying network behaviour (Jones *et al.* 1999; Xue *et al.* 1999).

Combining fMRI and electrophysiological techniques

Combining electrophysiological methods with fMRI promises to join the high temporal resolution of the former with the high spatial resolution of the latter (see Chapter 19). A fundamental limitation of EEG or MEG studies is that precise source localization is difficult. Unique maps of generators in the brain (based on the distribution of scalp potentials alone) cannot be calculated, particularly for EEG, where there is substantial spatial distortion of the potentials by the complex patterns of head conductivity. Both EEG and MEG share the problem that there is not a unique way of defining the numbers or localizations of neuronal generators that can give rise to any given activation pattern measured at the surface of the head. An attractive approach to minimizing these difficulties is to use fMRI to set limits on the number or localization of sources. In practice this has been achieved by assigning a higher probability to sources that co-localize with fMRI activation (Dale *et al.* 2000). For more routine electrophysiological methods which have little intrinsic spatial resolution such as ERP, fMRI can be used less directly to allow additional, neuroanatomically-based inferences (McCarthy 1999).

Animal fMRI

There have been increasing numbers of applications of fMRI in animal studies. Because of the smaller sizes of animal brains and the complexities of obtaining a good activation response with anaesthesia, animal fMRI can be much more challenging than similar studies on man. However, such studies offer potential, e.g. in dissecting fundamental phenomena regarding the nature of the BOLD response (as very high field systems can be used) or drug effects (Chen *et al.* 1997). Primate studies are of special interest because of the similarities of the monkey and the human brain and the potential for performing the studies of complex behaviours using trained animals without anesthesia. Animal studies allow fMRI to be combined with more invasive monitoring techniques (e.g. direct cortical electrophysiological recording and microdialysis) (Fig. 1.10) (Chen *et al.* 1997) or lesion studies.

1.10.2 Clinical applications of fMRI

Clinical applications of fMRI already are becoming common. Those conducted thus far may be summarized in three general areas (aspects of which are discussed further in Chapter 18, along with special problems associated with patient studies):

(1) Mapping of functional areas in the damaged brain;
(2) Providing state or trait markers;
(3) Defining mechanisms of reorganization or compensation from injury.

(a)   (b)   (c)

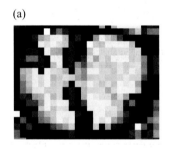 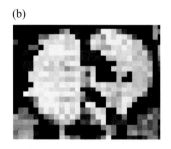 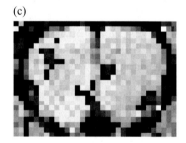

Fig. 1.10 Animal studies offer considerable scope for linking electrophysiological methods with fMRI. These images display activation patterns from direct cortical stimulation in the sensorimotor cortex using a carbon fibre electrode that was positioned through a small craniotomy hole directly on the cortex over the area of activation shown in the upper left of (a). Activation of cortex immediately beneath the stimulating fibre is apparent. In subsequent 2 mm sections immediately behind the area of stimulation (b, c) it is clear that activation occurs both in the area of stimulation and in more distant sides, particularly involving the deep basal ganglia. Such methods may allow functional definition of brain connectivities. (Image courtesy of Ms Vivienne Austen, MRC Clinical and Biochemical MRS Unit and FMRIB Centre, Oxford.) (See also colour plate section.)

A final application that likely could become important is the use of fMRI in monitoring the effects of drugs or other interventions.

Mapping functional areas in the damaged brain

One of the more important applications of clinical electrophysiological techniques (EEG, ERP) in critical care medicine and neurology has been to define the extent of undamaged cortex after severe insults. Like PET, recent work suggests that fMRI also could be used to define cortex that remains functional after brain injury (Cramer and Bastings 2000). A study of a patient with left inferior frontal damage after a stroke who subsequently recovered significant language function defined activation in brain areas closely adjacent to the damaged tissue, suggesting functional preservation of peri-infarct cortex (Calvert *et al.* 2000).

Localizing functional areas in chronic disease also can be important in planning treatment. Patients with intractable temporal lobe epilepsy may benefit from surgical excision of the ictal focus. However, removal of the temporal lobe must be planned carefully to ensure that temporal lobe tissue essential for language and memory functions is not removed. Current methods for lateralizing the activities associated with memory and language are rather crude, involving brief anaesthesia of each hemisphere in turn while performing psychological testing (the 'Wada test'). The potential for fMRI to be used as a non-invasive tool for identifying functional lateralization during language and memory tasks remains an attractive prospect (Fig. 1.11). Good agreement has generally been established between the non-invasive fMRI measures and those using Wada test (Desmond *et al.* 1995; Binder *et al.* 1996; Lehericy *et al.* 2000). A potential limitation of the fMRI studies is that while they identify regions of brain that are functionally active during the task, they do not specifically distinguish those for which activity is essential to the function in question. Damaging the latter is of course of particular concern in surgical treatment.

A similar problem is encountered in patients who need to have tumours or other lesions excised from the brain. If the lesion lies near functionally eloquent areas, there is a concern that removal of the lesion may impair critical functions subsequently. This is a particular

(a)   (b)   (c)

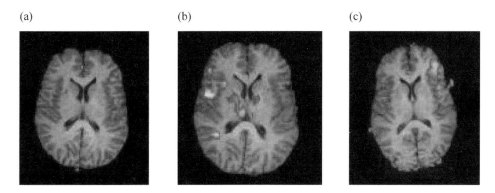

Fig. 1.11 The invasive Wada test is used to evaluate the lateralization of language and memory function in patients with temporal lobe epilepsy prior to possible surgery in order to minimize any potential for disability from the temporal lobe excision. There has been considerable interest in developing a non-invasive, fMRI-based method for lateralising language and memory functions. Here relative shifts in lateralization of brain activations in a verbal fluency task are illustrated. Each subject was presented with a visual letter cue and asked to recall as many words beginning with that letter during the active block of the fMRI paradigm. (a) A right-handed subject with right temporal lobe epilepsy demonstrates the pattern found in most healthy right- and left-handed controls showing almost entirely left-sided lateralization at this level of the brain, which includes Broca's area. (b) In contrast, a left-handed patient with left temporal lobe epilepsy demonstrates an almost complete shift in lateralization of activation to the right hemisphere. Here there is a more widely distributed pattern of activation at the same level, suggesting increased activation in more widely distributed nodes of the language network. (c) A right-handed patient with left temporal lobe epilepsy shows a bi-hemispheric pattern, suggesting that right hemispheric nodes in the putative language network become more active with damage to the left temporal lobe. (Images courtesy of Dr Jane Adcock, University of Oxford.) (See also colour plate section.)

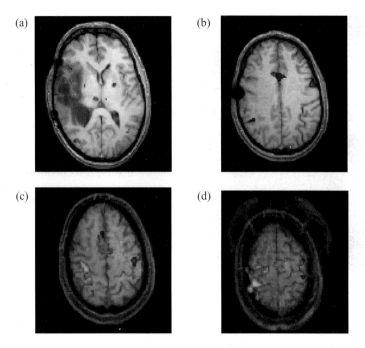

Fig. 1.12 Patterns of activation in patients with brain lesions may be useful in guiding neurosurgical excisions. This patient presented with a gliablastoma which was resected. With possible progression of the tumour the question of whether the excision margins could be extended arose. A concern was that the motor representation for movement of the contralateral (left) hand was too close to the excision margins to allow safe removal without subsequent disability. The patient then was studied using an FMRI paradigm involving simple movements of fingers of the left hand. The areas of significant activation are shown in blue. As can be seen particularly in images (b), (c) and (d), the patient (*blue*) shows predominantly ipsilateral cortical activation with movement of the hand. In contrast, healthy controls show predominantly contralateral sensorimotor cortex activation (*orange*). Panels (a) and (b) show loss of signal near the areas where the skull was interrupted by the craniotomy, a consequence of local magnetic susceptibility differences. (Images courtesy of Dr R. Pineiro, FMRIB Centre, Oxford.) (See also colour plate section.)

concern with many forms of brain tumour, for which prognosis may be improved by removing as much tissue from the adjacent brain as possible. A number of studies have explored the ability of fMRI to localize functional cortex adjacent to tumours, showing that the technique can distinguish functional and impaired brain tissue reliably (Fig. 1.12) (Atlas *et al.* 1996).

A related issue is to define *changes* in patterns of brain activation that are associated with functional recovery. An interesting illustrative example has been a study of a patient with blindsight (Sahraie *et al.* 1997). Blindsight patients have a loss of conscious visual awareness, yet can respond to at least a limited range of stimuli in the blind field without being consciously aware that they are present. The goal of this early study was to define the areas of the brain that are active when visual stimuli are unconsciously perceived with blind-

sight. Areas of frontal cortex activation as well as possible activation in the superior colliculus were demonstrated, suggesting that a secondary visual pathway was being used for processing of this information.

The capacity for the young brain to recover functionally even after major damage is well described and studies of animals have demonstrated a capacity for reorganization of the cortex in response to brain injury from both central and peripheral lesions (Nudo *et al.* 1996). A primary observation in the animal studies has been that *local* cortical functional representations can change. Interest has been generated by the demonstration of similar changes in the adult brain using fMRI. In motor studies with patients having tumours, for example, there are shifts in the cortical representation away from the tumours (Seitz *et al.* 1995). A consistent posterior shift in activation localization in the motor

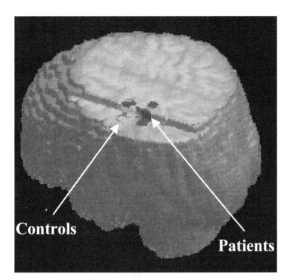

Fig. 1.13 Brain injury can lead to local adaptive changes in activation patterns from cortical 'plasticity' that can occur even in adults. This image illustrates a posterior shift in the centre of activation in the sensorimotor cortex for patients with established multiple sclerosis relative to a healthy control group. The yellow areas represent the mean centres of activation for a group of normal controls and the red areas shifted on average just under 1 cm more posterior) show similar centres of activation for a group of patients with established multiple sclerosis. Anatomically, this represents a shift in activation from the posterior wall of the pre-central gyrus in healthy controls to the anterior wall of the post-central gyrus in the patients. (Image courtesy of Drs H. Reddy and M. Lee, FMRIB Centre, Oxford.) (See also colour plate section.)

cortex has been reported in patients with multiple sclerosis and after strokes (Fig. 1.13) (Lee *et al.* 2000; Pineiro *et al.* 2001).

Longer distance functional changes also occur. Increased activation in the ipsilateral motor cortex also has been a consistent finding in studies of patients after brain injury or an 'unmasking' of uncrossed motor projection pathways that could contribute to recovery (Weiller *et al.* 1992; Cramer *et al.* 1997). A study of multiple sclerosis patients demonstrated a correlation between the lesion load and the extent of activation in the ipsilateral motor cortex, suggesting further that this functional change was related directly to the extent of brain injury (Lee *et al.* 2000).

Similar studies have been performed in patients with aphasia after left inferior frontal infarcts. Several groups have reported an increase in the relative extent

of activation in the right inferior frontal cortex for patients who show partial recovery of some speech (Thulborn *et al.* 1999) It has been argued that the right inferior frontal cortex may assume processing tasks performed previously by the injured left inferior frontal cortex. Alternatively, increased activity in the right inferior frontal cortex could otherwise compensate for lost functions, despite having distinct processing activities.

One confound of these and other studies after brain injury is that the tasks performed by patients and normal controls are difficult to match fully, as patients who are functionally impaired may find the tasks more difficult or may use different strategies to perform them. Differentiating adaptive reorganization from changes in strategy is difficult. In some instances a similar response can be elicited using a stimulus that can be provided in exactly the same way for both patients and controls, e.g. passive movement of the limb in a study of activation associated with hand movement. An alternative approach is to ensure behavioural matching of patients and controls. For example, in a study of multiple sclerosis, only patients with early disease who had no clinically significant disability in the limbs were studied (Reddy *et al.* 2000). Magnetic resonance spectroscopy provided a measure of white matter axonal damage. A strong correlation between the extent of axon injury in the white matter and the magnitude of ipsilateral motor cortex activation was established. The study was interpreted as demonstrating that the increased ipsilateral activation was not simply a response to altered task performance, but adaptive, allowing a normal level of function to be maintained despite accumulating injury. Alternatively, a task that can be matched between patients and controls and provides information relevant to the task of interest may be used, e.g. use of information from a passive movement task to define regions of brain active during voluntary, active movement (Fig. 1.14) (Weiller *et al.* 1996).

Another approach to task matching is to equalize the relative difficulty of tasks by having patients and controls perform the tasks at a rate or complexity that is a fixed proportion of the maximum individual rate. However, it may not be certain that there is a simple relationship between relative performance and brain activation.

A limitation of these fMRI studies of reorganization after injury is that, while areas of activation can be

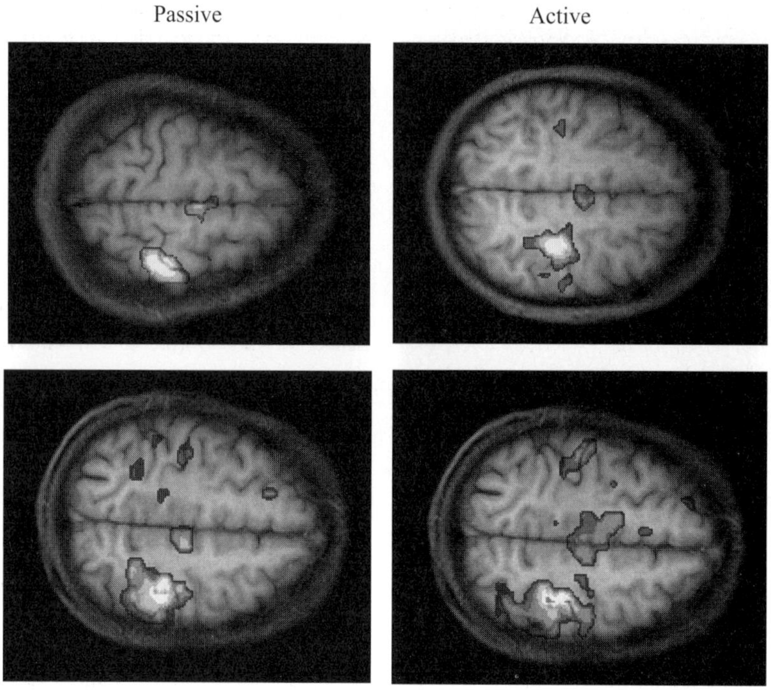

Passive   Active

Fig. 1.14 A major problem in studies of patients with disability from brain pathology is that of matching tasks between patients and controls to ensure that brain activation patterns represent responses to behaviourally comparable actions. One approach to the study of motor tasks may be to use the patterns of activation associated with passive movement of a limb. Because of the rich feedback from somatosensory and proprioceptive afferents to motor areas, activation patterns with passive movements generally recapitulate those accompanying active movement. Illustrated here are patterns of activation with either active (*upper panels*) or passive (*lower panels*) movements of a digit of the hand. (Images courtesy of Ms A. Floyer and Dr H. Reddy, FMRIB Centre Oxford.) (See also colour plate section.)

identified, it has yet to be demonstrated that the functionally more active areas are necessary for functional recovery, they could simply reflect responses to injury rather than be part of compensatory or adaptive mechanisms. To test this possibility, fMRI studies may need to be combined with other methods, such as repetitive transcranial magnetic stimulation (TMS), which allows transient interference with localized cortical functions (George *et al.* 1996; Pascual-Leone *et al.* 1994).

fMRI activation patterns as markers of state or trait

An exciting prospect for fMRI is that it may be used to define functional phenotypes, providing information not available either from the behavioural phenotype or structural imaging. A particularly intriguing example of how this could be possible has come from studies of dyslexia.

Patients with dyslexia appear to have difficulty reading at least in part because of defects in visual perceptual pathways. One clue as to how this might come about has come with the demonstration that patients with dyslexia have reduced or absent activation to moving stimuli in the motion-sensitive area (MT) of the extrastriate visual cortex (Eden *et al.* 1996). This result is consistent with the hypothesis that there is a developmental or acquired defect in the magnocellular visual processing pathway (which has relatively dense projections to the MT region). Subsequent work has extended this finding, suggesting that it identifies at least a subset of patients who have this complex behavioural phenotype (Demb *et al.* 1997). As clear clinical criteria for dyslexia has been difficult to achieve, the observation may contribute substantially to definition of the disease. In the future, fMRI studies could help to distinguish functional phenotypes in the syndrome in the search for genetic factors predisposing to dyslexia.

fMRI for drug and other treatment studies

The fMRI studies discussed thus far all have relied on comparisons between 'rest' and 'active' states produced by voluntary changes in cognitive activity or on stimulation of the cortex by sensory afferents. The neuroanatomical pattern of drug effects on brain activation or on regional blood flow can also be mapped (Leslie and James 2000). An early demonstration of this in an animal model showed appropriate lateralisation of activation changes in response to L-dopa after unilateral substantia nigra lesions (called pharmacological MRI or 'phMRI') (Chen *et al.* 1997). An issue in interpretation is to disambiguate direct effects on blood flow from effects on neuronal activity that are accompanied by a secondary haemodynamic response. Modulation of brain activation responses by drugs also can be probed. A study of alcohol showed a generally reduced activation response after ingestion (Levin *et al.* 1998). More specific drug

responses may also be altered as is demonstrated by an elegant study of opioid anaesthesia (Fig. 1.15). The drug remifentanil was shown to modulate activation of the somatosensory and limbic cortex associated with pain specifically, without effects on activation in the visual cortex (I. Tracey, unpublished).

A few practical considerations for clinical studies

In the interpretation of clinical studies, identifying *altered* activation (i.e. a new pattern or significant changes in the magnitude or extent of activation) is intrinsically more powerful than identifying *loss* of activation. The range of confounds to experimental paradigms such as movement during testing or poor compliance with the paradigm all tend to reduce signal, making loss of activation difficult to interpret. Clinical studies will also demand relatively unequivocal interpretations. Quantitative methods need to be developed with careful characterization of intra- and inter-patient reproducibility. Devising robust stimulation paradigms that can be performed easily and quickly to allow them to be integrated into busy imaging schedules, as well as rapid methods (e.g. real time fMRI) to allow immediate determination of the success of a study will be important.

(a)   (b)   (c)

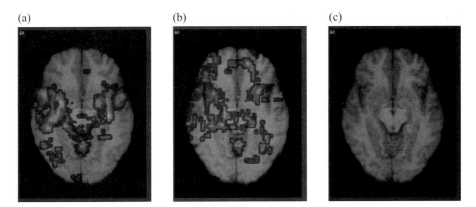

Fig. 1.15   One of the most exciting frontiers for fMRI is the objective description of subjective sensory experiences. A related area of excitement is the use of fMRI to assess the effects of pharmacological interventions. Here responses of the brain to a painful thermal stimulus are mapped using fMRI during intravenous infusion of a saline placebo (a). With infusion of 0.5 ng of the opiate analgesic remifentanil, there is small change in the pattern of activation, but the total volume of activation is little different from that with placebo and the subject reports little change in subjective pain perception (b). However, with infusion of 1 ng of remifentanil there is no subjective sensation of pain with the identical thermal stimulus. Associated with this is a loss of activation in this image slice, which includes the insula. (Images courtesy of Dr I. Tracey, FMRIB Centre, Oxford.) (See also colour plate section.)

1.11 BOLD fMRI in perspective

1.11.1 Limitations of the technique

BOLD-based fMRI is a powerful tool for basic and clinical neuroscience because it allows mapping of functional responses quantitatively using a technology that is non-invasive and already is widely disseminated. Particular excitement for its use in clinical applications comes in part from the fact that the technique can be integrated with other magnetic resonance-based techniques for a comprehensive investigation of pathological changes. However, there are important limitations of the technique that need to be recognized. The first is that the time resolution is limited by the rate of the haemodynamic response, which occurs over a time-course orders of magnitude slower than that of the primary neuronal response. The technique also both has intrinsically low signal-to-noise and contrast-to-noise, leading to the need for repetition of stimuli in order to decrease variance in results. Direct comparisons with PET studies also suggest that there is substantial variation in sensitivity to changes across the brain. Some of this is likely due to recognized artefacts, such as those from magnetic susceptibility changes in the temporal and frontal lobes. Finally, the unusual physical environment of the scanner and other constraints imposed on the experiment can be limiting.

1.11.2 The future of fMRI

Nonetheless, the future of fMRI looks bright. The technique has potential for answering a substantial and growing range of questions. In addition, developments in this active research area continue to promise greater capabilities.

A number of developments in hardware are promising. More flexible magnet designs, particularly short high field systems that would reduce problems of access to subjects during experiments may ease some experimental constraints. Particularly exciting also has been the introduction of extremely high field magnets (i.e. > 7T). These both promise increased signal-to-noise (which can be used to increase spatial resolution) and increased contrast-to-noise (allowing a greater variety of cognitive processes to be probed). Perhaps more importantly, work at such field strengths may allow more precise detection of activation solely in cortical tissue as opposed to the draining veins.

Image analysis currently is perhaps the most rapid growth area in functional imaging, however. Improved computational methods and the ever less expensive access to increased computer processing soon should allow true 'real time' fMRI. Not only would this potentially allow modulation of behaviour on the basis of the fMRI response, but it also should improve quality control by ensuring that experimenters or clinicians know whether a study has been successful before the subject ever leaves the magnet. While current fMRI experiments are constrained in their designs to a relatively rigid 'block' format or to less time-efficient, single event paradigms, there is every possibility that completely unconstrained experimental designs may be possible with flexible interleaving of multiple experiments involving the use of completely aperiodic stimuli. Advances particularly in model-free analysis methods (e.g. independent components analysis) may prove useful here. Other physiological measurements (e.g. perfusion, oxygen consumption or, ^{13}C-labelled metabolite turnover) may allow more quantitative imaging. Better methods for inter-modality registration of data and for using functional imaging data effectively in concert with electrophysiological data from techniques such as MEG will be important. Finally, substantial advances are being made in the nature of the structural data that is available, e.g. developing maps of cortical connectivities based on diffusion imaging (Mori *et al.* 1999).

Availability of such powerful methods for integrated analysis of images will make multi-modal functional imaging much more commonplace. This will enhance interpretations substantially by providing a multi-dimensional view of brain activities. An important goal will be to link efforts to model cognitive processing with empirical data from functional imaging. The hope is that functional imaging can substantially inform the development of such models. In turn, the models should be able to provide quantitative, testable hypotheses for functional imaging.

We fully expect that in coming years the potential of functional imaging will continue to expand and that fMRI will remain an important technique for neuroscience applications, despite growth of other functional imaging technologies. We hope that this book will provide a useful, practical guide to this new technology.

References

Amunts, K., Malikovic, A., Mohlberg, H., Schormann, T., and Zilles, K. (2000). Brodmann's areas, 17 and, 18 brought into stereotaxic space-where and how variable? *NeuroImage*, **11**, 66–84.

Amunts, K., Schleicher, A., Burgel, U., Mohlberg, H., Uylings, H.B., and Zilles, K. (1999). Broca's region revisited: cytoarchitecture and intersubject variability. *Journal of Comparative Neurology* **412**, 319–41.

Atlas, S.W., Howard, R.S., Maldjian, J., Alsop, D., Detre, J.A., Listerud, J., D'Esposito, M., Judy, K.D., Zager, E., and Stecker, M. (1996). Functional magnetic resonance imaging of regional brain activity in patients with intracerebral gliomas: findings and implications for clinical management. *Neurosurgery*, **38**, 329–38.

Bandettini, P.A., Kwong, K.K., Davis, T.L., Tootell, R.B., Wong, E.C., Fox, P.T., Belliveau, J.W., Weisskoff, R.M., and Rosen, B.R. (1997). Characterization of cerebral blood oxygenation and flow changes during prolonged brain activation. *Human Brain Mapping*, **5**, 93–109.

Belliveau, J.W., Kennedy, D.N., Jr., McKinstry, R.C., Buchbinder, B.R., Weisskoff, R.M., Cohen, M.S., Vevea, J.M., Brady, T.J., and Rosen, B.R. (1991). Functional mapping of the human visual cortex by magnetic resonance imaging. *Science*, **254**, 716–19.

Binder, J.R., Swanson, S.J., Hammeke, T.A., Morris, G.L., Mueller, W.M., Fischer, M., Benbadis, S., Frost, J.A., Rao, S.M., and Haughton, V.M. (1996). Determination of language dominance using functional MRI: a comparison with the Wada test. *Neurology*, **46**, 978–84.

Birn, R.M., Bandettini, P.A., Cox, R.W., and Shaker, R. (1999). Event-related fMRI of tasks involving brief motion. *Human Brain Mapping*, **7**, 106–14.

Brammer, M.J., Bullmore, E.T., Simmons, A., Williams, S.C., Grasby, P.M., Howard, R.J., Woodruff, P.W., and Rabe, H.S. (1997). Generic brain activation mapping in functional magnetic resonance imaging: a nonparametric approach. *Magnetic Resonance Imaging*, **15**, 763–70.

Buckner, R.L., Bandettini, P.A., O'Craven, K.M., Savoy, R.L., Petersen, S.E., Raichle, M.E., and Rosen, B.R. (1996). Detection of cortical activation during averaged single trials of a cognitive task using functional magnetic resonance imaging [see comments]. *Proceedings of the National Academy of Sciences* (*USA*), **93**, 14878–83.

Bullmore, E., Horwitz, B., Honey, G., Brammer, M., Williams, S., and Sharma, T. (2000). How good is good enough in path analysis of fMRI data? *NeuroImage*, **11**, 289–301.

Buxton, R.B. and Frank, L.R. (1997) A model for the coupling between cerebral blood flow and oxygen metabolism during neural stimulation. *Journal of Cerebral Blood Flow and Metabolism*, **17**, 64–72.

Calvert, G.A., Brammer, M.J., Morris, R.G., Williams, S.C., King, N., and Matthews, P.M. (2000). Using fMRI to study recovery from acquired dysphasia. *Brain and Language*, **71**, 391–9.

Carpenter, P.A., Just, M.A., Keller, T.A., Eddy, W., and Thulborn, K. (1999). Graded functional activation in the visuospatial system with the amount of task demand. *Journal of Cognitive Neuroscience*, **11**, 9–24.

Chen, Y.C., Galpern, W.R., Brownell, A.L., Matthews, R.T., Bogdanov, M., Isacson, O., Keltner, J.R., Beal, M.F., Rosen, B.R., and Jenkins, B.G. (1997a). Detection of dopaminergic neurotransmitter activity using pharmacologic MRI: correlation with PET, microdialysis, and behavioral data. *Magnetic Resonance in Medicine*, **38**, 389–98.

Cohen, M.S. and Bookheimer, S.Y. (1994) Localisation of brain functions usding magnetic resonance imaging *Trends in Neurological Science*, **17**, 268–77.

Cohen, M.S. and DuBois, R.M. (1999). Stability, repeatability, and the expression of signal magnitude in functional magnetic resonance imaging. *Magnetic Resonance Imaging*, **10**, 33–40.

Collins, D.L., Neelin, P., Peters, T.M., and Evans, A.C. (1994). Automatic 3D intersubject registration of MR volumetric data in standardized Talairach space. *Journal of Computer Assisted Tomography*, **18**, 192–205.

Cramer, S.C. and Bastings, E.P. (2000). Mapping clinically relevant plasticity after stroke. *Neuropharmacology*, **39**, 842–51.

Cramer, S.C., Nelles, G., Benson, R.R., Kaplan, J.D., Parker, R.A., Kwong, K.K., Kennedy, D.N., Finklestein, S.P., and Rosen, B.R. (1997). A functional MRI study of subjects recovered from hemiparetic stroke. *Stroke*, **28**, 2518–27.

Dale, A.M., Fischl, B., and Sereno, M.I. (1999). Cortical surface-based analysis. I. Segmentation and surface reconstruction. *NeuroImage*, **9**, 179–94.

Dale, A.M., Liu, A.K., Fischl, B.R., Buckner, R.L., Belliveau, J.W., Lewine, J.D., and Halgren, E. (2000). Dynamic statistical parametric mapping: combining fMRI and MEG for high-resolution imaging of cortical activity. *Neurone*, **26**, 55–67.

Demb, J.B., Boynton, G.M., and Heeger, D.J. (1997). Brain activity in visual cortex predicts individual differences in reading performance. *Proceedings of the National Academy of Sciences, (USA)*, **94**, 13363–6.

Desmond, J.E., Sum, J.M., Wagner, A.D., Demb, J.B., Shear, P.K., Glover, G.H., Gabriel, J.D., and Morrel, M.J. (1995). Functional MRI measurement of language lateralization in Wada-tested patients. *Brain*, **118**, 1411–19.

Detre, J.A., Zhang, W., Roberts, D.A., Silva, A.C., Williams, D.S., Grandis, D.J., Koretsky, A.P., and Leigh, J.S. (1994). Tissue specific perfusion imaging using arterial spin labeling. *NMR. in Biomedicine*, **7**, 75–82.

Devlin, J.T., Russell, R.P., Davis, M.H., Price, C.J., Wilson, J., Moss, H.E., Matthews, P.M., and Tyler, L.K. (2000). Susceptibility-induced loss of signal: comparing PET and fMRI on a semantic task. *NeuroImage*, **11**, 589–600.

Dirnagl, U., Niwa, K., Lindauer, U., and Villringer, A. (1994). Coupling of cerebral blood flow to neuronal activation: role of adenosine and nitric oxide. *American Journal of Physiology*, **267**, H296–H301.

Duncan, G.E. and Stumpf, W.E. (1991). Brain activity patterns: assessment by high resolution autoradiographic imaging of radiolabeled 2-deoxyglucose and glucose uptake. *Progress in Neurobiology*, **37**, 365–82.

Duncan, G.E., Stumpf, W.E., and Pilgrim, C. (1987). Cerebral metabolic mapping at the cellular level with dry-mount autoradiography of [3H]2-deoxyglucose. *Brain Research*, **401**, 43–9.

Eden, G.F., Van Meter, J.W., Rumsey, J.M., Maisog, J.M., Woods, R.P., and Zeffiro, T.A. (1996). Abnormal processing of visual motion in dyslexia revealed by functional brain imaging. *Nature*, **382**, 66–9.

Ernst, T. and Hennig, J. (1994) Observation of a fast response in functional MR. *Magnetic Resonance in Medicine*, **32**, 146–9.

Fischl, B., Sereno, M.I., and Dale, A.M. (1999). Cortical surface-based analysis. II. Inflation, flattening, and a surface-based coordinate system. *NeuroImage*, **9**, 195–207.

Friston, K.J., Zarahn, E., Josephs, O., Henson, R.N., and Dale, A.M. (1999). Stochastic designs in event-related fMRI. *NeuroImage*, **10**, 607–19.

Gati, J.S., Menon, R.S., Ugurbil, K., and Rutt, B.K. (1997). Experimental determination of the BOLD field strength dependence in vessels and tissue. *Magnetic Resonance in Medicine*, **38**, 296–302.

George, M.S., Wassermann, E.M., and Post, R.M. (1996). Transcranial magnetic stimulation: a neuropsychiatric tool for the 21st century. *Journal of Neuropsychiatry Clinical Neuroscience*, **8**, 373–82.

Geyer, S., Schormann, T., Mohlberg, H., and Zilles, K. (2000). Areas 3a, 3b, and, 1 of human primary somatosensory cortex. Part 2. Spatial normalization to standard anatomical space. *NeuroImage*, **11**, 684–96.

Gjedde, A. (1997). The relation between brain function and cerebral blood flow and metabolism. In *Cerebrovascular Disease*, (ed. H.H, Batjer, L.R., Caplan, L., Friberg, R.G., Greelee, T.A., Kopitnik, and W.L. Young), pp.23–40. Lippincott-Raven, Philadelphia.

Glendenning, K.K., Hutson, K.A., Nudo, R.J., and Masterton, R.B. (1985). Acoustic chiasm II: Anatomical basis of binaurality in lateral superior olive of cat. *Journal of Comparative Neurology*, **232**, 261–85.

Grinvald, A., Slovin, H., and Vanzetta, I. (2000). Non-invasive visualization of cortical columns by fMRI. *Natare Neuroscience*, **3**, 105–07.

Hashemi, R.H. and Bradley, W.G. (1997). *MRI: the basics*. Williams and Wilkins.

Hock, C., Muller, S.F., Schuh, H.S., Hofmann, M., Dirnagl, U., and Villringer, A. (1995). Age dependency of changes in cerebral hemoglobin oxygenation during brain activation: a near-infrared spectroscopy study. *Journal of Cerebral Blood Flow and Metabolism*, **15**, 1103–08.

Hoge, R.D., Atkinson, J., Gill, B., Crelier, G.R., Marrett, S., and Pike, G.B. (1999). Linear coupling between cerebral blood flow and oxygen consumption in activated human cortex. *Proceedings of the National Academy of Sciences (USA)*, **96**, 9403–08.

Hyder, F., Chase, J.R., Behar, K.L., Mason, G.F., Siddeek, M., Rothman, D.L., and Shulman, R.G. (1996). Increased tricarboxylic acid cycle flux in rat brain during forepaw stimulation detected with, 1H[13C]NMR. *Proceedings of the National Academy of Science (USA)*, **93**, 7612–17.

Hyder, F., Rothman, D.L., Mason, G.F., Rangarajan, A., Behar, K.L., and Shulman, R.G. (1997). Oxidative glucose metabolism in rat brain during single forepaw stimulation: a spatially localized, 1H[13C] nuclear magnetic resonance study. *Journal of Cerebral Blood Flow and Metabolism*, **17**, 1040–47.

Johansen-Berg, H., Christensen, V., Woolrich, M., and Matthews, P.M. (2000). Attention to touch modulates activity in both primary and secondary somatosensory areas. *Neuroreport*, **11**, 1237–41.

Jones, D.K., Simmons, A., Williams, S.C., and Horsfield, M.A. (1999). Non-invasive assessment of axonal fibre connectivity in the human brain via diffusion tensor MRI. *Magnetic Resonance in Medicine*, **42**, 37–41.

Karni, A., Meyer, G., Jezzard, P., Adams, M.M., Turner, R., and Ungerleider, L.G. (1995). Functional MRI evidence for adult motor cortex plasticity during motor skill learning. *Nature*, **377**, 155–8.

Kastrup, A., Li, T.Q., Takahashi, A., Glover, G.H., and Moseley, M.E. (1998). Functional magnetic resonance imaging of regional cerebral blood oxygenation changes during breath holding. *Stroke*, **29**, 2641–5.

Kim, S.G., Tsekos, N.V., and Ashe, J. (1997). Multi-slice perfusion-based functional MRI using the FAIR technique: comparison of CBF and BOLD effects [see comments]. *NMR in Biomedicine*, **10**, 191–6.

Kim, D.S., Duong, T.Q., and Kim, S.G. (2000). High-resolution mapping of iso-orientation columns by fMRI [see comments]. *Nature Neuroscience*, **3**, 164–9.

Kuschinsky, W. (1991). Coupling of function, metabolism, and blood flow in the brain. *Neurosurgical Review*, **14**, (3), 163–8.

Kuwabara, H., Ohta, S., Brust, P., Meyer, E., and Gjedde, A. (1992). Density of perfused capillaries in living human brain during functional activation. *Progress in Brain Research*, **91**, 209–15.

Lee, M., Reddy, H., Johansen-Berg, H., Pendlebury, S., Jenkinson, M., Smith, S., Palace, J., and Matthews, P.M. (2000). The motor cortex shows adaptive functional changes to brain injury from multiple sclerosis. *Annals of Neurology*, **47**, 606–13.

Lehericy, S., Cohen, L., Bazin, B., Samson, S., Giacomini, E., Rougetet, R., Hertz, P.L., Lee, B.D., Marsault, C., and Baulac, M. (2000). Functional MR evaluation of temporal and frontal language dominance compared with the Wada test. *Neurology*, **54**, 1625–33.

Leslie, R.A. and James, M.F. (2000). Pharmacological magnetic resonance imaging: a new application for functional MRI. *Trends in Pharmacological Sciences*, **21**, 314–18.

Levin, J.M., Ross, M.H., Mendelson, J.H., Kaufman, M.J., Lange, N., Maas, L.C., Mello, N.K., Cohen, B.M., and Renshaw, P.F. (1998). Reduction in BOLD fMRI response to primary visual stimulation following alcohol ingestion. *Psychiatry Research*, **82**, 135–46.

Liepert, J., Tegenthoff, M., and Malin, J.P. (1995). Changes of cortical motor area size during immobilization. *Electroencephalography and Clinical Neurophysiology*, **97**, 382–6.

Linden, D.E., Prvulovic, D., Formisano, E., Vollinger, M., Zanella, F.E., Goebel, R., and Dierks, T. (1999). The functional neuroanatomy of target detection: an fMRI study of visual and auditory oddball tasks. *Cerebral Cortex*, 9, 815–23.

Macaluso, E., Frith, C.D., and Driver, J. (2000). Modulation of human visual cortex by crossmodal spatial attention. *Science*, 289, 1206–08.

Magistretti, P.J. and Pellerin, L. (1996). The contribution of astrocytes to the, 18F-2-deoxyglucose signal in PET activation studies. *Molecular Psychiatry*, 1, 445–52.

Malonek, D., Dirnagl, U., Lindauer, U., Yamada, K., Kanno, I., and Grinvald, A. (1997). Vascular imprints of neuronal activity: relationships between the dynamics of cortical blood flow, oxygenation, and volume changes following sensory stimulation. *Proceedings of National Academy of Science (USA)*, 94, 14826–31.

Mathiesen, C., Caesar, K., Akgoren, N., and Lauritzen, M. (1998). Modification of activity-dependent increases of cerebral blood flow by excitatory synaptic activity and spikes in rat cerebellar cortex. *Journal of Physiology*, 512, 555–66.

McCarthy, G. (1999). Event-related potentials and functional MRI: a comparison of localization in sensory, perceptual and cognitive tasks. *Electroencephalography and Clinical Neurophysiology Supplement*, 49, 3–12.

McKeown, M.J. (2000). Detection of consistently task-related activations in fMRI data with hybrid independent component analysis. *NeuroImage*, 11, 24–35.

McKeown, M.J., Makeig, S., Brown, G.G., Jung, T.P., Kindermann, S.S., Bell, A.J., and Sejnowski, T.J. (1998). Analysis of fMRI data by blind separation into independent. spatial components. *Human Brain Mapping*, 6(3), 160–88.

Meek, J.H., Firbank, M., Elwell, C.E., Atkinson, J., Braddick, O., and Wyatt, J.S. (1998). Regional hemodynamic responses to visual stimulation in awake infants. *Pediatric Research*, 43, 840–43.

Menon, R.S. and Goodyear, B.G. (1999). Submillimeter functional localization in human striate cortex using BOLD contrast at 4 Tesla: implications for the vascular point-spread function. *Magnetic Resonance in Medicine*, 41, 230–5.

Mori, S., Crain, B.J., Chacko, V.P., and van Zijl, P. (1999). Three-dimensional tracking of axonal projections in the brain by magnetic resonance imaging. *Annals of Neurology*, 45, 265–9.

Nudo, R.J., Wise, B.M., SiFuentes, F., and Milliken, G.W. (1996). Neural substrates for the effects of rehabilitative training on motor recovery after ischemic infarct [see comments]. *Science*, 272, 1791–4.

O'Craven, K.M., Rosen, B.R., Kwong, K.K., Treisman, A., and Savoy, R.L. (1997). Voluntary attention modulates fMRI activity in human MT-MST. *Neurone*, 18, 591–8.

Ogawa, S., Lee, T.M., Kay, A.R., and Tank, D.W. (1990). Brain magnetic resonance imaging with contrast dependent on blood oxygenation. *Proceedings of the National Academy of Science (USA)*, 9868–72.

Ogawa, S., Menon, R.S., Tank, D.W., Kim, S.G., Merkle, H., Ellermann, J.M., and Ugurbil, K. (1993). Functional brain mapping by blood oxygenation level-dependent contrast magnetic resonance imaging. A comparison of signal charac-

teristics with a biophysical model. *Biophysical Journal*, 64, 803–12.

Ostergaard, L., Smith, D.F., Vestergaard, P.P., Hansen, S.B., Gee, A.D., Gjedde, A., and Gyldensted, C. (1998). Absolute cerebral blood flow and blood volume measured by magnetic resonance imaging bolus tracking: comparison with positron emission tomography values. *Journal of Cerebral Blood Flow and Metabolism*, 18, 425–32.

Palmer, J.T., de Crespigny, A., Williams, S., Busch, E., and van Bruggen, N. (1999). High-resolution mapping of discrete representational areas in rat somatosensory cortex using blood volume-dependent functional MRI. *NeuroImage*, 9, 383–92.

Pascual-Leone, A., Valls, S.J., Wassermann, E.M., and Hallett, M. (1994). Responses to rapid-rate transcranial magnetic stimulation of the human motor cortex. *Brain*, 117, 847–58.

Pauling, L. and Coryell, C. (1936). The magnetic properties and structure of hemoglobin, oxyhemoglobin, and carbon monoxyhemoglobin. *Proceedings of the National Academy of Sciences (USA)*, 22, 210–16.

Pineiro, R., Pendlebury, S., Johansen-Berg, H., and Matthews, P.M. (2001). FMRI detects posterior shifts in primary sensorimotor cortex after stroke: evidence for adaptive reorganization? *Stroke*, in press.

Ploghaus, A., Tracey, I., Gati, J.S., Clare, S., Menon, R.S., Matthews, P.M., and Rawlins, J.N. (1999). Dissociating pain from its anticipation in the human brain. *Science*, 284, 1979–81.

Ploghaus, A., Tracey, I., Clare, S., Gati, J.S., Rawlins, J.N., and Matthews, P.M. (2000). Learning about pain: the neural substrate of the prediction error for aversive events. *Proceedings of the National Academy of Sciences (USA)*, 97, (16), 9281–6.

Reddy, H., Narayanan, S., Arnoutelis, R., Jenkinson, M., Antel, J., Matthews, P.M., and Arnold, D.L. (2000). Evidence for adaptive functional changes in the cerebral cortex with axonal injury from multiple sclerosis. *Brain*, 123, 2314–20.

Rees, G., Friston, K., and Koch, C. (2000). A direct quantitative relationship between the functional properties of human and macaque V5 [see comments]. *Nature Neuroscience*, 3, (7), 716–23.

Roberts, D.R., Vincent, D.J., Speer, A.M., Bohning, D.E., Cure, J., Young, J., and George, M.S. (1997). Multi-modality mapping of motor cortex: comparing echoplanar BOLD fMRI and transcranial magnetic stimulation. Short communication. *Journal of Neural Transmission*, 104, 833–43.

Robitaille, P.M., Abduljalil, A.M., and Kangarlu, A. (2000). Ultra high resolution imaging of the human head at 8 Tesla: 2K × 2K for Y2K. *Journal of Computer Assisted Tomography*, 24, 2–8.

Sahraie, A., Weiskrantz, L., Barbur, J.L., Simmons, A., Williams, S.C., and Brammer, M.J. (1997) Pattern of neuronal activity associated with conscious and unconscious processing of visual signals. *Proceedings of the National Academy of Sciences (USA)*, 94, 9406–11.

Seitz, R.J., Huang, Y., Knorr, U., Tellmann, L., Herzog, H., and Freund, H.J. (1995). Large-scale plasticity of the human motor cortex. *Neuroreport*, 6, 742–4.

Sereno, M.I., Dale, A.M., Reppas, J.B., Kwong, K.K., Belliveau, J.W., Brady, T.J., Rosen, B.R., and Tootell, R.B. (1995). Functional MRI reveals borders of multiple visual areas in humans. *Science*, **268**, 889–93.

Servos, P., Zacks, J., Rumelhart, D.E., and Glover, G.H. (1998). Somatotopy of the human arm using fMRI. *Neuroreport*, **9**, 605–09.

Sibson, N.R., Dhankhar, A., Mason, G.F., Rothman, D.L., Behar, K.L., and Shulman, R.G. (1998). Stoichiometric coupling of brain glucose metabolism and glutamatergic neuronal activity. *Proceedings of the National Academy of Sciences (USA)*, **95**, 316–21.

Sobel, N., Prabhakaran, V., Desmond, J.E., Glover, G.H., Goode, R.L., Sullivan, E.V., and Gabrieli, J.D. (1998). Sniffing and smelling: separate subsystems in the human olfactory cortex. *Nature*, **392**, 282–6.

Talairach, J. and Tournoux, P. (1988). *Coplanar stereotactic atlas of the human brain: 3-dimensional system, an approach to cerebral imaging.* (1st edn). Stuttgart, New York: Georg Thieme Verlag.

Thulborn, K.R., Carpenter, P.A., and Just, M.A. (1999) Plasticity of language-related brain function during recovery from stroke. *Stroke*, **30**, 749–54.

Thulborn, K.R., Waterton, J.C., Matthews, P.M., and Radda, G.K. (1982). Oxygenation dependence of the transverse relaxation time of water protons in whole blood at high field. *Biochimica et Biophysica Acta*, **714**, 265–70.

Toni, I., Krams, M., Turner, R., and Passingham, R.E. (1998). The time course of changes during motor sequence learning: a whole-brain fMRI study. *NeuroImage*, **8**, 50–61.

Van, E.D. and Drury, H.A. (1997). Structural and functional analyses of human cerebral cortex using a surface-based atlas. *Journal of Neuroscience*, **17**, 7079–102.

Van, E.D., Drury, H.A., Joshi, S., and Miller, M.I. (1998). Functional and structural mapping of human cerebral cortex: solutions are in the surfaces. *Proceedings of the National Academy of Sciences (USA)*, **95**, 788–95.

Voyvodic, J.T. (1999). Real-time fMRI paradigm control, physiology, and behavior combined with near real-time statistical analysis. *NeuroImage*, **10**, 91–106.

Wagner, A.D., Koutstaal, W., and Schacter, D.L. (1999). When encoding yields remembering: insights from event-related neuroimaging. *Philosophical Transactions of the Royal Society of London Series B Biological Sciences*, **354**, 1307–24.

Weiller, C., Chollet, F., Friston, K.J., Wise, R.J., and Frackowiak, R.S. (1992). Functional reorganization of the brain in recovery from striatocapsular infarction in man. *Annals of Neurology*, **31**, 463–72.

Weiller, C., Juptner, M., Fellows, S., Rijntjes, M., Leonhardt, G., Kiebel, S., Muller, S., Diener, H.C., and Thilmann, A.F. (1996). Brain representation of active and passive movements. *Neuroimage*, **4**, 105–10.

Wong, E.C., Cox, R.W., and Song, A.W. (1995). Optimized isotropic diffusion weighting. *Magnetic Resonance in Medicine*, **34**, 139–43.

Wong, E.C., Buxton, R.B., and Frank, L.R. (1997). Implementation of quantitative perfusion imaging techniques for functional brain mapping using pulsed arterial spin labeling. *NMR Biomedicine*, **10**, 237–49.

Xue, R., van, Z.P., Crain, B.J., Solaiyappan, M., and Mori, S. (1999). *In vivo* three-dimensional reconstruction of rat brain axonal projections by diffusion tensor imaging. *Magnetic Resonance in Medicine*, **42**, 1123–7.

II | *Physics and physiology*

2 | Brain energy metabolism and the physiological basis of the haemodynamic response

Albert Gjedde

2.1 Understanding the haemodynamic response to neuronal activation

Under normal conditions the brain derives almost all of its energy from the oxidation of glucose: for this it needs a nearly constant supply of glucose and oxygen, delivered by the blood supply through a rich network of vessels. Although the brain accounts for only about 2 per cent of the total body mass, it consumes 20 per cent of the body's glucose and oxygen, and receives 20 per cent of its blood supply. A remarkable feature of brain metabolism, fundamental to many functional imaging methods, is that blood flow and energy metabolism are tightly linked to local neuronal activity. This implies that maps of local glucose consumption, local oxygen consumption, or local blood flow each provide information on neuronal activity. A good understanding of the mechanisms responsible for regulating these processes is needed in order to interpret such functional imaging data. However, as this chapter will emphasize, although the general principles of brain metabolism and the haemodynamic response to neuronal activity are known, the precise mechanisms responsible for the links between brain energy metabolism and brain work are not well defined.

To understand better the issues relating to local brain haemodynamic response, cellular energy production, and the electrochemical work associated with neuronal activation, it is useful to consider:

- the kind of work carried out in the brain;
- the cells which carry out the brain's work;
- oxidative and non-oxidative energy metabolism and the mechanisms determining their balance in brain cells;
- the mechanisms relating changes in local blood flow to changes in brain oxidative and non-oxidative metabolism.

2.2 The work of the brain: the energy cost of information transfer

The major work of the brain is the transfer and processing of information. An estimate of the energy cost of information transfer in the brain can be calculated from the concept of entropy, according to which information transfer locally reduces the entropy of a metabolic system such as the brain.

A general principle of thermodynamics is that energy input is needed to reduce entropy, a measure of information (the less entropy there is in a system, the better the state is defined). In the brain energy is used primarily for electrochemical work (Szilard 1929). The energy cost of information transfer therefore can be estimated from the total combustion of fuels measured during functional activity of the brain. According to one calculation, a single binary decision, i.e. a unity *bit*, requires a minimum energy supply of 3×10^{-24} kJ (Morowitz 1978). The hydrolysis of adenosine triphosphate (ATP), the primary energy 'currency' in the brain (as in all cells of the body), yields a free energy of about 30 kJ mol^{-1}. The brain tissue hydrolyses about 10 μmol ATP g^{-1} min^{-1}. Assuming an upper limit of thermodynamic efficiency of 50 per cent, brain tissue thus has the capacity to perform binary decisions at a rate of about 10^{18} g^{-1} s^{-1}.

2.3 *The nature of metabolic work for information transfer in the brain*

In order to understand the link between changes in energy metabolism affecting physiological parameters such as blood flow and neuronal activity, it is useful also to consider the nature of the metabolic work in more detail. In general, there are two ways in which information is transferred within the brain: through propagation of an altered membrane potential and through the release of chemical neurotransmitters, a process intimately coupled with their subsequent re-uptake. Both processes involve work coupled to ion transport (particularly of sodium and potassium ions) across the membranes of brain cells.

2.3.1 Ion transport

Cells in the brain actively maintain electrochemical membrane potentials and are able to change these potentials in a graded way. After depolarization to a critical threshold level, neurones can discharge repetitively. The electrochemical membrane potentials are established by specific ion channels in the plasma membranes that exchange free ions (e.g. sodium, potassium, chloride) between the intra- and extracellular spaces (Hodgkin and Huxley 1952). In order to maintain a stable membrane potential, the conductances for each of the ions must be matched by active transport of the ion against its concentration gradient (the sodium concentration is higher and the potassium concentration is lower outside of the cell). Pumping of ions *against* an electrochemical gradient is an energy-requiring process. A key membrane enzyme in brain cells therefore is the P-type ('phosphorylation-type') Na^+, K^+-ATPase (an ATPase is an enzyme that breaks down or hydrolyses ATP), which combines with the energy-rich molecule ATP, Mg^{2+}, Na^+, and K^+ to form an enzyme-substrate association during which the ATP is hydrolysed, releasing energy and inducing conformational changes in the enzyme to translocate Na^+ and K^+ in the appropriate directions (Skou 1960).

However, while maintaining the membrane potential makes a major contribution to brain energy utilization, other factors also are important. Whittam (1962) estimated that the metabolism of the brain associated with the transport of sodium and potassium represents only 40 per cent of normal energy consumption. Chemical work of 50–60 per cent of the average was found to remain when ion transport in isolated nervous tissue was blocked completely by inactivation of the Na^+, K^+-ATPase (Baker and Connelly 1966; Ritchie 1967; Hertz and Schousboe 1975; Mata *et al.* 1980).

2.3.2 Neuronal excitation

Neuronal excitation occurs when membrane channels with a voltage-dependent conductance open to allow the passive flow of sodium ions into the cytoplasm from the extracellular space. This leads to steady depolarization of the membrane that can trigger a spontaneous neuronal discharge if sufficiently great. Neuronal excitation thus leads directly to the need for metabolic work as the sodium ions that enter for membrane depolarization subsequently must be pumped out of the cell against an electrochemical gradient in order to restore the resting membrane potential. Not surprisingly, therefore, the energy metabolism of brain tissue in conditions of low activity (severed connections after injury, coma, persistent vegetative state, anesthesia) can be reduced to as much as half the normal average (McIlwain 1951; Shalit *et al.* 1970, 1972; Brodersen and Jørgensen 1974; Sokoloff *et al.* 1977; Levy *et al.* 1987). In line with this observation on the whole brain, the electrochemical work to maintain a 'resting' membrane potential in individual cells is only about half of that required for active depolarization. During excitation of brain tissue *in vivo*, local increases in metabolism can exceed 100 per cent of the metabolism of the resting state, depending on the intensity of stimulation (Bowers and Zigmond 1979; Yarowsky and Ingvar 1981; Kadekaro *et al.* 1985; Shulman and Rothman 1998) (Fig. 2.1).

2.4 *Biochemical pathways providing energy for brain work*

The energy 'currency' of brain cells, ATP, is the link between energy utilizing and energy producing processes. Brain energy metabolism normally maintains a constant concentration of this metabolite, as the processes that restore this metabolite are sensitive (directly or indirectly) to increased ATP utilization

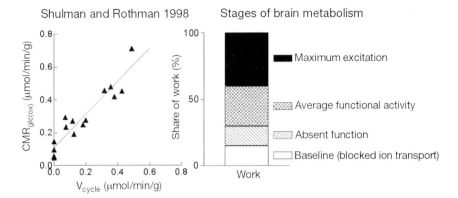

Fig. 2.1 Stages of brain activity and corresponding rates of brain oxidative metabolism versus rates of glutamate cycling measured by Shulman and Rothman (1998). A unitary slope is consistent with energy cost of glutamate cycling being 5 per cent of tissue total.

(feed-back). Observations in heart and brain suggest that even rapid variations in cellular work output by as much as 10-fold can be sustained with minimal changes in ATP concentration (Matthews *et al.* 1981; Balaban *et al.* 1986; Detre *et al.* 1990*a*, 1990*b*; Wyss *et al.* 1992)! This is possible because the biochemical pathways responsible for ATP synthesis are regulated by factors related to changes in its rate of utilization.

Both short- and longer-term regulatory mechanisms are used to maintain a constant concentration of ATP. A short-term mechanism for maintaining ATP concentration is by hydrolysis of phosphocreatine (PCr), a small, phosphorylated molecule unique to brain and muscle tissue. More sustained increases in rates of ATP utilization are balanced by increases in rates of *glycolysis*, the series of enzyme-catalysed reactions necessary for the orderly, energy-releasing breakdown of glucose to pyruvate and lactate, and *oxidative phosphorylation*, the oxygen requiring and energy-producing breakdown (or 'combustion') of pyruvate to generate carbon dioxide.

2.4.1 Hydrolysis of phosphocreatine

Creatine kinase (CK) occupies a pivotal role in the early buffering of the ATP concentration (Wyss *et al.* 1992). The 'low-energy' compound ADP is produced with energy-producing hydrolysis of ATP by ATPases. The enzyme CK catalyses the interconversion of ADP and PCr with ATP and creatine. One form of the enzyme is in the cytosol where it is active enough to maintain the reaction near equilibrium (i.e. [ADP][PCr] = [ATP][creatine] at a constant pH) (Roth and Weiner 1991; Mora *et al.* 1992). Thus, as [ADP] (the concentration of which is one–two orders of magnitude smaller than [ATP]) rises, [PCr] decreases to maintain [ATP] approximately constant.

Cytoplasmic PCr is replenished by a form of CK linked to mitochondrial ATP generation (Fedosov 1994). The advantage of this system for transfer of 'high energy' phosphate bonds in the cell is claimed to arise from the fact that PCr diffuses an order of magnitude faster than ATP (Wyss *et al.* 1992). However, under conditions of very high metabolic activity ATP homeostasis may not be maintained because of rate-limitation of the CK-transphosphorylation reaction in the mitochondria (Fedosov 1994).

2.4.2 Glycolysis

Glycolysis is the series of enzyme-catalysed reactions in the cytosol that are responsible for the breakdown of glucose to pyruvate and lactate with the generation of ATP. In the absence of oxygen anaerobic glycolysis occurs (at least as long as the end product lactate can be removed from the cell), but under normal conditions production of pyruvate and lactate is linked to their oxidation in the mitochondria (aerobic glycolysis). As glucose is the preferred energy substrate for the brain, understanding of the control of glycolysis is integral to the appreciation of how increased energy production and utilization are linked. Under condi-

Table 2.1   Selected brain metabolic reactions and metabolite transporters

Reaction or transporter	Equilibrium status	Activity [μmol g^{-1} min^{-1}]	Substrate concentration [μmol g^{-1}]	Time constant
[a]HK	Flux-generating	0.3	1.0	200 s
[b]PFK-1	Flux generating	0.3	0.1	20 s
[c]PDH	Flux-generating	0.3	0.01	2 s
[d]GLUT-1	Flux-limiting	2.0	5.0	150 s
[e]MCT (BBB)	Flux-limiting	0.2	0.1	30 s
[f]mMCT (mitochondria)	Flux-limiting	3.0	0.1	3 s
[g]GLUT-3	Near-equilibrium	1000	1.0	60 ms
[h]LDH	Near-equilibrium	2000	1.0	30 ms
[i]MCT (cell membranes)	Near-equilibrium	1000	0.1	6 ms

[a]hexokinase (Gjedde 1983); [b]phosphofructokinase-1 (Gjedde 1983); [c]pyruvate dehydrogenase complex (Katayama *et al.* 1998); [d]glucose transporter-1 (Gjedde 1992); [e]monocarboxylic acid transporters (Cremer *et al.* 1979); [f]mitochondrial monocarboxylic acid transport (Poole *et al.* 1993); [g]glucose transporter-3 (Diemer *et al.* 1985) ; [h]lactate dehydrogenase (Salceda *et al.* 1998); [i]monocarboxylic acid transporters (Desagher *et al.* 1997).

tions of maximal neuronal stimulation or in pathological states the rate glycolysis may be limited by the provision of glucose. Normally the rate is regulated by the reactions catalysed by the enzymes hexokinase and phosphofructokinase. Under aerobic conditions, most (but not all) of the glucose leaves the glycolytic chain as pyruvate, depending on the activity of the mitochondrial oxidative phosphorylation.

The main reactions of glycolysis and the time constants for these reactions are listed in Table 2.1 and their interactions are shown in schematic form in Fig. 2.2. The time constants dictate the half-times of change, i.e. the time it takes the system to reach halfway to a new steady-state after a change in concentration of a substrate. It is apparent from Table 2.1 that glycolysis can respond to change with time-constants of the order of milliseconds. This may be critical to maintaining bioenergetic homeostasis in response to rapid changes in cell energy utilization, e.g. with neuronal depolarization.

Glucose transport for glycolysis

Glucose is transported into neurones and astrocytes (a type of glial cell) by several members of the GLUT family of membrane spanning proteins (Gjedde 1992). In brain, the important transporters are GLUT-1 and GLUT-3 (Drewes 1999). The 55 kDalton GLUT-1 resides in the membranes of the capillary endothelium constituting the blood–brain barrier, while the slightly modified 45 kDalton GLUT-1 resides in the membranes of astrocytes and choroid plexus. The GLUT-3 protein resides in the membranes of neurones.

The transport capacities of GLUT-1 and GLUT-3 are known in some detail, and indicate that glucose provision itself is not normally rate-limiting to brain oxidative metabolism (Gjedde 1983, 1992). The maximum transport rate, T_{max}, of the endothelial GLUT-1 glucose transport is about 2–4 times the rate of unidirectional glucose transport, which is about twice the net transport of glucose (see Gjedde 1992). The T_{max} of the neuronal and glial glucose transporters GLUT-3 and GLUT-1 is 5000-fold higher (Diemer *et al.* 1985). Thus, under normal circumstances, glucose transport is not rate-limiting for glycolysis, and glucose concentrations in the different cellular compartments of brain tissue are likely to be similar. However, as the rate of transport of glucose is proportional to the difference between serum and cytoplasmic concentrations (Silver and Erecinska 1994), it could become rate-limiting in hypoglycemia. It also is possible that it could be rate-limiting under conditions of maximally stimulated glycolysis, unless blood flow changes are sufficient to continuously supply the glucose. For example, during physiological activation of rats, Silver and Erecinska (1994) demonstrated

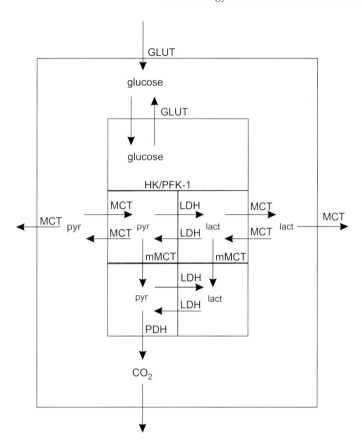

Fig. 2.2 A schematic model of the main metabolic reactions regulating glycolysis and oxygen consumption in brain. Symbols are defined in Table 2.1. Near-equilibrium reactions are shown with bidirectional arrows. Each compartment in the diagram represents a metabolic pool in the brain. The largest compartment is the brain, separated from systemic circulation by the blood–brain barrier. The next largest compartment is the 'brain cell', which metabolizes glucose to CO_2, lactate (lact) and pyruvate (pyr). Within the cell there are cytoplasmic pyruvate and lactate pools, interacting through catalysis by cytoplasmic lactate dehydrogenase (LDH), and mitochondrial pyruvate and lactate pools. The mitochondrial pyruvate pool provides the substrate for oxidative metabolism in the tricarboxylic acid cycle, the initial step of which is catalysed by pyruvate dehydrogenase (PDH).

slight decreases of the extracellular glucose concentration, by means of glucose-sensitive microelectrodes placed in the brain tissue.

Controlling the rate of glycolysis: hexokinase and phosphofructokinase

Two of the enzymes catalysing early steps in the glycolytic pathway are hexokinase and phosphofructokinase. Hexokinase (HK) is responsible for the phosphorylation of intracellular glucose to irreversibly commit it to breakdown by glycolysis. Phosphofructo-

kinase (PFK-1) catalyses a second phosphorylation step. Phosphate and citrate ions, AMP, ammonium and hydrogen ions, and PCr itself are among the classic regulators of theses two enzymes, whose activities are rate-limiting for glycolysis. The classical list of extrinsic regulators of these enzymes includes Mg^{++}, changes of the concentration of which may accompany increased ATP hydrolysis (as Mg^{++} binds to ATP). There is a net production of two moles of ATP for each mole of glucose metabolised to lactate.

Pyruvate and lactate production link glycolysis to oxidative metabolism

The enzyme *lactate dehydrogenase* (LDH) buffers changes in the concentration of pyruvate, which is a key bioenergetic intermediate linking glycolysis to oxidative metabolism. Pyruvate is a substrate for two competing reactions in brain tissue. It can be transported into mitochondria for oxidative metabolism, or reduced in the cytosol with conversion to lactate.

The link between glycolysis and oxidative metabolism in a cell is determined by metabolic competition for pyruvate. The kinetics of the alteration in pyruvate concentration thus provides a useful approach to understanding the overall kinetics of bioenergetic changes in the cell. The change of the cytosolic pyruvate concentration induced by an increase in the rate of glycolysis can be approximated by equations for the tissue contents of pyruvate (M_{pyr}) and lactate (M_{lact}), accounting for the three pathways available to pyruvate (export from cells, conversion to lactate, and transport into mitochondria) and the two pathways available to lactate (conversion to pyruvate and export from cells), as illustrated by the simplified model shown in Fig. 2.3. For pyruvate, the equation is

$$\Delta M_{pyr}(t) = \frac{2\Delta J_{glc}}{(1 + \Lambda)k}\left(1 - e^{-kt}\right) \qquad (2.1)$$

where ΔJ_{glc} is the increase of glycolysis, k is the lumped term $[\Pi k_{pyr} + \Lambda k_{lact}]/[1 + \Lambda]$ where k_{pyr} and k_{lact} represent the summed ratios $\Sigma T_{max}/K_t$, or clearances, of pyruvate and lactate import into the mitochondria and export across cell membranes (assuming M_{pyr} and M_{lact} always to be small relative to the so-called 'Michaelis constants', a measure expressing the relationship between enzyme rate and substrate concentrations, K_t of the transporters). The term Π (for 'pyruvate') is the fraction of mitochondria in the tissue which is 'active', i.e. stimulated to metabolize pyruvate. The term Λ (for LDH $= K^{lact}_m / K^{pyr}_m$) is the ratio between the Michaelis constants (K_m) of LDH towards lactate and pyruvate, which depends on the affinities of the prevailing isozymes (i.e. alternate enzymes catalysing the same reaction that have distinct characteristics) of LDH (LD_1–LD_5) towards its two substrates, as influenced by the $NAD^+/NADH$ ratio (a measure of relative oxidizing potential) and the pH. The ratio $\Pi k_{pyr}/(\Lambda k_{lact})$ is hence a measure of the tissue's oxidative

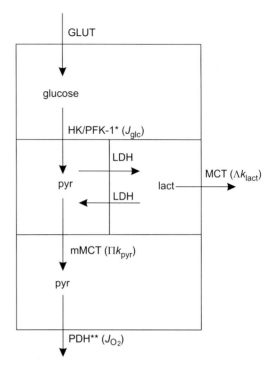

Fig. 2.3 A simplified model of the main metabolic reactions regulating glycolysis and oxygen consumption in brain, derived from the model shown in Fig. 2.2. Symbols are defined in Table 2.1. Metabolites linked by the near-equilibrium transport reactions shown with bidirectional arrows in Fig. 2.2 were assumed to form single kinetic compartments. Lactate and CO_2 productions are then regulated by prevailing LDH isozyme profile (Λk_{lact}) and rate of pyruvate entry into mitochondria (Πk_{pyr}). Eqns (2.1 and 2.2) were derived by simple solution of differential equations defined by the model.

capacity (ω), as influenced by the mitochondrial activity (Πk_{pyr}), the kinetic profile of LDH (Λ), and the blood–brain clearance of lactate (k_{lact}). With typical values for metabolite concentrations and transport clearances, the normal value of ω is 9 ([6/0.6]–1).

As Λ is generally known to be greater than 10 (see Table 2.5), the lumped rate constant k essentially is the product of the blood–brain barrier permeability–surface area (PS) product for lactate and the oxidative capacity of the tissue plus one: $k \approx PS(1 + \omega)/V_d$. This gives the rate constant a value of 0.4 min^{-1} for typical cortical tissue, with a half-time of change of less than about 2 min.

For lactate, the change of its tissue content is a function of the effective ratio of the affinities of LDH towards the two substrates,

$$\Delta M_{lact}(t) = \frac{2\Lambda \, \Delta J_{glc}}{(1 + \Lambda)k} (1 - e^{-kt}) \qquad (2.2)$$

where the ratio Λ varies with the isozyme subtype, such that the 'heart' form, LD_1 (H_4, adapted to function in an aerobic cell), has the lowest K_m^{lact} / K_m^{pyr} ratio and the 'muscle' form LD_5 (M_4, adapted to function in an anaerobic cell) has the highest (Kaplan and Everse 1972). These considerations lead to the important conclusion that the higher the ratio between LDH's 'affinities' or effective binding (i.e. the lower the ratio between the Michaelis constants) of lactate and pyruvate, the more rapid the approach to a new steady-state, with a time constant of $1/k$.

The brain has both H_4 (LD_1) and M_4 (LD_5). The equations show that with LD_1 pyruvate rises quickly for a given increase of glycolysis, while with LD_5 the pyruvate rises more slowly. These properties may have significance for cell physiology. For example, it is a common claim that the kinetic properties of LD_1 render this enzyme particularly useful for a tissue of high oxidative capacity because it allows rapid build-up of pyruvate, while LD_5 is more effective at buffering the increase of pyruvate in a tissue of lower oxidative capacity. Thus, some emphasis has been placed recently on the evidence that LD_1 and the messenger RNA (mRNA) for the subtype are found exclusively in neurones, while astrocytes appear to possess both LD_1 and LD_5 and their corresponding mRNA (Tholey *et al.* 1981; Bittar *et al.* 1996; Laughton *et al.* 2000). However, other factors are also important, e.g. the differences between the kinetics of the isozymes appear to be less pronounced at body temperature than at lower temperatures typically used for *in vitro* enzyme studies (Newsholme and Crabtree 1979). Therefore, it is probably incorrect to infer a net direction of the LDH reaction simply from the presence of a specific subtype in a population of cells and evidence for a relative compartmentation of LDH isozymes cannot be used to conclude that astrocytes and neurones use glycolysis in different ways (Van Hall 2000).

Transport of pyruvate and lactate out of cells

Pyruvate and lactate cross the membranes of neurones and astrocytes by means of proton-dependent transport catalysed by the so-called monocarboxylic acid transporter or MCT family of membrane spanning proteins (Oldendorf 1973; Halestrap 1975; Poole and Halestrap 1993; Halestrap and Price 1999). In brain tissue, the important transporters appear to be MCT-1 and MCT-2.

The MCT-1 protein spans the membranes of the capillary endothelium. Gerhart *et al.* (1997, 1998) claim that MCT-1 also resides on neurones, while the MCT-2 protein is found in astrocytes, apparently particularly their foot processes. In contrast, Broer *et al.* (1997) originally assigned MCT-1 to astrocytes and MCT-2 to neurones. As protons are transported with the monocarboxylic acids pyruvate and lactate, their transport is influenced by the pH of the cells and may thus decrease when pH rises. The MCT-2 is of higher affinity than the MCT-1, indicating that it is saturated by pyruvate and lactate at much lower concentrations than the MCT-1. For this reason, the MCT-2 may be more efficient at transporting pyruvate than MCT-1.

The maximal transport capacity (T_{max}) of the MCT-1 at the blood–brain barrier is 0.2 μmol g^{-1} min^{-1} (Pardridge 1981), with a Michaelis constant for lactate of about 5 mM (Halestrap and Price 1999), which is substantially higher than the normal lactate concentration in brain (Table 2.4). Under normal conditions the efflux rate is therefore only 25 per cent of the T_{max}. Since the T_{max} and K_t of the MCT-1 are about the same for pyruvate and lactate (Cremer *et al.* 1979), the export of pyruvate to the circulation is about one tenth that of lactate (Himwich and Himwich 1946). Considering the large surface area of neurones and glia, it is probable that the pyruvate and lactate exchange among the cell compartments of the brain is at near-equilibrium, as it is for glucose concentration.

Both pyruvate and lactate are transported into mitochondria by a specific mitochondrial monocarboxylic acid transporter, mMCT (Brooks *et al.* 1999a). The exact nature of mMCT is not known, but the bulk of the evidence suggests that it is related to MCT-2 (Halestrap and Price 1999), the high-affinity transporter, although its identity with MCT-1 has also been reported (Brooks *et al.* 1999a). The K_t of the mMCT is

0.5 μmol g^{-1}, i.e. somewhat higher than the cytosolic pyruvate concentration of 0.1–0.2 μmol g^{-1}, with a T_{max} of 3 μmol g^{-1} min^{-1} (LaNoue and Schoolwerth 1979; Nalecz *et al.* 1992), which is much higher than the average flux (0.6 μmol g^{-1} min^{-1}). Thus, the pyruvate rate of entry can rise five-fold in the absence of a change of the T_{max}.

The possibility that the mitochondrial mMCT causes the pyruvate concentration to be rate-limiting for oxidative metabolism in tissues other than brain was explored by Halestrap (1978). Halestrap and Armston (1984) concluded that this was not the case in liver. However, Shearman and Halestrap (1984) argued that pyruvate transport is rate-limiting for pyruvate oxidation by actively respiring heart mitochondria. This could also be true for the brain, although it is more usually accepted that mitochondrial pyruvate concentration is sufficient to saturate pyruvate dehydrogenase, the first enzyme in the pathway of oxidative phosphorylation, which is responsible for combustion of pyruvate in the mitochondrial.

2.4.3 Oxidative metabolism of pyruvate

At steady-state the brain almost completely oxidizes glucose via aerobic glycolysis (Himwich and Fazekas 1937; Gibbs *et al.* 1942; Himwich and Himwich 1946), so almost all pyruvate produced by glycolysis is subsequently oxidized in mitochondria. However, mitochondrial oxidative metabolism (i.e. oxidative phosphorylation, which proceeds from aerobic glycolysis) also is tightly regulated. There are two major sites for this regulation. The first is at the level of substrate provision by key enzymes of the tricarboxylic acid cycle responsible for oxidizing the three-carbon pyruvate into CO_2. A second level of control is in the transfer of the reducing equivalents (electrons) generated by these oxidation reactions to their final acceptor, molecular oxygen.

Mitochondrial dehydrogenases and control of the tricarboxylic acid cycle

As described above, mitochondria can import either pyruvate or lactate through their monocarboxylic acid transporter (Brooks *et al.* 1999a). Inside the mitochondria, any lactate is reconverted to pyruvate in another LDH-catalysed near-equilibrium reaction (Brandt *et al.* 1987; Brooks *et al.* 1999b). Electrons are then placed in a readily releasable storage for use with oxidation of pyruvate by the *pyruvate dehydrogenase* complex, the highly regulated, primary rate-controlling step for the mitochondrial tricarboxylic acid (TCA) cycle, which is the substrate provision arm of oxidative phosphorylation. Further storage of electrons released by oxidation comes with the enzymes *citrate synthase* and *oxoglutarate dehydrogenase*.

Cytochrome oxidase and control of the electron transport chain

The electrons produced with oxidation of pyruvate release a substantial amount of energy that can be used to synthesise ATP when transferred to an electron acceptor. This is done in the second arm of mitochondrial oxidative phosphorylation, known as the electron transport chain. The important terminal enzyme in this chain is cytochrome *c* oxidase (also known as the *cytochrome aa3* complex). Respiration is defined as the oxidation of cytochrome *c* by molecular oxygen, which serves as the ultimate electron acceptor. Transfer of electrons to oxygen by the enzyme complexes of the electron transport chain is linked to the pumping of protons across the mitochondrial membrane. This creates an electrochemical potential (the 'proton motive force') that can be harnessed to synthesise ATP by an F-type ATPase (working in this instance to *generate* rather than hydrolyse ATP) in the inner membrane of the mitochondrial cristae, named after its discoverer Ephraim ('F') Racker (Pullman *et al.* 1960), and now known commonly simply as the ATP synthase. Oxidative metabolism of glucose is much more efficient than anaerobic glycolysis alone: 38 moles of ATP are produced per mole of glucose oxidized in total.

Although the mitochondrial oxygen tension is a function of the relationship between the delivery of oxygen and the rate of cytochrome *c* oxidation, the influence of changes in oxygen tension on oxidative metabolism are poorly understood. Erecinska *et al.* (1974) and Erecinska and Wilson (1982) have assigned primary flux-generation and thus (under normal conditions) overall control of the rate of oxidative phosphorylation to the irreversible reaction between oxygen and cytochrome *c* (Wang and Oster 1998; Springett *et al.* 2000). To the extent that this holds, the ultimate maintenance of oxygen consumption depends on the regulation of oxygen delivery, particularly in the situations in which the mitochondrial oxygen tension threatens to drop below a minimum threshold. However, Erecinska and Wilson (1982) have argued that a 'near equilibrium' may exist such that the affinity of cytochrome *c* oxidase for oxygen may increase adaptively as the cellular energy state decreases in order to better maintain ATP homeostasis.

Using rat heart mitochondria as a model, LaNoue *et al.* (1986) confirmed that near-equilibrium of oxidative phosphorylation exists when respiration is very slow, but also provided direct evidence that mitochondrial ATP synthesis occurs far from equilibrium when respiration is active. Thus, the near-equilibrium model for regulation of oxidative metabolism fails in more rapidly respiring brain tissue. As a result of the imbalance between the delivery of oxygen and the cytochrome oxidase activity in these states, cytochrome *c* oxidase does not remain saturated when the mitochondrial P_{O2} declines relative to the average capillary P_{O2}. The imbalance can be expressed as a simple Michaelis–Menten relationship between the mitochondrial oxygen tension and the kinetic properties of the cytochrome oxidase,

$$J_{O2} = V_{max}^{cytox}\, \sigma_e \sigma_{O2} \qquad (2.3)$$

where J_{O2} is the net oxygen consumption, V_{max}^{cytox} is the maximum cytochrome *c* oxidase reaction rate, and σ_e and σ_{O2} are the cytochrome *c* oxidase saturation fractions ('occupancies') for electrons and oxygen, respectively. The oxygen tension in mitochondria (p_{O2}^{mit}) is the tension consistent with the observed oxygen consumption rate relative to the half-saturation tension (P_{50}^{cytox}),

$$P_{O2}^{mit} = \frac{P_{50}^{cytox} J_{O2}}{(\sigma_e V_{max}^{cytox}) - J_{O2}} \qquad (2.4)$$

from which it follows that the corresponding average capillary oxygen tension (P_{O2}^{cap}) driving the delivery is given by

$$\bar{P}_{O2}^{cap} = J_{O2}\left[\frac{1}{L} + \frac{P_{50}^{cytox}}{(\sigma_e V_{max}^{cytox}) - J_{O2}}\right] \qquad (2.5)$$

where *L* is the oxygen diffusion capacity.

The effect of these relationships on the mitochondrial oxygen tension is illustrated in Fig. 2.4, which plots the resulting mitochondrial oxygen tensions and rates of oxygen consumption for a range of cytochrome oxidase activities ($\sigma_e V_{max}^{cytox}$), given a constant capillary oxygen tension ($\bar{P}_{O2}^{cap}$), established by a constant oxygen extraction fraction, and hence a constant ratio between oxygen consumption and blood flow (linear flow-metabolism coupling). Figure 2.4 shows that the rate of oxygen consumption fails to rise above a certain threshold despite further increases of the cytochrome oxidase activity. The threshold is dictated by the mitochondrial oxygen tension and it is reached when the tension declines below the level associated with sufficient oxygen saturation of the cytochrome oxidase. Only elevations of the oxygen diffusion capacity (e.g. by capillary recruitment) or the mean capillary oxygen tension (e.g. by increased blood flow) allow the rate of oxygen consumption to rise above this threshold.

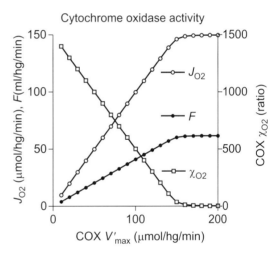

Fig. 2.4 Oxygen consumption threshold established by maximum oxygen delivery capacity $J_{O2}^{max} = L\bar{P}_{O2}^{cap} = 150\ \mu$mol hg^{-1} min^{-1}, $J_{O2}^{max} + J_{50}^{cytox} = L(\bar{P}_{O2}^{cap} + P_{50}^{hb}) = 150.1\ \mu$mol hg^{-1} min^{-1}, according to eqns (2.4 and 2.5). The rate of oxygen consumption, regulated by the cytochrome oxidase ("cox") activity ($V'_{max} = \sigma_e V_{max}^{cytox}$), cannot rise above the maximum oxygen delivery capacity, despite parallel increases of $J_{O2} = \omega k_{pyr} M_{pyr}$ and CBF. Further increases require increase of the oxygen delivery capacity, either by disproportionately large increases of CBF (raising $\bar{P}_{O2}^{cap}$) or by recruitment (raising *L*).

Modulation of substrate flux for oxidative phosporylation by calcium

Energy metabolism is modulated by a number of factors other than the provision of the carbon substrates and oxygen. Among the most important are calcium ions. Calcium ions play a role in the oxidation of pyruvate by activating the mitochondrial enzymes mediating non-equilibrium and flux-generating reactions (pyruvate dehydrogenase complex, citrate synthase, NAD^+-linked isocitrate dehydrogenase, and the 2-oxoglutarate dehydrogenase complex) which supply the NADH for oxidative phosphorylation (Denton and McCormack 1985).

In the resting state, mitochondria contain little calcium, but calcium accumulates with stimulation. The calcium entry is facilitated by the Ca^{++}-transporter in the mitochondrial membrane and driven by the mitochondrial membrane potential established by the H^+-extrusion mechanism. Rises in calcium concentration often occur as repeated spikes with steep upslopes and shallower downslopes which reach baseline during sustained excitation (Clapham 1995). Thus, a steady agonist level may induce pulsatile calcium release from calcium stores. The frequency of this calcium pulsation apparently depends on the agonist concentration.

2.5 Metabolic compartmentation and brain activation

Although brain bioenergetics thus far have been discussed with respect to a generic cell, brain tissue includes several populations of cells. Perhaps the most significant from the standpoint of bioenergetics are neurones and astrocytes, the metabolism of which are mutually interdependent. This section deals with the attempts to understand the role of astrocytes in the regulation of the metabolic response to neuronal excitation.

The cellular and subcellular sites of the increases of glucose and oxygen metabolism accompanying brain activation have been the subject of much investigation (Rose 1975; Muir *et al.* 1986; Bachelard *et al.* 1991; Poitry-Yamate and Tsacopoulos 1992; Magistretti *et al.* 1999). There is evidence that the major site for increased glycolysis with neuronal activity occurs in presynaptic structures (Eisenberg *et al.* 1993; Sokoloff *et al.* 1996; Sokoloff 1999) which also may be the predominant location of lactate dehydrogenase (Borowsky and Collins 1989). Mitochondria, on the other hand, have been observed to be particularly concentrated in the postsynaptic structures of neuropil (Ribak 1981; Gonzalez-Lima and Jones 1994), which stain weakly for the glycolytic enzyme hexokinase (Snyder and Wilson 1983). These observations suggest that the glycolytic and oxidative metabolism preferentially occur in separate cellular compartments (Aoki *et al.* 1987). This creates an apparent conundrum. As brain energy metabolism is predominantly aerobic (Hevner *et al.* 1995), this observation of relative metabolic compartmentation would suggest that the enhanced metabolism associated with brain activation should occur primarily in postsynaptic structures which are subject to direct-current (i.e. graded) depolarization during neuronal excitation. A key to resolving this problem may lie in understanding the metabolism of glutamate.

2.5.1 Interaction of neurones and astrocytes in the metabolism of glutamate

The main excitatory neurotransmitter in the brain is glutamate. Classically, discussion of the compartmentation of brain metabolism distinguishes between the larger and smaller pools of glutamate (Cremer 1976; Cremer *et al.* 1979). There is quantitative conversion of glutamine to glutamate catalysed by glutaminase in the large pool while the opposite process (catalysed by the glutamine synthetase and fueled by ATP) takes place in the small pool. The two pools of glutamate are now believed to be found in neurones (larger) and astrocytes (smaller). In mammalian cortex, the transfer of glutamate between the two pools occurs by neuronal release of glutamate during excitation and subsequent uptake predominantly by astrocytes. Shulman and Rothman (1998) claim that the amination of glutamate to glutamine (in the small compartment) is coupled linearly to the total tissue oxidative metabolism of glucose, i.e. one mol of glucose is metabolized oxidatively for each mol of glutamate released from neurones and aminated to glutamine in astrocytes (see Fig. 2.1), although studies *in vitro* have failed to show much stimulation of glial glycolysis by exposure to glutamate (Hertz *et al.* 1998).

Current evidence suggests that neurones are the major sites of oxidative phosphorylation of ADP to generate ATP, accounting for 70 per cent of the oxidative flux and 50 per cent of the glycolytic flux in brain tissue (Silver and Erecinska 1997; Shulman and Rothman 1998; Sokoloff 1999; Hassel and Bråthe, 2000). The oxidative capacity of astrocytes is low, not because of an innate preference for anaerobic glycolysis but rather because of their low rate of work. Silver and Erecinska (1997) have calculated that as much as 25 per cent of the metabolism of astrocytes is glycolytic. Taking into consideration that the import and amination of glutamate accounts for 5 per cent of the total oxidative metabolism (Shulman and Rothman 1998), this suggests that 20 per cent of the oxidative metabolism of astrocytes subserves the import and amination of glutamate. The estimated distribution of glycolytic and oxidative metabolism of neurones and astrocytes are shown in Fig. 2.5.

While astrocyte metabolism generally is low compared to neuronal metabolism, sustained stimula-

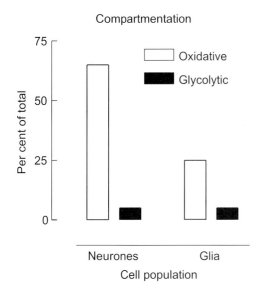

Fig. 2.5 Metabolic compartmentation of neurones and astrocytes: the relative proportions of oxidative and glycolytic metabolism in neuronal and glial tissue compartments are derived from measurements of oxygen-glucose indices (γ) for glial and neuronal compartments of 80 per cent and 93 per cent, respectively, reported by Silver and Erecinska (1994). Oxygen-glucose indices of this magnitude are consistent with an average oxidative capacity (ω) for glial cells that is only about 30 per cent of that for neurones ($\omega = \gamma/[1-\gamma]$).

tion of astrocyte metabolism could overtax their oxidative capacity (Alves *et al.* 1995). During some forms of excitation, for example, the neuronal firing frequency increases substantially and may require removal of excitatory neurotransmitters by astrocytes at rates incompatible with their oxidative capacity, which should lead to a net export of lactate.

Coupling of energy metabolism to glutamate transport

The presence of the LD_5 LDH subtype in astrocytes is consistent with a low metabolic rate but suggests that they could respond to large fluctuations in rate with brief, intense activations. In fact, astrocyte metabolism is closely coupled to highly variable neuronal firing rates as astrocytes have a critical role in the import of glutamate and potassium from the interstitial space surrounding the intrasynaptic clefts. Astrocytic processes surround the synapses and possess abundant excitatory amino acid (glutamate) transporters (EAAT-3 in humans [Vandenberg (1998)], GLAST and GLT-1 in rats [Rothstein *et al.* (1996)]). The transporters reside also on neurones (Vandenberg 1998), but recent gene knock-out studies suggest that the glial EAAT are indispensable for normal brain function, unlike the neuronal EAAT (Tanaka *et al.* 1997). One molecule of glutamate is symported from the extracellular space with three sodium ions. The transport increases the intracellular content of sodium and leads to an energy-requiring export of sodium ions coupled to import and astrocytic accumulation of potassium ions. The result is a net increase of potassium in the astrocytes.

Joint contribution of neurones and astrocytes to increased brain glucose utilization accompanying increased brain activity

The import of glutamate stimulates ATP hydrolysis by both the Na^+-K^+-ATPase and glutamine synthetase in astrocytes (Pellerin and Magistretti 1994; Magistretti *et al.* 1998). As the oxidative (aerobic) metabolism of glucose produces 19-fold more ATP than non-oxidative (anaerobic) metabolism, the fraction of total brain glucose metabolism ascribed to non-neuronal cells (30 per cent) is greater than the fraction ascribed to non-oxidative metabolism (10 per cent). If neuronal metabolism were entirely oxidative, glycolysis of glucose to pyruvate and lactate would be confined entirely to the non-neuronal cells, and the oxidative phosphorylation of pyruvate should occur only in neurones. This observation has led to the hypothesis that all or most of the glucose supplied to the brain undergoes anaerobic glycolysis to lactate in astrocytes which in turn supply some of their lactate to neurones which themselves consume little or no glucose directly (Magistretti *et al.* 1999). This attractive hypothesis has become popular, but also appears inconsistent with several observations.

The claim is a revival of an early speculation that the astrocytic processes serve to siphon glucose from the microvessels to the neurone terminals (Andriezen 1893). This earlier hypothesis was rejected initially when Brightman and Reese (1969) showed that the blood–brain barrier excludes the astrocytes' foot-processes (Reese *et al.* 1971). An important challenge to the more recent and compelling form of this hypothesis has come from a failure to demonstrate that glutamate import actually enhances glycolysis in astrocytes *in vivo* (Hertz *et al.* 1998). There also is no clear evidence that glycolytic and oxidative rates of metabolism are markedly ill-matched in astrocytes under normal physiological conditions *in vivo*, although the glycolytic fraction is somewhat higher than in neurones (20 per cent vs. 8 per cent in neurones, see Fig. 2.5).

There are other weaknesses of the hypothesis, as well. While neurones and astrocytes differ with respect to catabolic enzyme distribution and transporters, there is no evidence that glucose, pyruvate, and lactate are compartmentalized in distinct pools of neurones and glia. For example, unless pyruvate were strictly compartmentalized (which is ruled out by the abundance of MCT-1 and MCT-2), it is hard to appreciate how oxidative metabolism in neurones could prefer pyruvate of non-neuronal origin over pyruvate of neuronal origin (Poitry-Yamate *et al.* 1995). Of course, the two populations of cells may contribute differentially to the joint pyruvate and lactate pools when glycolysis is stimulated to a greater extent than oxidative metabolism, but this should only be a transient event in the normal brain.

The balance of glycolytic and oxidative metabolism in astrocytes and neurones is affected by the physio-

logical state. Substantial lactate generation would reflect the situation in which glutamate is released pre-synaptically but excitation is prevented because post-synaptic depolarization is limited by parallel inhibitory input. Mathiesen *et al.* (1998) showed that stimulation of cerebellar neurones in some cases led to increased blood flow despite inhibition of post-synaptic spiking activity by limiting the post-synaptic depolarization. Minimal post-synaptic depolarization would have two important consequences: (1) post-synaptic mitochondrial dehydrogenases would not be activated by calcium influx, but (2) astrocytes nevertheless would be stimulated to remove glutamate at a rate exceeding their oxidative capacity.

The removal of glutamate and the consequent hydrolysis and rephosphorylation of ATP in astrocytes must be sufficiently rapid to allow the frequent firing of excitatory neurones believed to underlie the functional integration of neurones in cerebral cortex (Joliot *et al.* 1994; Pedroarena and Llinas 1997). During non-steady state or otherwise uncommonly excited states it is possible that rapid removal of glutamate (Kojima *et al.* 1999) may generate pyruvate in astrocytes in excess of oxidative capacity. This could explain why astrocytes could react more glycolytically (i.e. produce more lactate) with stimulation than neurones. Thus, although recent measurements of the relative contributions of oxidative phosphorylation to the energy turnover in neurones and astrocytes suggest that 30 per cent of the total energy conversion of brain tissue takes place in astrocytes, the astrocytes may contribute significantly more to the increase of non-oxidative metabolism when excitation of post-synaptic neurones is prevented by parallel inhibition.

2.6 Understanding the quantitative relationship between work and energy metabolism

The precise link between increased work performed by brain tissue and an increased rate of metabolism is not known. Assuming the link is a signal from the changing concentration of a metabolite, the metabolite is not likely to be ATP. This sub-section deals with the attempts to identify an alternative regulator which changes in response to work and influences the rate of energy metabolism.

Table 2.2 Ion concentrations in nerve cells

| | Ion | | | | |
| Variable unit | Sodium | | Potassium | | Chloride |
	E&S	M	E&S	M	M
Equilibrium potential mV	+41	+40	−84	−100	−75
Intracellular concentration mM	27	30	80	140	8
Extracellular concentration mM	133	150	3	3	130

From Erecinska and Silver (1989) ('E&S'), McCormick (1990) ('M').

Table 2.3 Ion movements across nerve cell membranes

| | | Ion | | |
Variable	Unit	Sodium	Potassium	Chloride
Transmembrane leakage	μmol g^{-1} min^{-1}	15	10	5.0
PS product at −65 mV	ml g^{-1} min^{-1}	0.038	0.404	0.549
PS product at −55 mV	ml g^{-1} min^{-1}	0.044	0.285	0.246

From Gjedde (1993*b*), assuming 50% of ATP turnover dedicated to ion transport, calculated from the concentrations listed in Table 2.1 ('M'). To estimate the chloride permeability, it was necessary to use a simplified form of the equation.

As discussed above, increases of the intracellular concentration of Na$^+$ in neurones with an excitation-induced increase in neuronal membrane permeability stimulates membrane Na$^+$,K$^+$-ATPase activity. The energy released by the hydrolysis of 5 μmol g^{-1} min^{-1} ATP (half the ATP turnover) is sufficient to transport 15 μmol Na$^+$ g^{-1} min^{-1}. The resulting half-life of sodium in a stimulated neurone is less than a minute (and considerably less than the 20 min half-life of sodium in a stimulated squid axon!) (Hodgkin and Keynes 1956). This sodium ion flux through nerve membrane per unit tissue weight is one or more orders of magnitude greater than the sodium ion flux estimated from the average ATP turnover (Hurlbut 1970). This suggests that sodium flux occurs primarily in dendrites, rather than in the neuronal cell bodies or axons, where the density of sodium channels and (at least for the cell body) the ratio between the membrane surface area and intracellular volume is lower (Creutzfeldt 1975).

The apparent average sodium permeability-surface area product in the steady-state can be calculated from the sodium flux. With the concentrations listed in Table 2.2, as well as assumed values of an average steady-state membrane potential and corresponding sodium flux calculated from the measured ATP turnover, and the 3:2 ratio between the net sodium and potassium fluxes in the steady-state, the permeability-surface area products of sodium and potassium can be calculated by means of Goldman's flux equation (Goldman 1943; Hodgkin and Katz 1949) (Table 2.3). Details of this calculation are described elsewhere (Gjedde 1993*a*).

2.6.1 Average steady-state energy demand

Kety (1949) and Lassen (1959) first measured the magnitudes of resting brain energy metabolism and blood flow in human brain. More recently determined but similar steady-state values of energy metabolism and blood flow of the human brain are listed in Table 2.4, together with the steady-state turnover rates of ATP and lactate, calculated from the stoichiometric relationships,

$$J_{\mathrm{ATP}} = 2J_{\mathrm{glc}} + 6J_{\mathrm{O2}} \tag{2.6}$$

and

$$J_{\mathrm{lact}} = 2J_{\mathrm{glc}} - 1/3J_{\mathrm{O2}} \tag{2.7}$$

Table 2.4 Average physiological variables of human cerebral cortex

Somatosensory cortex	Average	Reference
J_{glc} [μmol g^{-1} min^{-1}]	0.30	—
J_{O2} [μmol g^{-1} min^{-1}]	1.60	Kuwabara et al. (1992)
CBF [ml g^{-1} min^{-1}]	0.45	—
ATP turnover [μmol g^{-1} min^{-1}]	10.0	Eqn (2.6)
Lactate flux [μmol g^{-1} min^{-1}]	0.05	Eqn (2.7)

where J_{ATP} is the ATP production, J_{glc} the glucose consumption, and J_{lact} the lactate production. Blood flow and metabolic rates were all measured by positron emission tomography (PET), blood flow after i.v. bolus injection of [^{15}O] water according to the method of Ohta et al. (1996), oxygen consumption after single-breath inhalation of [^{15}O] O_2 according to the method of Ohta et al. (1992), and glucose consumption after i.v. bolus injection of [^{18}F] fluoro-deoxyglucose according to the method of Kuwabara et al. (1990).

The molar oxygen–glucose ratio is 5.6, indicating that about 90 per cent of the glucose is fully oxidized (see also Himwich and Himwich 1946). At rest, total glucose consumption of cerebral cortex is about 30 μmol 100g^{-1} min^{-1}. The 10 per cent non-oxidative metabolism leads to a lactate production of about 5 μmol 100g^{-1} min^{-1}, of which 50 per cent is generated in neurones and 50 per cent is generated in glia (see Fig. 2.5). The lactate flux is about 25 per cent of the T_{max} of the blood–brain barrier MCT-1, consistent with a tissue lactate concentration of about 1.5 mM, as listed in Table 2.4. The corresponding ATP turnover calculated from eqn 2.6 is 10 μmol g^{-1} min^{-1}. Altogether, the brain tissue metabolite stores represent only about 1 min worth of energy consumption (Table 2.5).

2.6.2 Energy demands of neuronal excitation

Depolarization of neuronal membranes leads to increased oxygen uptake (Erecinska et al. 1991). This empirical finding is important, because cells in theory could depolarize without a change in ATP utilization if the increase of sodium conductance were coupled to substantial declines of potassium and chloride conductances (Gjedde 1993b). Table 2.3 illustrates this point by listing the identical ATP requirements at two different membrane potentials (−65 and −55 mV).

The Goldman–Hodgkin–Katz constant field equation predicts the changes of the membrane potential that occur when ion permeabilities change. Using the permeabilities calculated in Table 2.3, the corresponding membrane potentials were calculated as shown in Fig. 2.6. The membrane potentials reflect changes of both sodium and potassium (adjusted to preserve the 3:2 flux ratio required by the P-type Na$^+$-K$^+$-ATPase)

Table 2.5 Average metabolites in human brain

Metabolite	Cytosol		Glycolytic equivalents	
	Concentration (mM)	Content (μmol g^{-1})	ATP (μmol g^{-1})	Lactate (μmol g^{-1})
PCr	5.0	4.0	4.0	—
Glycogen	3.0	2.4	3.6	3.6
Glucose	1.2	1.0	2.0	2.0
ATP	2.2	1.7	1.7	—
ADP	1.2×10^{-2}	1.0×10^{-2}	5.0×10^{-3}	—
AMP	7.1×10^{-5}	5.6×10^{-5}	—	—
Pyruvate	0.16	0.13	—	0.1
Lactate	2.9 (0.75*)	2.3 (0.6*)	—	2.3
Total			11.3	8.0

From Olesen (1970), Roth and Weiner (1991). The 'glycolytic equivalent' is the ATP reserve that each metabolite would represent in case of complete depletion. *MRS measurements generally yield lower values of lactate in vivo (0.5–1 mM) but corresponding pyruvate values are not reported and the determination is indirect (see Prichard et al. 1991; Sappey-Marinier et al. 1992).

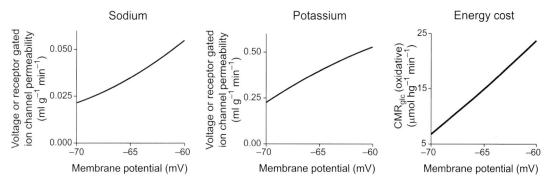

Fig. 2.6 The energy cost of depolarization (redrawn from Gjedde 1993b). *Left and centre panels*: steady-state neuronal membrane potential change as function of altered sodium and potassium ion membrane permeabilities at 0.549 ml g^{-1} min^{-1} constant chloride ion permeability. Ordinates: ion permeability [ml g^{-1} min^{-1}]. Abscissae: membrane potential [mV], calculated from the Goldman–Hodgkin–Katz constant field equation. *Right panel*: steady-state metabolism permitting membrane depolarization of the magnitude dictated by the increased sodium and potassium ion permeabilities. Abscissa: membrane potential [mV], calculated from the Goldman–Hodgkin–Katz constant field equation on the basis of chosen changes of sodium and potassium ion permeabilities. Ordinate: steady-state glucose consumption [μmol hg^{-1} min^{-1}], calculated from steady-state ion flux, assuming constant chloride ion permeability.

and chloride permeabilities. The resulting Na$^+$-K$^+$-ATPase activity was calculated as the flux required to preserve ion homeostasis. The glucose demand in turn was calculated as the nutrient delivery required to compensate for a steady-state ATPase activity of this magnitude by oxidative phosphorylation.

The fact that energy utilization is shown to rise with neuronal depolarization is an important confirmation of the hypothetical underlying mechanisms *in vivo*. Note that the values are intended as averages for a homogeneous tissue of cortical composition, in which no distinction is made between neurones and glia.

Figure 2.6 reveals the metabolic consequences of increased sodium and potassium permeability: even for a modest depolarization from −70 to −60 mV, the ATP turnover must increase four-fold from 2.5 to 9 μmol g^{-1} min^{-1} to preserve ion homeostasis. With a sodium-ion-transport-stimulated glucose metabolic rate of 0.15 μmol g^{-1} min^{-1}, the total glucose demand would be expected to increase from 0.2 to 0.4 μmol g^{-1}min^{-1} to fuel this turnover of ATP. For further depolarization to a firing level of −55 mV, the glucose supply would have to increase to as much as 0.6 μmol g^{-1} min^{-1} to fuel an ATP turnover of 20 μmol g^{-1} min^{-1}. In the absence of oxygen (or with no increase of oxygen consumption), the glucose supply would have to increase to as much as 10 μmol g^{-1} min^{-1}—a 30-fold increase—to cover the same need for ATP!

2.7 Balancing energy production and utilization

In order for cellular ATP concentrations to be maintained constant, it is necessary that rates of energy metabolism are tightly regulated to match rates of energy utilization. As described above, different pathways interact to make this possible. Rapid increases in ATP utlisation rates can be accommodated transiently by net breakdown of PCr. Increases in glycolytic rate have a slower time-constant. This can vary between cells and is important in regulating the rate of response of mitochondrial oxidative phosphorylation.

2.7.1 Hydrolysis of phosphocreatine

Hydrolysis of PCr buffers ATP concentrations at the expense of increased energy utilization. Protons are consumed by PCr hydrolysis and Erecinska and Silver (1989) have calculated that hydrolysis of 5 mM PCr may raise the pH of brain tissue by as much as 0.3 units at the prevailing buffering capacity. This prediction was confirmed by Chesler and Kraig (1987, 1989) who found that astrocytes become more alkaline when depolarized during brain activation. This may allow increased glycolytic flux, as activity of the rate-controlling glycolytic enzyme PFK is stimulated at higher pH.

In several kinds of cells a rise in pH correlates with an increase in metabolic activity (Kraig 1990).

2.7.2 Glycolysis

Increases in ADP concentration also stimulate glycolysis by activation of the glycolytic regulatory enzyme PFK (Connett 1987). Increases in the glycolytic rate by as much as 50 per cent were measured during functional activation of cerebral cortex (Fox *et al.* 1988; Ginsberg *et al.* 1988). When maximally stimulated, the rate of pyruvate generation can rise to 3–4 µmol g^{-1} min^{-1} (Robin *et al.* 1984; Gjedde 1984) which is several times the calculated maximum velocity of pyruvate oxidation, and close to the calculated T_{max} of the mMCT transporter in mitochondria. At these rates of pyruvate generation, the pyruvate concentration rises until the rate of pyruvate removal matches its rate of generation. The increase stimulates the pyruvate conversion to lactate, as well as its transport into the mitochondrial matrix and export to the circulation. The greater the equilibrium lactate/pyruvate ratio, the more slowly this rise occurs. For a pyruvate transport ratio ($k_{pyr} = \Sigma T_{max}/K_t$) of 6 min^{-1} (from the typical

values listed above) and assumed LDH affinity ratios (Λ) of 15 (as found for the LD$_1$ LDH sub-type), or 100 (LD$_5$ LDH). Eqns (2.1 and 2.2) yield the theoretical time-courses of the increase of tissue pyruvate during a 50 per cent augmentation of glucose consumption in the presence of LD$_1$ and LD$_5$, respectively, as shown in Fig. 2.7. The time-courses show that the half-time for approach of the pyruvate concentration to a new steady-state is approximately 2 min for an affinity ratio of 15 (LD$_1$), but as much as 15 min for an affinity ratio of 100 (LD$_5$). Lactate efflux through the capillary endothelium further increases the half-time for approach to a new equilibrium, as do decreases of the cytosolic oxidising potential (the NAD$^+$/NADH ratio).

As expected, Fig. 2.7 shows that the corresponding increase of the lactate concentration should be much greater for a cell with the LD$_5$ than with the LD$_1$ isozyme. The increase estimated for LD$_5$ is closer to the increase measured after glutamate receptor agonist (N-methyl-D-aspartate) administration to rat brain *in vivo* (Shram *et al.* 1998).

In the absence of an increase of oxidative phosphorylation, for an increase in total ATP flux of only 5 per cent there should be a 50 per cent increase of glucose

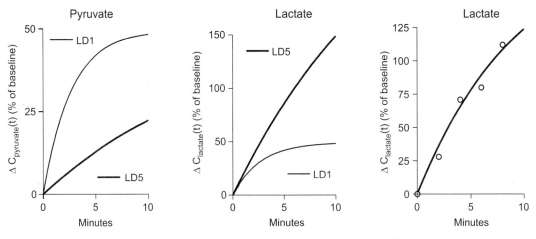

Fig. 2.7 Kinetics of lactate increase: estimation of rate of increase of lactate for two different rate constants dictated by different oxidative capacities, symbolized by subtype of lactate dehydrogenase, according to (eqns 2.1 and 2.2). The oxidative capacity associated with the LD$_1$ isozyme ('red' metabolism) was modeled with $k = 0.375$ min^{-1} and that for the LD$_5$ isozyme ('white' metabolism) with a rate constant, $k = 0.050$ min^{-1}. Abscissae: min. Ordinates: increase (per cent of baseline). *Left panel*: the increase of pyruvate is greater with LD$_1$ than for LD$_5$. *Centre panel*: conversely, the increase of lactate is greater for LD$_5$ than for LD$_1$. *Right panel*: estimation of the rate constant for lactate increases from measurements reported by Shram *et al.* (1998). A rate constant of 0.11 min^{-1} is consistent with oxidative capacity of 1.75 ([0.11/0.04]–1), which is below normal average of nine, and hence consistent with glycolytic (or 'white') metabolism. Note that low oxidative capacity can be due either to low mitochondrial activity or to a low LDH lactate/pyruvate affinity ratio.

Table 2.6 Neuronal activation of brain metabolism

Stimulus	Duration [min]	Supply			Products	
		ΔF	ΔJ_{glc}	ΔJ_{O2}	ΔJ_{ATP}	ΔJ_{lact}
		[%]			[μmol g^{-1} min^{-1}]	
Primary						
Somatosensory	1[a]	28	[17]	9*	0.96*	0.05
	1[b]	31	[18]	13*	1.35*	0.03
	1[c]	18	[8]	0	0.04	0.04
	20[d]	18	8	[0]	0.04	0.04
	20[c]	11	[8]	0	0.04	0.04
	45[e]	27	17	[0]	0.10	0.10
Visual (photic)	30[f]	43	27	0	0.15	0.15
	45[g]	49	51	5*	0.76*	0.26
Secondary						
Visual (checkerboard)	3–5[h]	25	[28]	28	2.83	0.008
	8–10[h]	26	[29]	29	2.93	0.009
	3–5[i] (1 Hz)	32	[10]	10	1.07	0.004
	3–5[i] (4 Hz)	38	[16]	16	1.71	0.006
	3–5[i] (8 Hz)	42	[6]	6	0.64	0.002
Thalamic stimulation	8[j]	88	[47]	47	5.02	0.019
Internal visualization	1[k]	31	[37]	37	3.95	0.015
Tactile learning	1[l]	23	—	—	—	—
Motor						
Hand grip	8[m]	30	[40]	40	4.27	0.016

From: [a]Fox and Raichle (1986); [b]Seitz and Roland (1992); [c]Fujita *et al.* (1999); [d]Kuwabara *et al.* (1992); [e]Ginsberg *et al.* (1988); [f]Ribeiro *et al.* (1993); [g]Fox *et al.* (1988); [h]Marrett and Gjedde (1997); [i]Vafaee and Gjedde (2000); [j]Katayama *et al.* (1986); [k]Roland *et al.* (1987); [l]Roland *et al.* (1989); [m]Raichle *et al.* (1976); values in brackets are estimates; * increase not significant.

phosphorylation (Table 2.6) with a seven-fold rise in lactate generation to 35 μmol 100g^{-1} min^{-1} and an increase in the fraction of non-oxidative metabolism from 10 per cent at baseline to as much as 40 per cent. When the rate of generation of lactate exceeds the T_{max} of the blood–brain barrier MCT-1, lactate concentration continues to rise (and the concentration of pyruvate rises with it) until the transport into mitochondria by the mMCT and oxidation by the pyruvate dehydrogenase complex match the rate of generation.

2.7.3 Oxidative phosphorylation

Recent measurements of oxygen consumption during simple primary somatosensory stimulation of human cerebral cortex are summarized in Table 2.6. They generally show little or no change of oxygen consump-tion (Fox and Raichle 1986; Fox *et al.* 1988; Seitz and Roland 1992; Ohta *et al.* 1999). With the single-inhalation method of measuring oxygen consumption, Fujita *et al.* (1999) compared changes of blood flow and oxygen consumption during 30 min of vibrotactile stimulation of the fingers of one hand. In primary sensory cortex, the blood flow change was 18 per cent at the onset of stimulation and still 11 per cent after 20 min of stimulation, but the oxygen consumption failed to increase for as long as 30 min.

The reason for this failure to observe an increase in oxygen consumption is not known. If this provocative observation accurately reflects the situation in acti-vated somatosensory cortex, it implies that the rate of oxidative phosphorylation cannot match the seven-fold increase of pyruvate production seen under the most extreme circumstances of glycolytic stimulation of the mammalian brain (van den Berg and Bruntink 1983). To increase the flux of pyruvate to mitochondria, cytosolic pyruvate concentration must increase (or mitochondrial pyruvate concentration must decline). Hence, insufficient accumulation of pyruvate because of conversion to lactate may prevent the activation of oxidative phosphorylation, while leading directly to oxidation of NADH in the cytosol. Connett *et al.* (1983, 1984) found that the lactate concentration in working dog skeletal muscle is directly rather than inversely proportional to the rate of oxygen consumption, as expected if a specific pyruvate level were required to sustain a given rate of oxygen consumption.

In contrast to the results showing no change of oxygen consumption with simple primary somatosensory stimulation, both motor stimulation and more complex stimulation of visual cortex with a reversing checkerboard pattern for 5 or 10 min caused significant increases of oxygen consumption (Raichle *et al.* 1976; Marrett and Gjedde 1997; Vafaee *et al.* 1998 1999, Vafaee and Gjedde 2000).

If pyruvate transport were indeed rate-limiting in state 3 activation (Shearman and Halestrap 1984), the consumption of oxygen would depend on the cytosolic pyruvate concentrations illustrated in Fig. 2.8 and hence on the rate of glycolysis as described by eqn 2.1:

$$\Delta J_{O2}(t) = \frac{6\Delta J_{glc}}{1 + [\Lambda k_{lact}/\Pi k_{pyr}]}(1 - e^{-kt}) \tag{2.8}$$

where k is the rate constant defined in eqns 2.1 and 2.2. Figure 2.8 predicts the time-course for the increase of oxygen consumption from eqn. 2.8, given the half-time of change as 2 min for a lactate-pyruvate ratio (Λ) of 15 (LD$_1$, $k = 0.375$) and 15 min for a ratio of 100 (LD$_5$, $k = 0.06$). Figure 2.8 illustrates that the increase of oxygen consumption measured by Marrett and Gjedde (1997) is consistent with the activation of a population of cells with an LDH kinetic profile consistent with that for LD$_1$.

Taken at face value, the data indicate activations of at least two different populations of cells, one with lower and one with higher oxidative capacity. The ratio between the rise of lactate and the rise of oxygen consumption can be quantified as the ratio between eqns 2.2 and 2.8,

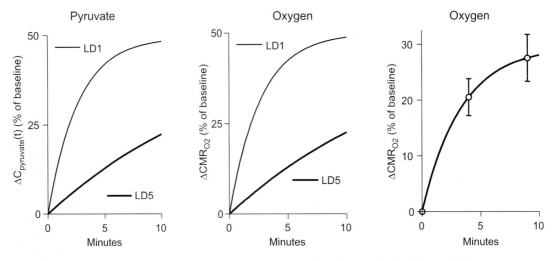

Fig. 2.8 Kinetics of CMRO$_2$ increase: estimation of rate of increase of oxidative metabolism for two different rate constants dictated by different subtypes of lactate dehydrogenase, according to eqns (2.1 and 2.2). The oxidative capacity associated with LD$_1$ isozyme ('red' metabolism) was modeled with $k = 0.375$ min^{-1} and that for the LD$_5$ isozyme ('white' metabolism) was modelled with rate constant $k = 0.050$ min^{-1}. Abscissae: min. Ordinates: increase (per cent of baseline). *Left Panel*: The increase of pyruvate is greater for LD$_1$ than for LD$_5$. *Centre Panel*: The increase of oxygen consumption also is greater for LD$_1$ than for LD$_5$. *Right Panel*: An estimation of the rate constant for increases of oxidative metabolism calculated from measurements reported by Marrett and Gjedde (1997). The rate constant of 0.44 min^{-1} is consistent with oxidative capacity of 10 ([0.44/0.04]−1), which is close to normal average, and hence consistent with the 'aerobic' (or 'red') metabolism. Note that high oxidative capacity can be due to both high mitochondrial activity and high LDH lactate-pyruvate affinity ratio.

$$\frac{\Delta M_{\text{lact}}(t)}{\Delta J_{O2}} = \frac{1}{3k_{\text{pyr}}}\left(\frac{\Lambda}{\Pi}\right) \qquad (2.9)$$

in which the ratio is seen to depend both on the prevailing LDH profile (Λ) and on the oxidative capacity (Π). The slow or absent rise during primary somatosensory stimulation could be a consequence of the slow rise of the pyruvate concentration in the presence of a substantial lactate sink. This behavior is to be expected when the bulk of the acceleration of metabolism occurs in cells of low oxidative capacity. The more substantial rise of oxygen consumption during more complex stimulation could be the consequence of activation of cells with a higher oxidative capacity.

It is apparent that Table 2.6 identifies two kinds of responses of oxidative metabolism to brain activation, i.e. a primary somatosensory response, in which the relative rise of oxygen consumption averages only 10 per cent of the relative rise of blood flow, and a motor and secondary somatosensory response, in which the rise of oxygen consumption averages 75 per cent of the rise of blood flow. The average primary somatosensory response shows a 3 per cent increase of $CMRO_2$ for each 29 per cent increase of CBF, while the average motor and secondary somatosensory response shows a 27 per cent increase of $CMRO_2$ for a 39 per cent increase of CBF, as illustrated in Fig. 2.9. This difference could have a substantial effect on the relationship

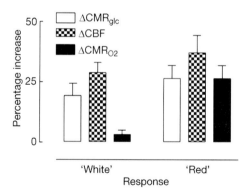

Fig. 2.9 Flow-$CMRO_2$ and flow-glycolysis coupling in stimulation of more relative less ('white') and relatively more ('red') highly oxidative tissue: relative increases of glycolysis, blood flow, and oxidative metabolism are estimated for two categories of the responses to stimulation (simple or primary somatosensory, 'white'; and complex or secondary somatosensory and motor, 'red') listed in Table 2.6. Note similar flow-glycolysis coupling in the two stimulations.

between BOLD fMRI contrast (determined by relative oxy-/dexoyhaemoglobin concentration changes in venous blood with activation and neuronal activity in different regions of the brain).

2.8 Local coupling of neuronal activity to the haemodynamic response

2.8.1 Relationship between increased oxidative metabolism and increased local blood flow

The measurements listed in Table 2.6 suggest that the relationship between a change of brain blood flow and a change in the rate of ATP generation is highly variable, with ratios of relative changes ranging from unity to 20. It is not known which specific aspect of neuronal excitation is most critically dependent on the blood flow increase but (perhaps surprisingly), the findings suggest that the blood flow changes are not related in a simple way to increased oxygen requirements for oxidative phosphorylation.

To rationalize this it is necessary to consider factors regulating the transfer of oxygen from blood to mitochondria in brain tissue. Gjedde *et al.* (1991) considered whether blood flow could sometimes fail to increase sufficiently to raise the rate of oxygen delivery to match needs for increased oxygen utilization. Initially interest in this proposal was limited to analyses of pathological flow restrictions with, e.g. stenosis of large vessels, as it has not been generally believed that the brain develops an (inappropriately named!) oxygen 'debt' immediately after periods of increased energy utilization as does skeletal muscle (Connett *et al.* 1985; Ye *et al.* 1990; McCully *et al.* 1991; Ohira and Tabata 1992; Reeves *et al.* 1992). In testing this notion directly in healthy volunteers, Kuwabara *et al.* (1992) found the cerebral oxygen consumption in brain to remain unchanged during vibrotactile stimulation of sensorimotor cortex, *despite* increased blood flow and increased capillary diffusion capacity. Because oxygen tension in the tissue must go up when blood flow rises if oxygen consumption does not increase in conjunction with increased flow, this experiment showed that a simple limitation of oxygen supply could not account for the failure of oxygen consumption in the brain to rise under these circumstances.

Possible clues to understanding the differences between the relative increases of oxygen consumption and blood flow in the brain come from studies of the kinetics of oxygen delivery (Gjedde 1996, 1997). Oxygen transport from blood to brain tissue is limited significantly by the haemoglobin binding (and possibly by factors such as diffusion resistance at the endothelium of brain capillaries) (Gjedde *et al.* 1991; Kassissia *et al.* 1995). The diffusion-limitation imposed by the haemoglobin binding renders oxygen transport, as reflected in the extraction fraction, somewhat insensitive to blood flow increases (Honig *et al.* 1992), so blood flow must increase disproportionately to raise oxygen transport. A blood flow/CMRO$_2$ coupling ratio of unity would imply that there would be a constant ratio between blood oxygen tension and the extraction fraction at all times and in all situations and hence no change of the oxygen tension gradient in the tissue. The key to understanding why this cannot occur lies in kinetic analysis of cytochrome oxidase activity (Fig. 2.4), which demonstrates that increases of blood flow above the increase of oxygen consumption are necessary for the delivery of additional oxygen during excitation.

When mitochondrial oxygen tension becomes low enough to begin to reduce the oxygen saturation of cytochrome oxidase, oxygen consumption becomes dependent directly on the mean capillary oxygen tension for a given capillary density (Gjedde *et al.* 1990). Brain activation above this threshold therefore demands disproportionately increased blood flow to maintain a sufficiently high mean capillary oxygen tension. Simple one-dimensional models of oxygen delivery to brain tissue based on these considerations (Buxton and Frank 1997; Gjedde 1997; Vafaee and Gjedde 2000) confirm that disproportionately increased blood flow delivers more oxygen during functional activation. The models assume that the mean capillary haemoglobin oxygen saturation is determined simply by the net extraction of oxygen and that oxygen is delivered similarly along the whole length of capillaries according to the equation,

$$\bar{S}_{O2} = 1 - \frac{E_{O2}}{2} \tag{2.10}$$

where $\bar{S}_{O2}$ is the average capillary oxygen saturation of haemoglobin and E_{O2} is the net oxygen extraction fraction. The mean capillary oxygen tension and haemoglobin saturation also are related by the equation for the oxygen dissociation curve,

$$\bar{S}_{O2} = \frac{1}{1 + [p_{50}^{hb} - P_{O2}^{cap}]^h} \tag{2.11}$$

where P_{50}^{hb} is the haemoglobin half-saturation oxygen tension. The resulting equation establishes the inverse correlation between the net extraction fraction and the average capillary oxygen tension,

$$\bar{P}_{O2}^{cap} = \sqrt[h]{\frac{2}{E_{O2}} - 1} \tag{2.12}$$

where h is the Hill coefficient (a measure of cooperativity in oxygen binding between the subunits of haemoglobin) and E_{O2} is the ratio $J_{O2}/(FC_{O2})$, in which F is the blood flow, and C_{O2} is the arterial oxygen concentration. The maximum delivery is proportional to the mean capillary oxygen tension for a given effective capillary density associated with a particular diffusion capacity L,

$$J_{O2}^{max} = L\bar{P}_{O2}^{cap} \tag{2.13}$$

where J_{O2}^{max} is the maximum oxygen delivery capacity and L is the tissue oxygen diffusion capacity for the mean distance between the capillary lumen and the mitochondria.

The maximum oxygen delivery capacity therefore determines an upper limit for oxygen consumption. It is reached when the mitochondrial oxygen tension is at the minimum level sufficient to sustain the cytochrome oxidase activity. Although conditions in which the average oxygen tension of capillary blood is the primary limit of oxygen consumption previously were thought to be approached only in situations of pathologically limited blood flow, they may in fact be the rule rather than the exception. The effect of the blood flow increase is then to raise the J_{O2}^{max}. When more oxygen is needed and blood flow rises disproportionately to satisfy this need, oxygen extraction decreases and raises the average capillary oxygen tension to a magnitude consistent with the pressure gradient required to drive an appropriate rate of oxygen delivery to the mitochondria.

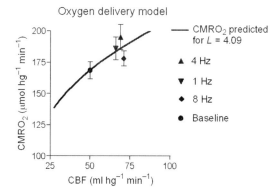

Fig. 2.10 Relationship between blood flow and oxygen delivery to brain tissue, reported by Vafaee and Gjedde (2000). Using measured values of blood flow and oxygen consumption, and P_{50}^{bb} equal to 26 mmHg, the average oxygen delivery capacity was 4.0 μmol mmHg^{-1} (100g brain)$^{-1}$ min^{-1}. This capacity was used to predict oxygen delivery in the range of blood flow values represented on the abscissa.

Eqns 2.10–2.13 were used to calculate the maximum oxygen delivery capacity as the function of blood flow shown in Fig. 2.10 for comparison with the blood flow and oxygen consumption values measured by Vafaee and Gjedde (2000) during stimulation of the visual cortex of healthy volunteers with a checkerboard stimulus reversing at several different frequencies. The empirical data show that blood flow and oxygen consumption both rise with stimulation but that blood flow rises more than the oxygen consumption, as predicted by the oxygen delivery model.

Blood flow into different branches of the extensive capillary network in the brain can be controlled by pre-capillary sphincters. In principle, these might be used to adjust the extent of the network that is perfused to match tissue metabolic demands. The relationship depicted in Figure 2.10 assumes that there is no 'absolute' recruitment of the capillary bed capable of increasing the diffusion capacity for oxygen by reducing the diffusion distance in the tissue, or increasing the intrinsic permeability of the capillary endothelial wall. It is the current consensus that recruitment of capillaries in brain tissue is 'relative', i.e. that it occurs by reduction of capillary transit times towards greater homogeneity of transit times and a lower average transit time, rather than by an absolute increase of the number of perfused capillaries (Kuschinsky and Paulson 1992). Because the capillary surface area remains the same, relative recruitment therefore does not contribute to increased transport of oxygen.

2.8.2 Physiological regulation of blood flow

If disproportionately greater blood flow increases are required to drive enough oxygen into brain tissue during functional activation, then it is important to understand the mechanisms responsible for these increases. Yet the detailed relationships among the possible contributing factors (e.g. synthesis of nitric oxide, accumulation of potassium, generation of lactate, acetylcholinergic activity) and the functionally induced blood flow changes of brain tissue remain unknown. The elucidation of these relations is among the most pressing items on the neuroscientific agenda of the future. Information concerning the three substances likely to play major roles is reviewed here.

Nitric oxide

Many blood flow stimulators (including acetylcholine, carbon dioxide and hydrogen ions) act by means of the endothelium-derived relaxation factor (EDRF) nitric oxide (NO) (Iadecola 1992; Iadecola *et al.* 1994; Fabricius and Lauritzen 1994; Villringer and Dirnagl 1995). NO causes vasodilatation of brain resistance vessels, in addition to other effects. It is synthesized in endothelial cells and neurones in proportion to the cytosolic concentration of unbound calcium. Brain NO is generated primarily in reactions catalysed by the cell-specific NO synthases (NOS) endothelial (eNOS) and neuronal (nNOS) or by the inducible iNOS. In the normal brain nNOS is by far the most abundant. Activation of eNOS is mediated by acetylcholine acting on muscarinic receptors of the M_5 subtype (Wang *et al.* 1994; Elhusseiny *et al.* 1999; Elhusseiny and Hamel 2000).

It is not clear to what extent eNOS activation is involved in functionally induced increases of cerebral blood flow. It is known that pharmacological blockade of the vascular receptors suspected of being involved in the synthesis of nitric oxide abolishes functionally induced blood flow increases, although the specificity of the blockade is in doubt. Focal changes of cortical blood flow induced by sensory stimulation can be eliminated by blocking endothelial acetylcholine receptors

(Ogawa *et al.* 1994), including those involved in mediating synthesis of NO, apparently without altering the underlying neuronal activation (Ogawa *et al.* 1994). Other evidence suggests that the cerebral vasodilatation associated with simple somatosensory stimulation in rodents is mediated by nNOS-derived NO (Ayata *et al.* 1996; Ma *et al.* 1996; Cholet *et al.* 1997). However, Reutens *et al.* (1997) stimulated NO synthesis with the precursor L-arginine in humans and found cerebral blood flow to be globally increased, while the regional blood flow increase in response to vibrotactile stimulation was unaffected, either because NO is not involved in the increase, or because the increase was already maximally stimulated by NO.

Potassium

As a consequence of increased permeability during the repolarisation phase of the action potential, neuronal excitation raises the extracellular potassium ion concentration, which drives the potassium into astrocytes by several non-energy-requiring routes, as well as in response to glutamate import.

Paulson and Newman (1987) speculated that excess potassium in glial cells is released perivascularly where it can relax smooth muscle cells and dilate resistance vessels. They reasoned that the time constant of delivery of potassium to the perivascular space is much lower when the potassium is siphoned to the vessels inside the foot processes (66 ms), rather than when the potassium is left to diffuse through the extracellular space (2.5 s). The lower time constant may assure a tighter regulation of the blood flow response.

The role of potassium ions in mediating functionally induced increases of blood flow in the brain was tested by Caesar *et al.* (1999), who found evidence for considerable heterogeneity in responses. The relative contributions of extracellularly applied potassium ions and adenosine to the blood flow regulation in cerebellum varied among the cell populations, NO, and potassium playing the greatest role in parallel fibre connections, NO and adenosine playing the greatest role in climbing fibre connections.

Removal of lactate

The observation that oxygen consumption may fail to increase despite adequately increased blood flow

(e.g. in response to vibrotactile stimulation), suggests either that additional factors prevent neurones from using the available oxygen or that additional oxygen is not needed. Increased blood flow has a number of consequences. It delivers substrates such as glucose and amino acids and removes substances such as water, hydrogen ions, lactate, and pyruvate. Therefore, it is possible that increased oxygen delivery is not the primary effect of increased blood flow. Skeletal muscle studies confirm that a correlation exists between the increase of blood flow and the increase of lactate (Connett *et al.* 1985). Laptook *et al.* (1988) showed that lactate may contribute to the regulation of cerebral blood flow.

The discrepancy between the results of the different types of sensorimotor stimulation listed in Table 2.5 and summarized in Fig. 2.7 suggests that the ultimate increase of oxygen consumption depends significantly on the biochemical peculiarities of the neuronal pathway mediating the response to the stimulus (Borowsky and Collins 1989). In brain (similar to the better-described situation in muscle cells), the cytochrome oxidase activity of populations of cells appears to be regulated by chronic energy utilization (Pette 1985; Hevner *et al.* 1995). Changing the maximal cellular oxidative capacity therefore requires sustained stimulation for an extended period of time. Transient increases of energy metabolism above typical levels may not be accompanied by commensurately increased oxygen consumption.

The ΔJ_{ATP}–ΔJ_{lact} ratio calculated from values listed in Table 2.5 distinguish metabolic responses to excitation into hypothetical 'red' and 'white' responses (based on the distinction between more oxidative and better perfused 'red' muscle and more glycolytic, less richly perfused 'white' muscle). Figure 2.11 illustrates that the primary somatosensory responses are 'white', while motor and secondary somatosensory responses are 'red'. These regions of course include heterogeneous cell populations. It is possible that neuronal metabolism is responsible for the 'red' components of these response, while astrocytes generate the 'white' response. Differences in patterns of synaptic activity also could influence bioenergetic characteristics of excitation. The two situations in which the 'white' response would be prominent are stimulation in excess of the capacity of oxidative metabolism and inhibition of post-synaptic depolarization. When there is little

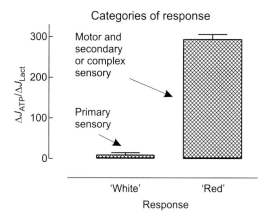

Categories of response

Fig. 2.11 'White' and 'red' responses of human brain tissue to stimulation *in vivo*. Based on ratio between ATP and lactate production during excitation, stimulus and/or cells fall into two metabolic categories, one with average ratio of less than 10 and one with average ratio of 300. Ordinate: ratio between change of ATP production and change of lactate generation.

increase of the oxidative capacity but increased glutamate uptake, the lactate generated is left to be exported across the blood–brain barrier and removed by the increased blood flow. This condition is associated with the low ATP/lactate flux ratio seen in the 'white' response to low oxidative capacity. Conversely, in the visual cortex stimulated by a complex checkerboard pattern, the energy demand rises greatly but lactate accumulation is kept at a minimum by the rise of oxygen consumption. In this case, the ATP/lactate flux ratio is in the high range. The increased oxygen supply establishes the increased ATP turnover characteristic of the 'red' response to high oxidative capacity.

2.9 Conclusions

Current evidence suggests that there is no rigid association *in vivo* between changes of oxygen consumption, glucose combustion, and blood flow in the human brain. The claim that increased blood flow must occur simply to satisfy the demands for oxygen and glucose during neuronal excitation therefore seems overly simplistic. It is important to note that Roy and Sherrington (1890) measured neither glucose nor oxygen consumption. They observed pial *vasodilatation* after adminis-

tration of post-mortem brain extracts to living animals. They surmised that a metabolite had caused the dilatation and that that metabolite might be lactate.

The theoretical analysis suggests that the cerebral energy demand reflects primarily the steady-state level of graded post-synaptic membrane depolarization. Substantial increases of net energy turnover are required neither for neuronal inhibition caused by increased chloride conductance, nor for increased action potential frequency *per se*. Increased energy turnover is not required to sustain hyperpolarization caused by decreased conductance of sodium or increased conductance of potassium. Increased energy supply is only required to maintain the graded dendritic and somatic depolarization of membranes with increased sodium and potassium conductances.

Glucose, lactate, and pyruvate most likely occupy single tissue compartments. For this reason, it is kinetically improbable that the properties of the LDH subtypes *in vivo* in different populations of cells cause great differences in steady-state bioenergetics. Instead, patterns may vary temporally, as dictated by the cytosolic redox potential and pH. Substantial lactate generation may occur when glutamate release is not followed by post-synaptic depolarization. In these cases, there may be a demand for glutamate removal at a rate exceeding the habitual oxidative capacity of the tissue. Although the resulting lactate accumulation is unrelated to the lactate export across the blood–brain barrier, the lactate thus accumulated can only be removed by the circulation. This conclusion suggests that the rapid ('white') response reflects inhibited or insufficient post-synaptic depolarization, while the bulk of the 'red' response reflects substantial mitochondrial activation of primarily post-synaptic origin. There is no evidence that lactate of glial origin preferentially is consumed in neurones *in vivo*.

The blood flow increase appears to be coupled to the rate of glycolysis, although there is little knowledge of the putative mechanism underlying such a flow-glycolysis coupling, as the blood flow increase has a moderate effect on glucose delivery if not accompanied by capillary recruitment. The evidence suggests that the increase of oxidative metabolism is coupled to the rise of pyruvate, as dictated by the prevailing kinetic profile of LDH (Λ) and the degree of mitochondrial activation (Π). The tissue lactate level at which this would occur would be under the control of the LDH isozyme profile and could therefore differ for different populations of cells. Under some circumstances, regional 'peaks' of increased blood flow and increased oxygen consumption could be dissociated by the differential activation of primary and secondary neuronal networks. The activations accompanying the most complex processing of information could be those with the tightest coupling between oxygen consumption and blood flow and hence with the least generation of lactate.

Acknowledgements

The author wishes to thank the Medical Research Councils of Canada and Denmark for support.

References

Alves, P.M., McKenna, M.C., and Sonnewald U. (1995). Lactate metabolism in mouse brain astrocytes studied by [13C] NMR spectroscopy. *Neuroreport*, 6, 2201–04.

Andriezen, W.L. (1893). The neuroglia elements in the human brain. *British Medical Journal*, ii, 227–30.

Aoki, C., Milner, T.A., Berger, S.B., Sheu, K.F., Blass, J.P., and Pickel, V.M. (1987). Glial glutamate dehydrogenase: ultrastructural localization and regional distribution in relation to the mitochondrial enzyme, cytochrome oxidase. *Journal of Neuroscience Research*, 18, 305–18.

Ayata C., Ma J., Meng W., Huang P., and Moskowitz M.A. (1996). L-NA-sensitive rCBF augmentation during vibrissal stimulation in type III nitric oxide synthase mutant mice. *Journal of Cerebral Blood Flow and Metabolism*, 16, 539–41.

Bachelard, H.S., Brooks, K.J., and Garofalo, O. (1991). Studies on the compartmentation of DOG metabolism in the brain. *Neurochemical Research*, 16, 1025–30.

Baker, P.F. and Connelly, C.M. (1966). Some properties of the external activation site of the sodium pump in crab nerve. *Journal of Physiology (London)*, 185, 270–97.

Balaban, R.S., Kantor, H.L., Katz, L.A., and Briggs, R.W. (1986). Relation between work and phosphate metabolites in the *in vivo* paced mammalian heart. *Science*, 232, 1121–23.

Bittar, P.G., Charnay, Y., Pellerin, L., Bouras, C., and Magistretti, P.J. (1996). Selective distribution of lactate dehydrogenase isoenzymes in neurones and astrocytes of human brain. *Journal of Cerebral Blood Flow and Metabolism*, 16, 1079–89.

Borowsky, I.W. and Collins, R.C. (1989). Metabolic anatomy of brain: A comparison of regional capillary density, glucose metabolism, and enzyme activities. *Journal of Comparative Neurology*, 288, 401–13.

Bowers, C. and Zigmond, R. (1979). Localization of neurones

in the rat superior cervical ganglion that project into different postganglionic trunks. *Journal of Comparative Neurology*, 185, 381–91.

Brandt, R.B., Laux, J.E., Spainhour, S.E., and Kline, E.S. (1987). Lactate dehydrogenase in rat mitochondria. *Archives of Biochemistry and Biophysics*, 259, 412–22.

Brightman, M.W. and Reese, T.S. (1969). Junctions between intimately apposed cell membranes in the vertebrate brain. *Journal of Cell Biology*, 40, 648–77.

Brodersen P and Jørgensen EO (1974). Cerebral blood flow and oxygen uptake, and cerebrospinal fluid biochemistry in severe coma. *Journal of Neurology, Neurosurgery and Psychiatry*, 37, 384–91.

Broer, S., Rahman, B., Pellegri, G., Pellerin, L., Martin, J.L., Verleysdonk, S., Hamprecht, B., and Magistretti, P.J. (1997). Comparison of lactate transport in astroglial cells and monocarboxylate transporter, 1 (MCT, 1) expressing Xenopus laevis oocytes. Expression of two different monocarboxylate transporters in astroglial cells and neurones. *Journal of Biological Chemistry*, 272, 30096–102.

Brooks, G.A., Brown, M.A., Butz, C.E., Sicurello, J.P., and Dubouchaud, H. (1999a). Cardiac and skeletal muscle mitochondria have a monocarboxylate transporter MCT1. *Applied Physiology*, 87, 1713–18.

Brooks, G.A., Dubouchaud, H., Brown, M., Sicurello, J.P., and Butz, C.E. (1999b). Role of mitochondrial lactate dehydrogenase and lactate oxidation in the intracellular lactate shuttle. *Proceedings of the National Academy of Sciences (USA)*, 96, 1129–34.

Buxton, R. and Frank, L.R. (1997). A model for the coupling between cerebral blood flow and oxygen consumption during neuronal stimulation. *Journal of Cerebral Blood Flow and Metabolism*, 17, 64–72.

Caesar, K., Akgoren, N., Mathiesen, C., and Lauritzen, M. (1999). Modification of activity-dependent increases in cerebellar blood flow by extracellular potassium in anaesthetized rats. *Journal of Physiology (London)*, 520, 281–92.

Chesler, M. and Kraig, R.P. (1987). Intracellular pH of astrocytes increases rapidly with cortical stimulation. *American Journal of Physiology*, 253, R666–70.

Chesler, M. and Kraig, R.P. (1989). Intracellular pH transients of mammalian astrocytes. *Journal of Neuroscience*, 9, 2011–19.

Cholet, N., Seylaz, J., Lacombe, P., and Bonvento, G. (1997). Local uncoupling of the cerebrovascular and metabolic responses to somatosensory stimulation after neuronal nitric oxide synthase inhibition. *Journal of Cerebral Blood Flow and Metabolism*, 17, 1191–201.

Clapham, D.E. (1995). Calcium signalling. *Cell*, 80, 259–68.

Connett, R.J. (1987). Glycolytic regulation during aerobic rest-to-work transition in dog gracilis muscle. *Journal of Applied Physiology*, 63, 2366–374.

Connett, R.J., Gayeski, T.E., and Honig, C.R. (1983). Lactate production in a pure red muscle in absence of anaoxia: Mechanisms and significance. *Advances in Experimental Medicine and Biology*, 159, 327–35.

Connett, R.J., Gayeski, T.E., and Honig, C.R. (1984). Lactate accumulation in fully aerobic, working dog gracilis muscle. *American Journal of Physiology*, 246, H120–8.

Connett, R.J., Gayeski, T.E., and Honig, C.R. (1985). Energy sources in fully aerobic rest–work transitions: A new role for glycolysis. *American Journal of Physiology*, **248**, H922–9.

Cremer, J.E. (1976). The influence of liver-bypass on transport and compartmentation *in vivo*. *Advances in Experimental Medicine and Biology*, **69**, 95–102.

Cremer, J.E., Cunningham, V.J., Pardridge, W.M., Braun, L.D., and Oldendorf, W.H. (1979). Kinetics of blood–brain barrier transport of pyruvate, lactate and glucose in suckling, weanling, and adult rats. *Journal of Neurochemicals*, **33**, 439–46.

Creutzfeldt, O.D. (1975). Neurophysiolcal correlates of different functional states of the brain. In Brain work: the coupling of function, metabolism and blood flow in the brain (ed. D.H. Ingvar and N.A. Lassen), pp.21–46, Alfred Benzon Symposium 7, Munksgaard, Copenhagen.

Denton, R.M. and McCormack, J.G. (1985). Ca transport by mammalian mitochondria and its role in hormone action. *American Journal of Physiology*, **249**, E543–54.

Desagher, S., Glowinski, J., and Premont, J.J. (1997). Pyruvate protects neurones against hydrogen peroxide-induced toxicity. *Neuroscience*, **17**, 9060–7.

Detre, J.A., Koretsky, A.P., Williams, D.S., and Ho, C. (1990a). Absence of pH changes during altered work in the *in vivo* sheep heart: a 31P-NMR investigation. *Journal of Molecular and Cellular Cardiology*, **22**, 543–53.

Detre, J.A., Williams, D.S., and Koretsky, A.P. (1990b). Nuclear magnetic resonance determination of flow, lactate, and phosphate metabolites during amphetamine stimulation of the rat brain. 3, 272–8.

Diemer, N.H., Benveniste, H., and Gjedde, A. (1985). *In vivo* cell membrane permeability to deoxyglucose in rat brain. *Acta Neurologica Scandinavica*, **72**, 87.

Drewes, L. (1999). Transport of brain fuels, glucose and lactate. Paulson OB, Knudsen GM and Moos T (eds.) In Brain barrier system pp.285–95, Copenhagen. Alfred Benzon Symposium 45, Munksgaard.

Elhusseiny, A., Cohen, Z., Olivier, A., Stanimirovic, D.B., and Hamel, E. (1999). Functional acetylcholine muscarinic receptor subtypes in human brain microcirculation: identification and cellular localization. *Journal of Cerebral Blood Flow and Metabolism*, **19**,794–802.

Elhusseiny, A., and Hamel, E. (2000). Muscarinic–but not nicotinic–acetylcholine receptors mediate a nitric oxide-dependent dilation in brain cortical arterioles: a possible role for the M5 receptor subtype. *Journal of Cerebral Blood Flow and Metabolism*, **20**, 298–305.

Eisenberg, H.M., Kadekaro, M., Freeman, S., and Terrell, M.L. (1993). Metabolism in the globus pallidus after fetal implants in rats with nigral lesions. *Journal of Neurosurgery*, **78**, 83–9.

Erecinska, M., Veech, R.L., and Wilson, D.F. (1974). Thermodynamic relationships between the oxidation-reduction reactions and the ATP synthesis in suspensions of isolated pigeon heart mitochondria. *Archives of Biochemistry and Biphysics*, **160**, 412–21.

Erecinska, M. and Silver, I. (1989). ATP and brain function. *Journal of Cerebral Blood Flow and Metabolism*, **9**, 2–19.

Erecinska, M. and Wilson, D.F. (1982). Regulation of cellular energy metabolism. *Journal of Membrane Biology*, **70**, 1–14.

Erecinska, M., Nelson, D., and Chance, B. (1991). Depolarization-induced changes in cellular energy production. *Proceedings of the National Academy of Sciences (USA)*, **88**, 7600–04.

Fabricius, M. and Lauritzen, M. (1994). Examination of the role of nitric oxide for the hypercapnic rise of cerebral blood flow in rats. *American Journal of Physiology*, **266**, H1457–64.

Fedosov, S.N. (1994). Creatine-creatine phosphate shuttle modeled as two-compartment system at different levels of creatine kinase activity. *Biochimica et Biophysica Acta/General Subjects*, **1208**, 238–46.

Fox, P.T. and Raichle, M.E. (1986). Focal physiological uncoupling of cerebral blood flow and oxidative metabolism during somatosensory stimulation in human subjects. *Proceedings of the National Academy of Sciences (USA)*, **83**, 1140–44.

Fox, P.T., Raichle, M.E., Mintun, M.A., and Dence, C.E. (1988). Nonoxidative glucose consumption during focal physiological activity. *Science*, **241**, 462–64.

Fujita, H., Kuwabara, H., Reutens, D.C., and Gjedde, A. (1999). Oxygen consumption of cerebral cortex fails to increase during continued vibrotactile stimulation. *Journal of Cerebral Blood Flow and Metabolism*, **19**, 266–71.

Gerhart, D.Z., Enerson, B.E., Zhdankina, O.Y., Leino, R.L., and Drewes, L.R. (1997). Expression of monocarboxylate transporter MCT1 by brain endothelium and glia in adult and suckling rats. *American Journal of Physiology*, **273**, E207–13.

Gerhart, D.Z., Enerson, B.E., Zhdankina, O.Y., Leino, R.L., and Drewes, L.R. (1998). Expression of the monocarboxylate transporter MCT2 by rat brain glia. *Glia*, **22**, 272–81.

Gibbs, E.L., Lennox, W.G., Nims, L.F., and Gibbs, F.A. (1942). Arterial and cerebral venous blood; arterial-venous differences in man. *Journal of Biological Chemistry*, **144**, 325–32.

Ginsberg, M.D., Chang, J.Y., Kelley, R.E., Yoshii, F., Barker, W.W., Ingento, G., and Boothe, T.E. (1988). Increases in both cerebral glucose utilization and blood flow during execution of a somatosensory task. *Annals Neurology*, **23**, 152–60.

Gjedde, A. (1983). Modulation of substrate transport to the brain. *Acta Neurologica Scandinavica*, **67**, 3–25.

Gjedde, A. (1984). On the measurement of glucose in brain. *Neurochemical Research*, **14**, 1667–71.

Gjedde, A. (1992). Blood–brain glucose transfer. In *Physiology and pharmacology of the blood–brain barrier*, Chapter 6a: *Handbook of experimental pharmacology*, (ed. M.W.B. Bradbury), pp.65–115. Springer-Verlag, Berlin Heidelberg.

Gjedde, A. (1993a). The energy cost of neuronal depolarization. In *Functional organization of the human visual cortex* (ed. B. Guly) Pergamon Press, Oxford.

Gjedde, A .(1993b). Interpreting physiology maps of the living human brain. In *Quantification of brain function. Tracer kinetics and image analysis in brain PET*, (ed. K. Uemura, N.A. Lassen, T. Jones and I. Kanno), pp.187–96 Elsevier, Amsterdam.

Gjedde, A. (1996). PET criteria of cerebral tissue viability in ischemia. *Acta Neurologica Scandinavica [Suppl]*, **166**, 3–5.

Gjedde, A. (1997). The relation between brain function and cerebral blood flow and metabolism. In *Cerebrovascular Disease*, (ed. H.H. Batjev), pp.23–40), Lippincott-Raven, New York.

Gjedde, A., Kuwabara, H., and Hakim, A. (1990). Reduction of functional capillary density in human brain after stroke. *Journal of Cerebral Blood Flow and Metabolism.*, 10, 317–16.

Gjedde, A., Ohta, S., Kuwabara, H., and Meyer, E. (1991). Is oxygen diffusion limiting for blood–brain transfer of oxygen? In *Brain Work and Mental Activity* (ed. N.A. Lassen, D.H. Ingvar, M.E. Raichle and L. Friberg), pp.177–84. Alfred Benzon Symposium 31, Munksgaard, Copenhagen.

Gjedde, A., Poulsen, P.H., and Østergaard, L. (1999). On the oxygenation of haemoglobin in the human brain. *Advances in Experimental Medicine and Biology*, 471, 67–81.

Goldman, D.E. (1943). Potential, impedance, and rectification in membranes. *Journal of General Physiology*, 27, 37–60.

Gonzalez-Lima, F. and Jones, D. (1994). Quantitative mapping of cytochrome oxidase activity in the central auditory system of the gerbil: a study with calibrated activity standards and metal-intensified histochemistry. *Brain Research*, 660, 34–49.

Halestrap, A.P. (1975). The mitochondrial pyruvate carrier. *Biochemical Journal*, 148, 85–96.

Halestrap, A.P. (1978). Stimulation of pyruvate transport in metabolizing mitochondria through changes in the transmembrane pH gradient induced by glucagon treatment of rat. *Biochemical Journal*, 172, 389–98.

Halestrap, A.P. and Armston, A.E. (1984). A re-evaluation of the role of mitochondrial pyruvate transport in the hormonal control of rat liver mitochondrial pyruvate metabolism. *Biochemical Journal*, 223, 677–85.

Halestrap, A.P. and Price, N.T. (1999). The proton-linked monocarboxylate transporter (MCT) family: structure, function and regulation. *Biochemical Journal*, 343, 281–99.

Hassel, B. and Bråthe (2000). A cerebral metabolism of lactate *in vivo*: evidence for neuronal pyruvate carboxylation. *Journal of Cerebral Blood Flow and Metabolism.*, 20, 327–36.

Hertz, L. and Schousboe, A. (1975). Ion and energy metabolism of the brain at the cellular level. *International Review Neurobiology*, 18,141–211.

Hertz, L., Swanson, R.A., Newman, G.C., Marrif, H., Juurlink, B.H., and Peng, L. (1998). Can experimental conditions explain the discrepancy over glutamate stimulation of aerobic glycolysis? *Developmental Neuroscience*, 20, 339–47.

Hevner, R.F., Liu, S., and Wong-Riley, M.T. (1995). A metabolic map of cytochrome oxidase in the rat brain: histochemical, densitometric and biochemical studies. *Neuroscience*, 65, 313–42.

Himwich, H.E. and Fazekas, J.F. (1937). Effect of hypoglycemia on metabolism of brain. *Endocrinology*, 21, 800–07.

Himwich, W.A. and Himwich, H.E. (1946). Pyruvic acid exchange of brain. *Journal of Neurophysiology*, 9, 133–6.

Hodgkin, A.L. and Katz, B. (1949). The effect of sodium ions on the electrical activity of the giant axon of the squid. *Journal of Physiology, (London)*, 108, 37–77.

Hodgkin, A.L. and Huxley, A.F. (1952). A quantitative description of membrane current and its application to conductance and excitation in nerve. *Journal of Physiology, (London)*, 117, 500–44.

Hodgkin, A.L. and Keynes, R.D. (1956). Experiments on the injection of substances into squid giant axons by means of a microsyringe. *Journal of Physiology (London)*, 131, 592–616.

Honig, C.R., Connett, R.J., and Gayeski, T.E. (1992). O_2 transport and its interaction with metabolism; a systems view of aerobic capacity. *Medicine and Science in Sports and Exercise*, 24, 47–53.

Hurlbut, W.P. (1970). Ion movements in nerve. In *Membranes and ion transport*, Vol. 2, (ed. E.E. Bittar), pp.95–143. Wiley-Interscience, New York.

Iadecola, C. (1992). Does nitric oxide mediate the increases in cerebral blood flow elicited by hypercapnia? *Proceedings of the National Academy of Sciences (USA)*, 89, 3913–16.

Iadecola, C., Pelligrino, D.A., Moskowitz, M.A., and Lassen, N.A. (1994). Nitric oxide synthase inhibition and cerebrovascular regulation. *Journal of Cerebral Blood Flow and Metabolism*, 14, 175–92.

Joliot, M., Ribary, U., and Llinas, R. (1994). Human oscillatory brain activity near 40 Hz coexists with cognitive temporal binding. *Proceedings of the National Academy of Sciences (USA)*, 91, 11748–51.

Kadekaro, M., Crane, A.M., and Sokoloff, L. (1985). Differential effects of electrical stimulation of sciatic nerve on metabolic activity in spinal cord and dorsal root ganglion in the rat. *Proceedings of the National Academy of Sciences (USA)*, 82, 6010–13.

Kaplan, N.O. and Everse, J. (1972). Regulatory characteristics of lactate dehydrogenases. *Advances in Enzyme Regulation*, 10, 323–36.

Kassissia, I.G., Goresky, C.A., Rose, C.P., Schwab, A.J., Simard, A., Huet, P.M., and Bach, G.G. (1995). Tracer oxygen distribution is barrier-limited in the cerebral microcirculation. *Circulation Research*, 77, 1201–11.

Katayama, Y., Tsubokawa, T., Hirayama, T., Kido, G., Tsukiyama, T., and Iio, M. (1986). Response of regional cerebral blood flow and oxygen metabolism to thalamic stimulation in humans as revealed by positron emission tomography. *Journal of Cerebral Blood Flow and Metabolism*, 6, 634–7.

Katayama, Y., Fukuchi, T., Mc Kee, A., and Terashi (1998). Effect of hyperglycemia on pyruvate dehydrogenase activity and energy metabolites during ischemia and reperfusion in gerbil brain. *Brain Research*, 788, 302–04.

Kety, S.S. (1949). The physiology of the human cerebral circulation. *Anesthesiology*, 10, 610–14.

Kojima, S., Nakamura, T., Nidaira, T., Nakamura, K., Ooashi, N., Ito, E., Watase, K., Tanaka, K., Wada, K., Kudo, Y., and Miyakawa, H. (1999). Optical detection of synaptically induced glutamate transport in hippocampal slices. *Journal of Neuroscience*, 19, 2580–88.

Kraig, R.P. (1990). Astrocytic acid-base homeostasis in cerebral ischemia. In *Cerebral ischemia and resuscitation*. (ed. A. Schurr and B.M. Rigor), pp.88–99. CRC Press, Boca Raton.

Kuschinsky, W. and Paulson, O.B. (1992). Capillary circulation in the brain. *Cerebrovascular and Brain Metabolism Reviews*, **4**, 261–86.

Kuwabara, H., Evans, A.C., and Gjedde, A. (1990). Michaelis–Menten constraints improved cerebral glucose metabolism and regional lumped constant measurements with [F] fluoro-deoxyglucose. *Journal of Cerebral Blood Flow and Metabolism*, **10**, 180–89.

Kuwabara, H., Ohta, S., Brust, P., Meyer, E., and Gjedde, A. (1992). Density of perfused capillaries in living human brain during functional activation. *Progress in Brain Research*, **91**, 209–15.

LaNoue, K.F. and Schoolwerth, A.C. (1979). Metabolite transport in mitochondria. *Annual Review of Biochemistry*, **48**, 871–922.

LaNoue, K.F., Jeffries, F.M., and Radda, G.K. (1986). Kinetic control of mitochondrial ATP synthesis. *Biochemistry*, **25**, 7667–75.

Laptook, A.R., Peterson, J., and Porter, A.M. (1988). Effects of lactic acid infusions and pH on cerebral blood flow and metabolism. *Journal of Cerebral Blood Flow and Metabolism*, **8**, 193–200.

Lassen, N.A. (1959). Cerebral blood flow and oxygen consumption in man. *Physiological Reviews*, **39**, 183–238.

Laughton, J.D., Charnay, Y., Belloir, B., Pellerin, L., Magistretti, P.J., and Bouras, C. (2000). Differential messenger RNA distribution of lactate dehydrogenase LDH-1 and LDH-5 isoforms in the rat brain. *Neuroscience*, **96**, 619–25.

Levy, D.E., Sidtis, J.J., Rottenberg, D.A., Jarden, J.O., Strother, S.C., Dhawan, V., Ginos, J.Z., Tramo, M.J., Evans, A.C., and Plum, F. (1987). Differences in cerebral blood flow and glucose utilization in vegetative versus locked-in patients. *Annals of Neurology*, **22**, 673–82.

Ma, J., Ayata, C., Huang, P.L., Fishman, M.C., and Moskowitz, M.A. (1996). Regional cerebral blood flow response to vibrissal stimulation in mice lacking type I NOS gene expression. *American Journal of Physiology*, **270**, H1085–90.

McCormick, D.A. (1990). Membrane properties and neurotransmitter actions. In *The Synaptic Organization of the Brain*, 3rd edn, (ed. G. Shepherd), pp.32–66. Oxford University Press, New York.

McCully, K.K., Kakihira, H., van den Borne, K., and Kent-Braun, J. (1991). Non-invasive measurements of activity-induced changes in muscle metabolism. *Journal of Biomechanics*, **24**, Suppl., 1, 153–61.

McIlwain, H. (1951). Metabolic response *in vitro* to electrical stimulation of section *Biochemical Journal*, **49**, 382–93.

Magistretti, P.J., Cardinaux, J.R. and Martin, J.L. (1998). VIP and PACAP in the CNS: regulators of glial energy metabolism and modulators of glutamatergic signaling. *European Journal of Neuroscience*, **10**, 272–80.

Magistretti, P.J., Pellerin, L., Rothman, D.L., and Shulman, R.G. (1999). Energy on demand. *Science*, **283**, 496–7.

Marrett, S. and Gjedde, A. (1997). Changes of blood flow and oxygen consumption in visual cortex of living humans. *Advances in Experimental Medicine and Biology*, **413**, 205–08.

Mata, M., Fink, D.G., Gainer, H., Smith, C.B., Davidsen, L., Savaki, H.E., Schwarts, W.J., and Sokoloff, L. (1980). Activity-dependent energy metabolism in rat posterior pituitary primarily reflects sodium pump activity. *Journal of Neurochemistry*, **34**, 213–15.

Mathiesen, C., Caesar, K., Akgoren, N., and Lauritzen, M. (1998). Modification of activity-dependent increases of cerebral blood flow by excitatory synaptic activity and spikes in rat cerebellar cortex. *Journal of Physiology*, **512**, 555–66.

Matthews, P.M., Bland, J.L., Gadian, D.G., and Radda, G.K. (1981). The steady-state rate of ATP synthesis in the perfused rat heart measured by 31P NMR saturation transfer. *Biochemical and Biophysical Research Communications*, **103**, 1052–9.

Mora, B.N., Narasimhan, P.T., and Ross, B.D. (1992). ^{31}P magnetization transfer studies in the monkey brain. *Magnetic Resonance in Medicine*, **26**, 100–15.

Morowitz, H.J. (1978). *Foundations of bioenergetics*. Academic Press, New York.

Muir, D., Berl, S., and Clarke, D.D. (1986). Acetate and fluoroacetate as possible markers for glial metabolism *in vivo*. *Brain Research*, **380**, 336–40.

Nalecz, K.A., Kaminska, J., Nalecz, M.J., and Azzi, A. (1992). The activity of pyruvate carrier in a reconstituted system: substrate specificity and inhibitor sensitivity. *Archives of Biochemistry and Biophysics*, **297**, 162–8.

Newsholme, E.A. and Crabtree, B. (1979). Theoretical principles in the approaches to control of metabolic pathways and their application to glycolysis in muscle. *Journal of Molecular and Cellular Cardiology*, **11**: 839–56.

Ogawa, S., Menon, R.S., Tank, D.W., Kim, S.G., Merkle, H., Ellermann, J.M., and Ugurbil, K. (1993). Functional brain mapping by blood oxygenation level-dependent contrast magnetic resonance imaging. A comparison of signal characteristics with a biophysical model. *Biophysical Journal*, **64**, 803–12.

Ogawa, M., Magata, Y., Ouchi, Y., Fukuyama, H., Yamauchi, H., Kimura, J., Yonekura, Y., and Konishi, J. (1994). Scopolamine abolishes cerebral blood flow response to somatosensory stimulation in anesthetized cats: PET study. *Brain Research*, **650**, 249–52.

Ohira, Y. and Tabata, I. (1992). Muscle metabolism during exercise: anaerobic threshold does not exist. *Annals of Physiological Anthropology*, **11**, 319–23.

Ohta, S., Meyer, E., Thompson, C.J., and Gjedde, A. (1992). Oxygen consumption of the living human brain measured after a single inhalation of positron emitting oxygen. *Journal of Cerebral Blood Flow and Metabolism*, **12**, 179–92.

Ohta, S., Meyer, E., and Gjedde, A. (1996). Cerebral [^{15}O]water clearance in humans determined by PET. I. Theory and normal values. *Journal of Cerebral Blood Flow and Metabolism.*, **16**, 765–80.

Ohta, S., Reutens, D.C., and Gjedde, A. (1999). Brief vibrotactile stimulation does not increase cortical oxygen consumption when measured by single inhalation of positron emitting oxygen. *Journal of Cerebral Blood Flow and Metabolism*, **19**, 260–5.

Oldendorf, W.H. (1973). Carrier-mediated blood–brain barrier transport of short-chain monocarboxylic organic acids. *American Journal of Physiology* 224, 1450–3.

Olesen, J. (1970). Total CO_2, lactate, and pyruvate in brain biopsies taken after freezing the tissue in situ. *Acta Neurologica Scandinavica*, 46, 141–8.

Pardridge, W.M. (1981). Transport of nutrients and hormones through the blood–brain barrier. *Diabetola,* 20, 246–54.

Paulson, O.B. and Newman, E.A. (1987). Does the release of potassium from astrocyte endfeet regulate cerebral blood flow? *Science*, 237, 896–8.

Pedroarena, C. and Llinas, R. (1997). Dendritic calcium conductances generate high-frequency oscillation in thalamo-cortical neurones. *Proceedings of the National Academy of Sciences (USA)*, 94, 724–28.

Pellerin, L. and Magistretti, P.J. (1994). Glutamate uptake into astrocytes stimulates aerobic glycolysis: a mechanism coupling neuronal activity to glucose utilization. *Proceedings of the National Academy of Sciences (USA)*, 91, 10625–29.

Pette, D. (1985). Metabolic heterogeneity of muscle fibres. *Journal of Experimental Biology*, 115, 179–89.

Poitry-Yamate, C.L. and Tsacopoulos, M. (1992). Glucose metabolism in freshly isolated Muller glial cells from a mammalian retina. *Journal of Comparative Neurology*, 320, 257–66.

Poitry-Yamate, C.L., Poitry, S., and Tsacopoulos, M. (1995). Lactate released by Muller glial cells is metabolized by photoreceptors from mammalian retina. *Journal of Neuroscience.*, 15, 5179–91.

Poole, R.C. and Halestrap, A.P. (1993). Transport of lactate and other monocarboxylates across mammalian plasma membranes. *American Journal of Physiology*, 264, C761–82.

Prichard, J., Rothman, D., Novotny, E., Petroff, O., Kuwabara, T., Avison, M., Howseman, A., Hanstock, C., and Shulman, R. (1991). Lactate rise detected by, 1H NMR in human visual cortex during physiologic stimulation. *Proceedings of the National Academy of Sciences (USA)*, 88, 5829–31.

Pullman, M.E., Penefsky, H.S., Datta, A., and Racker, E. (1960). Partial resolution of the enzymes catalyzing oxidative phosphorylation. I. Purification and properties of soluble dinitrophenol-stimulated adenosine triphosphatase. *Journal of Biological Chemistry*, 235, 3322–9.

Raichle, M.E., Grubb, R.L. Jr, Gado, M.H., Eichling, J.O., and Ter-Pogossian, M.M. (1976). Correlation between regional cerebral blood flow and oxidative metabolism. *In vivo* studies in man. *Archives of Neurology*, 33, 523–6.

Reese, T.S., Feder, N., and Brightman, M.W. (1971). Electron microscopic study of the blood–brain and blood-cerebrospinal fluid barriers with microperoxidase. *Journal of Neuropathology and Experimental Neurology*, 30, 137.

Reeves, J.T., Wolfel, E.E., Green, H.J., Mazzeo, R.S., Young, A.J., Sutton, J.R., and Brooks, G.A. (1992). Oxygen transport during exercise at altitude and the lactate paradox: Lessons from Operation Everest II and Pike's Peak. *Exercise and Sport Sciences Reviews*, 20, 275–96.

Reutens, D.C., McHugh, M.D., Toussaint, P.J., Evans, A.C., Gjedde, A., Meyer, E., and Stewart, D.J. (1997). ʟ-arginine

infusion increases basal but not activated cerebral blood flow in humans. *Journal of Cerebral Blood Flow and Metabolism*, 17, 309–15.

Ribak, C.E. (1981). The histochemical localization of cytochrome oxidase in the dentate gyrus of the rat hippocampal. *Brain Research*, 212, 169–74.

Ribeiro, L., Kuwabara, H., Meyer, E., Fujita, H., Marrett, S., Evans, A., and Gjedde, A. (1993). Cerebral blood flow and metabolism during nonspecific bilateral visual stimulation in normal subjects. In *Quantification of brain function: tracer kinetics and image analysis in brain PET* (ed. K. Uemura, N.A. Lassen, T. Jones, and I. Kanno, pp.217–24. Elsevier, Amsterdam.

Ritchie, J.M. (1967). The oxygen consumption of mammalian non-myelinated fibres at rest and during activity. *Journal of Physiology (London)*, 188, 309–29.

Robin, E.D., Murphy, B.J., and Theodore, J. (1984). Coordinate regulation of glycolysis by hypoxia in mammalian cells. *Journal of Cellular Physiology*, 118, 287–90.

Roland, P.E., Eriksson, L., Stone-Elander, S., and Widen, L. (1987). Does mental activity change the oxidative metabolism of the brain? *Journal of Neuroscience*, 8, 2373–89.

Roland, P.E., Eriksson, L., Widen, L., and Stone-Elander, S. (1989). Changes in regional cerebral oxidative metabolism induced by tactile learning and recognition in man. *European Journal of Neuroscience*, 7, 2373–89.

Rose, S.P. (1975). Cellular compartmentation of brain metabolism and its functional significance. *Journal of Neuroscience Research*, 1, 19–30.

Roth, K. and Weiner, M.W. (1991). Determination of cytosolic ADP and AMP concentrations and the free energy of ATP hydrolysis in huan muscle and brain tissues with ^{31}P NMR spectroscopy. *Magnetic Resonance in Medicine*, 22, 505–11.

Rothstein, J.D., Dykes Hoberg, M., Pardo, C.A., Bristol, L.A., Jin, L., Kuncl, R.W., Kanai, Y., Hediger, M.A., Wang, Y., Schielke, J.P., and Welty, D.F. (1996). Knockout of glutamate transporters reveals a major role for astroglial transport in excitotoxicity and clearance of glutamate. *Neurone*, 16, 75–86.

Roy, C.S. and Sherrington, C.S. (1890). On the regulation of the blood supply of the brain. *Journal of Physiology, (London)*, 11, 85–108.

Salceda, R., Vilchis, C., Coffe, V., and Hernandez-Munoz, R. (1998). Changes in the redox state in the retina and brain during the onset of diabetes in rats. *Neurochemical Research*, 23, 893–7.

Sappey-Marinier, D., Calabrese, G., Fein, G., Hugg, J.W., Biggins, C., and Weiner, M.W. (1992). Effect of photic stimulation on human visual cortex lactate and phosphates using, 1H and 31P magnetic resonance spectroscopy. *Journal of Cerebral Blood Flow and Metabolism*, 12, 584–92.

Seitz, R.J. and Roland, P.E. (1992). Vibratory stimulation increases and decreases the regional cerebral blood flow and oxidative metabolism: a positron emission tomography (PET) study. *Acta Neurologica Scandinavica*, 86, 60–7.

Shalit, M.N., Beller, A.J., Feinsod, M., Drapkin, A.J., and Cotev, S. (1970). The blood flow and oxygen consumption of the dying brain. *Neurology*, 20, 740–48.

Shalit, M.N., Beller, A.J., and Feinsod, M. (1972). Clinical equivalents of cerebral oxygen consumption in coma. *Neurology*, **22**, 155–60.

Shearman, M.S. and Halestrap, A.P. (1994). The concentration of the mitochondrial pyruvate carrier in rat liver and heart mitochondria determined with alpha-cyano-beta-(1-phenylindol-3-yl)acrylate. *Biochemical Journal*, **223**, 673–6.

Shram, N.F., Netchiporouk, L.I., Martelet, C., Jaffrezic-Renault, N., Bonnet, C., and Cespuglio, R. (1998). *In vivo* voltammetric detection of rat brain lactate with carbon fibre microelectrodes coated with lactate oxidase. *Analytical Chemistry*, **70**, 2618–22.

Shulman, R.G. and Rothman, D.L. (1998). Interpreting functional imaging studies in terms of neurotransmitter cycling. *Proceedings of the National Academy of Sciences (USA)*, **95**, 11993–8.

Silver, I.A. and Erecinska, M. (1994). Extracellular glucose concentration in mammalian brain: Continous monitoring of changes during increased neuronal activity and upon limitation in oxygen supply in normo-, hypo-, and hyperglycemic animals. *Journal of Neuroscience*, **14**, 5068–76.

Silver, I.A. and Erecinska, M. (1997). Energetic demands of the Na^+/K^+-ATPase in mammalian astrocytes. *Glia*, **21**, 35–45.

Skou, J.C. (1960). Further investigations on a Mg-Na-activated adenosine-triphospha- tase, possibly related to the active, linked transport of Na and K across the nerve membrane. *Biochimica et Biophysica Acta*, **42**, 6–23.

Snyder, C.D. and Wilson, J.E. (1983). Relative levels of hexokinase in isolated neuronal, astrocytic, and oligodendroglial fractions from rat brain. *Journal of Neurochemistry*, **40**, 1178–81.

Sokoloff, L. (1999). Energetics of functional activation in neural tissues. *Neurochemical Research*, **24**, 321–29.

Sokoloff, L., Reivich, M., Kennedy, C., DesRosiers, M.H., Patlak, C.S., Pettigrew, K.D., Sakurada, O., and Shinohara, M. (1977). The [^{14}C]deoxyglucose method for the measurement of local cerebral glucose utilization: Theory, procedure, and normal values in the conscious and anesthetized albine rat. *Journal of Neurochemistry*, **28**, 897–916.

Sokoloff, L., Takahashi, S., Gotoh, J., Driscoll, B.F., and Law, M.J. (1996). Contribution of astroglia to functionally activated energy metabolism. *Developmental Neuroscience*, **18**, 344–52.

Springett, R., Wylezinska, M., Cady, E.B., Cope, M., and Delpy, D.T. (2000). Oxygen dependency of cerebral oxidative phosphorylation in newborn piglets. *Journal of Cerebral Blood Flow and Metabolism*, **20**, 280–9.

Szilard, L. (1929). Uber die entropie verminderung in einem thermodynamischen system bei eingriffen intelligenter wesen. *Zeitsch Physik*, **53**, 840–56.

Tanaka, K., Watase, K., Manabe, T., Yamada, K., Watanabe, M., Takahashi, K., Iwama, H., Nishikawa, T., Ichihara, N., Kikuchi, T., Okuyama, S., Kawashima, N., Hori, S., Takimoto, M., and Wada, K. (1997). Epilepsy and exacerbation of brain injury in mice lacking the glutamate transporter GLT-1. *Science*, **276**, 1699–702.

Tholey, G., Roth-Schechter, B.F., and Mandel, P. (1981).

Activity and isoenzyme pattern of lactate dehydrogenase in neurones and astroblasts cultured from brains of chick embryos. *Journal of Neurochemistry*, **36**, 77–81.

Vafaee, M.S. and Gjedde, A. (2000). Model of blood–brain transfer of oxygen explains non-linear flow-metabolism coupling during stimulation of visual cortex. *Journal of Cerebral Blood Flow and Metabolism*, **20**, 747–54.

Vafaee, M.S., Meyer, E., Marrett, S., Evans, A.C., and Gjedde, A. (1998). Increased oxygen consumption in human visual cortex: Respond to visual stimulation. *Acta Neurologica Scandinavica*, **98**, 85–9.

Vafaee, M.S., Meyer, E., Marrett, S., Paus, T., Evans, A.C., and Gjedde, A. (1999). Frequency-dependent changes in cerebral metabolic rate of oxygen during activation of human visual cortex. *Journal of Cerebral Blood Flow and Metabolism*, **19**, 272–7.

Vandenberg, R.J. (1998) Molecular pharmacology and physiology of glutamate transporters in the central nervous system. *Clinical and Experimental Pharmacology and Physiology*, **25**, 393–400.

van den Berg, C.J. and Bruntink, R. (1983). Glucose oxidation in the brain during seizures: experiments with labeled glucose and deoxyglucose. In Hertz, L., Kvamme, E., McGeer, E.G., Schousboe, A. (ed.) *Glutamine, glutamate and GABA in the central nervous system Alan R Liss, New York*. pp. 619–24.

Van Hall, G. (2000). Lactate as a fuel for mitochondrial respiration. *Acta Physiologica Scandinavica*, **168**, 643–56.

Villringer, A. and Dirnagl, U. (1995). Coupling of brain activity and cerebral blood flow: basis of functional neuroimaging. *Cerebrovascular Brain Metabolism Reviews*, **7**, 240–76.

Wang, H. and Oster, G. (1998). Energy transduction in the F1 motor of ATP synthase. *Nature*, **396**, 279–82.

Wang, S.Z., Zhu, S.Z., and el-Fakahany, E.E. (1994). Efficient coupling of m5 muscarinic acetylcholine receptors to activation of nitric oxide synthase. *Journal of Pharmacology and Experimental Therapeutics*, **268**, 552–7.

Whittam, R. (1962). The dependence of the respiration of brain cortex on active cation transport. *Biochemical Journal*, **82**, 205–12.

Wyss, M., Smeitink, J., Wevers, R.A., and Wallimann, T. (1992). Mitochondrial creatine kinase: a key enzyme of aerobic energy metabolism. *Biochimica et Biophysica Acta*, **1102**, 119–66.

Yarowsky, P.J. and Ingvar, D.H. (1981). Neuronal activity and energy metabolism. *Fed. Proc.*, **40**, 2353–62.

Ye, J.M., Colquhoun, E.Q., Hettiarachchi, M., and Clark, M.G. (1990). Flow-induced oxygen uptake by the perfused rat hindlimb is inhibited by vasodilators and augmented by norepinephrine: a possible role for the microvasculature in hindlimb thermogenesis. *Can Journal of Physiology and Pharmacology*, **68**, 119–25.

3 | Principles of nuclear magnetic resonance and MRI

Peter Jezzard and Stuart Clare

3.1 Introduction

Nuclear magnetic resonance (NMR) has a long history dating back to the 1940s, when researchers at Harvard University and Stanford University simultaneously detected a resonance phenomenon in samples placed in a magnetic field (Bloch *et al.* 1946; Purcell *et al.* 1946). Edward Purcell at Harvard and Felix Bloch at Stanford later shared the 1952 Nobel Prize for Physics for their joint discovery. Over subsequent decades the NMR phenomenon has found substantial use in chemistry departments as an analytical chemistry technique, able to resolve chemical species and to provide information on bond lengths and dynamics. Imaging using NMR was first demonstrated in the 1970s, and has since seen huge application in diagnostic radiology.

3.2 The nuclear magnetic resonance phenomenon

NMR has been described using a number of formalisms and at a number of levels of complexity. A dedicated chemist using NMR for spectroscopic elucidation of a sample's chemical groups, bond angles, and inter-nuclear distances would require a detailed quantum mechanical explanation of the NMR phenomenon. Fortunately, most imaging experiments can be understood using the principles of classical physics, although some basic understanding of the underlying quantum effects can be useful. In this chapter a delicate path is traversed between unnecessary rigorous complexity and over-simplifying inaccuracy.

Before continuing, two common misconceptions about NMR should be cleared up immediately. The first is that whilst NMR is a nuclear effect, in the sense

that it is the constituents of the atomic nucleus that resonate, NMR does not involve radioactivity. Indeed, the word 'nuclear' has been dropped in medical circles to avoid patient concern, yielding the now familiar appellation 'magnetic resonance imaging' (MRI). The second confusion, repeated often, is that NMR (or MRI) involves radio waves. The confusion exists because the frequency of the nuclear magnetic resonance effect is often in the radio wave portion of the electromagnetic spectrum. But a well designed MRI system should detect all of its signal by electromagnetic induction (much in the way that a dynamo develops a current when a bar magnet is turned in a loop of wire), rather than by radio wave reception. Certainly a poorly designed MRI scanner may detect extraneous radio waves from external transmitters or machinery, which can appear as interference noise on the image or spectrum, but ideally the scan room is Faraday-shielded to eliminate this form of interference.

3.2.1 The nuclear moment

Consider the spinning top shown in Fig. 3.1. It is spinning with an angular frequency of ω radians per second (note that 2π radians equals 360°). Because the top is spinning about an axis it has no net linear momentum (the product of mass and velocity in a given direction). However, physicists define a quantity called 'angular momentum' that describes the fact that every point in the top is moving with some velocity about the axis of the spinning top, where the velocity depends on the radial position of the point. The direction of this angular momentum vector is defined to be pointing along the axis of the spinning top, with a magnitude that depends on the speed with which the top is spinning. This vector, **L**, is shown on the figure.

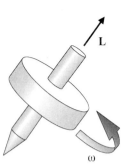

Fig. 3.1   A spinning top rotating with an angular frequency *ω* radians per second has an angular momentum **L** pointing along the axis of the top.

A fundamental physical property of protons and neutrons is that they also possess an angular momentum, which is often referred to as 'spin'. Because the protons and neutrons are sub atomic particles, quantum mechanical rules apply. Unlike a classical spinning top, the angular momentum of protons and neutrons is allowed only very specific 'quantized' values. Atomic nuclei, which comprise protons and neutrons, have a net angular momentum that is determined by the number of constituent protons and neutrons. Also, the fact that nuclei are charged (positively) creates a non zero nuclear magnetic moment if the angular momentum is non zero. In NMR it is the net nuclear moment of the nucleus (i.e. the net spin) that is of interest. Not all nuclei have a net spin, and hence a NMR signal. Specifically, any nucleus with an even atomic mass number and an even charge number has no spin. This means that nuclei such as carbon-12 and oxygen-16 are not visible in NMR experiments, which is unfortunate for biologists, since they must rely on the much less abundant isotopes of carbon-13 and oxygen-17 in order to study those elements. Fortunately, however, hydrogen-1 does have a nuclear moment (from its sole constituent proton), and it is therefore hydrogen-1 that is most commonly used in biological NMR and MRI experiments. Indeed, hydrogen-1 has one of the strongest of all nuclear moments, and so is an excellent candidate for biomedical spectroscopy and imaging.

Table 3.1 shows the natural abundance, nuclear spin and resonant frequency for a number of nuclei of biological interest. Note that hydrogen-1 has the highest resonant frequency in this list. This is because of its strong nuclear moment. Note also that some nuclei have a net quantum spin number of ½, while other nuclei have a net spin number which is greater than ½. The value of the spin number determines the complexity of the NMR spectrum of that nucleus, but does not predict the resonant frequency (which is dependent on the mass and charge of the nucleus). In the majority of this book only hydrogen-1 will be considered, and therefore all the following discussion will be directed towards this spin ½ nucleus.

3.2.2 Spin excitation

In a magnetic field the energy levels for a nucleus of spin number I will split into $(2I + 1)$ discrete energy levels. Thus, the energy level diagram for hydrogen $(I = ½)$ will consist of two levels. These may be thought of as representing the two possible relative orientations of the nuclear magnetic moment in the externally applied magnetic field. In the lowest energy state the nuclear moment is aligned parallel to the external magnetic field. In the higher energy state the nuclear magnetic moment is aligned anti-parallel to the external magnetic field. An analogy exists between a compass needle in the presence of the Earth's magnetic field. The lowest energy state for the compass needle is when it is aligned parallel to the external magnetic field. If the compass needle is manually turned to be anti-parallel to the external magnetic field then it will be in a higher energy state. Unlike the compass analogy, however, quantum mechanics dictates that for the hydrogen nucleus only the two (parallel and anti-parallel) energy states can exist, with no intermediate values.

In the absence of thermal agitation of the nuclei all spins would align with the magnetic field and the sample would be in its absolute minimum energy state. However, at physiological temperatures there is a great deal of thermal agitation of the nuclei, so much so that the thermal energy dominates the energy difference between the parallel and anti-parallel spins. As a consequence there is only a small imbalance within the sample between the number of spins pointing parallel to the field and the number of spins pointing anti-parallel to the field. As an example, at 1.5 Tesla, and at physiological temperatures, only 10 spins in every 1 000 000 contribute to the net magnetic moment of the sample. The other 999 990 effectively cancel one another out. Fortunately, there is a sufficient number

Table 3.1 NMR properties of biologically important nuclei. ³He and ¹²⁹Xe are included since they are being used in hyper-polarized gas form in humans. Fluorine can be used in drug studies, but has a negligible natural biological presence

Nucleus	Natural abundance (%)	Spin	Frequency/Tesla
¹H (hydrogen)	99.9	1/2	42.577 MHz
³He (helium)	0.00013	1/2	32.436 MHz
¹³C (carbon)	1.1	1/2	10.708 MHz
¹⁴N (nitrogen-14)	99.63	1	3.078 MHz
¹⁵N (nitrogen-15)	0.37	1/2	4.316 MHz
¹⁷O (oxygen)	0.037	5/2	5.774 MHz
¹⁹F (fluorine)	100	1/2	40.077 MHz
²³Na (sodium)	100	3/2	11.268 MHz
³¹P (phosphorus)	100	1/2	17.254 MHz
¹²⁹Xe (xenon)	26.44	1/2	11.843 MHz

density of spins in most samples that a signal can be detected from the net magnetic moment (or magnetization) of the ensemble.

The difference in energy levels between the parallel and anti-parallel states also leads to an important equation relating the magnetic field strength to the expected resonant frequency of the spins. If the sample is excited by an additional radiofrequency magnetic field then energy transitions can be induced between the two energy states, thus perturbing the net magnetization so that a signal can be detected. This relationship is given by the Larmor equation as follows:

$$\nu = \gamma B_0 \qquad (3.1)$$

where ν is the frequency in MHz ($= \omega/2\pi$), γ is the gyromagnetic ratio in MHz/Tesla for the spin under consideration (see Table 3.1) and B_0 is the magnetic field strength in Tesla. This is a very important equation in NMR since it also relates the frequency of the resulting signal to the static magnetic field strength. For example, hydrogen-1 will resonate at approximately 64 MHz in a 1.5 Tesla magnet, and at 128 MHz in a 3.0 Tesla magnet.

Figure 3.2 summarizes the sequence of events upon placement of a sample containing hydrogen-1 nuclei in a magnetic field. Initially, the individual nuclear magnetic moments are aligned in random directions (Fig. 3.2(a)). Gradually the nuclear magnetic moments tend to align along the direction of the magnetic field, defined as the z direction. Slightly more spins will align parallel to the field than anti-parallel to the field

(Fig. 3.2b), resulting in a net magnetization from the ensemble. The characteristic time constant describing the approach to magnetic equilibrium is known as T1 and will be described more thoroughly in Section 3.3.

When the net magnetization is at equilibrium no signal is detected in a conducting coil placed around the sample (since there is no time dependent change in

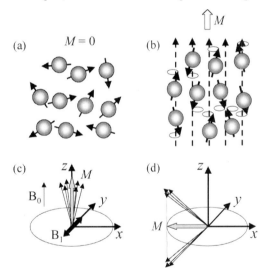

Fig. 3.2 Behaviour of a sample when placed in a strong magnetic field. (a) The nuclear magnetic moments are initially randomly oriented. (b) Gradually the moments align either with the field or against it. The slight preferential alignment along the direction of the field acts like a single magnetization vector **M**. (c) An oscillating B_1 magnetic field can change the orientation of some of the nuclear moments until there is a net magnetization vector in the x-y plane (d).

the net magnetization). In order to detect a signal in the receiver coil it is necessary to perturb the spins so that a vector component lies in the transverse (x, y) plane. This is done by applying an alternating magnetic field that is transverse to the main static (B_0) magnetic field and oscillates with the Larmor frequency of the spins (Fig. 3.2(c)). This additional oscillating magnetic field (oscillating at radio-frequencies to satisfy the Larmor equation) is known as the B_1 field. Fig. 3.2(d) shows how the B_1 field has perturbed the net magnetization of the sample and has created a 'coherence' along a direction in the x,y plane. Strictly speaking the transverse coherence is a quantum mechanical effect, but for the purposes of MRI it can be considered as a classical vector that lies in the x, y plane. The radio frequency (B_1) field is then switched off and a signal is seen in the receiver coil, since the net magnetization will precess about the main static field with a frequency given by the Larmor equation.

A further simplification that can be made to visualize more easily the precession of the magnetization vector in the transverse (x, y) plane is to view the spins in a frame of reference that rotates about the z-axis with a frequency equal to the demodulation frequency of the scanner. In the rotating frame, if the demodulation frequency of the scanner is set to be equal to the Larmor frequency of the spin of interest then, after a radiofrequency excitation pulse, the magnetization vector will appear to be stationary in the transverse plane. If, rather, the demodulation frequency of the scanner is set at a slightly different frequency to the Larmor value then the spin of interest will appear to precess about the z-axis at the difference frequency. In reality, of course, the transverse component of the magnetization vector is precessing about the z-axis at the Larmor frequency (many tens or even hundreds of MHz, depending on the field strength). But, since the scanner demodulates the signal and only stores the difference frequency between the Larmor frequency and the demodulation frequency, the rotating frame is a convenient reference frame in which to consider the evolution of the spins.

3.2.3 The free induction decay (FID)

The most basic NMR experiment is to perturb the nuclear magnetic moment into the transverse plane using a brief radiofrequency B_1 pulse, and then to observe the signal in a receiver coil. What will be observed is an oscillating signal that decays away under an exponential envelope. Figure 3.3 shows such a 'free induction decay' (FID) experiment. The signal collected by the scanner is the radiofrequency resonance signal from the precessing spins. However, this signal is demodulated down to audio frequency during digitization of the signal, since it is only the differences about the main static field that are of interest. (An analogy is a FM radio receiver in which the audio frequencies of interest are demodulated from a VHF carrier frequency.)

Since a classical vector representation of the net magnetization is entirely valid for almost all MRI experiments it will be used for the remainder of this book. Using this vector representation, the effect of a brief radiofrequency B_1 pulse can be visualized as tipping the net magnetization away from the equilibrium z-axis. Note once more that only when a vector component exists in the transverse plane will a signal be detected. Figure 3.4 shows the vector representation and resultant signal of a number of different FID experiments in which B_1 pulses of different duration were used. For a short duration pulse the net magnetization vector is tipped only a few degrees from the z direction, thus inducing only a small transverse component and a small signal. For a longer pulse duration a larger transverse component is induced, until a maximum signal is seen following a 90° tip away from the z axis. If a 180° pulse is used then no signal will be induced, since no transverse component will be generated. Note that between each of these FID experiments a delay must be inserted to allow for the equilibrium z-direction magnetization to be re-established. This delay is generally referred to as the 'scan repeat time' and is termed TR.

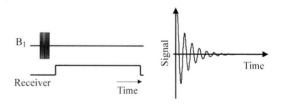

Fig. 3.3 A free induction decay experiment. A brief radio-frequency magnetic field pulse oscillating at the Larmor frequency is applied and the signal is then detected. The free induction decay, demodulated at the scanner frequency, shows a decay of the signal and audio frequency oscillations.

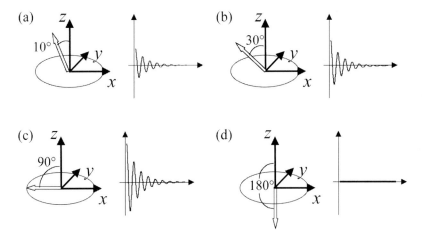

Fig. 3.4   Free induction decay experiments where a number of different pulse widths are used. (a) The short pulse tips the magnetization by 10° and a small FID is seen. (b) As the pulse length increases so does the tip angle and signal until (c) a 90° pulse is achieved and the FID signal is at a maximum. (d) If the pulse length is doubled the tip angle is now 180°, no component of the magnetization vector is in the *x-y* plane and no FID is seen.

If the detected signal is analysed for its frequency components then a spectrum of the chemical constituents of the sample may be displayed. This frequency analysis is typically performed by use of a Fourier transform (Bracewell 1986). The 1H NMR spectrum of water is shown in Fig. 3.5. It is a rather uninteresting spectrum consisting of a single resonant line that resonates at a frequency of $42.575 \times B_0$ MHz, where

B_0 is the static magnetic field in Tesla. It is this resonant line, however, that is used for almost all magnetic resonance imaging. Despite its apparent simplicity, it can richly report on the local physico-chemical environment of the water, as will be shown in the following sections.

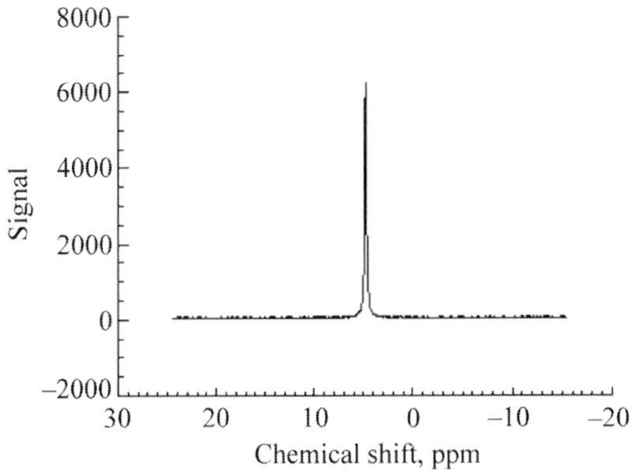

3.2.4 The spin echo

A simple extension to the FID experiment is to add a 180° refocusing pulse to the pulse sequence. This is shown in Fig. 3.6. The effect of the 180° pulse is to rotate the spins by 180 degrees about the axis of the B_1 field. Whereas the effect of a 180° pulse in Fig. 3.4(d) was to invert the magnetization vector, the effect of a 180° pulse in a spin echo sequence (i.e. following a 90° excitation pulse) is quite different. The utility of the 180° pulse is best appreciated in the case of a magnetization vector that is rotating at a frequency that is different to the demodulation frequency of the scanner. For such a magnetization vector, shown in the rotating frame in Fig. 3.7, the effect of the 90° excitation pulse at time $t = 0$ is to rotate the *z*-direction magnetization onto the transverse plane, as usual. After the 90° pulse the magnetization vector will precess in the transverse plane about the *z*-axis, accruing a phase angle, ϕ, relative to the *x*-axis which is proportional to the duration of free precession and the

Fig. 3.5   The hydrogen-1 spectrum of water. Note that the spectrum is shown on a parts per million (ppm) scale, referenced to tetra methyl silane. Also note that by convention the chemical shift scale runs right to left. The absolute resonant frequency of hydrogen-1 in MHz is given by $42.575 \times B_0$, where B_0 is the static magnetic field in Tesla.

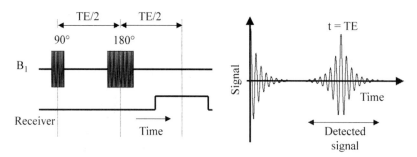

Fig. 3.6 A spin echo experiment. The 90° pulse is followed a time TE/2 later by a 180° refocusing pulse. This acts to refocus the magnetization at a time TE after the initial pulse.

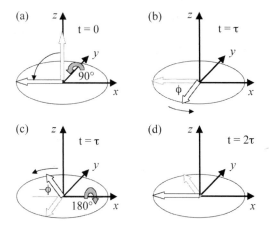

Fig. 3.7 Representation of the spin echo experiment in terms of the magnetization vector. (a) A 90° pulse tips the magnetization vector into the x-y plane. (b) The magnetization accrues a phase angle ϕ over the time τ. (c) A 180° refocusing pulse flips the magnetization about the x-axis. (d) The phase continues to change, but as it does it now acts to return the magnetization to its initial position until the phase is zero at time 2τ.

frequency difference of the spin. At time $t = \tau$, a 180° refocusing pulse is applied, which flips the magnetization vector to phase $-\phi$. The magnetization vector will then continue to accrue phase. Interestingly, at time $t = 2\tau$, the phase of the magnetization vector relative to the x-axis will be zero again, independent of the amount by which the frequency of the precession differs from the demodulation frequency of the scanner.

The particular benefit of the spin echo is in cases where imperfections in the uniformity of the static (B_0) magnetic field exist. This is in general the case, since

even modern super-conducting magnets will not have a totally homogeneous magnetic field, a problem that is often further degraded by the geometry and composition of the sample. In such cases, no single Larmor frequency satisfies all points in the sample, implying that the elemental magnetization vectors at different points in the sample will start to get out of phase with respect to one another after a 90° degree pulse. This will lead to destructive interference of the vectors across different parts of the sample, and hence to loss of signal. Application of a 180° pulse at time $t = \tau$ can lead to the phases (and hence the signal) being refocused at time $t = 2\tau$. This refocusing time is often known as the 'echo time', TE. In other words, the 180° refocusing pulse is transmitted at time $t = \tau = \text{TE}/2$, and the echo forms at time $t = 2\tau = \text{TE}$.

3.3 Nuclear magnetic relaxation times

Unlike many other medical imaging modalities, the contrast in a magnetic resonance image is strongly dependent upon the way the image is acquired. By adding radio frequency or gradient pulses, and by careful choice of timings, it is possible to highlight different components in the object being imaged. While it is generally true that MRI maps the distribution of water in the body, the useful contrast in MR images comes not just from the density of hydrogen-1 in a region but from contrast caused by fundamental NMR processes known as relaxation. There are three relaxation times that are of primary interest in MRI, namely T1, T2 and T2*.

Consider the simple free induction decay experiment described in Fig. 3.4 for the case of a 90° pulse. If we consider the vector components of the magnetization separately, the longitudinal (z-direction) magnetization is zero and the transverse (x, y) magnetization is a maximum immediately after the pulse. However, the system has been perturbed from equilibrium and thus two relaxation processes begin to restore the magnetization to its initial state. Recovery of the longitudinal magnetization back to its equilibrium value is termed T1 relaxation, and the decay of the transverse magnetization back to zero is termed T2 relaxation. Clearly, it is necessary that T1 > T2, since no transverse magnetization can remain after the longitudinal magnetization has been restored.

3.3.1 T1 relaxation

In Section 3.2.2 it was stated that when a sample is placed in a static magnetic field an equilibrium magnetization vector is established as the spins preferentially align with the static magnetic field. This magnetization vector does not form immediately, however, but requires random thermal processes to provide an energetic pathway to this state. In an analogous way to how an externally applied radiofrequency magnetic field can alter the energy state of the spins, the randomly fluctuating magnetic moments of neighbouring molecules can also affect the orientation of spins. Even though the resulting randomly fluctuating magnetic fields are small, they can have a component of motion that is at the same frequency as the Larmor frequency of the nuclei in the static field. It is these random molecular motions (translational, rotational, and vibrational modes of motion) that provide the fluctuating magnetic fields needed so that the spins can alter their energy state in order to preferentially orientate their magnetic moment along the longitudinal (z) direction.

In general there will be a broad spectrum of molecular motions over a wide frequency band. The strength of the randomly fluctuating magnetic field at the correct (Larmor) frequency determines the efficiency with which the nuclear magnetization can change its value. This explains how different tissues can have such different T1 relaxation times. If the local molecular motion has a high component at the Larmor frequency then the pathway to equilibrium will be rapid. Conversely, if there is only a very small component of the random tumbling at the Larmor frequency then the relaxation pathways will be slow. For example, the relatively free water in cerebro-spinal fluid (CSF) is tumbling at a rate far higher than the Larmor frequency at typical MRI field strengths, thus the T1 relaxation is relatively slow. The more restricted water that is in the white matter, however, has much faster T1 relaxation. A maximum T1 relaxation rate (shortest T1 time) is achieved when the characteristic tumbling time of the molecular motions is of similar value to the Larmor frequency. If the motions get so slow that they are below the Larmor frequency then a new regime is entered in which the T1 times get long once again. This is the case for many solids, which have very long T1 value since there is very little molecular tumbling with a component at the Larmor frequency. Note that the above discussion also explains why the T1 relaxation times are field strength dependent. For brain tissue, as the static magnetic field strength is increased (say from 1.5 Tesla to 3.0 Tesla) the Larmor frequency is also increased, and will correspond to less efficient relaxation pathways, resulting in longer T1 relaxation times for grey and white matter.

T1 relaxation is an exponential process. Whenever the magnetization vector is disturbed from its equilibrium value, the z-component of magnetization will recover in an exponential fashion, as shown in Fig. 3.8. This plot shows the recovery of longitudinal magnetization with time for the case of zero magnetization at time $t = 0$. This is, for example, the case corresponding to the initial insertion of a sample into a static magnetic field. The T1 relaxation time is defined through a set of equations known as the Bloch equations. The relevant equation for T1 processes is:

$$\frac{dM_z}{dt} = -\frac{M_z - M_0}{T1} \qquad (3.2)$$

Table 3.2 Average values of T1 and T2 in the human brain

Tissue	1.5T [1]	3.0T [2,3]	4.0T [4]
White matter T1	640	860	1040
Grey matter T1	880	1200	1410
White matter T2	80	80	50
Grey matter T2	80	110	50

[1] MacFall *et al.* (1987). *Magn. Reson. Imaging* 5, 209–220.
[2] Wansapura *et al.* (1999). *J. Magn. Reson. Imaging* 9, 531–538.
[3] Clare and Jezzard (2001). *Magn. Reson. Med.*, 45, 630–34.
[4] Duewell *et al.* (1996). *Radiology* 199, 780–86.

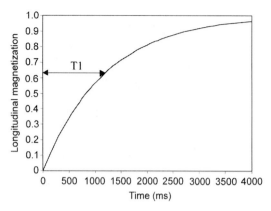

Fig. 3.8   Recovery of longitudinal magnetization M_z following a 90° pulse. This is an exponential process, the time constant for which is described by the longitudinal relaxation time T1. The recovery curve for the case $M_z(t = 0) = 0$ is shown.

In the case where the magnetization is zero at $t = 0$, this solves to give the simple exponential equation $M_z(t) = M_0(1 - e^{-t/T1})$, indicating a gradual approach to the equilibrium magnetization M_0 with time constant T1. Some typical values for T1 relaxation in the human brain are given in Table 3.2.

3.3.2   T2 relaxation

Whereas T1 relaxation is a recovery process of longitudinal magnetization, T2 relaxation is a decay process of transverse magnetization. Immediately following a 90° FID excitation pulse, all of the magnetization that was aligned along the z-axis is tipped into the transverse plane. In a perfect magnet and ideal sample all the nuclei will experience the same applied magnetic field, and hence the transverse magnetization will remain strong and coherent, rotating at the Larmor frequency, until T1 relaxation processes occur. In a real sample random tumbling of neighbouring nuclei affect this coherence via low frequency random fluctuations in the local field at the molecular level that cause the Larmor frequencies of different nuclei in a region to vary. Over time, these slight increases or decreases in Larmor frequency lead to a loss of bulk transverse magnetization as illustrated in Fig. 3.9, and to a loss of signal. Because T2 processes are highly sensitive to very slow molecular motions, as well as to motions at

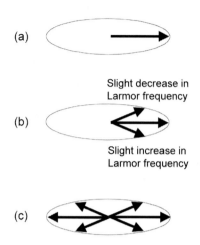

Fig. 3.9   Decay of transverse magnetization. (a) Initially all the signal is in phase. (b) Random field fluctuations mean that some nuclei lag behind the system resonant frequency and some lead ahead. (c) Eventually the spread of frequencies means that the signal is no longer coherently pointing along one direction and there is no signal detected.

the Larmor frequency, T2 is much less dependent on the static magnetic field strength than T1.

The T2 relaxation time is a measure of the rate of decay of transverse magnetization, and is also governed by an exponential process. The relevant Bloch equation for T2 decay is:

$$\frac{dM_{x,y}}{dt} = -\frac{M_{x,y}}{T2} \tag{3.3}$$

which solves to give a simple exponential equation $M_{x,y}(t) = M_{x,y}(0)e^{-t/T2}$. Table 3.2 also shows typical values of T2 in the human brain.

3.3.3   T2* relaxation

Perhaps of more significance to fMRI than T2 relaxation is what is termed T2* relaxation. The similarity in the nomenclature is due to the very similar way in which their effects are seen. However, the processes that drive T2* relaxation are rather different from those that drive T2 relaxation.

Consider a group of spins in a sample placed in the magnet. If the static magnetic field across that sample varies then the spins on one side will precess at a different frequency to those on the other side. Since the signal that is detected is the sum of all spins in the sample, the greater the variation in field that exists across the sample, the more rapidly the transverse magnetization will dephase and decay. T2* decay is distinct from T2 decay in that T2 decay is the result of random fluctuations in the Larmor frequency at the molecular level, whereas T2* decay results from larger scale variations in the applied static magnetic field. There are several such possible sources of variation in the applied field. First, the magnet may not be completely homogeneous over the sample, due to imperfections in the windings of the superconducting coil itself; this usually is a minimal effect. More serious is the effect of the geometry and composition of the sample being imaged on the local magnetic field.

In the human head, for example, there are regions of greatly varying magnetic susceptibility. That is, regions which respond differently to the applied magnetic field. This means that even if a perfectly uniform static magnetic field is applied to the head (i.e. the magnet itself is perfect), the nuclei in different regions within the head will not all experience the same field. This is particularly severe at the boundaries between sample components with very different magnetic susceptibilities, such as the air/tissue interfaces near the sinuses. These boundaries can cause very steep differences in the magnetic field across tissue in their vicinity and lead to very rapid local T2* relaxation. The magnetic susceptibility variations, while most prominent in the proximity of air/tissue interfaces, are also seen in blood vessels, where the level of deoxyhaemoglobin in the blood affects the T2* in tissue around the vessels. This effect is the basis of the BOLD contrast used in fMRI and is discussed in greater depth later in this chapter.

Another crucial difference between T2 and T2* relaxation is that T2* processes can be refocused using a 180° spin echo sequence, whereas T2 processes can not be refocused since they occur at the molecular level and are random. Figure 3.10 demonstrates the difference between T2 and T2* relaxation, showing how variations in the local magnetic field cause the net transverse magnetization to decay. Figure 3.10(a) shows a standard FID experiment in which signal is collected after a 90° pulse. The evolution of the phase of the spins at different locations in the sample is also shown. In Fig. 3.10(b) a 180° pulse is applied a short time, TE/2, after the excitation pulse, causing the

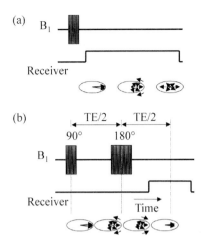

Fig. 3.10 Comparison of a gradient echo and spin echo experiment. (a) In a gradient echo experiment both T2 and T2* quickly dephase the signal. (b) In a spin echo experiment the T2* dephasing is refocused so that at the echo time (TE) the only loss in transverse magnetization is due to T2.

magnetization to be flipped through the transverse plane. The spins continue to lag behind or lead ahead of the Larmor frequency of the applied field and, after another TE/2 interval, the effects of T2* relaxation are fully refocused. Note that even the refocused magnetization has a reduced amplitude, this being due to unavoidable T2 processes. The effect of T2 cannot be refocused since the processes that drive T2 relaxation are random events at the molecular level and cannot be 'replayed' as the bulk effects can. Strictly speaking, T2* processes include the effect of T2 processes, since T2* can be written as $1/T2^* = 1/T2 + \gamma\pi\Delta B_0$, where ΔB_0 is the field variation across the sample (spectroscopy) or across a voxel (imaging). Thus, in the limit of a perfect magnetic field existing across the sample or voxel, the value of T2* can approach T2.

3.4 The concepts of spatial encoding and k-space

It should be evident from the preceding sections that NMR has a long history in helping to elucidate the chemical composition of samples via an analysis of their NMR spectra. In the 1970s it was realized that

NMR could also report on the spatial distribution of a particular nucleus by making the magnetic field, and hence its Larmor frequency, vary spatially (Lauterbur 1973; Mansfield and Grannell 1973; Damadian *et al.* 1977). Thus was born magnetic resonance imaging, which has since been refined to be able to report on many physiological, biochemical, and pathological parameters in tissue, in addition to simply reporting on the number density of the nucleus under observation.

3.4.1 Introducing spatial specificity

The crucial step in the development of MRI was the realization that a spatially resolved NMR signal could be obtained from a spatially varying magnetic field. Consider the Larmor equation described in eqn (3.1). If the magnetic field is made to vary in the z-direction, for example, then the Larmor equation will become:

$$v(z) = \gamma B_0(z) \tag{3.4}$$

In other words, the Larmor frequency of the spins will depend on their z position. The simplest spatial variation in magnetic field is a linear variation, such that the magnetic field in the z direction is directly proportional to the z coordinate. This is most simply achieved by passing current through a 'Maxwell Pair' of coils, as shown in Fig. 3.11. At the point exactly between these coils ($z = 0$) the additional magnetic field generated by each of the two coils of wire cancels, and so $v(0) = \gamma B_0$ (i.e. the Larmor frequency at the centre of the coils is equal to the static magnetic field of the magnet itself). In the $+z$ direction, however, the right-hand coil will slightly increase the local static magnetic field such that $v(+z) = \gamma B_0 + \gamma G_z z$, where G_z is the magnetic field gradient generated by the Maxwell Pair. Conversely, in the $-z$ direction, the left-hand coil will slightly decrease the local static magnetic field such that $v(-z) = \gamma B_0 - \gamma G_z z$.

Consider a sample of water placed in the magnet. If a current is passed through the Maxwell Pair immediately after an excitation pulse then the spins from different positions in the sample will precess about the static magnetic field according to their z position. The signal that is detected in the receiver coil is the summation of all these individual signals, and will therefore contain many different frequencies. By performing a frequency analysis of the detected signal one obtains

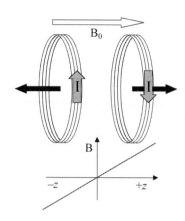

Fig. 3.11   Maxwell pair of coils for generating a field gradient that varies along the direction of the axis of the coils.

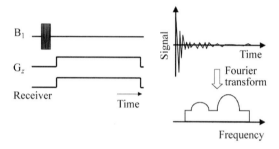

Fig. 3.12   Acquisition of signal in the presence of a field gradient. The frequency spectrum is a profile of the sample along the gradient direction.

a 'spectrum' which represents the number of spins contributing to each frequency interval. By application of eqn (3.4) it is therefore possible to plot the number of spins contributing to each positional interval along the z-axis. In effect, a one dimensional profile of the sample is obtained along the z-axis. This is shown schematically in Fig. 3.12.

It is also possible to wind a pattern of wire on a cylindrical surface that is able to generate a linear magnetic field gradient in the x or the y direction. Note, however, that the desired field variations are $\partial B_z/\partial x$ and $\partial B_z/\partial y$ rather than $\partial B_x/\partial x$ and $\partial B_y/\partial y$ (i.e. it is the magnitude of the static magnetic field, which points along the z-direction by convention, which is desired to vary in the x or y direction). If current is then passed through a coil that generates a magnetic field variation in the x direction then the Larmor frequency will vary according to $\nu(x) = \gamma B_0 + \gamma G_x x$. This will lead to a one dimensional profile of the sample along the x-axis. Repeating the procedure with a G_y coil yields a profile in the y direction.

3.4.2 2D back projection reconstruction imaging

The preceding section described how current which is passed through patterns of wire wound on a cylindrical surface can be made to generate a linear magnetic field gradient along the x ($G_x = \partial B_0/\partial x$), the y ($G_y = \partial B_0/\partial y$), or the z ($G_z = \partial B_0/\partial z$) direction. The structures that are able to generate these three field gradients are known as gradient coils, and reside inside the magnet bore, surrounding the sample. Figure 3.13 shows a block diagram of a magnetic resonance imaging scanner, showing the location of the gradient coil in relation to the sample and the radiofrequency transmit/receive coil.

It should also be evident that one dimensional profiles can be generated in turn along the x, y, and z directions by collecting signal following an excitation pulse in the presence of the relevant field gradient. In order to generate one-dimensional profiles of the sample at arbitrary orientations it is necessary to distribute the current between two or more of the three orthogonal gradients. For example, if a profile is

desired along the line $x = y$, then it is necessary to apply equal currents in the x and y gradient coils. In this fashion it is possible to collect profiles along any direction.

In the early days of MRI this was the way in which images were generated, as is shown in Fig. 3.14. A series of profiles was generated at a distribution of angles so that a full representation of the sample was obtained, viewed from all possible angles. Standard back projection algorithms could then be used to reconstruct a two- or even three-dimensional image, in an analogous way to how computed tomography (CT) and positron emission tomography (PET) images are reconstructed. Fairly rapidly, however, back projection methods for magnetic resonance image formation were replaced with Fourier imaging methods (described in Section 3.4.4).

3.4.3 Slice selection

In order to generate a two dimensional image it is necessary either to collect a 2D series of profiles from a selected slice, or to collect a full 3D series of profiles and to reconstruct all the slices. If the former approach is to be used then one must have a method for selecting signal only from a single slice from within a three dimensional object. This can be achieved using a slice selective excitation pulse. Such a pulse perturbs from

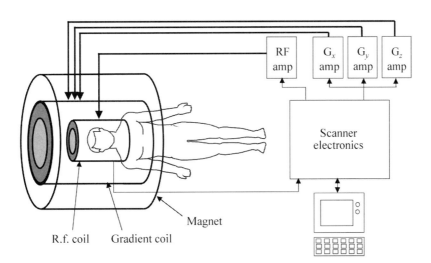

Fig. 3.13 Block diagram of an MRI scanner. The scanner electronics produce signals that are amplified before being sent to the gradient or RF coils. The detected signal is then digitized for processing by the computer.

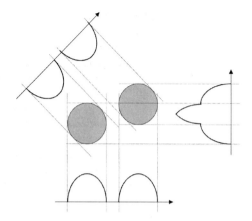

Fig. 3.14   Profiles obtained by gradients at different orientations around the sample can be used to form an image of the object using the back projection reconstruction algorithm.

their equilibrium position along the static field direction only those spins at specific points on a plane, and leaves unperturbed spins outside the selected plane. In practice this is done by playing out a shaped radiofrequency excitation pulse in the presence of a magnetic field gradient orientated in the direction normal to the desired plane.

Consider the 'sinc' excitation pulse envelope shown in Fig. 3.15(a). A property of a sinc modulated pulse is that the range of frequencies that it selects is approximated by a 'top hat' shape, as shown in Fig. 3.15(b). The central excitation frequency is given by the carrier frequency of the pulse, and the frequency width of the

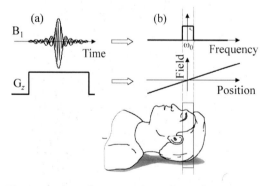

Fig. 3.15   Slice selection using a sinc ($\sin(x)/x$) modulated RF pulse and linear field gradient. The RF pulse excites only a specific band of frequencies. This corresponds to a plane through the sample when the field gradient is applied.

top hat is determined by the duration of the modulation envelope. When a sinc modulated excitation pulse is played out in the presence of a z-direction field gradient, as shown in Fig. 3.15, only those spins whose Larmor frequencies lie within the range of the top hat will be excited. The slice thickness can be adjusted by altering the strength of the field gradient, and the centre position of the slice can be adjusted by altering the carrier frequency of the excitation pulse (i.e. by altering the centre frequency of the top hat). In this way, any arbitrary plane of desired slice thickness and slice location can be excited, leaving all other spins unperturbed in their equilibrium (z-direction) state.

3.4.4   Fourier imaging

Although the method of slice selection described in Section 3.4.3 is the method still used in modern imaging sequences, back projection imaging is rarely used to provide the two dimensional encoding. This is largely because back projection methods are prone to unacceptable signal artefacts in the image. The method of choice for most modern scanners is the method of Fourier imaging. Fourier imaging results in fewer image artefacts, and is more suited to the modality of MRI.

To appreciate Fourier imaging it is necessary to understand the concept of the Fourier transform. The Fourier transform of a signal is the decomposition of that signal into a set of pure sine and cosine terms of differing frequency and amplitude (Bracewell 1986). This is shown schematically in Fig. 3.16, in which a one dimensional profile of an object is decomposed into a set of pure sine and cosine terms. By correctly adjusting the amplitude of the pure sine and cosine terms it is possible to reconstruct the original image by summing their contributions. Note that in order to correctly represent a profile consisting of N points it is necessary to employ sine and cosine pairs with N frequencies, given by $n2\pi/\text{FOV}$, where n takes the values $-N/2$ to $+N/2$, and FOV is the field of view of the object.

Given a signal or object, then, it is possible to specify the coefficients of the sine and cosine pairs that can be used to generate the object. This is shown in Fig. 3.17(a), which shows a one dimensional signal together with the coefficients that were determined by performing a Fourier transform of the signal (Fig.

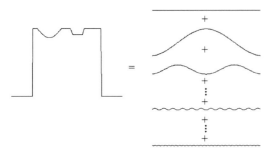

Fig. 3.16 Fourier demodulation of a complex shape splits the shape into a series of pure sine and cosine terms.

3.17(b)). The information content of the two graphs is identical—it is simply that one graph is recognisable as a profile of an object whereas the other graph shows the Fourier coefficients of the profile rather than the profile itself. It is possible to extend the principle of the Fourier transform to any number of dimensions. Figure 3.17(c) shows a two dimensional image together with its two dimensional Fourier coefficients (Fig. 3.17(d)). Remember that given the Fourier coefficients of a profile or an image it is possible to reconstruct the profile or image simply by summing the sines and cosines, having first multiplied them by the appropriate coefficients.

It may seem overly cumbersome to introduce the concept of Fourier imaging rather than the more intuitive back projection approach. However, in practice

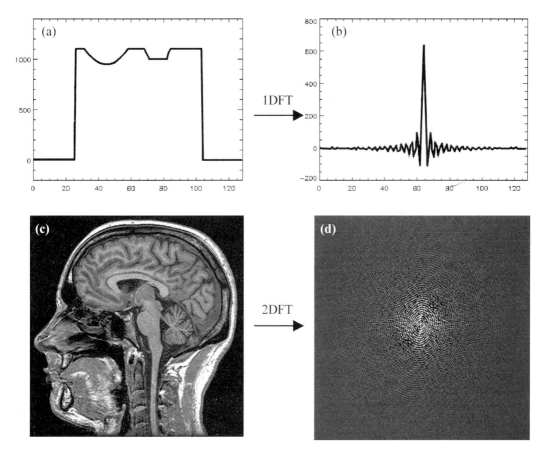

Fig. 3.17 (a) A one-dimensional shape can be Fourier transformed to yield its Fourier coefficients (b). (c) Similarly, a two-dimensional image can be 2D Fourier transformed (2DFT) to yield its 2D Fourier coefficients (d).

the Fourier coefficient concept is much better suited to MRI data, and enables elegant image acquisition methods to be developed that exhibit minimal artefact.

The object of Fourier imaging, therefore, is to measure the Fourier coefficients, so that an image can be reconstructed from them. In the case of a two-dimensional image, this requires the sampling of an $N \times M$ array of Fourier coefficients (where $N \times M$ is the matrix size of the desired image, e.g. 256×256). Only when the full 2D matrix of Fourier coefficients is known can an image be reconstructed.

3.4.5 K-space

The way in which the Fourier coefficients are measured is by use of appropriate magnetic field gradients following a radiofrequency pulse excitation. The principles and mathematics of this process are summarized in this section. It is not necessary for the general reader to include this section, unless he or she wishes to have a better understanding of how different MRI pulse sequences achieve their spatial encoding. However, the diagrammatic representation of k-space, which follows the mathematical background, may be of interest to readers who lack the grounding in mathematics but who nevertheless wish to better understand the concepts of Fourier imaging.

Mathematical background

We start by writing the Larmor equation for the frequency of an elemental volume of sample at the position (x,y), having first assumed that a plane at some location in z has already been excited. This is:

$$\nu(x, y) = \gamma B_0 + \gamma G_x x + \gamma G_y y \qquad (3.5)$$

Thus, upon excitation with a radiofrequency pulse, the elemental magnetization vector will start to accrue a phase relative to the x axis given by $\phi(x, y, t) = 2\pi\nu(x, y)t$, where t is the time after the excitation. The signal contribution that is induced in the receiver coil by the precessing elemental volume is a vector whose magnitude is equal to the number density of spins at position (x, y) multiplied by the size of the elemental pixel $dxdy$, and whose phase is equal to $\phi(x, y, t)$. The contribution to the signal from position (x, y) can therefore be written as:

$$dS(x, y, t) = \rho(x, y) \{\cos[2\pi(\gamma B_0 + \gamma G_x x + \gamma G_y y)t] + i \sin[2\pi(\gamma B_0 + \gamma G_x x + \gamma G_y y)t]\} \, dxdy \qquad (3.6)$$

where $\rho(x, y)$ is the number density of spins at location (x, y) and $dS(x, y)$ is the signal contribution from those spins. The 'i' reminds us that eqn (3.6) is a complex quantity, with a real part (the cos term) and an imaginary part (the sin term). i.e. the cos term is the contribution along the x axis, and the sin term is the contribution at 90° along the y axis.

Equation (3.6) does not account for the demodulation that is performed by the scanner during signal reception. This amounts to a transformation into the rotating frame, and so we can ignore the contribution from the static magnetic field. The signal that the scanner actually stores is therefore given by:

$$S(t) = \iint \rho(x,y) \{\cos[2\pi(\gamma G_x x + \gamma G_y y)t] + i \sin[2\pi(\gamma G_x x + \gamma G_y y)t]\} \, dxdy, \qquad (3.7)$$

in which we have also integrated (summed) the signal contribution from all points in the (x, y) plane to give a total signal $S(t)$.

At this point we introduce two definitions which simplify the form of the equation but do not alter it mathematically. The terms that are defined are the k-space terms that can be thought of as the area under the curve of the gradient versus time. For a constant gradient these terms are:

$$k_x(t) = 2\pi\gamma G_x t \qquad (3.8a)$$

$$k_y(t) = 2\pi\gamma G_y t \qquad (3.8b)$$

Slightly more complicated integral equations describe the general case. This allows the further simplification of the form of eqn (3.7) to:

$$S(t) = \iint \rho(x,y) \{\cos(k_x x + k_y y) + i \sin(k_x x + k_y y)\} \, dxdy \qquad (3.9)$$

Scholars of Fourier transform theory may recognize that eqn (3.9) is a Fourier equation with the signal S and the spin density ρ being a Fourier pair. Eqn (3.9) also reveals why measuring the Fourier coefficients of the image is so natural in an MRI pulse sequence. Indeed, the signal S, as expressed through eqn (3.9) can be thought of as the Fourier coefficients of the spin density, ρ. And a map of $\rho(x, y)$ is precisely what we are attempting to measure.

For completeness the pair of Fourier equations relating the MRI signal S and the spin density ρ are reproduced below. From them it should be clear that the signal that is measured can be thought of as the Fourier coefficients of the spin density, and that the spin density can be reconstructed from the measured Fourier coefficients via a simple Fourier transform.

$$S(k_x, k_y) = \iint \rho(x, y) \{\cos(k_x x + k_y y) +$$
$$i \sin(k_x x + k_y y)\} \, dx dy \qquad (3.10a)$$

$$\rho(x, y) = \iint S(x, y) \{\cos(k_x x + k_y y) -$$
$$i \sin(k_x x + k_y y)\} \, dk_x dk_y \qquad (3.10b)$$

Diagrammatic k-space representation

Figure 3.18 shows a schematic representation of the pair of Fourier equations represented by eqns 3.10a and 3.10b. The left-hand figure shows the value of the Fourier coefficients (S) of the image as a function of their k_x and k_y coordinates. The right-hand figure shows the value of the spin density (ρ) as a function of x and y. The recognizable spin density image on the right can be generated from the map of the Fourier coefficients on the left by a simple Fourier transform. The goal of Fourier imaging, therefore, is to collect the necessary information so as to fill up the $S(k_x, k_y)$

matrix. When sufficient information has been obtained an image can be generated via Fourier transformation.

The job of the particular pulse sequence that is employed, then, is to navigate through the necessary (k_x, k_y) coordinates so that a signal can be collected at each point in k-space. As was implied earlier, the way that this is done is by manipulating the magnitude and duration of the magnetic field gradients so that all locations in the (k_x, k_y) matrix can be sampled. The idea of analysing particular MRI pulse sequences in terms of how they sample points in k-space turns out to be a very powerful concept, and provides a great insight into how different pulse sequences work. To demonstrate this we provide two specific examples: the standard gradient echo sequence of FLASH (also known as SPGR and T1FFE, depending on the scanner vendor), and the gradient echo EPI sequence.

Figure 3.19 shows the pulse sequence for FLASH. At first sight it is rather daunting, but an analysis of how the FLASH sequence navigates k-space reveals its underlying simplicity. The pulse sequence itself consists of several time courses, one line for each time course. At the top is the time course of the radiofrequency excitation pulses, which are sinc-modulated pulses to enable a slice to be selected. This also requires a simultaneous slice selective magnetic field gradient, which in this case has been applied along the z-axis. The combination of the sinc-modulated radiofrequency pulse and the G_z field gradient enables a z-plane of spins to be excited. There is also a slice refocus gradient, which is required to ensure that the spins at the top of the slice and the spins at the bottom of the slice are returned to zero phase after slice selection

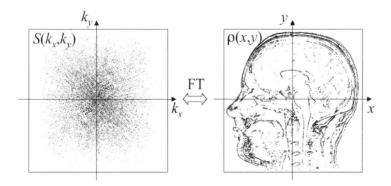

Fig. 3.18 Collection of the necessary Fourier coefficients as a function of their k_x and k_y coordinates enables the generation of a spin density image as a function of its x and y coordinates.

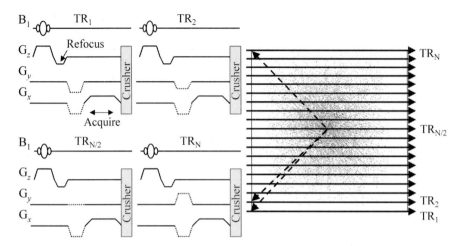

Fig. 3.19 Pulse sequence diagram (*left*) and *k*-space representation (*right*) of the FLASH pulse sequence. A gradient in the *x* direction (G_x) corresponds to collecting *k*-space information along k_x while a series of gradient pulses along the *y* direction with different amplitude (G_y) corresponds to collecting different lines in the k_y direction of *k*-space.

(some dephasing occurs in the slice direction during the radiofrequency excitation). Thus, the top two time courses of each TR interval are involved in selecting the desired slice, after which the 2D spatial encoding of the slice must be performed. This is the point at which we analyse the *k*-space trajectory of the G_x and G_y field gradients.

There are four basic rules to apply when assessing the *k*-space trajectory of a pulse sequence. They are:

(1) Immediately following slice selection the *k*-space coordinate of the signal for the slice is $k_x = k_y = 0$.
(2) Subsequently, the application of a G_x gradient for a time t moves the *k*-space coordinate along the k_x direction by an amount $2\pi\gamma G_x t$. The application of a G_y gradient for a time t moves the *k*-space coordinate along the k_y direction by an amount $2\pi\gamma G_y t$.
(3) If no G_x or G_y gradients are applied then the *k*-space coordinate remains stationary.
(4) The effect of a 180° spin echo pulse is to reflect the *k*-space coordinate through the point $k_x = k_y = 0$.

These rules are really just a re-statement of the fact that k_x and k_y have been defined as the area under the curve of G_x versus t and G_y versus t. It should be noted that the choice of a *z*-plane for the slice and therefore of *x* and *y* direction gradients for spatial encoding is

entirely arbitrary. Any plane orientation with the appropriate orthogonal in-plane spatial encoding gradients could be used. We simply use the *z*-plane as an example. Also, by convention, we use G_x to represent the 'read-out' direction of *k*-space, and G_y to represent the 'phase-encode' direction of *k*-space.

Application of these rules to the FLASH pulse sequence demonstrates how *k*-space is traversed. After the first slice selection during the TR_1 acquisition (Fig. 3.19) the signal has a *k*-space coordinate of (0, 0). A negative G_x and a negative G_y gradient are then applied (dashed lines) for a time τ which moves the *k*-space coordinate to the bottom left corner ($-k_x^{max}$, $-k_y^{max}$). The G_y gradient is then switched off and the G_x gradient is switched to be positive (solid line). This has the effect of driving the *k*-space coordinate across the bottom of *k*-space in the $+k_x$ direction. As this occurs, data points are collected to yield the k_x-direction line of points $S(k_x, -k_y^{max})$. During the first TR period (TR_1), therefore, a single line of *k*-space points is acquired along the bottom edge of *k*-space. Any remaining transverse magnetization is then dephased (crushed) before the next radio-frequency excitation pulse.

During the second TR period (TR_2) the next line in *k*-space is acquired. This is accomplished by using a slightly less negative G_y gradient during the τ period before the data points are acquired. During each TR period, therefore, a subsequent line in k-space is collected by using an appropriate G_y gradient. Figure 3.19 shows the gradient waveforms for a number of the TR periods. TR_1 represents the first phase encode step (maximum negative G_y). TR_2 represents the next most negative phase encode step. $TR_{N/2}$ represents the waveforms for the central line through k-space when G_y and hence k_y are zero. TR_N is the final TR period when the last (top) line in k-space is collected. Only when all the lines in k-space have been sampled can an image be reconstructed. Note that for an $N \times N$ pixel image, N individual phase encode (G_y) steps must be performed, each one yielding Nk_x (read-out) points on a line. The total duration of the image collection is therefore NTR s, where N is typically 256 and TR is typically 10 ms to 50 ms. This implies an imaging time of 2.5 s to 13 s per slice.

As a second example, we apply the principles of k-space to the echo planar imaging (EPI) sequence. EPI is particularly suited to functional MRI because of its great speed. This speed enables whole volume images of the brain to be acquired in 5 s or less, which is important in order to sample the fMRI signal regularly to maximize statistical significance. The speed of EPI arises from its ability to sample an entire two dimensional k-space matrix following a single radiofrequency excitation pulse. This can be appreciated schematically in Fig. 3.20(a), which shows a gradient echo EPI pulse sequence, along with the trajectory that is cast through k-space (Fig. 3.20(b)). The solid lines in Fig. 3.20(b) indicate the periods when data points are being acquired. The dashed lines indicate periods when the gradients are moving the k-space coordinate in preparation for the next acquisition of a line of k-space.

As for the FLASH sequence, following the slice selection (immediately after which the k-space coordinate is (0,0)) a negative G_x and negative G_y gradient are applied in order to position the k-space coordinate at the bottom left corner of k-space. A single k_x-direction line of k-space is then acquired, also as before. Unlike the FLASH sequence a short positive y-direction gradient is then applied (without re-exciting the spins) in order to move the k-space coordinate up a line, during which time no data points are collected. A negative G_x gradient then 'drives' the k-space coordinate backwards and sweeps out a second line of k-space, acquiring data as it goes. This process of using a short 'blip' of G_y gradient to bump the k-space coordinate up a line followed by a positive or negative G_x gradient to drive the trajectory forwards or backwards through k_x is repeated until all necessary points in k-space have been acquired.

Clearly there are constraints that affect the sorts of EPI pulse sequence that can actually be performed, since all image data must be acquired following a single excitation of the slice. Primarily, the fact that the signal is decaying with the time constant T2* during the k-space acquisition dictates that only a limited number of lines of k-space can be acquired. This in turn means that an image of only limited pixel resolution can be obtained. Typically, only 64×64 or at

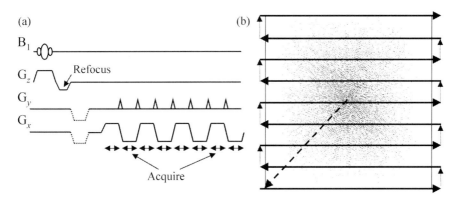

Fig. 3.20 Pulse sequence diagram (*left*) and k-space representation (*right*) of the EPI pulse sequence. A continually switching x gradient sweeps backward and forward in the k_x direction of k-space and the gradient blips in the y gradient move the k-space vector in steps progressively up the k_y direction.

most 128×128 pixel images are possible with the single-shot EPI pulse sequence, unlike a 256×256 or even 512×512 resolution that is possible with the FLASH sequence. This penalty in image resolution is compensated for with a significant improvement in temporal speed. Whereas a 256×256 FLASH image can take between 2.5 and 10 s to acquire (and a multi-slice volume of 24 slices between 60 and 240 s), a 64×64 or 128×128 pixel EPI image can be acquired in 30 to 50 ms, with a whole volume scan in 2 to 4 s. Ultimately, the limit on speed is the ability to rapidly switch the magnetic field gradients, which if fast enough can lead to peripheral nerve stimulation (usually a sense of being tickled or tapped on the arm, shoulder, or bridge of the nose). Although mild periph-eral nerve stimulation is not considered to be dangerous it may not be pleasant for an already nervous subject to experience!

The two examples above of FLASH and EPI repre-sent only two strategies for acquiring Fourier imaging data. Many other sequences exist, each with a different mechanism for covering k-space, but the principles remain the same. Either following a single spin excita-tion, or following several or many excitations, enough data must be acquired so that a full k-space matrix is filled. When this has been completed an image can be formed by Fourier transformation.

3.5 Image contrast

The most basic underlying source of image contrast in MRI is spin density contrast. For this contrast the image intensity is simply proportional to the local number density of spins contributing signal. Since almost all human MRI scans map the distribution of the single proton nucleus of hydrogen (^{1}H) this is often referred to as proton density contrast. In biomedical imaging, most of the proton signal comes from water which is bound in the tissue. Typical water concentra-tion values for various tissue types are shown in Table 3.3. Most notable is a very low water content in bone (which also has a very short T2 relaxation time). Additionally, there is not a great range in water content in other body tissue types. This means that, if relying on proton density alone, MRI images would show limited tissue contrast. Fortunately, it is possible to differentiate tissues in a number of other ways.

Table 3.3 Water content of various tissues in the human body

Tissue	Water content (%)
Brain, white matter	84.3
Brain, grey matter	70.6
CSF	97.5
Skeletal muscle	79.2
Heart	80.0
Bone	12.2

From Mansfield, P. (1988). *J. Phys. E.*, **21**, 18–30.

These include: exploiting relaxation time differences between tissue types; enhancing relaxation in certain tissues by injecting a contrast agent; relying on changes in physiology that affect the magnetic properties of the surrounding tissue; or sensitising the images to blood flow or molecular diffusion. Each of these contrast mechanisms is discussed in turn in this section.

3.5.1 Contrast based on relaxation times

Section 3.3 noted that different tissues in the head have different NMR relaxation times. It is possible to exploit these differences in order to provide image contrast that is derived from differences in T1, T2 or T2*. These are known as T1-weighted, T2-weighted and T2*-weighted images, respectively. Relaxation time contrast is most easily achieved by altering two of the fundamental sequence timing parameters: the repeat time between subsequent radiofrequency exci-tation pulses (TR), and the time to echo following the excitation pulse (TE). It is also possible to introduce relaxation time contrast by employing a 'preparation' module prior to the standard imaging sequence. The most common example is the inversion pulse used to generate T1 contrast.

T1-weighted contrast

T1-weighted contrast can be introduced by reducing the value of the repetition time between subsequent radiofrequency excitation pulses, TR. A conventional image (e.g. standard spin echo) is obtained using a series of radiofrequency pulses separated by a time TR. If TR is much greater than the T1 of the constituent tissues then the magnetization will completely recover between subsequent excitations of the spins and the

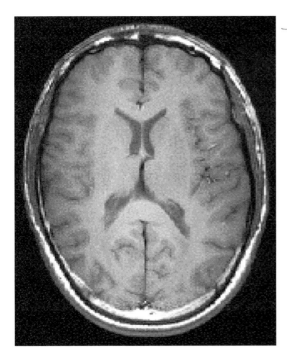

Fig. 3.21 A T1-weighted image of the brain.

contrast differences will be due to the proton (water) density of that tissue only. However, if TR is of comparable length to or shorter than the tissue T1 then the longitudinal magnetization will not have had sufficient time to recover fully from the previous excitation before the next one is executed. The signal seen in those regions of the image have a signal intensity that is modulated, or weighted, by a factor that depends on the ratio of TR and T1. An example of a T1-weighted image of the brain is the spin echo image shown in Fig. 3.21. The value of TR used was 300 ms, so the fluid filled ventricle regions, which have a T1 of over 3 s appear very dark. However, the white matter, which has a T1 of around 800 ms at 3 Tesla, is still relatively bright. Grey matter, which has an intermediate T1 value, is of intermediate intensity.

T1-weighting can also be obtained by the addition of an inversion pulse prior to the main imaging module. This pulse inverts the equilibrium magnetization from being aligned along the $+z$-axis to being aligned along the $-z$-axis (e.g. see Fig. 3.4(d)). The inversion pulse does not generate any transverse magnetization, but perturbs the spins away from their equilibrium state. Therefore, during the subsequent inversion recovery delay (TI) the spins begin to return to their equilibrium magnetization at a rate that depends on their T1 relaxation value. The form of the equation determining this process is given by:

$$M_z(t) = M_0 \{1 - 2 \exp(-TI/T1)\} \qquad (3.11)$$

Tissue with a short T1 will recover faster towards its equilibrium $+z$ magnetization than tissue with a long T1. After the time TI the image signal is collected. Clearly, if the value of TI is very long (TI > 5T1) then no T1 contrast will result, since all the spins will be fully recovered. But for moderate TI values it is possible to induce strong T1 contrast. Indeed, it is even possible to choose a TI such that the signal from a particular tissue is nulled (TI = ln(2) T1).

The amount of T1 weighting contained in the echo planar images typically used in fMRI is not usually very significant, since the time between successive radiofrequency excitation pulses is generally several s. However, there are two considerations that should be kept in mind when running fMRI experiments. The first is that unless the TR is very long (greater than ~8 s) the contrast will be slightly different in the first few images, before the longitudinal magnetization has reached a steady state recovery value. This difference in contrast is not insignificant and can heavily affect the result obtained from an fMRI analysis. Therefore, a few images should be acquired at the start of any fMRI run (or scanner dummy acquisitions should be run) and these images should be discarded prior to the subsequent analysis. The appropriate number of volumes to discard will depend upon the TR used, the T1 of the tissue and the flip angle used. However as a general rule of thumb 12 s worth of scans at the start should be discarded. The second issue is that of maximizing the signal-to-noise ratio at short repetition times. If the flip angle of a gradient echo sequence is kept constant, then reducing the TR will significantly degrade the signal-to-noise ratio of the images. However, some signal can be regained by changing the excitation flip angle to what is known as the Ernst angle. The Ernst angle, θ_E, is the optimum flip angle for maximizing signal-to-noise and can be calculated only for a particular combination of T1 and TR. It is given by the formula:

$$\cos(\theta_E) = \exp(-TR/T1) \qquad (3.12)$$

For example, in the case of a gradient echo fMRI experiment using a TR of 2000 ms then to maximize the signal in a tissue with T1 of 1400 ms a flip angle of 76°, rather than 90°, should be used.

T2-weighted contrast

Exploiting the variations in T2 over different tissues is another useful way of introducing contrast into images. T2-weighted contrast can be given to spin echo images by increasing the echo time delay, TE, which is the time between the initial excitation of the spins and the centre of the spin echo. At a short value of TE two tissues with different values of T2 but a similar proton density will have little contrast between them. However, for longer TE, the region with short T2 (i.e. rapid loss of transverse magnetization) will lose signal. Such conditions will result in good contrast between the two tissue types. For extremely long TE, though, the signal from the tissue with long T2 will also decrease until eventually no signal will result from

either tissue. Figure 3.22 shows an example of a T2-weighted spin echo image, collected with TR = 3s, TE = 80ms. In this image the CSF-filled ventricles, which have the longest T2 value, are brightest. Note that a long TR value is used to minimize unwanted T1 weighting.

T2*-weighted contrast

If a gradient echo sequence is employed then T2* weighting can result. T2* weighting is usually undesirable, since it is often more a secondary property of the geometry of the sample rather than a primary property of the tissue. But if it is desired then a gradient echo pulse sequence with a long TE will yield T2*-weighted contrast. In this case TE is the time between the initial excitation of the spins and the centre of the gradient echo. For long TE, tissue with a long T2* will have a higher signal compared with other tissue (note that since T2* is often much shorter than T2 it is not necessary to have such long TE times in gradient echo sequences compared with spin echo sequences). Figure 3.23 shows a gradient echo FLASH sequence with TE = 30ms at 3.0 Tesla. Excluding the bright CSF signal, the majority of the contrast in this image is caused by the strong intrinsic magnetic field gradients that are established at the interface between the frontal lobes of the brain and the frontal sinuses. This leads to a decreased signal in the frontal regions of the brain because of the large intrinsic field gradients across these voxels. This manifestation of T2* contrast is generally not of interest to the clinician or the neuroscientist. However, T2* contrast caused by the microscopic field gradients established around blood vessels containing exogenous contrast agent or endogenous blood are the basis behind blood volume mapping and BOLD imaging, respectively.

3.5.2 Exogenous contrast agent injection

In certain cases, intrinsic relaxation contrast alone is not enough to distinguish features in the image, particularly when subtle pathological contrast is desired. It is common, therefore, particularly in the imaging of tumours, to use an exogenous contrast agent to further shorten the relaxation times. The use of contrast agents is common in other imaging modalities, indeed some methods totally rely upon an injected agent for

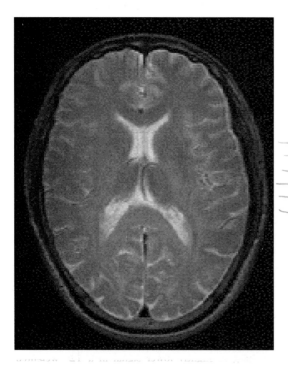

Fig. 3.22   A T2-weighted image of the brain.

their operation. MR contrast agents generally act to reduce the relaxation time of the substrate they are in, and are commonly based upon a strongly paramagnetic ion, such as gadolinium (Gd+). The unpaired electrons in Gd+ generate a very large magnetic moment, hundreds of times greater than the nuclear magnetic moment. This enhances transitions between spin states and reduces the T1 and T2 relaxation times considerably. However, such ions are highly toxic and therefore need to be bound into a large molecule to make them safe to administer to human subjects. The molecules used are typically large biological compounds such as the acid DTPA. Such molecules are too large to cross the blood–brain barrier, and so will show preferential uptake in areas that lack this barrier, such as brain tumours, or will remain intra-vascular. The presence of the bulky molecule around the ion reduces the magnetic effect that it has on its surroundings, but the ion still has a significant effect on the relaxation time of the surrounding tissue.

Some imaging studies require information on the first passage through the tissue of the contrast agent after it is injected in the form of a bolus, since once in the blood stream the agent will keep being recirculated until it is eventually excreted, predominantly by the kidneys. Following contrast injection the amount of signal change and its time course for a particular region can give a strong indicator as to pathology and can contain information on blood perfusion to the organ.

Whilst contrast agent-enhanced imaging is in common use in clinical MRI, it has less use in functional MRI studies. Contrast agents were used in the very early fMRI experiments to measure changes in cerebral blood volume (see Chapters 6 and 8), but it was soon established that blood itself could act as its own endogenous contrast agent. The so-called blood oxygenation level dependent (BOLD) contrast now forms the basis of most fMRI studies carried out.

3.5.3 Endogenous blood oxygenation contrast

As noted in Chapter 2, the activation of neurones and establishment of the ion potentials in the cells of the brain all require a supply of energy. This is supplied in the form of adenosine tri-phosphate (ATP) generated in the mitochondria within cells. Under normal condi-

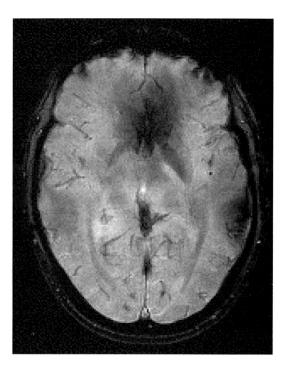

Fig. 3.23 A T2*-weighted image of the brain.

tions the formation of ATP via glucose consumption requires oxygen, and this oxygen is supplied by blood perfusing the tissue. Since oxygen is not very soluble in blood, it is transported bound to the large iron-containing molecule, haemoglobin. The presence of the iron atoms in the molecule mean that haemoglobin has magnetic properties, which in analogy to the contrast agents mentioned above, reduce the relaxation time of the blood.

The location of the oxygen binding sites on haemoglobin mean that, when oxygen is bound, the molecule alters from being paramagnetic (having a significant magnetic effect on its environment) to being diamagnetic (having little effect). Such oxygen dependence makes haemoglobin a sensitive magnetic marker to the level of blood oxygenation and consequently to neuronal activity. If the oxygenation level of the blood decreases (or more specifically, if the level of deoxy-haemoglobin increases) it causes the T2* of blood, and to a lesser extent the T2 of blood, to decrease also, resulting in slightly lower signal in a T2*-weighted image. Conversely, if the blood oxygenation level rises then the T2* value increases, resulting in higher signal in a T2*-weighted image. The details of the BOLD effect are dealt with in greater detail in Chapters 2 and 8, but one important feature is that the signal seen in MR images upon neuronal activation is a positive signal change, representing a decrease in the concentration of deoxyhaemoglobin.

This rather indirect coupling between neuronal activity and BOLD signal change in MRI has several significant features. First, since the signal change observed is as a result of a perfusion increase that is local to the tissue of interest but is generally on a larger spatial scale than the electrical activity, the site of the activation on an image may be somewhat larger than and distant from the site of the neural activity. Thus, even though the MR image can have a very high resolution spatially, the actual spatial resolution of the fMRI map may not be any greater than about 2–3 mm. Second, the delay in the onset of signal change as the blood flow and blood volume increase mean that, although it is possible to obtain MR images as fast as 10 frames per second, the actual temporal resolution of the BOLD haemodynamic response is somewhat poorer. For example, a brief burst of neural activity lasting only tens of milliseconds will result in a BOLD signal change that peaks after about 6 seconds, and does not return to baseline completely for approximately 12 seconds. That said, by approximating the BOLD signal change relative to the neuronal activity as a linear response function, deconvolution methods have been able to distinguish events that are as short as several hundred milliseconds apart. Chapter 7 deals with fMRI resolution in greater detail.

3.5.4 Other contrast mechanisms

All the contrast methods described above implicitly assume that the tissue being imaged is entirely stationary. While bulk movements of the tissue, such as during head motion, will introduce significant artefact to the image, effects such as molecular diffusion and blood flow have more subtle effects on image contrast. These effects can be exploited by use of special pulse sequences that give diffusion- or perfusion-weighted contrast, and can even provide semi-quantitative measurements of their values.

Perfusion imaging

Methods for perfusion imaging fall into two broad categories: contrast agent methods and arterial spin labelled methods. In the case of contrast agent methods, by injecting a bolus of contrast agent into the blood stream, the concentration time course for the bolus to perfuse a region of tissue can be obtained from the dynamics of the signal change in the MR images (Rosen *et al.* 1989). Unfortunately, because the injected bolus passes through the venous system and the heart before perfusing the brain its 'shape' is poorly defined. Without an accurate knowledge of the input time course of the volume of blood that contains the contrast agent, it is impossible to quantify perfusion. It is therefore necessary to attempt to determine the concentration-time course of the contrast agent in an artery located just before it perfuses the organ of interest.

Contrast agent injection is, of course, an invasive procedure. More recent methods have been proposed that allow MRI to measure perfusion with a non-invasive arterial spin labelling method. Instead of manipulating the image contrast by injecting an exogenous agent, a volume of blood in the arterial tree is 'tagged' by inverting the water spins in the blood prior to their arrival in the slice of interest. This can be accomplished using a slab-selective radiofrequency inversion pulse, or by use of a specialized 'adiabatic' inversion of all incoming blood spins. The tagged blood spins then continue to the slice of interest where they exchange with tissue water spins. By comparing the image thus obtained with one in which the arterial blood was not inverted, subtle changes in the signal intensity of the tissue image can be detected and related to blood perfusion. These methods have various names: CASL (Williams *et al.* 1992), FAIR (Kwong *et al.* 1992; Kim 1995), EPISTAR (Edelman *et al.* 1994), PICORE (Wong *et al.* 1997) and QUIPSS (Wong *et al.* 1998), for example.

Diffusion imaging

Diffusion contrast reports on the ability of water molecules in tissue to diffuse randomly through their surroundings (LeBihan 1995). The diffusion coefficient of water through normal tissue is on the order of 10^{-3} mm^2/s. Diffusion contrast can be introduced into images by the application of two large field gradient pulses between the excitation of the spins and the acquisition of the signal. The first gradient pulse causes a dephasing of the MR signal, where the phase is dependent on the position of the spins along the direction of the field gradient. A short time later, a second gradient pulse of equal shape and size but opposite polarity is played out (the second pulse should have the same polarity as the first if a spin echo sequence is used and the 180° pulse separates them). If the spins have not moved in the period between the two pulses then the effect of the second gradient pulse will be to completely rephase the effects of the first gradient pulse. Molecules that have diffused a distance along the direction of the field gradient will not be fully rephased by the second gradient and, due to the random nature of molecular motion, the result is a loss of signal in regions of molecular diffusion. The amount of diffusion weighting in the image will depend on the strength of the gradients applied, the delay between the two gradient pulses, and on the magnitude of the diffusion coefficient. Quantification of the diffusion coefficient is possible by acquiring several images with different gradient strengths and fitting a curve to the signal detected (LeBihan 1995).

In many cases the magnitude of diffusion is not the same in all directions. For example, the highly orientated axons in white matter allow less restricted diffusion of water along the direction of the axons, but more restricted diffusion perpendicular to them. By applying diffusion gradient pairs in a number of directions a full map of the diffusion coefficient in every direction is possible. Such information is known as the diffusion tensor, but, since it is difficult to visualize this three-dimensional information for each pixel, it is common to display simply a measure of the average diffusivity and a measure of the degree of anisotropy. The potential also exists to use diffusion anisotropy maps to follow white matter tracts in order to gain information on functional connectivity.

3.6 *Magnetic resonance spectroscopy*

For the purposes of imaging, it is generally assumed that the resonant signal of components in the object is purely dependent on the applied magnetic field. However, the resonant frequency of any particular nucleus is also dependent on the microscopic chemical environment that it is in. Nearby electrons and other nuclei have a small but significant effect on the resonant frequency, enabling chemists to use NMR to study the composition and, more importantly, the structure of molecules. NMR can be performed on any nuclei that possess a nuclear magnetic moment (see Section 3.2.1). In the case of biomedical MR spectroscopy, usually termed MRS, the most commonly studied nuclei are hydrogen, phosphorus and carbon.

3.6.1 Chemical shifts and nuclear coupling

Nuclei in molecules are never in isolation, but are surrounded by electrons. When placed in a magnetic field these charged electrons circulate around the nucleus as shown in Fig. 3.24. These circulating electrons, rather like the current in a wire, will themselves generate a magnetic field which opposes the main applied field, lightly shielding the nucleus from the external field. This shielding means that the effective magnetic field experienced by a nucleus placed in a field of strength B_0 is

$$B = (1 - \sigma)B_0 \tag{3.13}$$

where the shielding constant σ is a dimensionless quantity usually specified in parts per million (ppm). The shielding of electrons causes a frequency shift in the NMR spectrum dependent on the local electron distribution, given by a modified Larmor equation

$$\nu = \gamma (1 - \sigma)B_0. \tag{3.14}$$

Often, NMR spectra are displayed in units of chemical shift, where chemical shift is defined as the frequency shift relative to some reference chemical. Again, chemical shift is usually stated in ppm. The definition for the chemical shift scale is thus:

$$\delta = 10^6 \, (\nu_{sample} - \nu_{ref})/\nu_{ref}. \tag{3.15}$$

Figure 3.25 shows a low resolution ^1H spectrum of ethanol, with chemical structure $CH_3—CH_2—OH$, plotted on a chemical shift scale (note that increasing frequency is to the left on a chemical shift spectrum). The spectrum contains three groups of peaks corresponding to the different proton locations. The far right peak (lowest frequency) is due to the three protons on the CH_3 group. The two adjacent protons

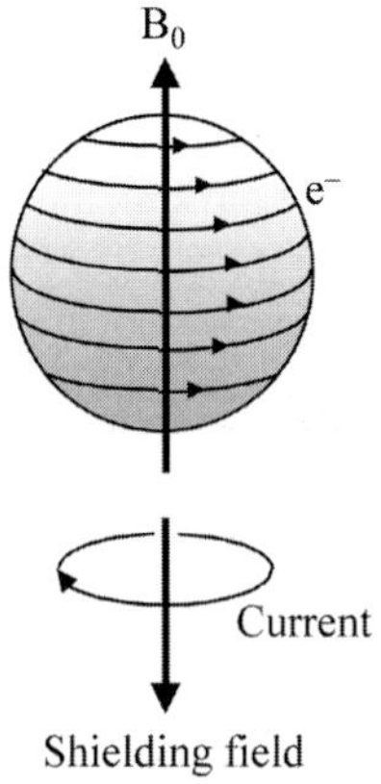

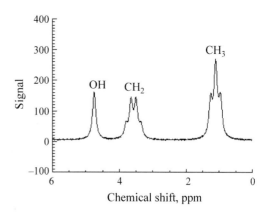

Fig. 3.24 The motion of electrons around a nucleus, induced by the static magnetic field B_0, acts like a current travelling in the opposite direction. This current produces a magnetic field in the opposite direction to the main applied field and acts to slightly shield the nucleus.

Fig. 3.25 Low resolution proton spectrum of ethanol, showing the three peaks corresponding to the CH_3, CH_2 and OH groups. Each has a different chemical shift due to the different chemical environment the protons are in. At this resolution the fine J-coupling is not well resolved.

to each ^1H nucleus on this group act to shield the field experienced by that nucleus quite strongly, thereby reducing B_0 and the resonant frequency. Next to the CH_3 group is the moderately shielded peak corresponding to the protons in the CH_2 group, followed at the highest field by the lightly shielded proton on the hydroxyl group. The area under the peaks is proportional to the number of protons in each environment.

The position of a peak in the spectrum is termed its chemical shift, usually expressed in ppm relative to a standard peak. The absolute magnitude of the frequency shift will depend on the B_0 field experienced by the molecule, which of course is not just dependent on the strength of the applied field but also on the local bulk susceptibility effects. When attempting to quantify chemical shift it is therefore necessary to have some standard with which to compare the spectrum. For example in the case of *in vitro* proton spectroscopy, methyl-silicon compounds such as tetra-methyl silane (TMS) or tri-methylsilyl propionic acid (TSP) are used.

It is not only the electrons that can have an effect on the resonant frequency of a particular nucleus. Most spectra will also display the effect of line splitting due to neighbouring nuclei. Such spin-spin coupling or J-coupling as it is termed, will split the peak of a nucleus in a particular chemical environment into $(2nI + 1)$ lines where I is the spin of the adjoining n nuclei.

Figure 3.26 shows a high resolution ^1H NMR spectrum of acetaldehyde. The right-hand peak corresponds to the methyl (CH_3) group. It is split into two by the proton on the adjoining aldehyde (CHO) group. Similarly, the aldehyde peak is split into a quartet by the three protons on the methyl group. The splitting of peaks by J-coupling is of particular use to chemists, since this reveals information about the structure of the molecule as well as its chemical composition. There are other nuclear interactions that modify the NMR spectrum that can be exploited by specially tailored pulse sequences.

3.6.2 Biomedical MR spectroscopy

The ability to perform MR spectroscopy on living tissue has given biochemists great potential to study cellular metabolism *in vivo* (Gadian 1995). Typically, biomedical MR is mostly concerned with ^{31}P, ^{13}C and ^1H nuclei, since these are the main NMR visible components of biological compounds. ^{13}C is not the naturally occurring isotope of carbon, making natural abundance NMR detection of this nucleus difficult. However it has proven a useful nucleus as a biological marker to study metabolism if ^{13}C enriched glucose is administered (usually only in animal experiments). The majority of biomedical MRS, however, involves phosphorus or hydrogen NMR. It is difficult to quantify

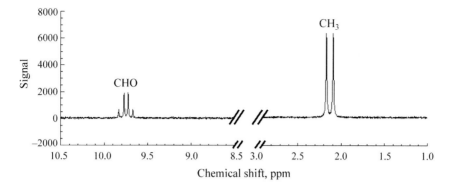

Fig. 3.26 Proton spectrum of acetaldehyde displaying the splitting of the two peaks into a doublet and a quartet as a result of *J*-coupling.

absolute levels of any particular metabolite from MR spectra, so it is usual to make relative comparisons. This is usually done by measuring the ratio of two peak (areas) at a particular spatial location. However, comparison of two spectra from different regions can also be used (e.g. left vs. right) or by performing dynamic studies to observe the change in a particular peak over time.

A list of compounds typically seen in a ^{31}P spectrum of the human brain is given in Table 3.4. The energy-providing ATP is seen as three peaks. Inorganic phosphate (Pi) is a sensitive marker for cellular pH via its chemical shift relative to phosphocreatine (PCr). A change in the acidity of the cell changes the electronic shielding of the phosphate ion and thus a pH dependent change in the chemical shift value occurs. The phosphorus NMR spectrum shows a relatively broad spread of chemical shifts (range < 25 ppm in most tissues), usually allowing good resolution of the constituent chemicals.

In contrast, the spread of the metabolites in a ^{1}H spectrum is quite compressed, spanning a chemical

shift range of less than 5 ppm. The dominant peak in any ^{1}H spectrum will be from water. This peak is so much stronger than any of the metabolites that its signal needs to be suppressed before the metabolite spectrum is acquired. This is achieved by using a frequency selective water saturation pulse prior to the main excitation pulse. The key compounds visible in ^{1}H spectroscopy are shown in Table 3.5. Glutamate and glutamine levels decrease upon ischaemic insult or hypoglycaemia, and this is coupled to an increase in aspartate. GABA, a neurotransmitter, has a relatively weak signal but an enhancement of its peak has been seen following the administration of anti-convulsant drugs. The above metabolites are very difficult to observe *in vivo*. A more abundant neurotransmitter, NAA, is observed to be depleted in the brains of patients suffering from neural degenerative diseases, such as multiple sclerosis, as well as in epilepsy.

Table 3.4 Some of the important components of a ^{31}P spectrum of the human brain and their chemical shifts (relative to PCr)

Compound	Peak	Typical label	Chemical shift (ppm)
Adenosine triphosphate	α	αATP	−7.5
	β	βATP	−16.0
	γ	γATP	−2.5
Phosphocreatine		PCr	0
Inorganic phosphate		Pi	~5

Table 3.5 Some of the important components of a ^{1}H spectrum of the human brain, and their chemical shifts (relative to TSP)

Compound	Typical label	Chemical shift (ppm)
Lactate	Lac	1.3, 4.1
Alanine	Ala	1.5, 3.8
γ-Aminobutyrate	GABA	1.9, 2.3, 3.0
N-Acetylaspartate	NAA	2.0, 2.5, 2.7, 4.4
Glutamate	Glu	2.1, 2.3, 3.8
Glutamine	Gln	2.1, 2.4, 3.8
Aspartate	Asp	2.7, 2.8, 3.9
Creatine/phosphocreatine	Cr	3.0, 3.9
Choline	Cho	3.2, 3.5, 4.1

Creatine and choline are involved in several metabolic pathways. It may also be possible to use MRS of lactate to test whether there is uncoupling of oxidative metabolism and blood flow in fMRI activations.

3.6.3 Localized spectroscopy and spectroscopic imaging

Spectroscopy of chemicals in solution or in extracted tissue samples is easily studied using NMR since the whole sample contains the compounds of interest. However, with *in vivo* spectroscopy it is not always desirable to sample the signal from the whole region of the coil. A degree of localization of signal is possible using radiofrequency coils that have a limited sensitive region. Such coils are usually surface coils, which for a circular winding of a particular radius have a sensitive volume reaching approximately that distance into the sample. Surface coils are useful when the region of interest is near the surface of the body, but to study deeper regions, such as the white matter of the brain, it is necessary to perform some other type of localization. This can be achieved by using magnetic field gradients. In a similar way to how an MRI slice select gradient and shaped RF pulse is used to excite only those spins in a thin slice, it is possible to excite only those spins in a discrete volume of interest. This usually involves applying three or more RF pulses, together with gradients. There are a variety of these sequences, such as PRESS, ISIS and STEAM (Gadian 1995).

Instead of limiting the spectroscopy to a single volume of interest, an alternative technique of magnetic resonance spectroscopic imaging (MRSI) introduces spectral information into MR images. The chemical shift domain essentially becomes a fourth dimension in the experiment by use of a spectral acquisition following suitable phase encoded spatial localization. For reasons of signal-to-noise and scan duration, spectroscopic imaging is usually limited to a relatively low resolution matrix (typically 16×16 or 32×32 pixels). However, the advantage over localized spectroscopy is that it is possible to bin the data into spectral intervals, and then plot these distributions over the sample. Thus, it is possible to produce maps of a particular metabolite. The combination of positional information with chemical composition is a powerful tool in biomedical MRS and as human scanner field strengths increase it is likely that spectro- scopic imaging will become increasingly useful as a research and ultimately a clinical tool.

References

Bloch, F., Hansen, W.W., and Packard, M. (1946). The nuclear induction experiment. *Physiological Reviews*, 70, 474–85.

Bracewell, R.N. (1986). *The Fourier transform and its applications*. McGraw-Hill, New York.

Damadian, R., Goldsmith, M., and Minkoff, L. (1977). NMR in cancer: XVI. FONAR image of the live human body. *Physiological Chemistry and Physics and Medical NMR*, 9, 97–100.

Edelman, R.R., Siewert, B., Darby, D.G., Thangaraj, V., Nobre, A.C., Mesulam, M.M., and Warach, S. (1994). Qualitative mapping of cerebral blood flow and functional localization with echo-planar MR imaging and signal targeting with alternating radio frequency. *Radiology*, 192, 513–20.

Gadian, D.G. (1995). *NMR and its applications to living systems*, (2nd edn). Oxford University Press, Oxford.

Kim, S.G. (1995). Quantification of relative cerebral blood flow change by flow-sensitive alternating inversion recovery (FAIR) technique: application to functional mapping. *Magnetic Resonance in Medicine*, 34, 293–301.

Kwong, K.K., Belliveau, J.W., Chesler, D.A., Goldberg, I.E., Weisskoff, R.M., Poncelet, B.P., Kennedy, D.N., Hoppel, B.E., Cohen, M.S., Turner, R., Cheng, H.M., Brady, T.J., and Rosen, B.R. (1992). Dynamic magnetic resonance imaging of human brain activity during primary sensory stimulation. *Proceedings of the National Academy of Sciences (USA)*, 89, 5675–9.

Lauterbur, P.C. (1973). Image formation by induced local interactions: examples employing nuclear magnetic resonance. *Nature*, 242, 190–1.

LeBihan, D. (1995). *Diffusion and perfusion magnetic resonance imaging*. Raven Press, New York.

Mansfield, P. and Grannell, P.K. (1973). NMR 'diffraction' in solids? *Journal of Physical Chemistry*, 6, L422–L426.

Purcell, E.M., Torrey, H.C., and Pound, R.V. (1946). Resonance absorption by nuclear magnetic moments in a solid. *Physical Reviews*, 69, 37–8.

Rosen, B., Belliveau, J.W., and Chien, D. (1989). Perfusion imaging by nuclear magnetic resonance. *Magnetic Resonance Quarterly*, 5, 263–81.

Williams, D.S., Detre, J.A., Leigh, J.S., and Koretsky, A.P. (1992). Magnetic resonance imaging of perfusion using spin inversion of arterial water. *Proceedings of National Academy of Sciences (USA)* 89, 212–6.

Wong, E.C., Buxton, R.B., and Frank, L.R. (1997). Implementation of quantitative perfusion imaging techniques for functional brain mapping using pulsed arterial spin labeling. *NMR Biomedicine*, 10, 237–49.

Wong, E.C., Buxton, R.B., and Frank, L.R. (1998). Quantitative imaging of perfusion using a single subtraction (QUIPPS and QUIPPS II). *Magnetic Resonance in Medicine*, 39, 702–08.

4 | Ultra-fast fMRI

Richard A. Jones, Jason A. Brookes, and Chrit T.W. Moonen

4.1 Introduction

Brain activation is known to lead to enhanced perfusion which, together with other physiological changes (e.g. blood volume, oxygen consumption), results in a decreased deoxyhaemoglobin concentration in regions of neuronal activity (Ogawa *et al.* 1990). This effect is referred to as the BOLD (blood oxygenation level dependent) effect and is by far the most commonly used method for fMRI studies and manifests itself as a slight increase in the strongly T2* (or T2) weighted MR images used for fMRI studies. BOLD signal changes occur both in the tissue (extra-vascular BOLD effect) and within the vasculature (intra-vascular BOLD effect). Non-BOLD related intra-vascular signal changes can also occur within larger vessels due to in-flow effects. The purpose of this chapter is to outline the acquisition methods for ultra-fast BOLD fMRI, in particular, to explain the basics of echo planar imaging (and alternative ultra-fast imaging techniques), and to discuss possible artefacts and pitfalls. In addition, promising recent developments will also be described.

4.2 Why ultra-fast fMRI?

The most widely used activation paradigm for fMRI is the so-called 'block' paradigm, which consists of alternated periods of activation (or task A) and rest (or task B). Each task is of roughly equal duration, typically in the range 20–30 s. The magnetic resonance (MR) acquisition methods used in conjunction with block

paradigms are designed to give both maximal signal-to-noise ratio and maximum BOLD contrast in conjunction with whole brain coverage. Recently, so-called 'single-event' paradigms, which employ much shorter periods of activation, alternated with longer periods of rest (sometimes of varying duration), have become popular (Buckner *et al.* 1996). For single event studies the MR acquisition methods are designed to measure the haemodynamic changes which occur over several seconds, and typically reach a maximum at about 6 s, after the start of the short activation.

Given these time scales, why does one need ultra-fast fMRI? The answer lies in signal stability over time. In particular, signal instabilities originating from the cardiac cycle, from respiratory motion and/or head motion effects can easily be of the same order as, or even overshadow, the BOLD effect (which has a maximum amplitude of only 2 or 3 per cent at 1.5 Tesla).

4.3 Requirements for BOLD fMRI acquisition methods

4.3.1 Echo time (TE) optimization

In a well shimmed magnetic field the phase of the MR signal of water changes with echo time (TE) due to changes in the local magnetic field caused by variations in the amount, and distribution, of deoxyhaemoglobin in the capillaries and veins. As a result the magnetic field alters microscopically within each volume element (voxel), leading to phase dispersions for the

---

This chapter is dedicated to the memory of our friend and colleague Jason Brookes who was killed in a mountaineering accident in the Pyrénées on 17 January 2000.

water magnetization across the voxel. This phase dispersion increases as the echo time is increased. When integrating over all water magnetization within one voxel, the net MRI signal will be observed to decay in amplitude as a function of TE with a time constant T2* (see Section 3.3.3). Thus, the value of T2* in a voxel is a measure of the extent and distribution of the local variations in the magnetic field over that voxel, together with a contribution from the nuclear transverse relaxation time T2. In order to determine the value of TE at which the maximum BOLD effect occurs, one can subtract the T2* decay curves in the activated and rest states. The optimum echo time (TE$_{opt}$) lies between the T2* value of the activated state (*a*) and the resting state (*b*) and can be calculated with eqn (4.1) (in which R2* is 1/T2*)

$$TE_{opt} = \frac{\ln [R2^*(a)] - \ln [R2^*(b)]}{R2^*(a) - R2^*(b)} \qquad (4.1)$$

Typical T2* values for voxels in the motor cortex at 1.5 Tesla are 72 and 70 ms during activation and rest, respectively. Hence, the maximum BOLD amplitude is obtained with a TE of 71 ms. However, the BOLD sensitivity does not depend critically on the TE, and TE values in the range 50–90 msec will produce acceptable results. It should be noted that methods with an extended signal acquisition period, such as echo planar imaging (EPI), will not have equal BOLD sensitivity for all acquired data points and thus the real resolution of a BOLD image may be less than the resolution of the original images. At higher field strengths the T2* values of the two states are shorter and hence the optimum TE is shorter (as is the range of suitable echo times).

4.3.2 The effect of field homogeneity on optimum TE values and BOLD signal

The T2* value for a voxel is determined not only by the microscopic field heterogeneity due to the presence of deoxyhaemoglobin, but also by the macroscopic field homogeneity (magnet shimming) and the T2 relaxation process. We can express the R2* (equal to 1/T2*) process as the sum of those effects:

$$R2^* = R2^d + R2_{mi'} + R2_{ma'} \qquad (4.2)$$

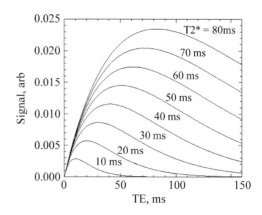

Fig. 4.1 Magnitude of the BOLD effect as a function of TE for different levels of macroscopic magnetic field inhomogeneity. The graph is obtained with simulations based on Eqns (4.1 and 4.2). The curves from top to bottom were calculated using T2* values for the resting state of 80, 70, 60, 50, 40, 30, 20 ms and 10 ms respectively. Note that the optimal echo time and the maximum BOLD effect decrease approximately linearly with decreasing T2* values in the resting state.

where R2^d reflects the T2 decay rate (including diffusion effects through microscopic field gradients), and R2$_{mi'}$ and R2$_{ma'}$ are the dephasing terms due microscopic (mi) and macroscopic (ma) susceptibility effects, respectively. The BOLD effect is expressed predominantly as a change in R2$_{mi'}$ (which decreases upon activation) accompanied by a smaller change in the R2^d term.

Figure 4.1 shows plots of the magnitude of the BOLD effect as a function of TE for different qualities of field homogeneity. It is evident that not only is the magnitude of the BOLD effect dependent on the field homogeneity, but also that the optimum TE value becomes shorter when the magnetic field becomes more inhomogeneous. Therefore, the point spread filter for acquisition methods with extended acquisition periods is a function of local field homogeneity. In these cases the actual resolution in BOLD fMRI data may vary locally as a function of field homogeneity.

The choice of voxel size has several consequences for EPI beyond the simple signal-to-noise ratio and resolution considerations common to all MRI sequences. First of all it should be noted that T2* itself is a function of voxel size and that increasing the voxel size

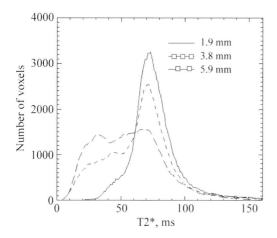

Fig. 4.2 Histograms of the number of voxels with a given T2* obtained from a thick slab through the brain of a volunteer at 1.5 Tesla. The histograms represent isotropic voxels with 1.9 mm (*solid line*), 3.8 mm (*short dashes*) and 5.7 mm (*long dashes*). Note the strong shift to lower T2* values at lower resolution.

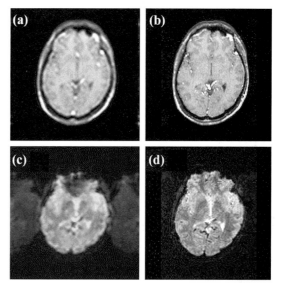

Fig. 4.3 Conventional spin echo (a and b) and gradient echo EPI images (c and d) with matrices of 64 × 64 (a and c) and 128 × 128 (b and d) corresponding to isotropic resolutions of 4 × 4 × 4 mm³ and 2 × 2 × 2 mm³ respectively. The EPI images were obtained using TE = 60 msec, TR = 3000 msec and EPI echo trains of 63 and 95 echoes respectively, with the field of view being adjusted in the phase direction to give the desired resolution. The low resolution EPI image exhibits a clear signal loss in the region of poor homogeneity in the pre-frontal cortex which is absent in the higher resolution EPI image and both spin echo images.

tends to shorten T2*, reducing both the magnitude of the BOLD effect and the range of echo times that give close to the maximal BOLD effect. Figure 4.2 shows whole brain histograms of T2* values obtained at 1.5 Tesla using a 3D FLASH sequence (a conventional gradient echo sequence which can also be used for BOLD fMRI) with a range of echo times and with isotropic resolutions of 1.9, 3.8, and 5.7 mm, respectively. The distribution of T2* values that is observed is rather narrow at 1.9 mm resolution. At 3.8 mm it is broadened and acquires a significant contribution from rather short T2* values (mainly originating from voxels in the cerebellum, frontal cortex and temporal lobes). At 5.7 mm resolution the histogram becomes very broad with 50 per cent of the voxels having a T2* of less than 50 msec and 20 per cent having a value below 30 msec. Thus, with 1.9 mm resolution, we have approximately equal BOLD sensitivity in all voxels, whereas at 3.8 mm the sensitivity decreases significantly in several regions of the brain. With 5.7 mm resolution the sensitivity is decreased significantly for most of the brain.

Figure 4.3 illustrates this point further by showing both conventional spin echo and gradient echo EPI data obtained with 4 mm (a and c) and 2 mm (b and d)

isotropic resolution. For the gradient echo EPI data a loss of signal in the region of poor field homogeneity in the pre-frontal cortex can be seen clearly in the low resolution (4 mm) image but is much less evident in the higher resolution (2 mm) image. No such effect is observed with the spin echo images since the spin echo refocuses (cancels) the effects of field inhomogeneity at time *t* = TE. The BOLD signal change, however, is also much attenuated for spin echo versus gradient echo EPI.

It should be noted that even though the tortuosity of the cortical ribbon makes cubic voxels the obvious choice for fMRI, for practical reasons many studies are carried out using multi-slice protocols with a slice thickness of 5–6 mm, despite a better in-plane resolution of 3.5 mm or better. The thick slice dimension leads to the sort of T2* shortening problems described above. Additionally, and for similar reasons, a higher spatial resolution will be required at higher field strengths in order to obtain a homogenous distribution of T2* values throughout the brain. This is a consequence of the fact that macroscopic susceptibility effects scale linearly with magnetic field strength.

4.3.3 Intra-scan motion: signal stability

Motion artefacts can manifest in a number of ways, including intra-image changes in position or more subtle inter-image effects such as those arising from the small phase changes in the brain that originate from gross magnetic susceptibility changes as the lungs expand and contract during the respiratory cycle. In single shot acquisitions the effect of the respiration-induced phase changes is relatively small, particularly for transaxial images, and the effect of intra-image changes in position can generally be addressed using image registration techniques. For MR acquisition sequences that use multiple excitations both bulk changes in position and phase changes are significant sources of instability. To minimize these effects independent 'motion-tracking' information, in the form of navigator signals or echoes (Ehman and Felmlee 1989) should be obtained. Navigator echoes can be very

simple, such as a single data point, indicating phase stability of the centre point of *k*-space, or more complex, such as a readout gradient without phase encoding, or even very complex, such as a two-dimensional navigator that describes a circle or spiral in *k*-space. The use of single point navigator information allows evaluation and correction of small displacements in the direction of the gradient used. The more complex navigator echoes allow evaluation of more than one head motion parameter. Figure 4.4 shows data acquired using a single point navigator which clearly depicts the fluctuations originating from cardiac and respiratory cycles.

As an alternative strategy, dedicated cardiac and/or respiratory monitoring hardware can be used, allowing fMRI scanning to be started at predetermined time points (gating). However, because variations in the duration of the cardiac cycle would then correspond to variations in the scan repetition time (TR), a varying level of signal saturation will occur. Unless a very long TR is used (at least three times the T1 of water), this in turn can lead to variations in signal intensity which can be comparable to or greater than those produced by the BOLD effect. Obviously, such a TR is inefficient, and thus gating methods are rarely used in fMRI. Nevertheless, monitoring of the cardiac and respiratory cycles during a study for the purpose of retrospective data correction has been used successfully by several groups to improve the quality of fMRI images (Hu *et al.* 1995; Guimaraes *et al.* 1998). Cerebrospinal fluid (CSF) motion can also be a cause of signal instability and suppression of the CSF may therefore be expected to improve the signal stability. However, methods such as inversion recovery in 2D methods, or the use of large flip angles in 3D methods (both methods use the long T1 time of CSF as a means of suppressing the CSF signal) either cost too much time or lead to other signal instabilities. As a final example of sources of instability, if the eyes are within the imaged volume then eye movement can lead to increased signal instabilities in a region which is displaced from the eyes by some fraction of the field of view in the phase encoding direction. A careful choice of the orientation of the images can reduce this problem by causing the artefact to occur outside the brain. Alternatively, spatial saturation can be used to suppress the signal from the eyes (Chen and Zu 1997).

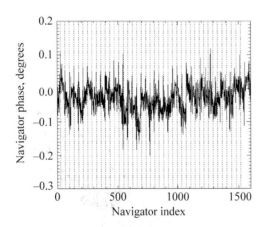

Fig. 4.4 Phase fluctuations of the centre point of *k*-space as a function of time during 42 s with one data point per 26 ms (every fourth point is plotted here for clarity). The evolution of this zero order navigator signal was measured using the PRESTO method for the full brain. Note the sharp deviations (spikes) associated with the cardiac cycle and the slower rolling evolution with the respiratory cycle.

4.4 Gradient echo methods

The signal generated following a radiofrequency pulse is dephased by the presence of the imaging gradients and has to be reformed at a time TE after the radiofrequency excitation pulse through the use of either a gradient echo or a spin echo. The gradient echo relies on designing an appropriate form for the gradient waveforms such that at the echo time (TE) all applied gradient effects are refocused and an attenuated echo of the signal is formed. This is illustrated in Fig. 4.5 where the measurement (readout) gradient is initially negative, causing a dephasing of the spins. The gradient is then reversed causing the spins to rephase into an echo at the centre of the readout window at a time TE after the excitation pulse. Although the gradient echo removes the effects of the imaging gradients it affects neither chemical shift effects nor the dephasing produced by the $R2_{mi'}$ and $R2_{ma'}$ terms in eqn (4.2). Thus, the signal amplitude of the gradient echo at time $t = \text{TE}$ is given by $S(t) = S_0\exp(-\text{TE}/T2^*)$ where S_0 is the transverse magnetization present immediately after the radiofrequency excitation pulse.

4.4.1 FLASH sequences

The FLASH sequence (Haase *et al.* 1986) is a 2D-FT gradient echo sequence which uses low flip angle excitation pulses to improve the signal-to-noise ratio. Using a pulse angle θ where $\theta < 90°$ might, at first sight, seem to be counter-productive since the fraction of the magnetization rotated into the transverse plane ($M_0\sin(\theta)$) will be reduced. However, at short TR repetition times the fraction of magnetization left in the z direction ($M_0\cos(\theta)$) also has to be considered. The reason for this is that the component remaining in the z direction is utilised by subsequent excitation pulses. When a 90° excitation pulse is used the z direction magnetization is zero immediately afterwards, meaning that the z-component of magnetization prior to the subsequent excitation pulse would consist solely of magnetization which has recovered during the repetition time. For lower flip angles, however, the z magnetization is less disturbed by each pulse, meaning that more longitudinal magnetization may be available for subsequent excitation pulses. In fact, the flip angle that provides the optimum magnetization can be found. For a given T1 and TR the flip angle, θ_E, which gives the maximum signal-to-noise ratio for a gradient echo sequence is known as the Ernst angle (Ernst and Anderson 1966). See also Section 3.5.1.

Figure 4.6 illustrates the dependence of the signal from a FLASH sequence with a TR and TE which are typical for fMRI studies. The Ernst angles can be clearly seen to be around 20° and 25° for grey matter and white matter brain tissue, respectively. The absolute signal levels are less than 10 per cent of the maximum available signal (M_0). An additional problem with running FLASH sequences at or greater than the Ernst angle is that the magnetization in the blood vessels is constantly replenished by the blood flowing from outside the slice. Since the inflowing spins have not experienced the preceding RF pulses (the RF pulses being slice selective), the inflowing spins have full magnetization (M_0 rather than $M_0\cos(\theta)$), leading to an artefactually strong signal from the vessels (Duyn *et al.* 1994). To attenuate this effect it is necessary to reduce the flip angle to around 10° (Frahm *et al.* 1994), which has the unfortunate side effect of further reducing the signal-to-noise ratio, or to use 3D techniques (see Section 4.4.4).

For an echo time of 60 ms the minimum achievable TR will be around 70 msec (the weak signal level means that a relatively low sampling bandwidth per pixel has to be used in order to maximize the SNR). Thus the time required to acquire 64 lines of data is approximately 4.5 s. For an individual scan duration of 4.5 s the total imaging time for a series of images long enough to allow a robust detection of BOLD induced signal changes is already rather long and, in addition, each image in the series is subject to the

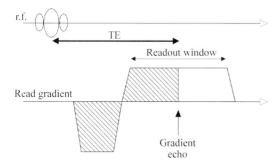

Fig. 4.5   The formation of a gradient echo. The initial negative lobe and the shaded area of the subsequent positive lobe have equal area leading to the formation of a gradient echo at the point indicated in the figure.

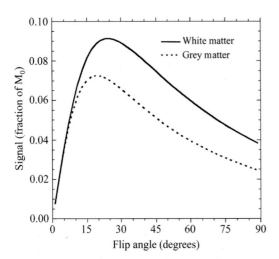

Fig. 4.6   A simulation of the dependence of the signal on the flip angle for a FLASH sequence with TR = 70 and TE = 60 ms. The relaxation times used for the simulation were 750 and 1200 ms for the T1 values of white and grey matter, respectively. The T2* of both tissues was assumed to be 70 ms.

refocused. This process can be repeated as long as there is appreciable transverse magnetization present (e.g. after echo times equal to T2* and 3 × T2* the signal will have decayed to $0.37S_0$ and $0.05S_0$, respectively). For a train of n echoes, each echo provides one line of k-space for each of n images, with each image having a different degree of T2* weighting. The T2* value can be calculated on a pixel by pixel basis by fitting the signal decay to an exponential function, provided sufficient echoes are available. In order to obtain more echoes for a given TR the sampling bandwidth can be increased which reduces the measurement time (and, unfortunately, the signal-to-noise ratio) per echo, allowing more echoes to be collected within a given time period.

4.4.2   Echo planar imaging

The multiple echo FLASH sequence described above increases the amount of information derived from each RF excitation pulse but does not address the problem of the long acquisition time. To reduce the acquisition time per image one can retain the concept of deriving multiple echoes from a single excitation pulse, but rather than using each of n echoes to encode one line of k-space for each of n images, the pulse sequence can be altered such that the n echoes encode n lines of k-space in a single image. For a low resolution (64 × 64) image 64 echoes can be acquired after an excitation pulse and the complete image can thus be derived from a single excitation pulse (Section 3.4.5).

There are several ways of modifying the pulse sequence to achieve this goal. The most commonly used method is echo planar imaging based on the sequence originally proposed by Mansfield which sampled half of k space using a zigzag trajectory (Mansfield 1977). Today virtually all echo planar imaging is performed using a sequence of the type shown in Fig. 4.7 which depicts a blipped EPI scheme which samples all of k-space in a rectilinear fashion (Johnson *et al.* 1983). As in the multiple echo FLASH schemes, repeated reversals of the measurement (read-out) gradient repeatedly refocuses the transverse magnetization to yield a train of gradient echoes. The crucial difference is the form of the phase encoding gradient. In the multiple echo FLASH sequence a single phase encoding gradient is applied prior to the first echo such that all the echoes are identically phase

variations produced by physiologically induced changes in the signal discussed above. If multiple slices are required, which is generally the case for neuroscience applications, then the total imaging time becomes unacceptable. In practice, this means that FLASH studies are restricted to one or two slices unless either a suitable interleaving of the slices is performed in order to increase the efficiency of the sequence (Loenneker *et al.* 1996) or echo shifting techniques are utilised to permit the use of TR < TE by shifting the gradient echo into the following TR period (Moonen *et al.* 1992; Liu *et al.* 1993). While both of these modifications increase the efficiency of FLASH type sequences they also tend to increase the dephasing experienced by the spins in the vasculature, resulting in a reduced intravascular BOLD effect.

A development of the FLASH sequence, which has proved useful in the study of the mechanisms underlying the BOLD effect and the relative sizes of the intra- and extravascular components of the BOLD effect, is to extend the sequence to measure a series of gradient echoes (Menon *et al.* 1993). This is accomplished by reversing the polarity of the read gradient for alternate echoes, which leads to the formation of a train of gradient echoes with each gradient echo representing a point where the net applied read gradient is

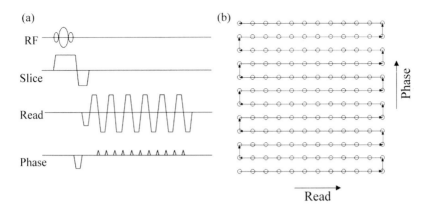

Fig. 4.7 A blipped EPI pulse sequence (a) and *k*-space traversal diagram (b) for a 12 × 12 point gradient echo image. The initial phase gradient moves the acquisition to the edge of *k*-space in the phase encoding direction. The alternating read gradient then causes a train of gradient echoes to be formed and the subsequent gradient 'blips' on the phase axis serve to step the acquisition through *k*-space in the phase encode direction. The combination of the readout and phase encode gradients yields a rectilinear array of data points in *k*-space with the direction of the readout gradient being switched for alternate lines.

encoded. In the EPI sequence a large initial phase encode gradient is used to place the first echo at the periphery of *k*-space, and the subsequent blips of the phase encode gradient serve to increment the acquired echoes through *k*-space. The blips serve to progressively reduce the net phase gradient to zero and then to increment the phase gradient until it reaches the opposite side of *k*-space (see Fig. 4.7). In contrast to multiple echo FLASH, the effect of other parameters, such as field inhomogeneity, susceptibility effects, and chemical shift, which influence the evolution of the phase during the echo train, will affect the resulting image more severely and thus will impose a number of limitations on EPI sequences.

4.4.3 Limitations of EPI sequences

Two types of 'off-resonance' effects need to be dealt with in EPI :

(1) Off-resonance effects of fat spins.
(2) Off-resonance effects of water spins.

The resonance frequencies of the signals from ^{1}H protons in water and fat tissue, respectively, are separated by 3.44 ppm (i.e. 220 Hz at 1.5 Tesla, 440 Hz at 3 Tesla, etc.). This difference in resonance frequency causes the signals from fatty tissues to be displaced in the readout direction in all MRI sequences (producing what is known as the chemical shift artefact). The size of displacement depends on the sampling bandwidth in the readout direction and since EPI sequences use a large readout bandwidth (typically 1500–3000 Hz/pixel) the chemical shift in this direction is negligibly small. However, with EPI sequences (unlike conventional sequences) a chemical shift also accumulates in the phase encode direction, and since the imaging bandwidth in that direction is rather low (typically 20–30 Hz/pixel) this component of the chemical shift can cause substantial displacements of the fat signal. For this reason several fat suppression techniques have been developed to remove the fat signal, one of which should always be used in conjunction with single shot EPI techniques. The fat suppression techniques use a frequency selective RF pulse to selectively excite either the fat signal (the resulting signal is then dephased by a strong 'crusher' gradient pulse) or the water signal to give images which are free of any signal originating from fatty tissue.

Off-resonance artefacts of water spins are principally generated by inhomogeneities in the main magnetic field, resulting from poor shimming and susceptibility effects, and induce geometric distortion in the images. While good shimming can help to reduce the overall level of inhomogeneity there is little that can be done to alleviate the effects on the acquired data of highly localized changes in susceptibility, other than by reducing the sensitivity of the sequence to such effects. However, characterizing the field inhomogenities with a B_0 field map allows the use of post-processing techniques to correct for the geometric distortion (Jezzard and Balaban 1995). The parameter which has the most influence on the amount of geometric distortion is the interval between successive echoes (IEI—inter echo interval). The greater the IEI the more time spins have to accumulate phase shifts originating from sources other than the desired phase encoding gradient. Several measures can be taken to reduce the IEI and these are tabulated in Table 4.1. Increasing the sampling bandwidth (in the readout direction) reduces the IEI at the expense of also reducing SNR but this approach becomes counter productive once the ramp times start to dominate the IEI. In such situations the use of ramp sampling, in which the signal is sampled both on the flanks as well as on the plateau of the alternating readout gradient, is a better option. Increasing the number of shots (i.e. interleaving the k-space acquisition) reduces the IEI, but the increased scan time means that the signals are more likely to be affected by signal fluctuations of physiological origin. Hence, such sequences may actually be less suitable for fMRI studies unless navigator echoes are simultaneously collected to enable post-acquisition correction of these fluctuations.

The final type of artefact that will be discussed arises from the alternation in the polarity of the readout gradient between successive lines of k-space. The alternating polarity produces an alternation in the direction of the shift in the echo position that will be induced by the presence of any small gradient imperfections or eddy currents between alternate lines. When the image is reconstructed, the artefactually alternating signal leads to a lower intensity 'ghost' of the image appearing, which is shifted by half the field of view in the phase encode direction (also known as a Nyquist ghost). Evidence of such a ghost can be seen in Fig. 4.3(c), in which the phase encode direction is left–right. More complex ghosting patterns are observed when interleaved EPI is used. The ghosting can in theory be eliminated by very precise adjustment of the system. However, the most widely used strategy is to acquire a non-phase encoded data set (often referred to as the reference data set) prior to acquiring the EPI images themselves. The shifts in echo position can then be measured from the reference data and the raw data can be corrected accordingly prior to reconstruction of the EPI images (Bruder 1992). Alternatively, the required corrections can be derived from the image data set itself (Buonocore 1997).

Multiple-slice EPI fMRI studies are generally run using a relatively long repetition time (TR = 2–3 s) which allows a large number of slices to be collected (such techniques are often able to provide whole brain coverage). The longer TR also renders the sequence relatively insensitive to macrovascular inflow effects (Howseman 1999) but results in a relatively strong signal from CSF. This latter effect may lead to fluctuations in the signal level in regions of the brain where the CSF is pulsatile (such as the cerebellum) due to temporally varying partial volumes of CSF within the voxel.

Table 4.1   The effect of system and imaging parameters on EPI images for a sequence with a fixed field of view

Parameter	Echo spacing	Resolution	SNR	Geometric distortion
Increase gradient slew rate	Reduced	—	—	Reduced
Increase sampling bandwidth	Reduced	—	Reduced	Reduced
Increase the number of shots	Reduced	—	Increased	Reduced
Use of ramp sampling	Reduced	—	—	Reduced
Increase the read matrix	Increased	Increased	Reduced	Increased
Increase the phase encode matrix	—	Increased[1]	Reduced	—
Increase the field strength	—	—	Increased	Increased

[1] Increasing the phase encode matrix increases the nominal resolution in the phase encode direction (phase encode field of view/number of phase encode steps). However, the actual resolution is less than the nominal resolution due to the 'filtering' effect of the signal decay during the echo train. Increasing the phase encode matrix increases this effect so the increase in the actual resolution can be fairly modest.

4.4.4 3D gradient echo methods

For most neuroscience studies three-dimensional fMRI information is required. While contiguous multi-slice methods can provide such information, pure 3D methods would appear to have some advantages. Notably, the same (large) volume is excited by every RF pulse in 3D methods (and is subsequently spatially encoded in all three directions). Because the entire volume is excited by all RF pulses the saturation of the nuclear magnetization is spatially homogeneous which means that 3D fMRI methods generally avoid confounding inflow effects. In addition, true three dimensional images are more easily corrected for small head motions between the images than multi-slice acquisitions. Also the signal intensity can be optimized for the entire volume using the minimum TR and Ernst angle acquisition which generally results in a higher signal per unit time for 3D methods.

For fMRI studies 3D imaging is usually carried out using an EPI sequence in which the slice selection gradient is replaced with a second phase encoding gradient (Johnson *et al.* 1983). Because of the ringing effect (propagation of signal from one slice into the adjacent slices) experienced for reconstruction with a small number of slices, the minimum number of slices for a 3D technique is around 16. Unless the whole brain is to be imaged, the exclusion of 'wrap around' artefacts in the slice phase encode dimension requires that a thick slab is selected and then subdivided, using phase encoding, into the required number of slices. In practice, the slab profile of the excited volume is imperfect, necessitating that the encoded volume be slightly larger than the excited slab. The outer slices are then discarded after the FFT reconstruction in the slice direction (once again to exclude 'wrap around' artefacts). Consequently, of any 20 encoded slices typically four or six outermost slices will have to be discarded. Thus the minimum number of slice direction phase encode steps is approximately 20 so that, assuming a single shot EPI acquisition with TE = 60 ms, the minimum measurement time per volume is around 1.7 s.

One important consideration that should be borne in mind with true 3D acquisitions is that they have a different sensitivity to physiological noise than their multi-slice equivalents. Whereas pure 'white' noise can be expected in single shot 2D EPI images, physiological effects arising from the cardiac and respiratory cycles tend to be major sources of 'physiological noise' in acquisitions lasting for one or more seconds and these effects constitute the main drawback of 3D methods. If the inherent advantages of 3D methods are to be realized either 3D methods need to become even faster or better artefact correction schemes need to be employed to reduce the effect of the physiological motion on the inter-scan stability. The former requirement can be addressed either by using echo shifting principles (TR < TE) in conjunction with EPI as in the PRESTO method (Van Gelderen *et al.* 1995) or by employing other methods, such as half Fourier imaging (see Section 4.7), to shorten the total imaging time.

4.5 *Spin echo methods*

A spin echo uses a second radiofrequency pulse in the pulse sequence, rather than relying solely on changing the polarity of the readout gradient, to refocus the signal into an echo. The most important difference between a spin echo and a gradient echo is that at the centre of the spin echo there are no additional phase shifts due to macroscopic field inhomogeneities, resulting in less signal loss in the image. Additionally, the attenuation of the signal with increasing echo time is determined by T2, rather than T2*, and the optimum BOLD effect is obtained with TE = T2. Since the second RF pulse complicates the recovery of the magnetization following the excitation pulse Ernst angle excitation no longer yields the maximum signal-to-noise per unit time and longer repetition times are necessary, compared to gradient echo sequences. In addition, as well as entirely removing the effects of the $R2_{ma'}$ term, the presence of the refocusing RF pulse also reduces the contribution of the $R2_{mi'}$ term to the BOLD effect, causing spin echo sequences to exhibit a smaller BOLD effect, for a given TE, than a gradient echo sequence. In particular, the extra-vascular component of the BOLD effect around larger vessels is much weaker for spin echo sequences (though the intravascular component of the BOLD effect from these vessels remains). Hence, spin echo sequences would appear to offer few advantages for fMRI studies. However, in regions (or at field strengths) where T2* is short (20–30 msec) the reduced sensitivity of the gradient echo means that spin echo sequences may provide comparable performance with fewer image artefacts.

Further, the weak extra-vascular contribution from large vessels means that, provided the intra-vascular contribution from larger vessels is suppressed, the sequence is more specific for activation in and around capillaries and smaller venules. Unfortunately, these components of the BOLD effect are relatively weak and higher field strengths would appear to be necessary to reliably detect them. The intra-vascular signal can be suppressed either through the use of bipolar gradients to dephase moving spins (Boxerman *et al.* 1995) or, at very high fields, the short T2 of the vascular protons causes the vascular signal to be greatly attenuated at the optimum echo time even when no spoiling gradients are used (Lee *et al.* 1999). Two basic types of spin echo sequences have been employed for fMRI studies, namely multiple echo sequences and spin echo EPI.

4.5.1 Multiple echo sequences

In the same way that one can employ multiple reversals of the readout gradient to convert a FLASH sequence into a multiple echo FLASH sequence, a conventional spin echo experiment can be converted into a multiple echo experiment by applying a series of 180° refocusing pulses, with each TE interval containing a readout acquisition. If each echo is identically phase encoded then *n* echoes contribute one line of *k*-space to each of *n* images with different T2 weighting. M excitations, each acquiring *N* data points per echo, are required to produce the required *M* phase encode steps for a series of images of resolution $N \times M$. The resulting images show increasing T2 weighting with increasing echo time and can be used to calculate T2 maps. Alternatively, instead of using each echo to contribute one line of *k*-space to each of *n* images, each echo can be separately phase encoded such that the *n* echoes contribute *n* *k*-space lines to a single image. This approach was first described by Hennig *et al.* (1986) who used the term RARE to describe this kind of sequence. The RARE sequence is now widely used as a multiple shot technique for clinical studies with typically eight echoes being derived from each excitation pulse. When using this technique at its limit to derive a complete low resolution image from a single excitation pulse several problems are encountered, notably image blurring and high RF power deposition. The former problem is caused by the T2 decay during the lengthy echo train (the requirement of having an RF refocusing pulse for every readout interval means that the IEI is much greater than for gradient echo sequences). The latter problem is due to the large number of closely spaced 180° refocusing RF pulses. The most commonly used approach for single-shot multiple echo imaging is the FLARE sequence (Norris *et al.* 1992) which uses a reduced flip angle for refocusing. The FLARE sequence results in less blurring in the final image (since the time for which the signal persists becomes a function of both T1 and T2) and to reduced RF power deposition. The use of multiple refocusing pulses means, however, that the BOLD sensitivity is even less than that of a classic spin echo experiment, due to the repeated refocusing of the transverse magnetization. One approach to counteracting this reduced sensitivity, while retaining some of the advantages of a spin echo sequence, is to use a preparation sequence to offset the echo train to give a degree of T2* weighting. Since the imaging is still performed using a multiple echo sequence the restrictions imposed on gradient echo EPI by short T2* values are avoided. However, this technique suffers from a significant SNR penalty since only half the available signal can generally be used (Niendorf 1999).

Another multiple echo sequence that has been applied to fMRI is the BURST sequence (Jakob *et al.* 1998), which uses a series of closely spaced, low flip angle RF pulses to generate a train of spin echoes. While this technique is much less demanding on the imaging hardware than either EPI or other multiple echo sequences it is unlikely to become popular due to its very poor SNR and poor BOLD sensitivity.

4.5.2 Spin echo EPI

The term spin echo EPI is something of a misnomer since EPI is fundamentally a gradient echo technique. But by applying a 180° refocusing pulse prior to the gradient echo train, and arranging for the centre of the gradient echo train to coincide with the centre of the spin echo, spin echo weighting will result. Under these conditions the image contrast is less affected by macroscopic field inhomogeneities, although the limitations imposed by the IEI on image distortion (as described in Section 4.4.3) remain. In terms of the BOLD signal the image contrast reflects characteristics of the spin echo and hence extra-vascular BOLD changes around large vessels are largely absent leading to a weaker BOLD effect and, in general, the points raised in Section 4.5.1 apply also to spin echo EPI. The GRASE sequence, in which a number of gradient echoes are acquired for each refocusing RF pulse (Oshio and Feinberg 1991), represents a compromise between the multiple echo sequences described in Section 4.5.1 and gradient echo EPI. In general, the same comments apply to GRASE as apply to the FLARE sequence, although the train length is shorter. Due to the incorporation of gradient echoes the signal decay is now a mixture of T2 and T2* which leads to a significant degradation of the actual resolution of the sequence. A controllable degree of T2* weighting can be introduced for the GRASE sequence in the same way as was described for the FLARE sequence, with the same disadvantage as was noted for the FLARE sequence, namely a reduction in the SNR of 50 per cent for single shot acquisition (Jovicich and Norris 1999).

The main applications for spin echo EPI are probably either where local susceptibility effects cause the T2* to be rather short or at higher fields where the BOLD signal changes are strong enough to permit the use of spin echo sequences in which the microvascular BOLD contribution is dominant.

4.6 Alternative *k*-space trajectories for fast MRI

The methods discussed so far traverse *k*-space in a rectilinear fashion. A number of alternative strategies have been described in the literature, of these only the two most relevant for fMRI will be described here.

4.6.1 Spiral trajectories

A circular *k*-space can be efficiently covered with a spiral trajectory, either from the centre outwards, or from the outer part inwards. A major advantage is that data acquisition occurs in a continuous process at regular intervals along the spiral. Reconstruction of the image is generally achieved by first resampling the data ('regridding') onto a Cartesian sampling pattern similar to that acquired directly using rectilinear trajectories. Fourier transformation again results in the image. A few points should be noted:

- Artefacts arising from intra-scan instabilities in a spiral trajectory are quite different to those

obtained with rectilinear trajectories. Whereas 'streaking' patterns arise in the phase encode direction for the latter, the former leads to circular artefacts.

- Continuous acquisition along a spiral is time-efficient. However, the symmetry of the (simple archimedean) spiral leads to a square field of view (FOV). The fact that the left–right FOV in axial fMRI maps is generally smaller than the anterior-posterior FOV leads to some loss of efficiency for spiral trajectories compared to rectilinear trajectories.

- A circular *k*-space gives the same resolution as a square *k*-space for the same 'surface' of *k*-space. For example, a 112×112 square matrix is comparable in image resolution to a circular matrix with a diameter of 128 points (Van Gelderen 1997).

- When using a spiral starting from the centre, the first data point can be used as a navigator signal (Yang *et al.* 1996).

- A spiral trajectory is not compatible with half-Fourier techniques unless a third dimension is included with conventional phase encoding.

- Correction for off-resonance effects is slightly more complicated for spiral scans.

4.6.2 Projection reconstruction

The name projection reconstruction (PR) originates from computed tomography (CT) techniques and refers more to image processing than to MR acquisition methods. The name is generally used in MR to indicate that *k*-space is covered by a series of straight lines which are rotated about the centre of *k*-space with each line crossing the centre of *k*-space, creating a star-like pattern in *k*-space (see Section 3.4.2). This *k*-space trajectory leads to a longer acquisition time per image because of the higher density of data-points towards the centre of *k*-space (oversampling). However, PR methods are often advantageous when high signal stability is required since the image reconstruction is based on signal intensity and is unaffected by changes in the phase of the signal. In addition, the apparent temporal resolution can be improved when using image processing with a sliding window in *k*-space. For example, the last 25 per cent of image *i* can be taken together with the first 75 per cent of image

$i + 1$ in order to interpolate a 'new' image n at time $t_n = 0.25t_i + 0.75t_{i+1}$. Of course, the actual temporal resolution is unchanged with such procedures. However, the fact that each k-space line includes the centre renders the sliding window procedure in PR methods smoother than methods based on recti-linear k-space sampling. A similar advantage applies to multi-shot spiral trajectories.

4.7 Advanced fMRI methods with reduced k-space coverage

Because of the importance of the cardiac and respiratory cycles for multi-shot 2D and 3D studies much effort has gone towards reducing the size of the data matrix to be acquired by reducing the k-space coverage. In addition, the same techniques are often the only way of obtaining higher spatial resolution at higher field strengths where the shorter T2* values exclude the direct acquisition of higher resolution matrices (Jesmanowicz *et al.* 1998). At first sight reduced k-space coverage would appear to lead to reduced resolution but the use of prior information (in the form of reference images) or special data processing methods may, in some cases, allow the resolution to be retained by estimating the data for the 'missing' sections of k-space. In general, reduced k-space coverage leads to a reduced ratio of signal to white noise. However, this disadvantage may be more than compensated for by the potential of these techniques to reduce the scan time (and hence reduce other signal instabilities), or to increase the spatial resolution (thus increasing the specificity by means of reduced partial volume artefacts).

4.7.1 Keyhole fMRI techniques

In keyhole procedures a full k-space image (referred to as the reference image) is acquired prior to starting the dynamic fMRI activation study. Subsequently, during the fMRI activation protocol, only the central part of k-space is acquired for each image. Prior to data processing the sections of k-space not measured in the fMRI study (i.e. the high spatial frequencies) are filled with data from the reference image. The fMRI images are then reconstructed and have the appearance of

high-resolution images, but have been obtained in a much reduced total imaging time. The problem with this approach is that no high spatial frequency information is obtained for the BOLD series and thus the activation patterns depicted in the fMRI images actually have low spatial resolution, despite their anatomical appearance. Several improvements have been suggested including measuring separate reference images for the rest and activation phases and slowly updating the high spatial frequencies. Despite these modifications, the fundamental problem of reduced spatial resolution for the functional changes remains.

4.7.2 Half-Fourier

Another significant gain in speed can be obtained by partial k-space scanning. This method takes advantage of the natural redundancy that is inherent in the two halves of k-space data (either a top/bottom redundancy or a left/right redundancy). For this technique the complex conjugate of the acquired k-space data can be substituted for the missing data. In principle, a gain of almost 50 per cent in speed can be obtained. In its simplest form typically 60 per cent of the full k-space data are acquired, which cover one half of k-space in its entirety and the low spatial frequency region of the other half of k-space. The central 20 per cent, covering the low spatial frequencies, can then be used to calculate the necessary phase correction map that enables the missing data to be estimated from the complex conjugate of the acquired data (McGibney *et al.* 1993). This approach works well for conventional spin echo techniques, FLASH sequences with short echo times and for spin echo, but does not work so well for long TE FLASH images or gradient echo EPI images (see Fig. 4.8). In these latter cases the main problem is the quality of the phase correction and this can be improved by acquiring a full k-space phase reference map (Stenger *et al.* 1998). Because of the importance of reducing the size of the data matrix for multi-shot 2D methods (by reducing the number of shots) and 3D fMRI datasets (by reducing the scan time per imaged volume) it is hoped that partial k-space methods will become available for gradient echo fMRI studies.

4.7.3 Sensitivity encoding (SENSE)

Sensitivity encoding (SENSE) (Pruessmann *et al.* 1999), and the related technique of simultaneous acquisition of spatial harmonics (SMASH) (Sodickson and Manning 1997), are recent techniques that hold much promise for fMRI. Both techniques are based on the use of multiple surface coils with the signal from each surface coil being independently acquired. Since each of the surface coils has a unique spatial distribution for its intensity profile it is possible to determine the origin of the signal in situations which would usually lead to fold-over artefacts and hence reduce the number of acquired phase encoding steps. The SENSE method is more general since it is not restricted to particular combinations of the arrangement of the surface coils. In the SENSE technique calibration maps are calculated using full *k*-space images acquired with

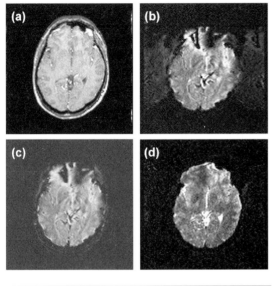

Fig. 4.8 Half Fourier images reconstructed using an approach where the central 20 per cent of *k*-space is used to estimate the phase correction required to insert the missing data by complex conjugation. This approach was applied to a conventional spin echo image (a), a gradient echo EPI with TE = 60 ms (b), a FLASH image with TE = 60 ms (c) and a spin echo EPI with TE = 120 ms (d). This simple approach works well for conventional spin echoes and gives acceptable results for spin echo EPI but gives poor results for long TE gradient echo sequences in regions of poor field homogeneity, such as the pre-frontal cortex. For all images the phase encoding was applied left–right and in the gradient echo EPI image the correction for the alternating read gradient was not completely successful and a residual ghost image, which has been shifted by half the field of view, can be seen.

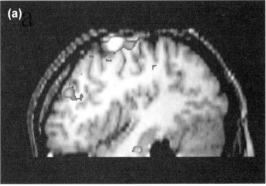
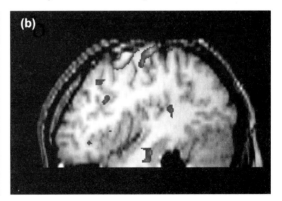

Fig. 4.9 PRESTO fMRI data, acquired with and without SENSE, overlaid on T1-weighted images acquired using the same resolution as the functional scan in order to demonstrate the spatial resolution of the functional sequence. The PRESTO parameters were TR = 24 ms, TE = 40 ms, θ = 9° and a voxel size of $3.5 \times 3.5 \times 3.5$ mm³. Using a synergy coil consisting of two 20 cm surface coils placed on either side of the head both a two shot conventional PRESTO sequence: (a) matrix = $64 \times 48 \times 30$, 80 per cent rFOV, EPI Factor = 23, acquisition time = 2s, and a single shot PRESTO-SENSE sequence; (b) matrix $64 \times 24 \times 30$, 40 per cent rFOV, EPI Factor 23, acquisition time = 1 s, SENSE factor = 2, were acquired. The coil sensitivities needed for the SENSE reconstruction were obtained by using the body coil to acquire an image with the same parameters. The fMRI paradigm consisted of finger-to-thumb opposition, with three activation periods interleaved with 3 resting periods, each of 20 s, leading to a total scan time of 2 min for both imaging sequences (60 or 120 dynamic scans respectively). All volumes were registered and spatially smoothed with a 6 mm Gaussian filter; *t* maps were then calculated and thresholded at p < 0.05. (Images courtesy of Xavier Golay, ETH, Zurich).

the surface coil array. These are then used to calculate sensitivity maps for each surface coil which are in turn used to generate an unfolding matrix from which a non-artefacted image can be calculated. The reduction in the number of phase encoding steps (by a factor R) can be used either to reduce the scan time for conventional imaging techniques or to reduce the echo train length for EPI and related techniques. The total imaging time per image can, in theory, be reduced by a factor equal to the number of independent surface coils. However, in practice a reduction factor greater than $R = 2$ is not trivial to attain, even with multiple surface coils, although it is possible to achieve a factor of $R = 4$ for certain 3D acquisitions. At these larger values of R one tends to observe worse than the expected SNR decrease of $\sqrt{R}$. A comparison of fMRI data acquired with and without SENSE (the latter acquired with half the number of dynamic scans) is shown in Fig. 4.9. It should be noted that the SENSE approach can be further combined with half k-space techniques and echo-shifting principles (see also Golay *et al.* 2000) for additional gains in speed.

4.7.4 UNFOLD

The UNFOLD (Unaliasing by Fourier-Encoding the Overlaps using the temporal Dimension) method is yet another recent technique with reduced k-space coverage per image (Madore *et al.* 1999). Here, the 'trick' is that prior information (most of the image details do not change with time) is combined with a particular k-space coverage which varies as a function of the dynamic scan number. For example, in the case of rectilinear k-space coverage, every fourth k-space trajectory might be acquired starting with line 1 in image 1 (acquisition order 1, 5, 9, 13, etc.). In image 2 acquisition starts with line 2, followed by 6, 10, 14, etc., and in images 3 and 4, acquisition starts with line 3 and 4, respectively. This specific example of an acquisition matrix leads to a factor of four reduction in time per image. However, aliasing of course would occur due to the missing data points (and hence reduction of FOV). The recovery of the missing data points (unaliasing) is based on the fact that the fMRI signal variations can be expected to occur only at the paradigm frequency (and its harmonics). Other frequency terms in signal variations originate (ideally) from aliasing and can be zeroed during data processing. The reader is referred to

the original UNFOLD paper for further processing details and a discussion of possible artefacts.

4.8. Concluding remarks

Apart from requirements of high SNR, high BOLD contrast, and minimal artefacts, imaging speed is an important factor in fMRI. The reason is only partly related to the need for a high temporal resolution (1 to 2 s would be sufficient to characterize the haemodynamic response). A temporal resolution well below 1 s helps to suppress instabilities related to cardiac and respiratory cycles. Because of its short acquisition time (about 75 ms per slice) and good sensitivity, multi-slice gradient echo EPI has a very good performance for BOLD imaging and is therefore the most widely used fMRI method. Ultra-fast 3D methods are under development that will potentially provide better SNR and BOLD contrast per unit time than EPI, and which are also less sensitive to inflow effects. However, 3D imaging speed needs to be improved if this potential is to be realized.

Acknowledgements

The authors would like to thank the European Union for grants to JAB (TMR) and RAJ (BIOMED) and the Conseil Régional d'Aquitaine for support.

References

Boxerman, J.L., Bandettini, P., Kwong, K.K., Baker, J., Davis, T., Rosen, B., and Weisskoff, R.M. (1995). The intravascular contribution to fMRI signal change. Monte-carlo modelling and diffusion weighted studies *in vivo*. *Magnetic Resonance in Medicine*, **34**, 4–10.

Bruder, H., Fischer, H., Reinfelder, H.E., and Schmitt, F. (1992). Image reconstruction for echo planar imaging with non-equidistant k-space sampling. *Magnetic Resonance in Medicine*, **20**, 311–23.

Buckner, R.L., Bandettini, O'Craven, K.M., Savoy, R.L., Petersen, S.E., Raichle, M.E., and Rosen, B.R. (1996). Detection of cortical activation during averaged single trials of a cognitive task using functional magnetic resonance imaging. *Proceedings of the National Academy of Sciences (USA)*, **93**, 14878–83.

Buonocore, M.H. and Gao, L. (1997). Ghost artefact reduction for echo planar imaging using image phase correction. *Magnetic Resonance in Medicine*, **38**, 89–100.

Chen, W. and Zu, X.H. (1997). Suppression of physiological eye movement artefacts in functional MRI using slab pre-saturation. *Magnetic Resonance in Medicine*, 38, 546–50.

Duyn, J.H., Moonen, C.T.W., de Boer, R.W., van Yperen, G.H., Luyten, P.R. (1994) Inflow versus deoxyhemoglobin effects in BOLD functional MRI using gradient echoes at, 1.5T. *NMR in Biomedicine*, 7, 83–88.

Ehman, R.L. and Felmlee, J.P. (1989). Adaptive technique for high definition MR imaging of moving structures. *Radiology*, 173, 255–63.

Ernst, R.R. Anderson, W.A. (1966). Application of Fourier transform spectroscopy to magnetic resonance. 37, 93–102.

Frahm, J., Merboldt, K.D., Hänicke, W., Kleinschmidt, A., and Boecker, H. (1994). Brain or vein—oxygenation or flow? On signal physiology in functional MRI of human brain activation. *NMR in Biomedicine*, 7, 45–53.

Golay, X., Pruessmann, K.P., Weiger, M., Crelier, G.R., Folkers, P.J.M., Kollias, S.S., Boesiger, P. (2000). PRESTO-SENSE: An ultra-fast, whole-brain fMRI technique. *Magnetic Resonance in Medicine*, 43, 779–86.

Guimaraes, A.R., Melcher, J.R., Talavage, T.M., Baker, J.R., Ledden, P., Rosen, B.R., Kiang, N.Y.S., Fullerton, B.C., and Weisskoff, R.M. (1998). Imaging subcortical auditory activity in humans. *Human Brain Mapping*, 6, 33–41.

Haase, A., Frahm, J., Matthaei, D., Hanicke, W., and Merboldt, K.D. (1986). FLASH imaging: Rapid NMR imaging using low flip angles. *Journal of Magnetic Resonance*, 67, 217–22.

Hennig, J., Nauerth, A., and Friedburg, H. (1986). RARE imaging : a fast imaging method for clinical MRI. *Magnetic Resonance in Medicine*, 3, 823–33.

Howseman, A.M., Grootoonk, S., Porter, D.A., Ramdeen, J., Holmes, A.P., and Turner, R. (1999). The effect of slice order and thickness on fMRI activation data using multislice EPI. *Neuroimage*. 9, 363–76.

Hu, X., Le, T.H., Parrish, T., and Erhard, P. (1995). Retrospective estimation and correction of physiological fluctuations in functional MRI. *Magnetic Resonance in Medicine*, 34, 201–12.

Jakob, P.M., Schlaug, G., Griswold, M., Lovblad, K.O., Thomas, R., Ives, J.R., Matheson, J.K., and Edelman, R.R. (1998). Functional BURST imaging. *Magnetic Resonance in Medicine*, 40, 614–21.

Jesmanowicz, A., Bandettini, P.A., and Hyde, J.S. (1998). Single shot half *k*-space high resolution gradient recalled EPI for fMRI at 3 Tesla. *Magnetic Resonance in Medicine*, 40, 754–62.

Jezzard, P. and Balaban, R.S. (1995). Correction for geometric distortion in echo planar images from B_0 field variations. *Magnetic Resonance in Medicine*, 34, 65–73.

Johnson, G., Hutchison, J.M.S., Redpath, T.W., and Eastwood, L.M. (1983). Improvements in performance time for simultaneous three dimensional NMR imaging. *Journal of Magnetic Resonance*, 54, 374–9.

Jovicich, J. and Norris, D.G. (1999). Functional MRI of the human brain with GRASE based BOLD contrast. *Magnetic Resonance in Medicine*, 41, 871–6.

Lee, S.P., Silva, A.C., Ugurbil, K., and Kim, S.G. (1999). Diffusion-weighted spin echo fMRI at 9.4T : microvascular / tissue contribution to BOLD signal changes. *Magnetic Resonance in Medicine*, 42, 919–28.

Liu, G., Sobering, G., Duyn, J., Moonen, C.T.W. (1993). A functional MRI technique combining principles of echo-shifting with a train of observations (PRESTO). *Magnetic Resonance in Medicine*, 30, 764–8.

Loenneker, T., Hennel, F., and Hennig, J. (1996). Multislice interleaved excitation cycles (MUSIC): an efficient gradient echo technique for functional MRI. *Magnetic Resonance in Medicine*, 35, 870–4.

McGibney, G., Smith, M.R., Nichols, S.T., and Crawley, A. (1993). Quantitative evaluation of several partial Fourier reconstruction algorithms used in MRI. *Magnetic Resonance in Medicine*, 30, 51–9.

Madore, B., Glover, G.H., Pelc, N.J. (1999). Unaliasing by Fourier-encoding the overlaps using the temporal dimension (UNFOLD), applied to cardiac imaging and fMRI. *Magnetic Resonance in Medicine*, 42, 813–28.

Mansfield, P. (1977). Multi-planar image formation using NMR spin echoes. *Journal of Physical Chemistry*, 10, L55–8.

Menon, R.S., Ogawa, S., Tank, D.W., and Urgurbil, K. (1993). Four Tesla gradient recalled echo charactheristics of photic stimulation induced changes in the human primary visual cortex. *Magnetic Resonance in Medicine*, 30, 380–6.

Moonen, C.T.W., Liu, G., van Gelderen, Sobering, G. (1992). A fast gradient-recalled MRI technique with increased sensitivity to dynamic susceptibility effects. *Magnetic Resonance in Medicine*, 26, 184–9.

Niendorf, T. (1999). On the application of susceptibility weighted ultra-fast low angle RARE experiments in functional MR imaging. *Magnetic Resonance in Medicine*, 41, 1189–98.

Norris, D.G., Börnert, P., Reese, T., and Leibfritz, D. (1992). On the application of ultra-fast RARE experiments. *Magnetic Resonance in Medicine*, 27, 142–64.

Ogawa, S., Lee, T.M., Ray, A.R., Tank, D.W. (1990). Brain magnetic resonance imaging with contrast dependent on blood oxygenation. *Proceedings of National Academy of Sciences (USA)*, 87, 9868–72.

Oshio, K. and Feinberg, D.A. (1991). GRASE (gradient and spin echo) imaging: a novel fast MRI technique. *Magnetic Resonance in Medicine*, 20, 344–9.

Pruessmann, K.P., Weiger, M., Scheidegger, M.B., and Boesiger, P. (1999). SENSE : sensitivity encoding for fast MRI. *Magnetic Resonance in Medicine*, 42, 952–62.

Sodickson, D.K. and Manning, W.J. (1997). Simultaneous acquisition of spatial harmonics (SMASH): ultra-fast with radio-frequency coil arrays. *Magnetic Resonance in Medicine*, 38, 591–603.

Stenger, V.A., Noll, D.C., and Boada, F.E. (1998). Partial Fourier reconstruction for three dimensional gradient echo functional MRI; comparison of phase correction methods. *Magnetic Resonance in Medicine*, 40, 481–90.

Van Gelderen, P. (1997). Comparing true resolution in square versus circular k-space sampling. Proceedings of the International Society of Magnetic Resonance in Medicine, Sydney, Australia, p. 424.

Van Gelderen, P., Ramsey, N.F., Liu, G., Duyn, J.H., Frank, J.A., Weinberger, D.R., and Moonen, C.T.W. (1995). Three dimensional functional MRI of human brain on a clinical,

1.5T scanner. *Proceedings of the National Academy of Sciences (USA)*, **92**, 6906–10.

Yang, Y., Glover, G.H., Van Gelderen, P., Mattay, V.S., Santha, A.K.S., Sexton, R., Ramsey, N.F., Moonen, C.T.W., Weinberger, D.R., Frank, J.A., and Duyn, J.H. (1996). Fast 3D fMRI at, 1.5T with Spiral Acquisition. *Magnetic Resonance in Medicine*, **36**, 620–6.

5 | Hardware for functional MRI

Gary H. Glover

5.1 Introduction: Requirements for fMRI hardware

Task-driven changes in neuronal metabolism during a functional magnetic resonance imaging (fMRI) experiment result in relatively small signal modulations, typically only a few per cent at 1.5 Tesla (Ogawa *et al.* 1990). Analysis of the data generally compares (in a statistical sense) the signal levels resulting from a sensory or cognitive task with those obtained during a baseline condition. Changes in the signal that result from system drift, physiological functions, basal metabolism fluctuations, and other sources add noise to the comparison process and reduce the significance of the results. Because the neuronal signal modulations are small, it is important that the scan technique is optimized to maximize the signal levels and reduce these spurious sources of noise as much as possible.

A major component of noise derives from physiological sources, including both respiration and circulation (Noll and Schneider 1994). Even when the subject's head is immobilized, cardiovascular-induced brain pulsatility causes phase shifts from expansion and dilation of the brain (Poncelet *et al.* 1992; Noll and Schneider 1994; Glover and Lee 1995). Similarly, respiration causes shifts in the static magnetic field that extend spatially as far as the brain. Conventional gradient-recalled echo (GRE) methods require 64 or more 'shots' to acquire all of k-space, and are sensitive to phase perturbations because the lack of phase coherence between k-space lines causes misplaced signal, or ghosting. The degree of ghosting depends on the timing of the breathing and cardiac cycles relative to collection of the centre of k-space in each time frame, and therefore has variable amplitude from image to image (Glover and Lee 1995).

While navigator echo methods have been developed that reduce such ghosting in GRE methods (Hu and Kim 1994), the most effective method of diminishing the effects of physiological motion is to use single-shot or few-shot acquisitions such as echo planar imaging (EPI) (Kwong *et al.* 1992) or Spiral (Noll *et al.* 1995; Glover and Lai 1998; Yang *et al.* 1998). However, such techniques require the use of high performance imaging hardware for single shot implementation. Scanners capable of EPI acquisitions must incorporate gradients that achieve high slew rate and high amplitude, and receivers with wide bandwidth sampling. Thus, the need for rapid imaging is the first basic requirement of the hardware for fMRI.

The second attribute desired for fMRI scanner hardware is that the systematic drift and noise should be small compared to the remnant physiological noise. Such drift and noise can arise from a variety of sources in the scanner itself or from stimulus equipment in the magnet room.

A third characteristic is that the signal levels must be as large as possible. This requires high field strength (B_0), at least 1.5 Tesla, and careful attention to radiofrequency (RF) coil selection and deployment.

The rest of this chapter describes MR imaging hardware optimized for fMRI with reference to these basic requirements.

5.2 The magnet and spectrometer

5.2.1 Block diagram of a MRI system

The nuclear magnetic resonance (NMR) process requires a static magnetic field to polarize hydrogen spins, radio frequency coils for producing a rotating magnetic field at the Larmor frequency (e.g. ~128 MHz for 3 Tesla) and a receiver to record the NMR signal. For imaging, gradients are utilized to encode spatial information into the signal by inducing controlled phase shifts. Figure 5.1 shows the elements of a MRI scanner and their relationship to one another.

(a)

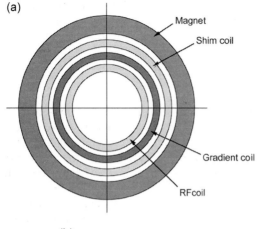

Magnet

Solenoidal magnets capable of achieving high field strengths and having a bore large enough to accommodate human subjects are invariably constructed with superconducting technology in order to achieve sufficient currents. In the superconducting state wire resistance drops to zero, enabling large currents without energy dissipation. The wire must be kept at low temperatures in order to maintain the superconducting state by immersing the windings in liquid helium (LHe), which boils at 4K ($-269°C$). This necessitates a cryostat for containing the helium, a radiation shield and other insulation, and structures capable of supporting the weight of the internal components without

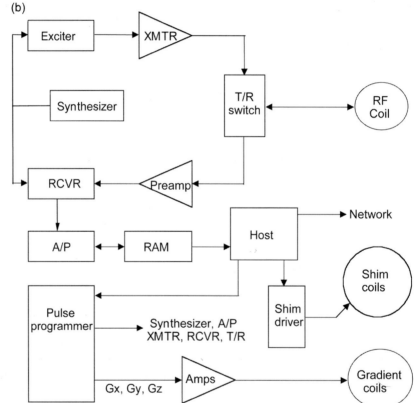

Fig. 5.1   MRI scanner pictorial diagram, showing (a) end view of magnet; (b) supporting electronics.

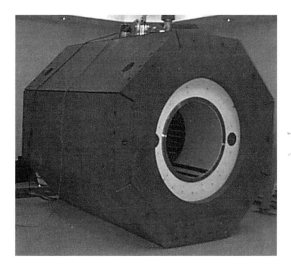

Fig. 5.2 Photograph of a 3 Tesla magnet (white) inside passive iron shielding. Magnetic shielding reduces the area of the magnetic 'footprint'. Passive shim trays can be seen inside the magnet bore.

incurring significant heat losses. Some magnet designs also use a liquid nitrogen jacket (77K, $-196°C$) as an intermediate step in reducing the LHe boil off, and/or may use cryogenic refrigerators to reliquify gaseous helium. Even with the use of such refrigerators, however, all magnets require periodic replenishment of the cryogens, with re-fill periods typically once or twice per year. The magnet is brought up to field ('charged') by an external power supply that ramps up the current at a rate that is slow enough to avoid 'quenching' (see Section 5.2.3). After the desired current (field strength) is obtained the charging supply is removed.

Magnetic shielding

Unshielded MRI magnets have fringe fields that can extend many metres, depending on the field strength and bore size. Shielding can be employed in the magnet room or within the magnet itself to reduce these fringing fields. Room shielding requires many tons of iron encasing the room that houses the magnet. Alternatively, magnet shielding can be used: either active, in which additional superconducting current windings are placed outside the main field windings in such a way as to severely reduce the fringing fields, or passive, in which iron cladding tightly encloses the

magnet, as shown in Fig. 5.2. In either case, shielding can make it easier to place stimulus equipment in the magnet and control rooms, and can have safety advantages (see Section 5.2.3).

Shims

Shimming is a process whereby the static magnetic field is made more homogeneous over the region of interest. Magnetic field homogeneity is critical to successful fMRI because rapid imaging uses a small effective bandwidth per pixel, so that small field perturbations can cause local image distortions or blurring. Several forms of shims are used, including superconducting shims, passive shims, and resistive shims. Superconducting shims are auxiliary windings in the magnet that produce specific field patterns, often based on spherical harmonic functions up to third order or even higher. Passive shims utilize pieces of ferromagnetic metal (typically washer-shaped) arranged in trays within the warm bore of the magnet. Generally, the passive and superconducting shims are adjusted in an iterative process, using a plotting fixture to measure the field at many points on the surface of a sphere in the magnet bore, together with software that calculates the amount and placement of metal as well as the superconducting shim currents. Often many iterations are required to achieve satisfactory homogeneity (typically 1–2 ppm over a specified spherical volume). This process is time consuming and boils off LHe due to the room temperature connections required to the shim windings. Consequently, 'supercon-shimming' is performed only when the magnet is installed and thereafter only if a major change is made to the magnetic environment of the magnet.

Resistive shims are installed in the warm bore of the magnet, as shown in Fig. 5.1. Because these windings consume electrical power, the correction capability is much smaller than that of the superconducting and passive shims. However, the room temperature (RT) shims have the major advantage in that they are always available (no special connections are required, as is the case for the superconducting shims), and the currents can be adjusted under computer control. This makes it possible to tailor the shim for each individual subject by collecting field maps with phase contrast magnetic resonance imaging (e.g. Schneider and Glover 1991; Webb and Macovski 1991). Some manufacturers of high field MRI scanners include automated software that allows shimming over a selected region of interest within the brain. RT-shimming is usually necessary for optimum fMRI results, and is performed as part of the setup for the study before the activation scans are obtained.

Spectrometer

The spectrometer consists of a synthesizer which sets the operating (Larmor) frequency, a transmitter with pulse modulator, a receiver with digitizer and array processor, and a pulse sequence controller that schedules all aspects of the acquisition, including generating RF waveforms for the transmit modulator, control bits for the receiver and analogue-to-digital converter(s), and waveforms for the gradient axes (Fig. 5.1). The RF system also includes a transmit/receive (T/R) switch that connects the RF coil alternately to the transmitter during excitation and the receiver preamp during the reception phase. For fMRI, it is critical that the stability of the spectrometer is very high, since drifts in frequency, amplitude or phase of either the transmitter or receiver can cause additional noise in the images. The noise figure of the RF system (a measure of noise added (Javid and Brenner 1963)) determines the limiting signal-to-noise ratio (SNR) of the system, and is set by the T/R switch and preamplifier, with typical values of 0.5 dB or less. The array processor performs image reconstruction and must have enough memory to hold raw data and images for the acquisition, typically 256 Mbytes or more.

5.2.2 Choice of magnetic field strength, B_0

The choice of the fMRI scanner's magnetic field strength must consider several tradeoffs, which include B_0-dependent changes in SNR, NMR relaxation times T1 and T2*, RF power deposition, and acoustic noise of the gradients.

Signal-to-noise ratio (SNR)

The thermal SNR increases approximately linearly with the magnetic field strength in the absence of relaxation effects. As the raw SNR increases, the T2*-weighted BOLD contrast/noise ratio (CNR) also increases approximately linearly (Gati *et al.* 1997).

However, as B_0 increases, the longitudinal relaxation time T1 becomes longer and the transverse relaxation time T2* becomes shorter. This causes the net gain in CNR to be less than linear.

The image SNR is given by:

$$\text{SNR} \propto B_0 \Delta v f \sqrt{T_{AD}} \Psi(\text{T1,T2*,TR,TE,}\theta), \qquad (5.1)$$

where Δv is the volume of the image voxel, T_{AD} is the total duration of the data acquisition ('readout'), $0 < f < 1$ is a parameter that depends on the k-space trajectory ($f = 1$ for constant velocity trajectories, i.e. with constant gradients, $f = \sim 0.9$ for EPI sinusoidal readout) and Ψ depends on the RF pulse structure, repetition time TR, echo time TE, and excitation flip angle θ. For gradient-recalled-echo (GRE) acquisitions with TR > 2 T1, eqn (5.1) becomes approximately

$$\text{SNR} \propto B_0 \Delta v f \sqrt{T_{AD}} \exp(-\text{TE/T2*}). \qquad (5.2)$$

Generally TE is chosen as ~T2*, so that the exponential factor in eqn (5.2) is independent of field. For conventional GRE methods such as GRASS or FLASH for which $T_{AD} \ll$ T2*, the SNR is then expected to scale linearly with B_0 as predicted from eqn (5.2). However, for rapid imaging methods the readout duration T_{AD} can become long enough (~T2*) that T_{AD} must decrease as T2* decreases in order to avoid blurring and image distortion (Farzaneh *et al.* 1999). This in turn requires increased gradient strength and is equivalent to increasing the bandwidth. In this limit, therefore, the SNR varies as $B_0\sqrt{\text{T2*}}$. A reasonable model for calculating T2* is $1/\text{T2*} = 1/\text{T2} + cB_0$ (Farrar and Becker 1971), where c is a constant and T2 is assumed to be independent of field here. In the rapid imaging case, the SNR is then given by

$$\text{SNR} \propto B_0 \Delta v f \sqrt{1/(1/\text{T2} + cB_0)} \qquad (5.3)$$

Using T2* values measured for cortical grey matter at 0.5 Tesla, 1.5 Tesla and 3 Tesla, one finds T2 = 95 ms and $c = 4.8$ (s-T)$^{-1}$. The normalized SNR using these values is plotted in Fig. 5.3 for both conventional imaging ($T_{AD} \ll$ T2*) and rapid imaging ($T_{AD} \sim$ T2*) cases. The crossover between these cases depends on the imaging resolution and gradient characteristics since these parameters determine T_{AD}, so that for a given set of choices the SNR curve falls between the

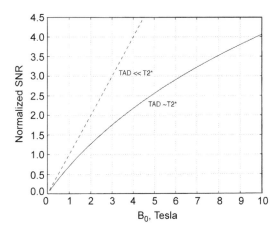

Fig. 5.3 Plots of normalized signal-to-noise ratio (SNR) for the two limiting cases when the readout duration T_{AD} is small compared to T2* (dashed) and when T_{AD} is limited by T2* and is proportional to it (solid). The first case occurs with conventional multi-shot imaging, while the second can occur with single shot rapid methods. In practice, the SNR gain from higher field falls between the two curves, but can be substantially less than expected from the field itself. The T2* dependence was calculated with parameters described in the text.

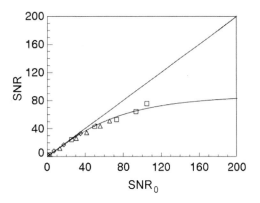

Fig. 5.4 Total SNR as a function of thermal SNR (SNR_0) in fully relaxed GRE images in resting state human brain. Data points show measurements made on seven normal volunteers at 1.5 Tesla (triangles) and 3.0 Tesla (squares), fitted to eqn (5.5) (solid line). Straight line is theoretical line of identity if only thermal noise is present. As the signal (and SNR_0) is increased, physiological noise becomes a larger fraction of the total noise and begins to dominate, limiting further gains in SNR.

two in Fig. 5.3. For example, T2* in cortical grey matter is ~65 ms at 1.5 Tesla and ~48 ms at 3 Tesla. The bandwidth (and gradient strength) would need to be increased by 1.35× to maintain the same T_{AD}/T2* at 3 Tesla, and the increased bandwidth would imply an SNR loss factor of 0.86.

Thus the gains in thermal SNR with increasing B_0 are tempered by the need for higher bandwidth and higher readout gradient strength. In BOLD fMRI, the thermal SNR is not the entire story, however. The brain is richly perfused by blood and is constantly undergoing physiological motion of regions and surfaces, including pulsatility of cortical surfaces in synchronization with the cardiac cycle (Poncelet *et al.* 1992). In addition, normal fluctuations in basal metabolism in cortical grey matter cause fluctuations in the NMR signal, and these fluctuations have an amplitude proportional to the NMR signal itself. As the field increases, the physiological noise components therefore can become comparable to, or even larger than, the thermal noise. When this occurs the total SNR improvements with field increases are further compromised.

The total noise σ in an fMRI experiment includes thermal and system noise σ_0 as well as physiological noise σ_p:

$$\sigma = \sqrt{(\sigma_0^2 + \sigma_p^2)}. \tag{5.4}$$

Noting that σ_p is proportional to the signal, the observed SNR is given by

$$SNR = SNR_0/\sqrt{(1 + \lambda^2 \, SNR_0^2)}, \tag{5.5}$$

where λ is a constant. Equation (5.5) is plotted in Fig. 5.4 using data obtained at 1.5 Tesla and 3.0 Tesla to fit λ (Kruger *et al.* 2001). As this figure demonstrates, when physiological noise is present there are limitations to improvements in SNR that can be achieved by increases in the field strength because the physiological noise increases at the same rate as the signal strength.

Radio-frequency considerations

As the static (B_0) field increases, the power deposited in the subject by the B_1 RF field increases also. For $B_0 < 3$ Tesla, the increase is approximately square law with B_0, but increases less rapidly at higher fields (Collins *et al.* 1998). The US Food and Drug Administration

(FDA) has issued guidelines for the amount of power that can be deposited during an MRI examination in terms of the Specific Absorption Rate (SAR), that include 3.2 W/kg or less averaged over the head. The practical result of these limits is that some types of imaging, notably spin echo and RARE (e.g. Fast Spin Echo or Turbo Spin Echo), are limited at the higher B_0 values because of the 180° pulses, which each deposit four times the energy of a 90° pulse. The limits are manifested as a reduced number of slices that may be acquired for a given TR.

As B_0 increases, substantial B_1 heterogeneity effects occur, especially at 3 Tesla and higher. These effects result because brain tissue acts as a lossy dielectric, which foreshortens the wavelength and causes RF eddy currents (Collins *et al.* 1998). Ignoring the conductive component, the half wavelength for 3 Tesla is approximately 13 cm, which is comparable to the size of the head. At 4 Tesla it is approximately 10 cm. As a result, a 'hot spot' can occur near the centre of the head at > 4 Tesla, due to standing wave effects.

Thus, fMRI at very high fields is challenging because of the two-pronged RF issues of SAR limitations and B_1 heterogeneity.

Acoustic noise

Gradient coils generate acoustic noise because of the interaction between the currents (I) within the coils and the B_0 field. The ($I \times B_0$) forces established during pulsing cause flexure of the gradient coil former and result in generation of air pressure waves (Hedeen and Edelstein 1997). The force per unit current increases linearly with field. However, as discussed above, the gradient strength also increases with B_0 in order to overcome reduced T2*. Thus, the acoustic pressure tends to increase superlinearly with B_0 for the same imaging resolution. Typical measured sound levels at 1.5 Tesla are 115 dB (A-weighted) (Shellock *et al.* 1998).

Thus, the improved image SNR from higher field strengths must be weighed against increased gradient noise. Many of the concerns with increased noise in auditory-cued tasks can be alleviated with clustered acquisitions, in which dead time is provided for the stimuli presentation before each time frame is gathered (Elliott *et al.* 1999). However, the increased gradient

noise itself can still be problematic for studies with subjects having hyperacute hearing (e.g. fragile-x syndrome (Pimentel 1999)).

5.2.3 Safety implications of high magnetic fields

As with any MRI application, safety must be a consideration in fMRI experiments. The primary issues include biological effects of static, RF and pulsed magnetic fields, and concerns about injury from projectiles (attraction of ferromagnetic objects by the magnetic field). A review of the biological effects is beyond the scope of this chapter, and the interested reader is referred to Shellock and Kanal (1996) and to their web site at http://kanal.arad.upmc.edu/MR_Safety/. However, at the time of writing there is little objective evidence that high static fields are harmful.

Injury from projectiles is a concern of particular importance to fMRI applications, however, because of two factors. First, many magnets are being installed in sites other than the traditional radiology department, where access to, and operation of the MRI scanner is generally limited to trained technologists. In many brain mapping centres, fMRI experiments are conducted by the investigators without assistance from centre staff. In such cases, adequate safety awareness for all users must be a responsibility of the centre. This should include mandatory safety training for all investigators with access to the magnet and the use of suitable screening forms for the subjects. Second, fMRI utilizes a substantial amount of auxiliary equipment for stimulus presentation, subject monitoring and response recording. This equipment must be carefully qualified for safety (as well as compatibility; see Section 5.5.2). Before bringing a new piece of equipment into the magnet room, it should be tested for magnetic attraction using a hand held magnet. If found to have ferromagnetic components, the device should be anchored or tethered in such a way that it does not present a hazard, especially to individuals not familiar with the device or its potential danger. It is wise to remember that the attractive forces tend to rise at least quadratically as the magnet is approached, and rise even more rapidly when the magnet is self-shielded.

5.3 Gradient coils

5.3.1 Overview of gradient coils

The purpose of the gradient coils is to produce magnetic fields directed along the axis of the magnet (*z* direction) that vary linearly with *x*, *y*, or *z*. Figure 5.5 shows a schematic diagram of transverse (G_x or G_y) gradients and the longitudinal gradient, G_z. In practice, the transverse gradients are often constructed as printed circuit boards that are wrapped around a former containing the G_z windings. The assembly may also contain resistive shim windings as well as coolant pipes and is potted for rigidity.

Generally, whole body gradient coil assemblies include an active shield coil, as shown in Fig. 5.6, in order to confine the gradient fields as much as possible to the scan volume and exclude them from the rest of the magnet and cryostat. Without such shielding, eddy currents are generated that oppose the desired fields, causing significant image degradation in rapid imaging techniques such as EPI. The shield coil receives the same current as the main coil, and is designed to cancel the fields outside the shield at the cost of increased drive power for the main coil. A typical shielded gradient coil may reduce the eddy currents by a factor of 15–20. Remaining eddy currents are compensated by prefiltering the drive waveforms (Wysong *et al.* 1994).

Parameters that are important in the design of gradient coils and their driver amplifiers include maximum gradient amplitude G^0 (mT/m), slew rate S^0 (T/m/s) or rise time τ (minimum time to reach full scale, μs), and duty cycle. In general, fast imaging

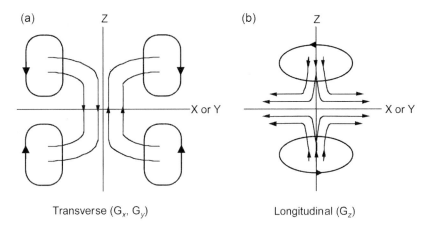

Transverse (G_x, G_y)   Longitudinal (G_z)

Fig. 5.5 Simplified pictorial diagram of transverse (a) and longitudinal (b) gradients. In this design, the transverse gradients use four current loops to generate a magnetic field along the *z* direction that varies and changes sign from left to right. The longitudinal gradient uses two current loops whose B_z fields are in opposition and cancel at *z* = 0 (the B_x and B_y components play no role). By careful design of the current distributions, the variations can be made linear within a limited imaging volume centred at the origin of the gradient system (isocentre).

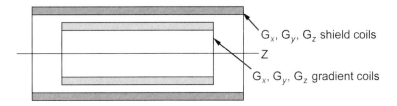

Fig. 5.6 Shielded gradient coils use outer windings to reduce the gradient fields outside the shield to a small fraction of the unshielded configuration. This reduces eddy current effects by excluding time varying fields from the shim coils and magnet cryostat.

sequences require high G^0 and high S^0 in order to achieve the resolution desired with T_{AD} short enough to avoid blurring. Typical values for these parameters for a whole body system with high performance gradients capable of performing EPI are 22–40 mT/m, 150–200 mT/m/s, 50–100 per cent duty cycle. In some cases, the specifications are not simultaneously met; for example, a gradient system may only sustain maximum gradient amplitude and slew rate at 50 per cent duty cycle, but may achieve one or the other at a higher duty cycle.

5.3.2 Biological considerations for fast gradient switching

Rapidly switched gradient fields can induce magnetostimulation effects in humans by creating local electric potentials. In some cases, the potentials may be large enough to cause nerve membrane depolarization, which leads to 'twitching' from muscle contractions, peripheral nerve stimulation, or magnetophosphenes manifested as flashing lights from excitation of the optic nerve. The magnetic field changes are zero at the gradient isocentre and increase until a radius near the edge of the imaging field of view at which the gradient fields fall off. The effects depend on the peak amplitude of the B fields created by the gradients $B = rG$ (r is the radius from isocentre) and the slew rate $dB/dt = rS^0$, as well as the anatomic position and tissue orientation relative to the maximum gradient field (Harvey and Mansfield 1994). The magnitude of magnetostimulation effects can range from imperceptible to painful in different individuals undergoing the same scan protocol (Chronik and Rutt 1999). However, the potential for such effects is greater for gradient coils that cover a larger imaging volume (larger r). For further information, consult Shellock and Kanal (1996).

5.3.3 Whole body, insertable or head dedicated?

There are several tradeoffs to be considered when choosing between whole body gradients and insertable, head only gradient coils. Similar considerations apply to the choice of a head-only scanner.

Whole body gradients

The advantage of a whole body scanner is that the gradient coils do not physically intrude in the patient space, and are always in place. This allows ease of setup and greater flexibility in choice and placement of RF coils and stimulus delivery apparatus. It also allows flexibility when the scanner is used in a multi-purpose environment for which fMRI is not the only application. The disadvantage of gradients capable of whole body coverage is that the potential for magnetostimulation effects is greater than with localized gradients, because larger volumes are accompanied by larger peak field swings (see Section 5.3.2).

Insertable gradient coils

Scanners without high performance gradient systems capable of single-shot EPI can be equipped with insertable gradient coils that, by virtue of their small size, can achieve adequate G^0 and S^0 using the scanner's existing gradient driver amplifiers. Besides enabling EPI acquisitions, such coils have a further advantage that G^0 and S^0 can often be increased considerably over that available with a whole body gradient set. This results because the B and dB/dt generated by the gradients can be kept small because of the small radii over which the gradients act. This makes the use of such devices attractive even for EPI-equipped scanners because of the benefits of having very high performance gradients for rapid scanning.

The disadvantage of such coils is that they are cumbersome and require setup time in order to connect the wires and cooling hoses. This may be a major factor if the scanner is used for multiple purposes and must be reconfigured often. In addition, there may be questions of reproducibility in re-establishing the mounting of the coil assembly on the patient table. Moreover, the coil assembly can interfere with stimulus delivery and may limit RF coil choices. Finally, there is growing interest in fMRI of the spinal cord, which would be precluded by some of the existing insertable designs.

Head-only scanners

Using small superconducting magnets and specially-designed gradient coils, head-only scanners are becoming available. These scanners can be expected to have lower cost both in terms of capital investment as well as in siting costs. Smaller magnets weigh less and have smaller magnetic 'footprints', which allows for a reduction in the size of the examination room. Furthermore, the gradient performance may significantly exceed that of a whole body scanner for the reasons given above for insertable coils. A disadvantage of such scanners is that there may be little flexibility in RF coil choice or stimulus placement because of the small inner bore size. In addition, cervical spine imaging would be compromised or impossible.

5.4 Radiofrequency coils

NMR requires a radio frequency (RF) coil to generate the oscillating magnetic field (often denoted 'B_1') rotating at the Larmor frequency in order to cause transitions between spin states during the 'excitation' (or 'transmit') phase of the pulse sequence. The same or a different coil is used to receive the echo signal. There are a number of variations on volume and surface coils, and careful choice is important because the image SNR is strongly affected by the RF coil.

5.4.1 Volume head coils

Transmit/receive (T/R) coils

Generally, the head coils supplied by scanner manufacturers use the same coil for transmit and receive functions. Coil designs can use either 'linear' or 'quadrature' drive, although most commercial volume coils are of the quadrature variety, because this provides a factor of two reduction in transmit power and $\sqrt{2}$ advantage in SNR over linear drive (Glover *et al.* 1985). With quadrature drive, two independent resonant modes are excited in time and space, and this eliminates one of two counter-rotating B_1 components, leaving only the component rotating in the proper direction to excite the NMR process. Quadrature drive also reduces B_1 heterogeneity effects that are caused by interaction of the B_1 field with the lossy dielectric tissue in the head, manifested as standing wave and eddy current effects. These effects are more severe when the cranial size becomes comparable to a half wavelength at the RF frequency, which occurs at the higher fields.

Receive-only coils

In this case, the body coil is used for transmit, during which time the head coil is disabled, with the opposite

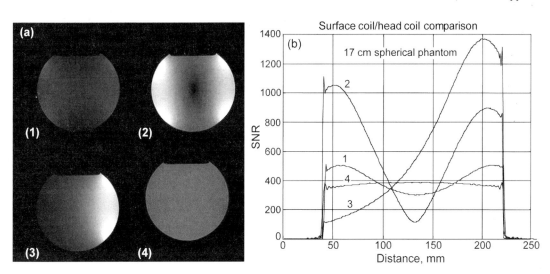

Fig. 5.7 (a) Images obtained at 1.5T using 17 cm diameter spherical phantom and: (1) two 12.5 cm surface coils aligned in phase; (2) two 12.5 cm surface coils aligned in phase opposition; (3) single 12.5 cm surface coil; (4) head coil. (b) Plots of SNR profiles along horizontal line through each image. Careful choice of coil configuration can have major effect on SNR. If volume coverage is not needed, surface coils can be highly beneficial.

conditions used during receive. The advantage of this technique is that the body coil can often produce more uniform B_1 field within the head because the coil elements are distant from the head and there are no 'hot spots', as can occur close to the coil. However, at the time of writing > 3 Tesla scanners do not have body coils, so this method is limited presently to the lower fields.

5.4.2 Surface coils

The advantage of a volume coil is that coverage of the entire brain is obtained with relatively uniform signal intensity. However, when less coverage is required, significant SNR advantages can be obtained by using surface coils. The benefits result from the reduction in sensitive volume, which limits the noise contribution that is picked up to a smaller fraction of the head. An example is shown in Fig. 5.7, in which the SNR of volume and of surface coils in three arrangements are compared. If a surface coil can be used, it may be seen that large gains can be made.

Like volume coils, surface coils can be either receive-only or transmit/receive. Generally it is preferable to use receive-only mode for surface coils because the severe B_1 heterogeneity effects are further compounded when transmitting with the surface coil.

A disadvantage of surface coils is that they must be placed so that their B_1 field is largely perpendicular to B_0. For a loop coil, the B_1 field passes through and is perpendicular to the plane of the loop. Thus loop coils may be placed posterior, anterior, left or right of the brain, but not on the top of the head (Fig. 5.8). The coil(s) must be secured so that no motion is possible, because otherwise image artefacts can be generated.

5.4.3 Safety considerations of RF coils

As with any MRI examination, care must be taken that SAR limits are not exceeded (see Section 5.2.2). Similarly, caution should be used with surface coils that the cables do not form loops and do not touch the subject as burns can result (Shellock and Kanal 1996).

For fMRI, however, additional considerations may apply because of the wide variety of stimulus and monitoring equipment in use. Any equipment placed in the RF field (e.g. eye trackers in a head coil, or a finger response button box in the active body coil) may be

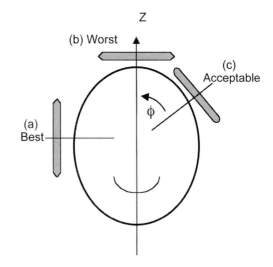

Fig. 5.8 Sketch showing possible surface coil orientations. The NMR signal is maximized when the B_1 field is perpendicular to the z-directed B_0 field, as in (a). If the coil is oriented at ϕ degrees the maximum signal is reduced by a factor $\sin(\phi)$.

subjected to substantial RF fields. This can cause large induced RF currents to flow on the outside of the device and its cables, and is a potential concern for causing burns from high RF voltages. The induced currents may also have a deleterious effect on the device and any equipment connected to it, although the latter may be protected by filters (e.g. in passing through the screened room wall). Particular care must be taken if electrodes are connected to the subject for recording EEG, ECG, or other physiological functions. Usually, high impedance leads must be used to reduce the RF effects.

5.5 *Special considerations for fMRI*

5.5.1 Data throughput

Data handling

Functional imaging generates large amounts of image data, and it is important that data handling does not impede scan operations, both from the standpoint of efficiency as well as cognitive aspects of the experiment. There are two considerations in data handling, including image reconstruction/storage and image transfer.

Many scanners are capable of gathering images from an EPI sequence at a rate faster than can be reconstructed. If this is the case, the scanner may impose a suspension of further scanning after the scan finishes until the reconstruction queue is empty. Depending on the scanner and its available array processor options, the post-scan reconstruction time can be many s to min. There may be alternatives, including delayed reconstruction or storing the raw data for reconstruction on an off-line computer, and some manufacturers offer such features as options. A related issue is that the scanner may impose a limit on the total number of images that can be created in a scan, and that can be a handicap for many experiments. This limitation is removed by off-line reconstruction, at the expense of additional processing steps and time. It is important that large amounts of data storage are available on the scanner in RAM and hard disk, for image data and/or raw data, in order to avoid scan limitations while waiting for data transfer. It may be desirable to install an auxiliary hard disk (> 4 Gbytes) to augment the available data storage, if possible.

A second aspect of data handling is retrieval of the images from the scanner. With several thousand images in a typical fMRI scan, the transfer time can be lengthy. Many scanners use DICOM for the image format, and many analysis packages are capable of directly importing such images. In some cases, the images are stored in proprietary format, and vendor-supplied software may be needed to retrieve the images. Some investigators have developed transfer programmes that perform more efficiently than the manufacturer's software.

A severe limitation that often applies on scanners that are shared between neuroscience applications and clinical duties is the existence of firewalls that limit network access to scanners. In such cases, it will be necessary to install a workstation on the local network for efficient transfer of the data from the scanner. The workstation may be equipped with the fMRI analysis and display software, or it may have archival means such as a CD ROM burner or DAT drive. In most cases, archiving the images from the scanner and transferring them manually is only acceptable for low volume fMRI situations.

Hardware limitations

A data throughput limitation can arise indirectly if the duty cycle of the gradient system is inadequate. When examining specifications for a scanner prior to purchase, it is important to understand the actual number of images/second that can be acquired with a typical sustained fMRI protocol. Some scanners have 'burst' modes, that allow higher collection rates for a short period of time, while others may have duty cycles that depend on slice orientation (oblique planes can be more limiting), field of view, resolution, or other parameters.

5.5.2 Stimulus considerations

Most fMRI experiments require some form of sensory cueing to the subject in the form of a visual, auditory or other stimulus, and many experiments also require measurement of subject responses. These systems must neither affect nor be affected by the MRI. Thus, mirrors, goggles, headphones and other devices placed within or close to the RF coil must not be magnetic nor affect the RF coil. Video projectors and finger response button boxes must not inject noise in the images. It is imperative that imaging tests be conducted to ascertain that the equipment is benign before its use can be certified.

A typical test sequence is the following. First, perform baseline scans with the stimulus equipment absent using a phantom with size, NMR and electrical loading characteristics similar to a head and with all RF coils that will be used with the equipment. Imaging sequences should include typical anatomic and functional scans in order to cover different bandwidths, and ultimately to expose the equipment to realistic gradient and RF ambient conditions. In addition to normal scans, disable the transmitter so that only noise images are reconstructed, if possible. Next, repeat the scans with the equipment in place and operating. Ascertain that the equipment functions normally during the functional scans. The images should be compared both for signal changes as well as the presence of discrete 'zipper' artefacts and/or more diffuse noise. In the opinion of this author, *no* additional noise or reduced signal is acceptable, and the equipment must be modified or rejected if found otherwise.

5.5.3 System tests

Systems used extensively for fMRI experiments should be tested periodically to establish benchmark performance measures for long-term quality control (QC). This can take the form of scans performed on a weekly basis with records kept. The important characteristics for fMRI are the SNR and system stability. Stability is critical because noise added by the system, if comparable to physiological noise components, directly compromises the statistical relevance of small BOLD signal changes, thereby reducing z-scores.

The QC scan should use a typical functional protocol that covers at least 5 min of scanning. A phantom that has size, NMR and electrical loading characteristics similar to a head should be used. The image time series can be analysed in several ways. Using a region of interest (ROI), the time series amplitude can be plotted. The root-mean-squared variation after linear trend removal should be recorded as a percentage of the mean signal, as well as the percentage of linear drift over the scan. Next, the noise is calculated by separately averaging the even-numbered images and the odd-numbered images, and then subtracting the two averaged images. The resulting difference image should have zero mean and should not show structures of the phantom. The noise is obtained from this image as the standard deviation in an ROI within the region of the phantom, divided by $\sqrt{2}$ (Weisskoff 1996; Glover and Lai 1998). The advantage of this procedure over the more commonly employed ROI in a region of the image outside the phantom is that the procedure incorporates a tacit stability test. Finally, it may be beneficial to record other system settings such as transmitter and receiver gains and centre frequency, as well as other parameters that may vary in the site such as room temperature. An example is shown in the table below, where the table records the root-mean-squared fluctuation of the mean signal, the linear drift (expressed as a percentage of the

mean), the signal-to-noise ratio (SNR), the signal-to-fluctuation-noise ratio (SFNR), the transmitter gain value (TG), the receiver gain value (R1) and the centre frequency.

Another simple test that requires no analysis software is to gather scans as a function of the number of signals averaged (NSA), and plot the SNR versus $\sqrt{NSA}$, with the noise measured as the standard deviation in an ROI outside the phantom (which does not contain any ghosting artefact). This test measures system amplitude and phase stability because the raw data are averaged as complex measurements, so that phase incoherence over the averaging period will prevent optimum summation. Deviations in the resulting plot from a straight line indicate instability.

The value of such long-term QC procedures is that system changes may be gradual enough that degradation may go unnoticed without objective data. Having such data is also beneficial as a monitor of before/after performance when the hardware or software is upgraded.

5.6 Future developments in MRI hardware

5.6.1 Head only scanners

Functional MRI was developed and is almost exclusively practiced using whole body scanners at the time of writing. However, the explosive growth in fMRI has caused several instrument vendors to develop dedicated head-only scanners. The advantages for such scanners are reduced size and siting costs, and higher performance gradients. Disadvantages at present are reduced magnetic field homogeneity from the shorter magnet and reduced access to the subject for stimulus presentation. These systems will continue to evolve and will eventually include integrated analysis and stimulus generation software.

Scanner ID: _____

Date	Coil	RMS Fluct, %	Linear Drift, %	SNR	SFNR	TG	R1	Freq., MHz
10/31/99	Head_0	0.06	0.2	325	204	60	9	127.701 712

5.6.2 Very high performance gradients

Presently, the amplitude and slew rate of whole-body and insertable gradients are limited by physiological considerations associated with the need to avoid magnetostimulation (see Section 5.3.3). However, it may be possible to reduce the area of the body outside the head subtended by the gradient flux by careful design of the gradients (Chronik and Rutt 1999). If that is the case, the gradient amplitudes and slew rates should be capable of achieving much higher levels than current designs. This would make possible higher spatial and temporal resolution and higher SNR, as well as improved diffusion tensor imaging.

5.6.3 Real-time fMRI

With the continued evolution of high performance scanners and array processors, it is now possible to perform real-time fMRI, in which the image reconstruction and a limited analysis such as a correlation or t-test are performed concurrently with scanning. The results are displayed as a continuously updated activation map. One potential for such systems lies in providing a rapid method for functional localization to optimize the acquisition. This may be important in surgical planning, especially for imaging-guided interventions. A second application for real-time fMRI may be for providing biofeedback to subjects in plasticity experiments and rehabilitation after surgery or trauma.

Present commercial systems are limited in the data rate and number of slices that can be processed, and have no motion correction steps in the processing pipeline. However, there are no conceptual barriers to eliminating these deficiencies, and future equipment may be available with full real-time processing incorporated.

5.7 Concluding remarks

Functional neuroimaging places strong demands on the MR imaging hardware because of the need for rapid acquisition, high signal-to-noise ratio, and exceptional system stability. In many cases, these requirements are in conflict, and tradeoffs must be made when choosing instrumentation.

For example, the thermal SNR increases roughly linearly with B_0, which augers for high field strength.

However, increased B_0 is accompanied by the need for stronger gradients, which increases the acoustic noise during imaging and causes greater proclivity for peripheral nerve stimulation. In turn, the stronger gradients result in reduced SNR gains because of increased bandwidth. In addition, physiological noise components increase at the same rate as signal increases, further limiting potential gains in BOLD CNR from higher field. Moreover, the RF power deposited in the head by the NMR process increases with field, and regulatory guidelines may impose limits on the number of slices that can be obtained at a given imaging speed with some pulse sequences. Siting of magnets is also more expensive for higher fields.

Thus, the choice of field strength for routine cognitive neuroscience is influenced by numerous factors. At the present stage of development, 7 Tesla and 8 Tesla magnets capable of human neuroimaging are becoming available. While there are exciting research opportunities that are enabled by such systems, instruments with fields in this range do not appear to be suitable for *routine* fMRI because many of the limitations described above come into play. A field strength of 3 Tesla offers significant SNR advantages over 1.5 Tesla (Kruger *et al.* 2001) and is not severely impacted by RF, acoustic or physiological noise limits. Thus, 3 Tesla magnets are now in common use for fMRI. The further BOLD CNR gains in moving from 3 Tesla to 4 Tesla appear to be modest (Fig. 5.4), but may be worth the effort for many research programs, particularly when spectroscopic studies are contemplated.

Other choices involve head versus whole body scanners, and again tradeoffs must be made depending on cost and the need to perform other studies (besides fMRI).

In all cases, once the scanner is installed, it is important to establish and maintain a good quality monitoring program so that trends in scanner performance can be noted and deleterious (but often gradual) reductions in SNR or system stability can be caught before longitudinal studies are compromised.

References

Chronik, B. and Rutt, B. (1999) In *Predicting magnetostimulation by central and edge gradient coils*. p.472, Proceedings, ISMRM Seventh Scientific Meeting, Philadelphia.

Collins, C.M., Li, S., and Smith, M.B. (1998). SAR and B1 field distributions in a heterogeneous human head model within a birdcage coil. Specific energy absorption rate. *Magnetic Resonance in Medicine*, 40, 847–56.

Elliott, M.R., Bowtell, R.W., and Morris, P.G. (1999). The effect of scanner sound in visual, motor, and auditory functional MRI. *Magnetic Resonance in Medicine*, 41, 1230–5.

Farrar, T. and Becker, E. (1971). *Pulse and Fourier transform NMR*. Academic Press, New York.

Farzaneh, F., Riederer, S.J., and Pelc, N.J. (1990). Analysis of T2 limitations and off-resonance effects on spatial resolution and artifacts in echo-planar imaging. *Magnetic Resonance in Medicine*, 14, 123–39.

Gati, J.S., Menon, R.S., Ugurbil, K., and Rutt, B.K. (1997). Experimental determination of the BOLD field strength dependence in vessels and tissue. *Magnetic Resonance in Medicine*, 38, 296–302.

Glover, G.H. and Lai, S. (1998). Self-navigated spiral fMRI: interleaved versus single-shot. *Magnetic Resonance in Medicine*, 39, 361–8.

Glover, G.H. and Lee, A.T. (1995). Motion artifacts in fMRI: comparison of 2DFT with PR and spiral scan methods. *Magnetic Resonance in Medicine*, 33, 624–35.

Glover, G., Hayes, C., Pelc, N., Edelstein, W., Mueller, O., Hart, H., Hardy, C.J., O'Donnell, M., and Barber, W.D. (1985). Comparison of linear and circular polarization for magnetic resonance imaging. *Journal of Magnetic Resonance*, 64, 255–70.

Harvey, P.R. and Mansfirld, P. (1994). Avoiding peripheral nerve stimulation: gradient waveform criteria for optimum resolution in echo-planar imaging. *Magnetic Resonance in Medicine*, 32, 236–41.

Hedeen, R.A. and Edelstein, W.A. (1997). Characterization and prediction of gradient acoustic noise in MR imagers. *Magnetic Resonance in Medicine*, 37, 7–10.

Hu, X. and Kim, S.G. (1994). Reduction of signal fluctuation in functional MRI using navigator echoes. *Magnetic Resonance in Medicine*, 31, 495–503.

Javid, M. and Brenner, E. (1963). In *Analysis, transmission, and filtering of signals*. McGraw-Hill Book Co., New York.

Kruger, G., Kastrup, A., and Glover, G. (2001). Neuroimaging at, 1.5T and 3.0T: comparison of oxygen-sensitive magnetic resonance imaging. *Magnetic Resonance in Medicine*. 45, 594–604.

Kwong, K.K., Belliveau, J.W., Chesler, D.A., Goldberg, I.E., Weisskoff, R.M., Poncelet, B.P., Kennedy, D.N., Hoppel, B.E., Cohen, M.S., Turner, R., Cheng H.M., Brady, T.J., and Rosen, B.R. (1992). Dynamic magnetic resonance imaging of human brain activity during primary sensory stimulation. *Proceedings of National Academy of Sciences (USA)*, 89, 5675–9.

Noll, D.C. and Schneider, W. (1994). In *Theory, simulation and compensation of physiological motion artifacts in functional MRI*. pp.40–4, IEEE International Conference on Image Processing, Austin.

Noll, D., Cohen, J., Meyer, C., and Schneider, W. (1995). Spiral *k*-space MR imaging of cortical activation. *Magnetic Resonance Imaging*, 5, 49–57.

Ogawa, S., Lee, T.M., Kay, A.R., and Tank, D.W. (1990). Brain magnetic resonance imaging with contrast dependent on blood oxygenation. *Proceedings of National Academy of Sciences (USA)*, 87, 9868–72.

Pimentel, M.M. (1999). Fragile X syndrome (review). *Int. J. Mol. Med.*, 3, 639–45.

Poncelet, B.P., Wedeen, V.J., Weisskoff, R.M., and Cohen, M.S. (1992). Brain parenchyma motion: measurement with cine echo-planar MR imaging. *Radiology*, 185, 645–51.

Schneider, E. and Glover, G. (1991). Rapid *in vivo* proton shimming. *Magnetic Resonance in Medicine*, 18, 335–47.

Shellock, F. and Kanal, E. (1996). *Magnetic resonance bioeffects, safety, and patient management*, 2nd edn. Lippincott-Raven, Philadelphia.

Shellock, F.G., Ziarati, M., Atkinson, D., and Chen, D.Y. (1998). Determination of gradient magnetic field-induced acoustic noise associated with the use of echo planar and three-dimensional, fast spin echo techniques. *Magnetic Resonance Imaging*, 8, 1154–7.

Webb, P. and Macovski, A. (1991). Rapid, fully automatic, arbitrary-volume *in vivo* shimming. *Magnetic Resonance in Medicine*, 20, 113–22.

Weisskoff, R.M. (1996). Simple measurement of scanner stability for functional NMR imaging of activation in the brain. *Magnetic Resonance in Medicine*, 36, 643–5.

Wysong, R.E., Madio, D.P., and Lowe, I.J. (1994). A novel eddy current compensation scheme for pulsed gradient systems. *Magnetic Resonance in Medicine*, 31, 572–5.

Yang, Y.H., Glover, G.H., van Gelderen, P., Patel, A.C., Mattay, V.S., Frank, J.A., and Duyn, J.H. (1998). A comparison of fast MR scan techniques for cerebral activation studies at 1.5 Tesla. *Magnetic Resonance in Medicine*, 39, 61–7.

6 | *Selection of the optimal pulse sequence for functional MRI*

Peter A. Bandettini

6.1 Introduction

Since its inception in 1991, functional MRI (fMRI) has experienced an explosive growth in the number of users and a steady widening in its range of applications. A recent (2000) search of the National Library of Medicine database for articles with 'fMRI' or 'BOLD' in the title revealed over 1000 citations. The rapid rate of improvement in pulse sequence design, data processing, information content, data interpretation, and paradigm design can be overwhelming to the novice and even to the advanced user. This chapter is written to assist the fMRI user in making an informed decision regarding the choice of functional MRI pulse sequence. A second goal is to present the pulse sequence choices against a wider backdrop of relevant variables, ranging from paradigm timing to available hardware. The hope is to build a broader perspective of what the limits and possibilities of fMRI are.

Most fMRI experimental planning can be reduced to an iterative optimization between what is practically possible and what is ideally desired from the experiment—both factors being inter-dependent. They drive both the development of the methodology and the sophistication of the questions that can be asked. The following sections describe the variables that can be optimized in typical functional MRI experiments. These factors include information content, sensitivity, acquisition speed, image resolution, brain coverage, and anatomical image quality. Summaries and discussions of the tradeoffs regarding the variables described are included.

6.2 Information content

Several types of physiological information can be mapped using fMRI. This range of information includes the following: baseline cerebral blood volume (Rosen *et al.* 1989; Moonen *et al.* 1990; Rosen *et al.* 1991), changes in blood volume (Belliveau *et al.* 1991), baseline and changes in cerebral perfusion (Detre *et al.* 1992; Williams *et al.* 1992; Edelman *et al.* 1994b; Kwong *et al.* 1994; Kim 1995; Wong *et al.* 1997), and changes in blood oxygenation (Ogawa *et al.* 1990; Turner *et al.* 1991; Bandettini *et al.* 1992; Frahm *et al.* 1992; Kwong *et al.* 1992; Ogawa and Lee 1992; Haacke *et al.* 1997). Recent advances in fMRI pulse sequence and experimental manipulation have allowed quantitative measures of oxygen metabolism ($CMRO_2$) changes and dynamic non-invasive measures in blood volume with activation to be extracted from fMRI data (Kim and Ugurbil 1997; Davis *et al.* 1998; van Zijl *et al.* 1998; Hoge *et al.* 1999a,b). A detailed treatment of the MRI techniques available to map these physiological parameters, in particular $CMRO_2$ estimation, is provided in Chapter 8. Table 6.1 provides a summary of the tradeoffs involved with the use of each of the above mentioned contrast mechanisms and the types of information that can be obtained from each. Also, a brief overview of the basic principles is given below.

6.2.1 Blood volume

In the late 1980s, the use of rapid MRI allowed tracking of transient signal intensity changes over time. One application of this utility was to follow the T2* or T2-weighted signal intensity changes as a bolus of intravascular paramagnetic contrast agent passed through the tissue of interest (Rosen *et al.* 1989). As it passes through, the bolus induces susceptibility-related signal dephasing which then recovers as the bolus washes out. The area under the signal attenuation curve is proportional to the relative blood volume. In 1990, Belliveau and colleagues took this approach one

Table 6.1   Summary of the practical advantages and disadvantages of pulse sequences that have contrast based on BOLD, perfusion, volume, and CMRO$_2$

	Advantages	Disadvantages
BOLD	• highest functional activation contrast by a factor of 2 to 4 over perfusion • easiest to implement • multislice trivial • can use very short TR	• complicated non-quantitative signal • no baseline information • susceptibility artefacts
Perfusion	• unique and quantitative information • baseline information • easy control over observed vasculature • non-invasive • no susceptibility artefacts	• low functional activation contrast • longer TR required • multislice is difficult • slow mapping of baseline information
Volume	• unique information • baseline information • multislice is trivial • rapid mapping of baseline information	• invasive • susceptibility artefacts • requires separate rest and activation runs
CMRO$_2$	• unique and quantitative information	• semi-invasive • extremely low functional activation contrast • susceptibility artefacts • processing intensive • multislice is difficult • longer TR required

step further when they mapped blood volume during rest and during activation (Belliveau *et al.* 1991). Indeed, the first maps of brain activation using fMRI were demonstrated with this technique. Soon after its demonstration, contrast agent fMRI was rendered largely obsolete (for brain activation imaging) by the endogenous oxygen-sensitive contrast agent haemoglobin. Recently, non-invasive methods for dynamic measurement of blood volume have been introduced (Liu *et al.* 2000).

One advantage of blood volume mapping is that the information that is derived is directly interpretable, and that baseline information on blood volume and perfusion (which can be derived by taking into consideration the measured tissue transit time) can be obtained. It also has the advantage that multi-slice imaging is trivial and a very short scan repeat time (TR) can be used, if desired. The total time required for the acquisition of data required for a blood volume measurement is also quite short (approximately 2 min).

Blood volume mapping with a bolus injection of a susceptibility contrast agent has its drawbacks, how-ever. Even though the contrast agents are non-toxic at the doses given, the technique is considered invasive. Larger doses or repeated doses would become toxic. All brain activation maps obtained with this technique involve separate runs of about 2 min each: the first being a rest state, and the second an activated state. Since the number of repeated doses is limited, a constraint is placed on what types of cognitive question can be asked with the use of this technique. Because of the limited number of brain activation studies that have been performed with this technique, it is difficult to draw a conclusion regarding the relative contrast-to-noise ratio provided by its functional activation maps.

6.2.2 Blood oxygenation

As early as the 1930s it was known that deoxyhaemoglobin was paramagnetic and oxyhaemoglobin was diamagnetic (Pauling and Coryell 1936). In 1982 it was discovered that decreases in blood oxygenation lead to a decrease in the T2 NMR relaxation time of blood (Thulborn *et al.* 1982), and also lead to decreases in T2*. It was not until 1989 that this knowledge was used to image *in vivo* changes in blood oxygenation in rat. Blood oxygenation level dependent contrast, coined BOLD by Ogawa (Ogawa *et al.* 1992), was used to image the activated human brain for the first time in 1991, and the first results using BOLD contrast for imaging brain function were published in 1992 (Bandettini *et al.* 1992; Kwong *et al.* 1992; Ogawa *et al.* 1992). The basic concept behind this contrast mechanism is described in detail elsewhere in this book. The effect of neuronal activity is to produce an increase in T2 and T2*, and thus to cause a small signal increase in T2 and T2*-weighted images. Because of its improved sensitivity and ease of implementation, gradient echo (T2*-weighted) BOLD imaging has emerged as being the most commonly used fMRI method. Asymmetric spin echo techniques, used extensively by one of the first groups to perform fMRI (Kwong *et al.* 1992), have similar contrast as gradient echo techniques and have been implemented with similar results.

With BOLD contrast, several distinct advantages exist. First, the technique is of course completely non-invasive. Second, the functional contrast-to-noise ratio is at least a factor of 2 to 4 greater than that of perfusion imaging (i.e. the functional maps are much less noisy). Third, it is easiest to implement since it only requires, typically, a gradient echo sequence with an echo time (TE) of 30 to 40 ms. Fourth, it is trivial to perform multi-slice whole brain echo planar imaging (EPI). All that is required is that the repetition time (TR) be long enough to accommodate all of the slices desired in each volume. Typically, with a TE of about 40 ms, the total time for acquiring a single-shot echo planar image is about 60 to 100 ms, which translates to a maximum rate of 10 to 16 slices per second. If a reduced number of slices is sufficient, then a very short TR can be utilized for fine temporal mapping of the dynamics of the BOLD signal change, though the signal-to-noise ratio can be compromised under such conditions due to incomplete T1 recovery of magetisation between subsequent slice excitations.

Despite some clear advantages, several disadvantages do, however, exist in regard to BOLD contrast imaging. First, as is described in Chapters 2 and 8, the physiology underlying BOLD contrast is extremely complicated, involving the interplay of perfusion, $CMRO_2$, and blood volume changes, and is further modulated by the heterogeneity of the vasculature and neuro-vascular coupling over time and space. This problem leads to limits of interpretation in the location, magnitude, linearity, and dynamics of the BOLD contrast signal. In addition, it makes comparisons over populations, clinical mapping, and mapping of the effects of pharmacologic intervention extremely challenging. Also, unlike the perfusion and volume mapping methods, no baseline oxygenation information can, as yet, be obtained since resting state T2* and T2 times are dominated by the type of tissue rather than by its oxygenation state. If resting state oxygenation information is required, considerable assumptions have to be made regarding blood volume and vessel geometry, among other things. Another problem with BOLD contrast in general is that the same susceptibility weighting that allows for the observation of the functional contrast also contributes to many of the artefacts in the images used. These artefacts include signal dropout at tissue interfaces and at the base of the brain. This problem becomes greater at higher field strengths.

6.2.3 Blood perfusion

An array of new techniques exists for mapping cerebral blood *perfusion* in humans. For a recent review, please refer to Wong (1999). Perfusion MRI techniques based on arterial spin labeling, abbreviated as ASL techniques, are conceptually similar to other modalities such as positron emission tomography (PET) and single photon emission computed tomography (SPECT) in that they involve tagging of inflowing blood, and then allow flow of the tagged blood into the imaging plane. In MRI a radiofrequency (RF) tagging pulse is used, which is usually a 180° pulse that 'inverts' the arterial blood magnetization.

ASL techniques can be subdivided into those that use continuous arterial spin labeling, which involves continuously inverting arterial blood flowing into the slice of interest, and those that use pulsed arterial spin labeling, which involves periodically inverting a 'plug' of arterial blood and measuring the arrival of that blood into the imaging slice. Examples of these techniques include 'echo planar imaging with signal targeting and alternating RF' (EPISTAR) (Edelman *et al.* 1994*a*) and 'flow-sensitive alternating inversion recovery' (FAIR) (Kim 1995; Kwong *et al.* 1995).

Recently, a pulsed arterial spin labeling technique known as 'quantitative imaging of perfusion using a single subtraction' (QUIPSS), has been introduced (Wong *et al.* 1998).

The primary advantage of perfusion mapping is that quantitative maps of perfusion changes can be obtained, at least in principle. The changes in signal are simply due to perfusion effects and not based on any complicating interactions of neurovascular coupling and blood volume dynamics. Also, quantitative maps of resting state or baseline perfusion are obtained by default in every time series. With modulation of the timing parameters such as the inversion time (TI) specific parts of the vasculature may be isolated based on their flow rates. Since the tagging of in-flowing spins involves only the use of an RF pulse, the technique is non-invasive. Lastly, since the basis of the contrast is not susceptibility, an extremely short TE can be used, significantly reducing larger scale suscep-tibility artefacts. For this reason, this technique might be the method of choice for mapping activation near the problematic tissue interfaces and at the base of the brain.

Perfusion imaging has several potentially prohibi-tive disadvantages, however. First, the functional contrast-to-noise ratio is lower than BOLD contrast by a factor of about 2 to 4, leading to the requirement of more temporal averaging (by a factor of 4 to 16) to achieve similar quality activation maps. Second, because of the time (TI) required to allow the tagged blood to perfuse into the tissue of interest, a relatively long TR is required. The minimum TR that can be used is typically 2 s. Nevertheless, techniques are emerging that allow for a shorter TR to be used (Liu and Gao 1999; Duyn *et al.* 2000; Wong *et al.* 2000b) or

that provide other solutions (Buxton *et al.* 1998a,b) by using periodically divisible TR and stimulus timing intervals. Third, because the tagged blood spins undergo signal decay from the moment they are tagged (dictated by the T1 of blood), all the images have to be acquired in a very short time, putting a limit on the number of slices that can be obtained. Under such multi slice conditions, each slice also has a different TI associated with it, making quantification slightly more difficult. The typical upper limit of slices is in the range of 5 to 10. Finally, in a clinical setting where mapping of baseline perfusion information may be critical, ASL requires more scanning time to create a usable perfu-sion map than does the currently used method involving dynamic imaging following the injection of a bolus of contrast agent. Although such contrast injec-tion methods are better able to measure relative blood volume, perfusion maps can also be obtained if the tissue transit times are available.

For mapping baseline information, ASL is slower than such dynamic contrast agent methods by a factor of at least 3, which is potentially critical when deter-mining compromised perfusion in acute stroke, for instance.

6.2.4 Haemodynamic specificity

Each of the MRI techniques outlined above relies on the ^{1}H nuclei within water molecules to provide its signal. These water spins are in a number of vascular and tissue environments and, depending on the details of the MRI pulse sequence used, each environment may contribute more or less of the signal. Importantly, a poor choice of sequence parameters may introduce signals from unwanted environments that may affect

---

Fig. 6.1 The vascular tree, including (*left to right*) arteries, arterioles, capillaries, venules, and veins. The figures illustrate the signal seen from the vessels and from surrounding tissue for different classes of MRI pulse sequence. In the case of arterial spin labeled perfusion sequences (a) signal is detected from the water spins in the arterial–capillary region of the vasculature and from water in tissue surrounding the capillaries. The relative sensitivity of these contributions can be controlled by adjusting the TI inversion time and by incorporation of velocity nulling (also known as diffusion weighting) gradients. A small amount of velocity nulling and a TI of approx. 1 s makes ASL perfusion techniques selectively sensitive to capillaries and tissue and less sensitive to large vessel effects (*lower figure*). Gradient echo BOLD techniques (b) are sensitive to susceptibility perturbers of all sizes, and are therefore sensitive to all intravascular and extravascular effects in the capillary-venous portion of the vasculature. Spin echo BOLD techniques (c) are sensitive to susceptibility perturbers about the size of a red blood cell or capillary, making them predominantly sensitive to intravascular water spins in vessels of all sizes and to extravascular (tissue) water surrounding capillaries. Use of velocity nulling gradients reduces the contribution of signal from larger vessels (venules and veins). If a very short TR scan repeat time is used, then GE-BOLD methods may additionally show signal originating from arterial inflow, which can be removed by using a longer TR and/or outer volume saturation.

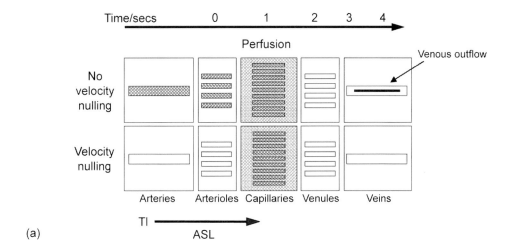

(a)

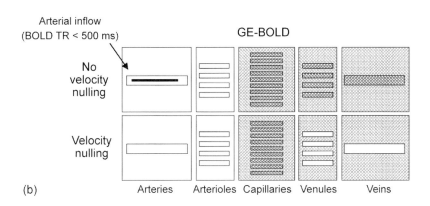

(b)

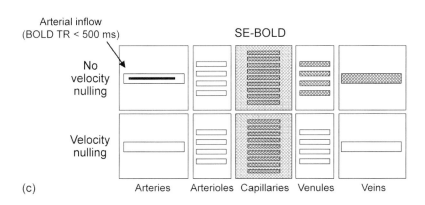

(c)

the interpretation of the data. It is, therefore, crucial to understand the effect of particular sequence parameters on the signal that is measured. The current section attempts to provide a summary of which vascular and tissue environments contribute the predominant signal to the MRI approaches discussed above. Figure 6.1 shows a schematic depiction of pulse sequence sensitization to specific vascular components. It shows the amount of signal contribution from both the intravascular (i.e. water spins that are in the blood vessels) and extravascular (i.e. water spins that are in the tissue) compartments. The shaded regions of the figures show those compartments that contribute signal to (a) perfusion, (b) gradient echo BOLD, and (c) spin echo BOLD pulse sequences. Note that blood volume maps typically use a gradient echo pulse sequence, and therefore have a profile similar to that of (b). The more lightly shaded regions surrounding the vessels depict extravascular (tissue) contributions, versus the darker shaded regions depicting the vessels. The functional contrast in the tissue signal is derived from blood water spins exchanging with tissue water spins in the case of ASL perfusion, and from spin dephasing effects (in the presence of extravascular field gradients) in the case of BOLD. Broadly, Fig. 6.1 shows that perfusion techniques show predominantly signal contrast either from within or around arterial—capillary vessels, whereas BOLD (and blood volume) techniques show predominantly signal contrast from within or around capillary—venous vessels. In both cases the use of some velocity nulling field gradients can have the beneficial effect of minimizing unwanted signal changes from within the very large vessels.

Regarding susceptibility contrast (BOLD) imaging, Fig. 6.1 shows that spin echo sequences are more sensitive to small susceptibility compartments (capillaries and red blood cells) whereas gradient echo sequences are sensitive to susceptibility compartments of all sizes (Ogawa *et al.* 1993; Weisskoff *et al.* 1993; Kennan *et al.* 1994; Bandettini and Wong 1995; Boxerman *et al.* 1995*b*). A common mistake is to assume that spin echo sequences are sensitive to capillaries only. Since red blood cells also are also 'small compartments' spin echo sequences are in fact selectively sensitive to intravascular signal arising from small *and* large vessels (Boxerman *et al.* 1995*a*). Since BOLD contrast is highly weighted by the resting state blood volume in the voxel it is important to consider the vascular content of voxels showing significant BOLD activation. For example, it is likely that many voxels having pial vessels running through them will have at least 50 per cent blood volume. These voxels are therefore likely to show the largest gradient echo *and* spin echo signal changes unless specific steps are taken to eliminate the signal from within the large blood vessels.

Flowing spins may also present a problem for BOLD sequences, since flow changes in macroscopic arterial vessels may contribute signal changes in an fMRI experiment and these arterial effects may be some distance upstream of the active tissue. These so called 'inflow' effects are particularly pronounced when a short scan repeat time (TR) is used in conjunction with a high excitation flip angle (e.g. 90°). Outer volume radio-frequency saturation can remove inflowing spins (Duyn *et al.* 1994), and can thus reduce such non-susceptibility related inflow changes when using sequences with short TR. Reduction of the flip angle can also help to remove these unwanted effects. Finally, diffusion weighting, or 'velocity nulling', involving the use of diffusion gradients with b-values of 50 s²/mm or greater (see LeBihan 1995, for a discussion of diffusion weighting and b-values) can also help. These gradients effectively dephase rapidly moving intravascular signal (Boxerman *et al.* 1995*a*), therefore reducing but not eliminating large vessel effects in gradient echo fMRI and all large vessel effects in spin echo fMRI. Note that intravascular effects are removed but extravascular effects will remain. A significant caveat to this approach is that, at 1.5 Tesla, application of this amount of diffusion weighting reduces the BOLD signal change by about 60 per cent (Boxerman *et al.* 1995*a*) which is prohibitive under even the most optimal circumstances. This also implies that at 1.5 Tesla up to 60 per cent of the BOLD signal originates from intravascular water and not from water better localized in tissue experiencing modulation of magnetic field gradients around smaller vessels.

Performing BOLD contrast fMRI at high field strengths (> 3 Tesla) certainly has many advantages, one being that it has the same benefits as diffusion weighting in its effect on susceptibility-based contrast. This is because the T2* and T2 relaxation times of venous blood become progressively shorter than the T2* and T2 values of grey matter as a function of increasing static field strength. Therefore, proportionately less signal will arise from intravascular water at higher field strengths (Menon *et al.* 1993). This unique characteristic of imaging at high field strengths can be put to use in the creation of high resolution venograms (Menon *et al.* 1993).

6.3 *Sensitivity*

Extraction of a 1–5 per cent signal change against a backdrop of thermal noise, physiological fluctuations, head motion, and system instabilities requires careful consideration of the variables which influence signal detectability. These range from factors that optimize the fMRI contrast, increase the signal, reduce physiological fluctuations, and minimize artefactual signal changes.

6.3.1 Optimizing fMRI contrast

Figure 6.2 shows three varieties of BOLD contrast EPI pulse sequences: gradient echo, spin echo, and asymmetric spin echo. The optional modules to generate perfusion contrast are also shown (*boxed*). Note that the readout acquisitions in the figures are abbreviated, since each sequence typically has at least 64 frequency encoding lobes and phase encoding blips. With regard to BOLD contrast, gradient echo (or asymmetric spin echo) sequences are typically used because they produce the largest activation-induced signal changes by a factor of 2 to 4 over other contrast sensitizations. Gradient echo images are collected during the free induction decay of the signal after an initial RF pulse is applied. This signal decay can be described by an exponential function with a decay rate $R2^* = 1/T2^*$ or a characteristic decay time of $T2^*$. During activation, this decay rate decreases slightly (i.e. $T2^*$ increases slightly).

Approximate values for resting decay times and activation-induced changes in rate are shown in Table 6.2 for two field strengths. Figure 6.3 is a comparison of the signal intensity, functional contrast, and activation-induced percent signal change for spin echo, asymmetric spin echo and gradient echo sequences at 1.5 Tesla and 3 Tesla with the values shown in Table 6.2. The TE that optimizes contrast when performing gradient echo fMRI is that which maximizes the difference between two exponential decay rates (the value for $1/T2^*$ during rest versus the value for $1/T2^*$ during activation). This maximization occurs at TE ≈ resting $T2^*$. When performing spin echo fMRI, since changes

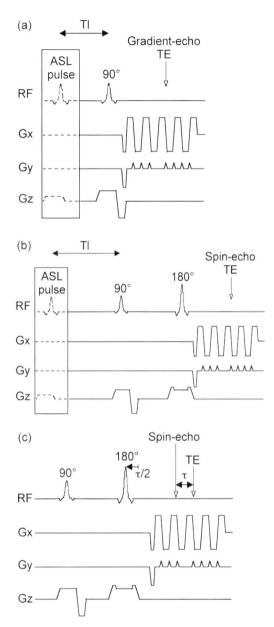

Fig. 6.2 Pulse sequence diagram of (a) gradient echo, (b) spin echo, and (c) asymmetric spin echo EPI. The TE is shown here to occur at the centre of the abbreviated 9 line *k*-space. Typically, the readout window includes at least 64 blips or readout lobes. In the asymmetric spin echo sequence the τ value is the amount of time that the centre of *k*-space is removed from when the spin echo occurs. The additional pulses required to generate ASL perfusion contrast are also indicated schematically.

Table 6.2 Approximated values for grey matter relaxation times and activation-induced relaxation rate changes. These values are used specifically for the illustration of contrast and per cent change curves in Figure 6.3

	1.5T	3T
T2	100 ms	80 ms
T2*	60 ms	50 ms
T2'	150 ms	133.3 ms
$\Delta R2 = \Delta(1/T2)$	-0.2 s^{-1}	-0.4 s^{-1}
$\Delta R2^* = \Delta(1/T2^*)$	-0.8 s^{-1}	-1.6 s^{-1}
$\Delta R2' = \Delta(1/T2')$	-0.6 s^{-1}	-1.2 s^{-1}

in T2 rather than T2* are observed, the optimal TE ≈ resting T2. Note from Fig. 6.3 that the percentage signal change increases linearly with TE while the contrast has a well defined peak.

In the case of the asymmetric spin echo sequence, BOLD contrast is generated when the image is collected at a time, τ, from the spin echo. To maximize BOLD contrast, τ should also be approximately equal to the T2* of the tissue.

For arterial spin labeling sequences the basic EPI readout module is still used, but an ASL tagging pulse is added a time TI before the EPI readout. It is desirable to tailor the pulse sequence parameters such that the perfusion maps show only tissue perfusion with no signal seen in larger arteries from tagged blood that is

destined for more distal slices. This can be accomplished by careful choice of tagging pulse parameters and by use of flow-crushing gradient pulses. The rationale is to optimize quantification or information content (Wong *et al.* 1998; Wong 1999). If full control for quantification is not necessary, and some contamination from blood which is flowing through the slice is acceptable, then maps having greater functional contrast by at least a factor of 2 can be obtained by relaxing some of the above constraints.

While not directly improving perfusion contrast itself, one simple method for improving ASL signal-to-noise ratio without compromising quantification is the use of as short a TE as possible. For example, in single shot-imaging, starting at the centre of k-space, as with spiral imaging, allows for an extremely short TE (as short as 3 ms), yielding higher signal-to-noise ratio in the raw images.

Methods exist that are able to collect both BOLD contrast and perfusion contrast in a single experimental run. These include techniques that collect perfusion images and BOLD images during separate segments of the same run (Hoge *et al.* 1999a), those that use the same images for perfusion and BOLD contrast calculations (Wong and Bandettini 1999), and those that employ a double echo sequence—using the first echo (short TE: no T2*-weighting) for optimally obtaining perfusion information and the second echo (long TE: high T2*-weighting) for optimally obtaining BOLD information.

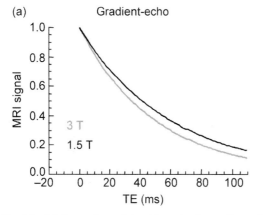
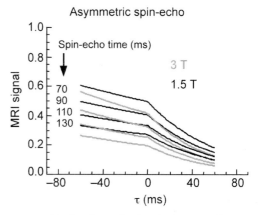

Fig. 6.3 (a) Comparison of signal intensity for gradient echo, asymmetric spin echo, and spin echo sequences for approximated decay rates of grey matter for 1.5 Tesla and 3 Tesla. The values from Table 6.2 were used. Note that the spin echo sequence corresponds to $\tau = 0$.

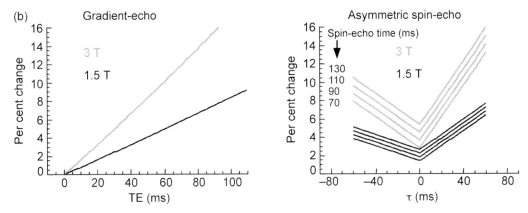

Fig. 6.3 (b) Comparison of the percent signal change with brain activation for gradient echo, asymmetric spin echo, and spin echo sequences for approximated activation-induced relaxation rate changes for 1.5 Tesla and 3 Tesla (taken from Table 6.2). With gradient echo sequences and with increasing τ for the asymmetric spin echo sequence, and for the spin echo ($\tau = 0$) the percent signal change has an approximately linear relationship with TE.

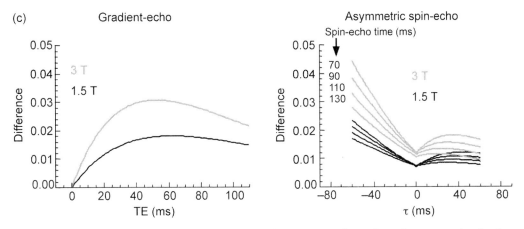

Fig. 6.3 (c) Comparison of the signal difference or contrast with brain activation for gradient echo, asymmetric spin echo, and spin echo sequences for approximated activation-induced relaxation rate changes for 1.5 Tesla and 3 Tesla (taken from Table 6.2). Note that there is a peak in contrast for gradient echo sequences at TE $\approx$ T2* and with asymmetric spin echo sequences for $\tau \approx$ T2*. Also note that spin echo sequences ($\tau = 0$) have the lowest contrast.

6.3.2 Maximizing signal

Field strength and sequence parameters

Imaging at higher static field strength increases both the anatomical image signal-to-noise ratio and also the magnitude of the activation-induced signal change for BOLD and perfusion contrast (Menon *et al.* 1993; Ugurbil *et al.*, 1993). MRI signal-to-noise ratio increases linearly with field strength because the net mag-

netization (or proton magnetic moment) increases in proportion to field strength. BOLD contrast calculations are slightly more complicated (Moonen and van Gelderen 1999). The magnitude of the BOLD signal change increases in a manner that is approximately linear with field strength due to a greater stratification in precession frequencies for a given change in blood oxygenation. Regarding functional *contrast*, BOLD contrast, as mentioned above, is maximized with TE $\approx$ T2* of grey matter. At 1.5 Tesla, T2* is about 50 to 60 ms. At 3 Tesla, T2* is about 30 to 40 ms, depending typically on the quality of the shim, and sometimes on the spatial resolution (T2* tends to increase with improved resolution—see Chapter 4). Activation-induced changes in T2* increase at least linearly with field strength. An interesting point is that if the activation-induced T2* change increased as a function of field strength at the same rate that the resting state T2* decreased then there would be no improvement in functional contrast at higher field strength. Fortunately, the resting state T2* does not decrease with field strength as rapidly as the increase in activation-induced changes in T2*. It should be noted that when using susceptibility contrast, issues related to susceptibility problems, such as shimming and distortion, are more prominent at higher field strengths. This becomes most significant when imaging the base of the brain or regions near interfaces of susceptibility, such as near the sinuses or ear canals.

The choice of TR to use is usually dictated by the number of slices that are required and by the acquisition speed of the scanner (10 to 16 per second as mentioned above). If this is not an issue (e.g. when one is only collecting a few slices), it is important to take into consideration the effect of a reduction in TR on the signal intensity and to use the appropriate flip angle which maximizes signal at a given TR, known as the Ernst angle (see Chapter 3). It follows that a longer TR increases signal, but decreases the number of samples in a time series. As a rule of thumb, it is usually found that the functional contrast drops off dramatically when using a TR less than 500 ms. The reasons for this, while perhaps related to noise autocorrelation, are as yet somewhat unclear.

When performing arterial spin labeling, functional perfusion contrast also increases at higher field strengths. The T1 or longitudinal relaxation time of blood increases with field strength, resulting in more signal from the tagged inflowing blood.

An important point discussed in Section 6.3.3 is that an increase in image signal-to-noise ratio or functional contrast does not necessarily translate to higher functional contrast-to-noise ratio since functional images are created from time series data. Noise in time series data contains physiological fluctuations as well as artefactual signal changes which reduce the quality of the functional images (Jezzard 1999). To reap the full benefits from increasing the signal intensity and signal-to-noise ratio of individual images, it is critical to minimize the effects of physiological fluctuations and artefactual signal changes.

Imaging at higher field strength has some other disadvantages which include greater susceptibility artefacts, and greater RF power deposition. RF power deposition only becomes a problem when performing high resolution anatomical imaging that involves multiple 180° pulses, for example with fast spin echo. Some arterial spin labeling techniques, particularly continuous labeling techniques, are also limited by RF power deposition at higher field strengths.

Radio frequency coils

RF coils are used both for exciting the spins and for receiving signal from the spins. Regarding the use of RF coils to receive signal, the smaller the coil, the less tissue to which it couples. This gives a higher signal-to-noise ratio but results in less brain coverage. Larger RF coils allow for more brain coverage but have a lower signal-to-noise ratio than smaller coils. Where sensitivity is critical, a surface coil in a specific region may be desirable. A brain-specific RF coil should be generally as close to the head as possible so that it couples only to brain tissue. Where whole brain imaging is required, a whole brain quadrature RF coil is likely to be optimal. It should be noted here that typical whole *head and neck* coils used clinically are sub optimal for whole brain fMRI, since they couple also to the face and neck regions (only adding noise), and they are generally not as close as possible to the head.

Regarding the use of RF coils for excitation, the larger the coil the more uniform the excitation distribution. This is desirable for maintaining uniform contrast. Obtaining uniform excitation with a small coil usually requires the use of specialized RF pulses. Thus, the optimal solution is to use a large RF coil for excitation of the spins, and a separate smaller coil for signal reception. When multiple RF receiver channels are available with the appropriate bandwidth for high speed imaging, multiple smaller RF coils can be used simultaneously as receive coils and a larger coil for excitation. In this manner, the advantages of each coil size are combined.

At high field strengths, because of RF power deposition issues, it has been difficult to use whole body

RF coils for excitation. Currently at field strengths of 3 Tesla and above, excitation coils are limited to brain RF coils.

Voxel size

The signal-to-noise ratio in an MR image is directly proportional to voxel volume. Functional contrast-to-noise ratio is optimized by matching the volume of the active region to the voxel volume. This matching of voxel volume to activated region minimizes the partial volume averaging of inactive tissue while maximizing the signal-to-noise ratio. Since functional region sizes are not well characterized, and are likely to vary widely over space and across experimental question, the optimal voxel size is difficult to predict. Recent work suggests that the optimal voxel volume dimensions are $1.5 \times 1.5 \times 1.5$ mm^3 (Hyde *et al.* 2000). Matching the voxel volume to the cortical thickness—about 3 mm—is also a common practice. The issue becomes more complicated when one takes into consideration physiological noise, which is nearly independent of voxel volume. More work must be done to characterize this.

One other advantage to imaging with smaller voxels is that, particularly in regions of poor shim, T2* tends to increase as voxel volume is reduced, providing higher signal at a given TE and, subsequently, more functional contrast (see also Chapter 4). Because the voxel size dependence is so much dependent on the shim, the precise relationship between voxel size and T2* cannot be simply predicted. Methods for decreasing the voxel volume include using a longer readout window with more points, using partial *k*-space reconstruction techniques, and using multi-shot techniques – all are discussed in Section 6.4.

6.3.3 Reducing physiological fluctuations

In most fMRI studies which use snap shot imaging, a large contribution to the temporal stability of the images over the time scale of min, as opposed to the typical 30 ms acquisition time per snap shot image, is from physiological processes. The brain pulsates with every heart beat (Poncelet *et al.* 1992; Dagli *et al.* 1999). Also, the effect of the lungs filling with air with every breath changes the magnetic field profile passing through the brain. This change in magnetic field profile causes changes in image placement and geometry. Breathing also modulates the cardiac frequency. Additionally, physiological fluctuations in the 0.1 to 0.2 Hz range have been observed in MRI data. Some have attributed these low frequency oscillations to vasomotion (Mayhew *et al.* 1996). Others have attributed them to spontaneous brain activity (Biswal *et al.* 1995; Lowe *et al.* 1998). Aside from the fact that they are interesting in themselves, these physiological fluctuations, when not the topic of study, should be removed to reap full sensitivity. These fluctuations are less of a hindrance at extremely high spatial resolution or when using a pulse sequence with a low contrast sensitivity, in which case random thermal noise effects are similar in magnitude to the physiological fluctuations, and tend to dominate.

Filtering

Filtering out frequencies associated physiological processes can reduce the temporal fluctuations or at least make their noise contribution closer to a Gaussian distribution so that standard parametric statistical tests can be applied. Filtering is also a relatively easy post-processing step. It should be noted that if the frequencies do not overlap with the frequency spectrum of the haemodynamic impulse response function, then they are inconsequential to the data quality and do not need removing, particularly when performing regression or correlation analysis with a realistic reference function that contains all the frequencies that are of interest.

One major difficulty in filtering out the effects of physiological processes from the MRI data itself is that it is necessary to sample the processes at a rate at least double that of the highest fluctuation frequency in order to remove them. To properly filter cardiac frequencies, for example, it is required that the scan TR be very short since the frequencies of fluctuations induced by the cardiac cycle can be much higher than the heart rate itself. Because the sampling rate for most fMRI studies is typically in the range of 2 s per sampling of the same slice, the cardiac frequencies typically cannot be removed by analysis of the MRI data alone. Strategies have been used, with limited results, to work around this undersampling problem (Frank *et al.* 1999; Lowe 1999).

Filtering of respiration related fluctuations is easier since the respiration frequency is well within the sampling rate of most time series. One method for filtering involves applying to the data a band-stop filter in the range of the respiration frequencies. Another method, which is generally more accurate, involves using the respiration time course, obtained from direct measurement using a billows in the scanner, as a regressor or reference function in data analysis. This function can then be subtracted out of or orthogonalized to the data. The regions that appear the most affected by respiration are similar to those most affected by cardiac fluctuations—typically at the base of the brain.

Pulse sequence strategies

Standard multi-shot techniques suffer from significantly more physiological-related noise than do EPI techniques or single and multi-shot spiral imaging (Glover and Lee 1995; Noll *et al.* 1995). This is because standard multi-shot images take several s to acquire, during which time physiological processes evolve, introducing 'ghosting' into the images. The magnitude of the ghosts in single and multi-shot imaging depends on how well individual lines of *k*-space are registered. With multi-shot imaging the *k*-space lines are acquired over, say, 3 s. The relative phase of each *k*-space line (or its 'placement') is particularly dependent on when in the cardiac cycle it is collected, so one can imagine that no multi-shot image will have precise placement of *k*-space lines due to the non-repeatability of the phase of the cardiac cycle relative to the timing of data collection. This leads to non-repeatable ghosting which adds an order of magnitude more temporal instability to the time series. The lines near the centre of *k*-space contribute most to the image intensity, so it is primarily important to have those lines registered across all images. Multi-shot *spiral* techniques perform better since they always start data acquisition at the centre of *k*-space, therefore oversampling this region. Manifestation of any differences in the phase of the cardiac cycle near the centre of *k*-space tends to get reduced with multi-shot spiral techniques because of this oversampling. Regardless, multi-shot techniques should generally be used only if extremely high resolution is desired (Menon and Goodyear 1999) either for imaging small activated regions or for minimizing signal dropout. Unwanted fluctuations associated with single shot imaging are much more readily corrected than those associated with multi-shot techniques.

For snap shot EPI, each image is essentially captured in 30 to 40 ms, 'freezing' any physiological process and making each line within an individual image consistently 'registered' relative to all other lines. Ghosting may occur, but it does not significantly fluctuate over time.

Another solution to the instability problem of multi-shot techniques is the application of navigator pulses or retrospective correction (Stenger *et al.* 1999; Hu and Kim 1994; Glover and Lai 1998). Navigator pulses can also be useful for correction of head motion when using single shot techniques (Lee *et al.* 1996).

While discussing ghosting, it is worth mentioning that ghosts from blood vessels are also created, due to fluctuations in the flow velocity. With EPI, one can see these as small ghosting variations propagating from the vessel in the phase encode direction as the blood velocity changes with the cardiac cycle between images. These are easily recognized as a small smear of artefact in one direction, with spiral sequences the artefact appears differently. Because of the way in which single-shot spiral scans are collected (centre-out in *k*-space as opposed to bottom-up or top-down), the vessel ghost is no longer a linear smear, but instead is a ripple in all directions, which can be more problematic for functional imaging near these pulsatile vessels since this ripple causes changes throughout the brain.

Finally, while gradient echo and asymmetric spin echo techniques have similar contrast weightings, asymmetric spin echo sequences are somewhat less sensitive to rapidly flowing blood and to the artefacts induced by changes in the velocity of rapidly flowing blood (Baker *et al.* 1993). The reason for this is that asymmetric spin echo sequences involve the application of two RF pulses: the 90° excitation pulse and then, about 40 ms later, a 180° refocusing pulse. Rapidly flowing blood that has experienced the initial 90° pulse has mostly flowed out of the imaging plane by the time that the 180° pulse is applied, therefore not contributing to the signal. With a gradient echo sequence, only the excitation pulse is applied, therefore including this rapidly flowing and pulsatile blood.

Gating

Gating of the data acquisition to the cardiac cycle would seem to be a simple solution to the problems of cardiac-induced signal fluctuation. However, the technique presents a serious drawback. Gating involves triggering of the scanner to the heart beat so that an image is always collected at a specific phase of the cardiac cycle. This is advantageous because a primary source of physiological noise is the collection of images at varying phases of the cardiac cycle causing head misregistration (the brain moves with every heart beat) and pulsatile flow artefacts. Image collection at a single cardiac phase would eliminate this misregistration, thereby reducing the noise and potentially increasing the spatial resolution of fMRI (i.e. the brain would be imaged at a single position for every acquisition). The drawback to gating is that if the heart rate changes during the collection of images, the MR signal intensity also changes, depending on the tissue T1 and the average TR used. This generally causes even larger fluctuations in the data—making gating relatively worthless in the context of fMRI. A technique has recently been developed to correct the global fluctuations that occur with changes in heart rate, therefore making gating a feasible option in fMRI (Guimaraes *et al.* 1995; Guimaraes *et al.* 1998). Gating would be especially useful for identifying activation in structures at the base of the brain since that is where pulsatile motion is greatest, where activation is most subtle, and where activated regions are the smallest—requiring the most consistent image to image registration.

Cardiac gating and subsequent T1 correction is cumbersome to implement. A precise record of the timing of each heart beat must be maintained and used in the correction. Also, the TR is variable, which leads to more difficulty in properly binning the data relative to the brain activation timing. In addition, the minimum TR is limited to the average cardiac cycle. One unique advantage to this technique is that a map of T1 can be derived from the correction data at no additional cost, perhaps useful for subsequent cortical parcellation. Also, gating is the only means by which it is certain that the tissue content in each voxel will remain constant. This may be critical when imaging small structures at the base of the brain.

6.3.4 Minimizing temporal artefacts

Temporal artefacts are less cyclic signal changes introduced into the time series by means other than physiological fluctuations (which are thought of here as being more cyclic). Temporal artefacts can be caused by, among other things, scanner instabilities and subject motion. The methods for reducing sensitivity to these effects are described below.

Brain activation paradigm timing

The choice in fMRI timing is usually determined by the sluggishness of the haemodynamic response (it is usually not useful to go much faster than an on-off cycle of 8 s on and 8 s off), by the particular brain system that is being activated, and by the predominant frequency in the power spectrum of the noise. As a rule-of-thumb, the goal is to maximize both the number of on–off cycles and the amplitude of the signal response during each cycle in order to optimize the power of the post-processing techniques. This is particularly true when using correlation analysis to extract functional information since much of the artefactual signal change energy (from signal drift or slow motion) is in the lower frequencies. Generally, contrast-to-noise ratio is maximized and artefact is minimized by cycling the activation at the highest rate with which the haemodynamics can keep up and by having a time series no longer than about 3 to 4 min in duration.

A second strategy has recently proven effective for separating activation-induced signal changes from artefact. Activation related to overt word production has been successfully imaged using fMRI (Birn *et al.* 1999), this being previously thought problematic due to head motions during overt speech. The strategy uses the knowledge that the artefactual signal changes associated with moving the jaw have a very different time course than the haemodynamic response of the desired signal changes associated with brain activation. The action of speaking introduces a rapid signal change that lasts only as long as the jaw is out of its resting position. The positive BOLD response to a brief task only begins to increase after 2 s, peaks about 5 s later, and takes an additional 6 s to return to baseline. If an event-related overt word production paradigm is used, the artefactual signal can be easily separated from the BOLD signal change and removed from the time series.

Post processing

Motion correction methods have been developed for fMRI and are used on a routine basis (Woods *et al.* 1992; Eddy *et al.* 1996; Cox and Jesmanowicz 1999). These have been further refined by methods to correct for non-equilibrium signal induced by through-plane motion (Friston *et al.* 1996). Limits do exist as to how robustly these techniques perform. First, for most fMRI acquisition sequences the slices in the volume are not collected simultaneously, so the assumption of rigid motion cannot be made. Second, motion beyond a few voxels typically causes most of these methods to fail in practice.

Real time fMRI

It is often more efficient to re-collect a poor run rather than spend time trying to perform motion correction and artefact reduction afterwards. This approach is only possible if the anatomical and functional data quality can be monitored as it is collected. Several groups have developed methods by which EPI data are collected, reconstructed, and repeatedly analysed in 'real time', allowing for quality assessment (Cox *et al.* 1995; Cox and Hyde 1997; Cox and Jesmanowicz 1999). In the context of clinical fMRI, this immediate feedback can be critical since the information needs to be correct in one pass. One can also imagine cognitive and other experiments that are iterative in nature, being performed in a branching manner depending on the previously obtained results. In addition, many experiments may require 'tuning' the stimulus quality or slice location to optimize the results. All of these methods would benefit from 'real-time' fMRI.

Physical restraint

Methods of physical restraint of the head to prevent motion include packed foam padding, a simple tape across the nose or forehead for feedback, a bite bar, a head vice, a face mask, and a head-neck cast. All methods used to date have found limited success which depends not only on effectiveness of immobilization but also critically on the motivation and comfort of the volunteer. Even with the most motivated and comfortable volunteer, sub-voxel motion still occurs. In addition, physiological fluctuations—brain, blood, and CSF motion—remain.

Pulse sequence strategies

Many pulse sequence strategies exist for reducing the impact of subject head motion. These include clustered volume acquisition, phase encode direction adjustment, slice orientation adjustment, image contrast manipulation, and the application of crusher gradients.

A novel image collection timing scheme, called clustered volume acquisition, was first introduced by Talavage *et al.* (1998) to alleviate the problem of artefactual auditory activation arising from the scanner noise (Bandettini *et al.* 1998) when performing auditory activation experiments (Melcher *et al.* 1999). Typically with EPI on clinical scanners the individual slice acquisitions are spaced evenly within a TR. For example, if 10 slices are specified with a TR of 2 s, then the acquisition of each slice is spaced 200 ms apart. With clustered volume acquisition, the ten slices are collected as rapidly as possible, followed by a period of silence during the remainder of the TR interval. Since the positive BOLD haemodynamic response lags temporally from the brain activity, it is not necessary to collect images during the immediate time of stimulation. Rather, after waiting a time from 4 to 6 s after auditory stimulation, the imaging gradients may be applied to collect the images without introducing artefactual activation. This technique lends itself well to presenting auditory stimuli without contamination from the 100–130 dB EPI scanner noise. In addition, it lends itself to having subjects give brief overt responses (which might otherwise cause motion artefacts) without any time series contamination. An important further issue in clustered volume acquisition is that for the effects of the scanner noise on the haemodynamic response to be *completely* eliminated there must be a sufficient period of silence to allow for the signal from cortex activated by scanner noise to return to baseline. This will add about 6 s on to the necessary TR, making the scan prohibitively long for many types of experiment.

Some amount of image ghosting invariably exists in EPI images, and these ghosts often overlap with the main image. The ghosts are usually stable over time and do not contaminate the time series. However, if they vary, as can be the case with subtle eye movements, then instability in the ghost can introduce instability in the main image. A common strategy is to set the phase encoding direction of the EPI acquisition such that the ghosts minimally overlap with brain tissue. In this manner any artefactual signal changes that occur in the ghosts or that cause the ghosts to change slightly will be clearly identified as such since they occur outside the brain.

The motion correction schemes mentioned above benefit substantially from having the entire volume collected as rapidly as possible. The use of clustered volume acquisition, 3D fMRI techniques (Yang *et al.* 1996), and PRESTO (Liu *et al.* 1993; Ramsey *et al.* 1996; Ramsey *et al.* 1998; Golay *et al.* 2000), allow for simultaneous volume acquisition, and are therefore beneficial to motion correction algorithms that assume rigid body motion.

When images in the volume cannot be collected simultaneously, it is through-plane motion that is hardest to correct properly. It is therefore useful to chose the imaging plane along which the most motion is expected to occur. Most head motion during fMRI runs is typically a head-bobbing motion. For this reason, the choice of a sagittal plane for slice collection usually allows for better motion correction results.

Since artefactual signal changes originating from head motion only arise if adjacent voxels have differing signal intensities, a flatter time series image contrast will reduce the effects of small sub-voxel motion. Typically, a flat contrast is achieved with gradient echo (T2*-weighted) EPI using a TR that is less than 2 s.

It has been shown that when using a short TR the existence of magnetization remaining in the transverse plane can enter into the time series during subsequent RF pulses. This results in variably periodic 'stimulated echoes' that add to the temporal instability. Simple application of 'crusher gradients' (a gradient pulse at the end of the TR period lasting for ≈ 10 ms) effectively removes this 'left over' transverse magnetization and increases temporal stability (Zhao *et al.* 2000).

Stimulus equipment

Many stimulus and subject interface devices, such as projectors, joysticks, and button boxes, emit RF noise.

If these devices are used in the scanning room or wires from them are passed through wave guides into the magnet room, it is important to make sure that they are properly shielded. Ideally, all wires should pass through a filtered penetration panel. Otherwise, this 'RF noise' can significantly contaminate image temporal stability. One method for checking this is by inspecting the high resolution anatomical images. If these have any prominent stripes passing through them, then there exists RF contamination that should be removed.

6.4 Issues of resolution and speed

The following section considers some of the issues relating to selection of the possible and the optimal temporal resolution and spatial resolution in fMRI experiments. These issues are dealt with in greater detail in Chapter 7.

6.4.1 Acquisition speed

The image acquisition rate is limited ultimately by how rapidly the signal can be digitized by the scanner and by how rapidly the imaging gradients can be switched. As discussed above, MR imaging can be divided into single-shot and multi-shot techniques. In single-shot imaging, spins are excited with a single excitation pulse and all the data necessary for creation of an image are collected at once. Echo planar imaging is the most common single shot technique. (With one echo train an entire image 'plane' is acquired). Multi-shot techniques are the most commonly used method for high resolution anatomical imaging. Usually, a single 'line' (in *k*-space) of raw data is acquired with each excitation pulse. Because of the relatively slow rate at which the magnetization returns to equilibrium following excitation (determined by the T1 of the tissue), a certain amount of time is required between shots, otherwise the signal would rapidly be saturated. Because of this required recovery time (at least 150 ms), multishot techniques are typically slower than single shot techniques. For a 150 ms TR, a fully multi-shot image with 128 lines of raw data would take 150ms × 128 = 19.2 s.

In the case of echo-planar imaging, the entire data set for a single plane is typically acquired in about 20 to 40 ms. For a BOLD experiment, the time to echo (TE) is about 40 ms. Along with some additional time for applying other necessary gradients, the total time for an image to be acquired is about 60 to 100 ms, allowing 10 to 16 images to be acquired in a second. Improvements in digital sampling rates and gradient slew rates will allow small further gains in this figure, but essentially this is about the upper limit for imaging humans.

In the context of an fMRI experiment with echo planar imaging, the typical image acquisition rate is determined by how many slices can temporally fit into a TR time. For whole brain imaging, approximately 20 slices (5 mm thickness) are required to cover the entire brain. This would allow a TR of about 1.25 to 2 s at minimum. This sampling rate is more than adequate to capture most of the details of the slow and dispersed haemodynamic response. Even with a relatively long TR or image acquisition rate, the temporal resolution may be improved by spacing the image timing unevenly with the task timing, therefore sampling a different part of each on-off cycle.

6.4.2 Image resolution

The spatial resolution is also primarily determined by the gradient strength, the digitizing rate, and the time available. For multi shot imaging, as high resolution as desired can be achieved if one is willing to wait: one can keep on collecting lines of data with more RF pulses. For snap-shot echo planar imaging, the free induction decay time, $T2^*$, plays a significant role in determining the possible resolution (Jesmanowicz *et al.* 1998). One can only sample for so long before the signal has completely decayed away. For this reason, echo planar images are generally lower resolution than multi-shot images. To circumvent the problem of decaying transverse signal, two strategies are commonly used (Cohen and Weisskoff 1991; Cohen 1999). The first strategy is multi-shot EPI, in which a larger k-space data set is acquired in multiple interleaved passes (but still with many fewer passes than for conventional clinical multi-shot imaging). The second strategy is to perform an operation called conjugate synthesis, which involves making use of the fact that due to a symmetry in the full k-space data, half of the data that conventionally is collected is redundant. By only measuring the minimum lines required, the uncol-

lected lines of k-space can be calculated using the symmetry properties. This allows a gain of at most twice the spatial resolution, with some cost in signal-to-noise ratio and image quality. The procedure is also known as partial k-space EPI.

Multi-shot EPI suffers from some of the same temporal stability problems as other multi-shot techniques, mentioned in Section 6.3.4 above. Navigator echoes can be used to effectively correct these k-space misregistration problems. With partial k-space acquisition, the image quality tends to suffer because complete phase information is not obtained, causing the phase correction accuracy for all lines of k-space to be degraded. A further advantage of multi-shot EPI is that if the resolution is kept the same as with single-shot imaging, the effective readout echo intervals are shorter, reducing image distortion.

6.4.3 Brain coverage

All MRI sequences can give full brain coverage. The goal is to achieve the most uniform brain coverage as rapidly as possible. Single shot EPI or spiral sequences can achieve complete brain coverage within 2 s. Many 3D sequences, including PRESTO, are becoming increasingly popular in fMRI applications (Yang *et al.* 1996; Liu *et al.* 1993; Ramsey *et al.* 1996; Golay *et al.* 2000). Other than the temporal resolution and simultaneity issues in regard to brain coverage, a key concern is making sure that specific areas in the brain, such as near the base, orbits, and ear canals, are covered. This issue is discussed in the following section.

6.5 Structural and functional image quality

Even though it is the time series stability that gives the most difficulty, the anatomical image quality, for both EPI time series images and the high resolution structural images on which the functional images are registered, is critical for functional localization.

6.5.1 Functional time series image quality

Image quality issues that are the most prevalent in time series image collection are image warping (Jezzard and Clare 1999) and signal dropout (Glover 1999). While much can be written on this subject, the description here is kept to the bare essentials.

Image warping or distortion is fundamentally caused by one or both of two things: B_0 field inhomogeneities and gradient non-linearities. A non linear gradient will cause non-linearities in spatial encoding, causing the image to be distorted. This is primarily a problem when using small (e.g. head-only) gradient coils that have a small region of linearity that drops off rapidly at the base and top of the brain (Wong *et al.* 1992). With the growing prevalence of whole body gradient-coils for performing echo planar imaging, this problem is less often a major issue.

If the B_0 field is inhomogeneous, as is typically the situation with imperfect shimming procedures—particularly at higher field strengths—the spins will precess at a different frequency than is expected in their particular location. This leads to image deformation in those areas of poor shim—particularly with an imaging procedure that requires a long readout window (e.g. snap-shot EPI). A solution to this is to shorten the readout window, achieve a better shim (Glover 1999; Constable *et al.* 2000), or map the B_0 field and perform a correction based on this map (Weisskoff and Davis 1992; Jezzard and Balaban 1995).

Another potential solution is the use of a spiral readout window instead of EPI. Because of its radial path through k-space, spiral imaging manifests off-resonance effects as radial blurring while EPI manifests off-resonance effects as image warping. Spiral readout windows are also typically shorter in duration and more efficient than corresponding EPI readout windows. So, the user performing single shot imaging for fMRI needs to decide if blurring or warping is less problematic.

Signal dropout in gradient echo acquisitions is also caused by localized B_0 field inhomogeneities, typically at the interfaces of tissues having different magnetic susceptibilities. If, within a voxel, the B_0 inhomogeneities are on a smaller scale than the voxel itself, then instead of the voxel being shifted (causing warping) the spins within the voxel will precess at different frequencies and their varying phases will cancel each other out. Several strategies exist for reducing this problem. One is, again, to shim as well as possible at the desired location. Higher order localized shimming is an automated procedure on many scanners, although a full correction of all inhomogeneities

is not possible with the available shim terms. Another method is to reduce the voxel size (increase the resolution), thereby having less of a stratification of frequencies within a voxel and therefore less destructive dephasing. A third method is to choose the slice orientation such that the smallest voxel dimension is orientated perpendicular to the largest B_0 gradient. Since in many studies the slice thickness is greater than the in-plane voxel dimension, the slice dimension should *not* be parallel to the direction of highest intrinsic B_0 gradient. Because of this, many studies are performed using sagittal or coronal slice orientations since a prominent gradient in B_0 is in the inferior-superior direction at the base of the brain.

6.5.2 High resolution structural image quality

A technique that should not be overlooked is the necessity for collection of a high resolution anatomical MRI scan that shows good grey-white discrimination. The primary concerns regarding high resolution anatomical image collection include maximizing signal-to-noise ratio, resolution, and image contrast while minimizing the amount of time it takes to collect an entire high resolution data set.

Some groups have aimed to match the degree of geometric warping induced in the high resolution anatomical scan with that of the functional time series data (Sereno *et al.* 1995; Tootell *et al.* 1996, 1998). This has been performed by using T1-weighted, high resolution, multi-shot EPI techniques which have a similar readout window duration as the functional time series images, therefore matching the degree of warping. The warped high resolution anatomical scan can then be unwarped onto a standard high resolution image. This procedure guarantees that precise functional-anatomical registration is achieved.

Practically, it is important to create the highest quality (high resolution, high grey-white matter contrast, and high signal-to-noise ratio) images in about 10 min. While not necessarily optimal, a typical pulse sequence used for this purpose is a 3D spoiled gradient echo sequence (e.g. 3D-FLASH, 3D-SPGR). Typical spoiled gradient recalled parameters used at 1.5 Tesla are: TE = 5 ms, TR = 10 ms, Flip angle = 15°.

At higher magnetic field strengths, maintaining image quality while keeping acquisition time low is an ongoing challenge. The main reason for this challenge is that, with an increase in static field strength, grey and white matter T1 times become longer, and T2 times decrease (Jezzard *et al.* 1996). This causes the anatomical contrast to flatten out somewhat and requires some adjustment in the timing parameters. Typical spoiled gradient echo pulse sequences and parameters used at 3.0 Tesla are: TE = 4 ms, TR = 9 ms, Flip angle = 12°.

New pulse sequences for performing high resolution structural imaging are still being developed (Deichmann *et al.* 2000; Norris 2000; Wong *et al.* 2000a), and may turn out be critical in enabling more precise automatic image segmentation.

6.6   *Conclusion*

The breadth of knowledge and experience necessary to practice fMRI well has become overwhelming—even for the expert! This chapter has focussed on providing information that is helpful in choosing the optimal pulse sequence and sequence parameters. Of course, this quickly expands into a multi-variable and multi-level optimization problem—ultimately unsolvable. The overall goal of this chapter was of course not to leave the reader overwhelmed, but to give the reader a practical feel for what is important and what is possible: to decide for themselves what variables are critical, and then figure out what they will have to trade-off to achieve a given goal. The potential solutions to any fMRI paradigm/hardware/pulse sequence problem are many. The details or references to details are presented here to aid the reader in choosing the most satisfying solution. Lastly, it is hoped that a sense of excitement in the possibilities of fMRI has also been conveyed. Functional MRI hardware, the understanding of contrast mechanisms, processing techniques, and neuroscience questions continue to co-evolve at a very high rate.

References

Baker, J.R., Hoppel, B.E., Stern, C.E., Kwong, K.K., Weisskoff, R.M., and Rosen, B.R. (1993). In *Dynamic functional imaging of the complete human cortex using gradient-echo and asymmetric spin-echo echo-planar magnetic resonance imaging.* p. 1400, Proceedings of SMRM 12th Annual Meeting, New York.

Bandettini, P.A. and Won, E.C. (1995). Effects of Biophysical and physiologic parameters on brain activation-induced R2* and R2 changes: simulations using a deterministic diffusion model. *International Journal of Imaging Systems Technology.* 6, 134–52.

Bandettini, P.A., Wong, E.C., Hinks, R.S., Tikofsky, R.S., and Hyde, J.S. (1992). Time course EPI of human brain function during task activation. *Magnetic Resonance in Medicine,* 25, 390–7.

Bandettini, P.A., Jesmanowicz, A., Van Kylen, J., Birn, R.M., and Hyde J.S. (1998). Functional MRI of brain activation induced by scanner acoustic noise. *Magnetic Resonance in Medicine,* 39, 410–6.

Belliveau, J.W., Kennedy, D.N., McKinstry, R.C., Buchbinder, B.R., Weisskoff, R.M., Cohen, M.S., Vevea, J.M., Brady, T.J., and Rosen, B.R. (1991). Functional mapping of the human visual cortex by magnetic resonance imaging. *Science,* 254, 716–19.

Birn, R.M., Bandettini, P.A., Cox, R.W., and Shaker, R. (1999). Event-related fMRI of tasks involving brief motion. *Human Brain Mapping,* 7, 106–14.

Biswal, B., Yetkin, F.Z., Haughton, V.M., and Hyde, J.S. (1995). Functional connectivity in the motor cortex of resting human brain using echo-planar MRI. *Magnetic Resonance in Medicine,* 34, 537–41.

Boxerman, J.L., Bandettini, P.A., Kwong, K.K., Baker, J.R., Davis, T.L., Rosen, B.R., and Weisskoff, R.M. (1995a). The intravascular contribution to fMRI signal change: Monte Carlo modeling and diffusion-weighted studies *in vivo.* *Magnetic Resonance in Medicine,* 34, 4–10.

Boxerman, J.L., Hamberg, L.M., Rosen, B.R., and Weisskoff, R.M. (1995b). MR contrast due to intravascular magnetic susceptibility perturbations. *Magnetic Resonance in Medicine,* 34, 555–66.

Buxton, R.B., Luh, W.M., Wong, E.C., Frank, L.R., and Bandettini, P.A. (1998a). In *Diffusion-weighting attenuates the BOLD signal change but not the post-stimulus undershoot.* p. 7, Proceedings ISMRM 6th Annual Meeting, Sydney.

Buxton, R.B., Wong, E.C., and Frank, L.R. (1998b). Dynamics of blood flow and oxygenation changes during brain activation: the balloon model. *Magnetic Resonance in Medicine,* 39, 855–64.

Cohen, M.S. (1999). Echo planar imaging and funcational MRI. In *Functional MRI* (ed. C.T.W. Moonen and P.A. Bandettini), pp.137–48, Springer, London.

Cohen, M.S. and Weisskoff, R.M. (1991). Ultra-fast imaging. *Magnetic Resonance Imaging,* 9, 1–37.

Constable, R.T., Carpentier, A., Pugh, K., Westerveld, M., Oszunar, Y., and Spencer, D.D. (2000). Investigation of the human hippocampal formation using a randomized event-related paradigm and Z-shimmed functional MRI. *NeuroImage,* 12, 55–62.

Cox, R.W. and Hyde, J.S. (1997). Software tools for analysis and visualization of fMRI data. *NMR in BioMedicine,* 10, 171–8.

Cox, R.W. and Jesmanowicz, A. (1999). Real-time 3D image registration for funcational MRI. *Magnetic Resonance in Medicine* 42, 1014–8.

Cox, R.W., Jesmanowicz, A., and Hyde, J.S. (1995). Real-time functional magnetic resonance imaging. *Magnetic Resonance in Medicine* 33, 230–6.

Dagli, M.S., Ingeholm, J.E., and Haxby, J.V. (1999). Localization of cardiac-induced signal change in fMRI. *NeuroImage*, 7, 407–15.

Davis, T.L., Kwong, K.K., Weisskoff, R.M., and Rosen, B.R. (1998). Calibrated functional MRI: Mapping the dynamics of oxidative metabolism. *Proceedings of the National Academy of Sciences (USA)*, 95, 1834–9.

Deichmann, R., Good, C.D., Josephs, O., Ashburner, J., and Turner, R. (2000). Optimization of 3-D MP-RAGE sequences for structural brain imaging. *NeuroImage*, 12, 112–27.

Detre, J.A., Leigh, J.S., Williams, D.S., and Koretsky, A.P. (1992). Perfusion imaging. *Magnetic Resonance in Medicine*, 23, 37–45.

Duyn, J.H., Moonen, C.T.W., van Yperen, G.H., de Boer, R.W., and Luyten, P.R. (1994). Inflow versus deoxyhemoglobin effects in BOLD functional MRI using gradient-echoes at, 1.5 T. *NMR in Biomedicine*, 7, 83–8.

Duyn, J.H., Tan C.X., van der Veen, J.W., van Gelderen, P., Frank, J.A., Ye, F.Q., and Yongbi, M. (2000). In *Perfusion-weighted 'single-trail' fMRI*, p.55, Proceedings of ISMRM 8th Annual Meeting, Denver.

Eddy, W.F., Fitzgerald, M., and Noll, D.C. (1996). Improved image registration by using Fourier interpolation. *Magnetic Resonance in Medicine*, 36, 923–31.

Edelman, R., Siewert, B., and Darby, D. (1994a). Qualitative mapping of cerebral blood flow and functional localization with echo planar MR imaging ans signal targeting with alternating radiofrequency (EPISTAR). *Radiology*, 192, 1–8.

Edelman, R.R., Siewert, B., Wielopolski, P., Pearlman, J., and Warach, S. (1994b). Noninvasive mapping of cerebral perfusion by using EPISTAR MR angiography. *Magnetic Resonance Imaging*, 4(P) [Abstr.], 68.

Frahm, J., Bruhn, H., Merboldt, K.-D., Hanicke, W., and Math, D. (1992). Dynamic MR imaging of human brain oxygenation during rest and photic stimulation. *Magnetic Resonance Imaging*, 2, 501–05.

Frank, L.R., Buxton, R.B., and Wong, E.C. (1999). In *Detection of physiological noise fluctuations from undersampled multi-slice fMRI data*. p.277, Proceedings, ISMRM 7th Annual Meeting, Philadelphia.

Friston, K.J., Williams, S., Howard, R., Frackowiak, R.S.J., and Turner, R. (1996). Movement related effects in fMRI time-series. *Magnetic Resonance in Medicine*, 35, 346–55.

Glover, G.H. (1999). 3D z-shim method for reduction of susceptibility effects in BOLD fMRI. *Magnetic Resonance in Medicine*, 42, 290–9.

Glover, G.H., and Lai, S. (1998). Self-navigated spiral fMRI: interleaved versus single-shot. *Magnetic Resonance in Medicine*, 39, 361–8.

Glover, G.H. and Lee, A.T. (1995). Motion artifacts in fMRI: comparison of 2DFT with PR and spiral scan methods. *Magnetic Resonance in Medicine*, 33, 624–35.

Golay, X., Pruessmann, K.P., Weiger, M., Crelier, G.R., Folker, P.J., Kollias, S.S., and Boesiger, P. (2000). PRESTO-SENSE: an ultrafast whole-brain fMRI technique. *Magnetic Resonance in Medicine*, 43, 779–86.

Guimaraes, A.R., Baker, J.R., and Weisskoff, R.M. (1995). In *Cardiac-gated functional MRI with T1 correction*, p.798. Proceedings of SMR 3rd Annual Meeting, Nice.

Guimaraes, A.R., Melcher, J.R., Talavage, T.M., Baker, J.R., Ledden, P., Rosen, B.R., Kiang, N.Y., Fullerton, B.C., and Weisskoff, R.M. (1998). Imaging subcortical auditory activity in humans. *Human Brain Mapping*, 6, 33–41.

Haacke, E.M., Lai, S., Reichenbach, J.R., Kuppusamy, K., Hoogenraad, F.G.C., Takeichi, H., and Lin, W. (1997). *In vivo* measurement of blood oxygen saturation using magnetic resonance imaging: a direct validation of the blood oxygen level-dependent concept in functional brain imaging. *Human Brain Mapping*, 5, 341–46.

Hoge, R.D., Atkinson, J., Gill, B., Crelier, G.R., Marrett, S., and Pike, G.B. (1999a). Investigation of BOLD signal dependence on cerebral blood flow and oxygen consumption: the deoxyhemoglobin dilution model. *Magnetic Resonance in Medicine*, 42, 849–63.

Hoge, R.D., Atkinson, J., Gill, B., Crelier, G.R., Marrett, S., and Pike, G.B. (1999b). Stimulus-dependent BOLD and perfusion dynamics in human V1. *NeuroImage*, 9, 573–85.

Hu, X. and Kim, S.-G. (1994). Reduction of signal fluctuations in functional MRI using navigator echoes. *Magnetic Resonance in Medicine*, 31, 495–503.

Hyde, J.S., Biswal, B.B., and Jesmanowicz, A. (2000). In *Optimum voxel size in fMRI*, p.240, Proceedings, ISMRM 8th Annual Meeting, Denver.

Jesmanowicz, A., Bandettini, P.A., and Hyde, J.S. (1998). Single-shot half *k*-space high-resolution gradient-recalled EPI for fMRI at 3 Tesla. *Magnetic Resonance in Medicine*, 40, 754–62.

Jezzard, P. (1999). Physiological noise: strategies for correction. In *Functional MRI* (ed. Moonen, C.T.W. and Bandettini, P.A.), pp.173–81, Springer, Berlin.

Jezzard, P. and Balaban, R.S. (1995). Correction for geometric distortion in echo planar images from B_0 field distortions. *Magnetic Resonance in Medicine*, 34, 65–73.

Jezzard, P. and Clare, S. (1999). Sources of distortion in functional MRI data. *Human Brain Mapping*, 8, 80–5.

Jezzard, P., Duewell, S., and Balaban, R.S. (1996). MR relaxation times in human brain: measurement at 4 T. *Radiology*, 199, 773–9.

Kennan, R.P., Zhong, J., and Gore, J.C. (1994). Intravascular susceptibility contrast mechanisms in tissues. *Magnetic Resonance in Medicine*, 31, 9–21.

Kim, S.-G. (1995). Quantification of relative cerebral flood flow change by flow-sensitive alternating inversion recovery (FAIR) technique: application to functional mapping. *Magnetic Resonance in Medicine*, 34, 293–301.

Kim, S.-G. and Ugurbil, K. (1997). Comparison of blood oxygenation and cerebral blood flow effects in fMRI: estimation of relative oxygen consumption change. *Magnetic Resonance in Medicine*, 38, 59–65.

Kwong, K.K., Belliveau, J.W., Chesler, D.A., Goldberg, I.E., Weisskoff, R.M., Poncelet, B.P., Kennedy, D.N., Hoppel, B.E., Cohen, M.S., Turner, R., Cheng, H.M., Brady, T.J., and Rosen, B.R. (1992). Dynamic magnetic resonance imaging of human brain activity during primary sensory stimulation.

Proceedings of the National Academy of Sciences (USA), **89**, 5675–9.

Kwong, K.K., Chesler, D.A., Weisskoff, R.M., and Rosen, B.R. (1994). In *Perfusion MR imaging*, p.1005, Proceedings, SMR, 2nd Annual Meeting, San Francisco.

Kwong, K.K., Chesler, D.A., Weisskoff, R.M., Donahue, K.M., Davis, T.L., Ostergaard, L., Campbell, T.A., and Rosen, B.R. (1995). MR perfusion studies with T1-weighted echo planar imaging. *Magnetic Resonance in Medicine*, **34**, 878–87.

LeBihan, B. (ed.) (1995). *Diffusion and perfusion magnetic resonance imaging*. Raven Press, New York.

Liu, H.L. and Gao, J.H. (1999). Perfusion-based event-related functional MRI. *Magnetic Resonance in Medicine*, **42**, 1011–3.

Liu, G., Sobering, G., Duyn, J. and Moonen, C.T. (1993). A functional MRI technique combining principles of echo-shifting with a train of observations (PRESTO). *Magnetic Resonance in Medicine*, **30**, 764–8.

Lee, C.C., Jack, C.R. Jr., Grimm, R.C., Rossman, P.J., Felmlee, J.P., Ehman, R.L., and Riederer, S.J. (1996). Real-time adaptive motion correction in functional MRI. *Magnetic Resonance in Medicine*, **36**, 436–44.

Liu, T.T., Luh, W.-M., Wong, E.C., Frank, L.R., and Buxton, R.B. (2000). *A method for dynamic measurement of blood volume with compensation for T2 changes*, p.53. Proceedings, ISMRM 8th Annual Meeting, Denver.

Lowe, M.J., Mock, B.J., and Sorenson, J.A. (1998). Functional connectivity in single and multislice echoplanar imaging using resting-state fluctuations. *NeuroImage*, **7**, 119–32.

Lowe, M.J. (1999). In *Gram-Schmidt orthogonalization to reduce aliased physiologic noise in low sampling rate fMRI*, p.1711, Proceedings, ISMRM 7th Annual Meeting, Philadelphia.

Mayhew, J.E.W., Askew, S., Porrill, J., MaxWestby, G.W., Redgrave, P., Rector, D.M., and Harper, R.M. (1996). Cerebral vasomotion: a 0.1 Hz oscillation in reflected light imaging of neural activity. *NeuroImage*, **4**, 183–93.

Melcher, J.R., Talavage, T.M., and Harms, M.P. (1999). Functional MRI of the auditory system. In *Functional MRI*, (ed. C.T.W. Moonen and P.A. Bandettini), p.393–406, Springer, Berlin.

Menon, R.S. and Goodyear, B.G. (1999). Submillimeter functional localization in human striate cortex using BOLD contrast at 4 Tesla: implications for the vascular point-spread function. *Magnetic Resonance in Medicine*, **41**, 230–5.

Menon, R.S., Ogawa, S., Tank, D.W., and Ugurbil, K. (1993). 4 Tesla gradient recalled echo characteristics of photic stimulation—induced signal changes in the human primary visual cortex. *Magnetic Resonance in Medicine*, **30**, 380–6.

Moonen, C.T.W. and van Gelderen, P. (1999). Optimal Efficiency of 3D and 2D BOLD gradient echo fMRI Methods. In *Functional MRI*, (ed. C.T.W. Moonen and P.A. Bandettini), pp.161–72, Springer, Berlin.

Moonen, C.T.W., van ZIJL P.C.M., Frank, J.A., LeBihan, D. and Becker, E.D. (1990). Functional magnetic resonance imaging in medicine and physiology. *Science*, **250**, 53–61.

Noll, D.C., Cohen, J.D., Meyer, C.H., and Schneider, W. (1995). Spiral k-space MR imaging of cortical activation. *Journal of Magnetic Resonance Imaging*, **5**, 49–56.

Norris, D.G. (2000). Reduced power multislice MDEFT imaging. *Journal of Magnetic Resonance Imaging*, **11**, 445–51.

Ogawa, S. and Lee, T.M. (1992). Functional brain imaging with physiologically sensitive image signals. *Journal of Magnetic Resonance Imaging*, **2**(P)-WIP supplement [Abstr.], S22.

Ogawa, S., Lee, T.M., Kay, A.R., and Tank, D.W. (1990). Brain magnetic resonance imaging with contrast dependent on blood oxygenation. *Proceedings of the National Academy of Sciences (USA)*, **87**, 9868–72.

Ogawa, S., Tank, D.W., Menon, R., Ellermann, J.M., Kim S.-G., Merkle, H., and Ugurbil, K. (1992). Intrinsic signal changes accompanying sensory stimulation: functional brain mapping with magnetic resonance imaging. *Proceedings of the National Academy of Sciences (USA)*, **89**, 5951–55.

Ogawa, S., Menon, R.S., Tank, D.W., Kim, S.-G., Merkle, H., Ellerman, J.M., and Ugurbil, K. (1993). Functional brain mapping by blood oxygenation level—dependent contrast magnetic resonance imaging: a comparison of signal characteristics with a biophysical model. *Biophysical Journal*, **64**, 803–12.

Pauling, L. and Coryell, C.D. (1936). The magnetic properties and structure of hemoglobin, oxyhemoglobin, and carbon-monoxyhemoglobin. *Proceedings of the National Academy of Sciences (USA)*, **22**, 210–16.

Poncelet, B.P., Wdeen, V.J., Weisskoff, R.M., and Cohen, M.S. (1992). Brain parenchyma motion: measurement with cine echo planar MR imaging. *Radiology*, **185**, 645–51.

Ramsey, N.F., Kirkby, B.S., Van Gelderen, P., Berman, K.F., Duyn, J.H., Frank, J.A., Mattay, V.S., Van Horn, J.D., Esposito, G., Moonen, C.T., and Weinberger, D.R. (1996). Functional mapping of human sensorimotor cortex with 3D BOLD 4MRI correlates highly with H2(15)O PET rCBF. *Journal of Cerebral Blood Flow and Metabolism*, **16**, 755–64.

Ramsey, N.F., van den Brink, J.S., van Muiswinkel, A.M., Folkers, P.J., Moonen, C.T., Jansma, J.M., and Kahn, R.S. (1998). Phase navigator correction in 3D fMRI improves detection of brain activation: quantitative assessment with a graded motor activation procedure. *NeuroImage*, **8**, 240–8.

Rosen, B.R., Belliveau, J.W., and Chien, D. (1989). Perfusion imaging by nuclear magnetic resonance. *Magnetic Resonance Quarterly*, **5**, 263–81.

Rosen, B.R., Belliveau, J.W., Aronen, H.J., Kennedy, D., Buchbinder, B.R., Fischman, A., Gruber, M., Glas, J., Weisskoff, R.M., Cohen, M.S., Hochberg, F.H., and Brady, T.J. (1991). Susceptibility contrast imaging of cerebral blood volume: human experience. *Magnetic Resonance in Medicine*, **22**, 293–9.

Sereno, M.I., Dale, A.M., Reppas, J.B., Kwong, K.K., Belliveau, J.W., Brady, T.J., Rosen, B.R., and Tootell, R.B. (1995). Borders of multiple visual areas in humans revealed by functional magnetic resonance imaging. *Science*, **268**, 889–93.

Stenger, V.A., Peltier, S., Boada, F.E., and Noll, D.C. (1999). 3D spiral cardiac/respiratory ordered fMRI data acquisition at 3 Tesla. *Magnetic Resonance in Medicine*, **41**, 983–91.

Talavage, T.M., Edminster, W.B., Ledden, P.J., and Weisskoff, R.M. (1998). Comparison of impact of fMRI sequence acoustics on auditory cortex activation. In *6th Proceedings of the International Society of Magnetic Resonance in Medicine*, p.1503.

Thulborn, K.R., Waterton, J.C., Matthews, P.M., and Radda, G.K. (1982). Oxygenation dependence of the transverse relaxation time of water protons in whole blood at high field. *Biochemica et Biophysica Acta*, **714**, 265–70.

Tootell, R.B., Dale, A.M., Sereno, M.I., and Malach, R. (1996). New images from human visual cortex. *Trends in Neurosciences*, **19**, 481–9.

Tootell, R.B.H., Hadjikhani, N.K., Vanduffel, W., Liu, A.K., Mendola, J.D., Sereno, M.I., and Dale, A.M. (1998). Functional analysis of primary visual cortex (V1) in humans. *Proceedings of the National Academy of Sciences (USA)*, **95**, 811–17.

Turner, R., LeBihan, D., Moonen, C.T.W., Despres, D., and Frank, J. (1991). Echo-planar time course MRI of cat brain oxygenation changes. *Magnetic Resonance in Medicine*, **22**, 159–66.

Ugurbil, K., Garwood, M., Ellermann, J., Hendrich, K., Hinke, R., Hu, X., Kim, S.-G., Menon, R., Merkle, H., Ogawa, S., and Salmi, R. (1993). Imaging at high magnetic fields: initial experiences at 4 T. *Magnetic Resonance Quarterly*, **9**, 259–77.

van Zijl, P.C.M., Eleff, S.M., Ulatowski, J.A., Oja, J.M.E., Ulug, A.M., Traystman, R.J., and Kauppinen, R.A. (1998). Quantitative assessment of blood flow, blood volume, and blood oxygenation effects in functional magnetic resonance imaging. *Nature Medicine*, **4**, 159–16.

Weisskoff, R.M. and David, T.L. (1992). In *Correcting gross distortion on echo planar images*, p.4515, Proceedings, SMRM, 11th Annual Meeting, Berlin.

Weisskoff, R.M., Boxerman, J.L., Zuo, C.S., and Rosen, B.R. (1993). Endogenous susceptibility contrast: principles of relationship between blood oxygenation and MR signal change. In *Functional MRI of the Brain*, pp.103, Society of Magnetic Resonance in Medicine, Berkeley.

Williams, D.S., Detre, J.A., Leigh, J.S., and Koretsky, A.S. (1992). Magnetic resonance imaging of perfusion using spin-inversion of arterial water. *Proceedings of the National Academy of Sciences (USA)*, **89**, 212–16.

Wong, E.C. (1999). Potential and pitfalls of arterial spin labelling based perfusion imaging techniques for functional MRI. In *Functional MRI*, (ed. C.T.W. Moonen and P.A. Bandettini), p.63–70, Springer, Berlin.

Wong, E.C. and Bandettini, P.A. (1999). Simultaneous acquisition of multiple forms of fMRI contrast. In *Functional MRI* (ed. C.T.W. Moonen and P.A. Bandettini), pp.183–92, Springer, Berlin.

Wong, E.C., Bandettini, P.A. and Hyde, J.S. (1992). In *Echo planar imaging of the human brain using a three-axis local gradient coil*, pp. 105, Proceedings SMRM, 11th Annual Meeting, Berlin.

Wong, E.C., Buxton, R.B., and Frank, L.R. (1997). Implementation of quantitative perfusion imaging techniques for functional brain mapping using pulsed arterial spin labeling. *NMR Biomedicine*, **10**, 237–49.

Wong, E.C., Buxton, R.B., and Frank, L.R. (1998). Quantitative imaging of perfusion using a single subtraction (QUIPSS and QUIPSS II). *Magnetic Resonance in Medicine*, **39**, 702–8.

Wong, E.C., Luh, W.-M., Buxton, R.B., and Frank, L.R. (2000a). In *Single slab high resolution 3D whole brain imaging using spiral FSE*, p.683. Proceedings, ISMRM 8th Annual Meeting, Denver.

Wong, E.C., Luh, W.-M., and Liu, T.T. (2000b). In *Turbo ASL: arterial spin labeling with higher SNR and temporal resolution*, p.452. Human Brain Mapping Meeting, San Antonio.

Woods, R.P., Cherry, S.R., and Mazziotta, J.C. (1992). Rapid automated algorithm for aligning and reslicing PET images. *Journal of Computer Assisted Tomography*, **115**, 565–87.

Yang, Y., Glover, G.H., van Gelderen, P., Mattay, V.S., Santha, A.K., Sexton, R.H., Ramsey, N.F., Moonen, C.T., Weinberger, D.R., Frank, J.A., and Duyn, J.H. (1996). Fast 3D functional magnetic resonance imaging at, 1.5 T with spiral acquisition. *Magnetic Resonance in Medicine*, **36**, 620–6.

Zhao, X., Bodurka, J., Jesmanowicz, A., and Li, S.-J. (2000). B_0-fluctuation-induced temporal variation in EPI image series due to the disturbance of steady-state free precession (SSFP). *Magnetic Resonance in Medicine*, **44**, 758–65.

7 | *Spatial and temporal resolution in fMRI*

Ravi S. Menon and Bradley G. Goodyear

7.1 *Introduction*

Most functional MRI studies to date have used relatively low resolution, both in space and time, to interrogate brain function. Typically, an in-plane resolution of 3–4 mm is used, in conjunction with slice thicknesses of 5–10 mm. This means that the typical volume element (voxel) being interrogated is on the order of 100 mm³. Additionally, a temporal resolution of several s is usually employed, due to the need to allow for T1 signal recovery between acquisitions and because of the sluggish nature of the haemodynamic response. Many brain processes occur on spatial scales that are smaller than can be readily accessed with fMRI and with temporal scales that are much faster than the haemodynamic response time. This chapter addresses the limitations imposed by the fMRI technique and suggests some strategies to improve both resolutions.

7.2 *Limits to spatial resolution in fMRI*

7.2.1 Overview of the spatial scale of human brain function

Numerous electrophysiological, autoradiographic, and blood flow studies have demonstrated that the human brain is segmented into many distinct areas that are functionally specialized (for a review, see Churchland and Sejnowski 1988). However, the spatial scale of this functional specialization varies. Some brain functions are distributed throughout an entire hemisphere. Speech and language are good examples, which are each part of a distributed network

located primarily within the left hemisphere. Other functions, such as vision and motor control, have their cortical representations located within both hemispheres, and are localized within gyri and sulci tens of millimeters in size. These sensory cortices are subdivided into a number of functionally specialized areas, each several millimetres in size. The visual cortex is perhaps the best-studied example of cortex that is organized into multiple specialized areas, namely areas V1 through V8, all of which have been successfully demonstrated using BOLD fMRI (Sereno *et al.* 1995; DeYoe *et al.* 1996; Tootell *et al.* 1996; Tootell *et al.* 1998). However, the segmentation of brain function into specialized areas can occur at an even finer resolution. A considerable amount of early sensory processing is accomplished by a complex interaction of sub-units that are less than a millimetre in size. For example, processes such as object recognition and binocular vision are both believed to be organized on a submillimetre spatial scale. Also, the segregation of visual input based on the originating eye occurs within groups of neurones arranged in columnar structures known as ocular dominance columns, which are less than a millimetre in cross-section.

Since its inception, fMRI has been used extensively to investigate the hemispherical and gyral organization of human brain function. As has been shown in the preceding chapters, BOLD fMRI is not a direct measure of neural activity, but rather is an indicator of oxygenation within the responding vasculature. It is further assumed that this haemodynamic response is co-localized to the site of neural activity. Using appropriate fMRI techniques, as discussed in Chapter 6 and highlighted in upcoming sections of this chapter, this assumption is generally valid, at least at the spatial resolution most often used in fMRI where image voxel volumes are in the range of tens of cubic millimetres. Hence, one reason for the success of fMRI in investigations of hemispherical and gryal organization of human brain function is that the fMRI response is quite robust at low spatial resolution in cases where the increases in neural activity take place on a similar spatial scale. One of the challenges of fMRI, however, is to explore the function of the human brain at submillimetre resolution. This would allow researchers to investigate the complex interactions between the functional sub-units that underlie many functions of the human brain and allow the link to be made between single-unit recording in animals and the corresponding human behaviour.

There are a number of factors to consider in order to achieve high spatial resolution with fMRI, not the least of which is minimizing signal contributions from larger vessels and localizing the source of the fMRI signal to the capillaries nearest the site of neural activity. Of course, even if the fMRI response *is* localized to the site of neural activity, it is not possible to distinguish if the underlying neural processes are excitatory or inhibitory, or whether a single BOLD activation comprises both excitatory and inhibitory components, since they are both energy-consuming. Some recent evidence suggests that inhibitory activity will not result in a BOLD signal at the site of inhibition (Waldvogel *et al.* 2000). In that case, one probably needs to look proximal to the site of inhibition at the active neurones responsible for the inhibition, or distal to the inhibited neurones to see a decrease in synaptic activity in the region where the inhibited neurones project to. This implies that the brain needs to be evaluated as a network or, at the very least, one has to know something about the relevant functional connectivity (Friston 1997). Additionally, the contributions of spiking and sub-threshold action potentials to the fMRI signal within a region are unknown. This could potentially be important for spatial localization, because subthreshold activity often extends further in space than the active spiking (Das and Gilbert 1995).

Attempts to use conventional fMRI techniques for high spatial resolution applications will most likely fail due to technical limitations of the MR scanner and the spatial limitations of the haemodynamic response to prolonged episodes of stimulation (> 6 s, say). Rather, fMRI methodology must be improved to increase the task-induced fMRI signal change while decreasing signal fluctuations unrelated to the task (i.e. increase the contrast-to-noise ratio, CNR). Further, as mentioned above, larger vessel contributions to the BOLD fMRI signal must be minimized, and the haemodynamic response must be spatially specific to the site of neural activity, which ideally should be accurate to less than a millimetre in cross-section. Within the spatial context of this chapter, these issues will be addressed within two categories. First, the spatial resolution of the haemodynamics will be discussed. Since the haemodynamics are the source of the fMRI signal, we will discuss how different sources contribute to the fMRI signal and we will review current opinion on how well localized the haemodynamic response actually is. Second, we will review fMRI techniques that can be used to eliminate unwanted contributions to the measured signal and thereby increase the CNR of the fMRI signal directly related to submillimetre neural activity. Finally, we will show an example of the high spatial resolution capabilities of fMRI in human visual cortex at 4 Tesla.

7.2.2 Spatial resolution of the haemodynamics

As discussed above, a major complication for high spatial resolution BOLD fMRI is the need to optimize sensitivity to haemodynamic responses that are co-localized to the site of neural activity. The haemodynamics that give rise to observed fMRI signal changes originate from a number of sources on both the supply (arterial) side and the draining (venous) side. The desired response is that of the capillaries embedded within the cortex which are well co-localized with the site of neural activity. On the arterial side, there are large increases in blood flow to the cortical region of increased brain activity, but these flow increases are regulated by arterial vessels that can be a centimetre or more away from the active site. Because most fMRI is not done in a fully T1 relaxed NMR state, there exists the potential that the in-flow effects in these arterioles brought about by an increased supply of unsaturated magnetization may result in signal increases that masquerade as activation changes but which are not co-localized to the neural activity. Arterial in-flow effects have been demonstrated to contaminate BOLD fMRI images under rapid RF pulsing conditions (Duyn *et al.* 1994; Kim *et al.* 1994; Frahm *et al.* 1994).

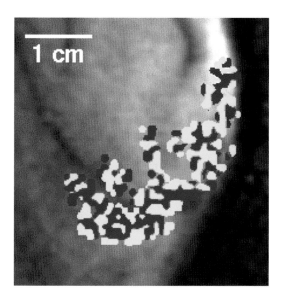

Fig. 1.7 The local perfusion changes in the brain extend beyond the aggregate of neurones activated, prompting the metaphor that the brain 'waters the entire garden for the sake of one flower'. Spatial resolution for defining activation changes on the basis of a haemodynamic response can be maximized by contrasting the haemodynamic responses from adjacent aggregates of neurones with a subtraction procedure. Common areas of activation that are non-specifically perfused by the haemodynamic response in adjacent territories are nulled, highlighting activations very local to the areas recruited. This is nicely demonstrated by results from this study in which the visual cortical activation with stimulation of alternate eyes was subtracted, yielding high spatial resolution maps of the ocular dominance columns. (Image courtesy of Dr Ravi Menon, University of Western Ontario).

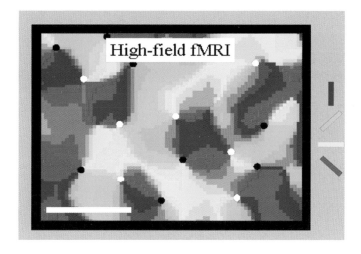

Fig. 1.8 The time course for the haemodynamic response in the visual cortex begins with a decrease in signal over approximately the first second after stimulation. By comparison of the time course of a gradient echo MRI sequence with that from optical imaging studies in animals, it has been suggested that this early decrease in signal is related to a transient increase in oxygen extraction fraction from blood in capillaries local to the area of neuronal activation occurring as a direct result of the increase in oxidative metabolism. It is argued that because such an increase in oxygen extraction can occur only within oxygen diffusion distance of activated cells, mapping the cortical volume that shows this decreased signal provides a more localized measure of the region of cotical activation than does the later increase signal resulting from the subsequent hyperaemia. This image shows cortical columns in the cat visual cortex mapped out on the basis of the early negative response in BOLD fMRI using a 4.7 Tesla imaging system. Cats were exposed to moving grating stimuli with different orientations, as illustrated in the colour boxes to the *right*. The composite angle map was attained through pixel-by-pixel vector addition of the four single orientation maps to display the resulting orientation preference at each cortical location. There is an interruption of the smooth changes in preferred orientations along the cortical surface at so-called 'orientation pinwheels', where cortical columns for different orientations are arranged in a circular manner. These generate two types of topological singularities based on their rotational symmetries. White and black circles represent clockwise and counter-clockwise pinwheels, respectively. The scale bar shown represents 1 mm. (Image courtesy of Dr D.S. Kim, T.Q. Duong and S-G. Kim of the University of Minnesota.)

(a) (b) (c)

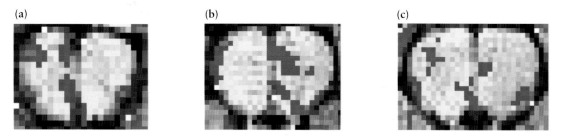

Fig. 1.10 Animal studies offer considerable scope for linking electrophysiological methods with fMRI. These images display activation patterns resulting from direct cortical stimulation in the sensorimotor cortex using a carbon fibre electrode that was positioned through a small craniotomy hole directly on the cortex over the area of activation shown in the upper left of (a). Activation of cortex immediately beneath the stimulating fibre is apparent. In subsequent 2 mm sections immediately behind the area of stimulation (b, c) it is clear that activation occurs both in the area of stimulation and in more distant sides, particularly involving the deep basal ganglia. Such methods may allow functional definition of brain connectivities. (Image courtesy of Ms Vivienne Austen, MRC Clinical and Biochemical MRS Unit and FMRIB Centre, Oxford.)

(a) (b) (c)

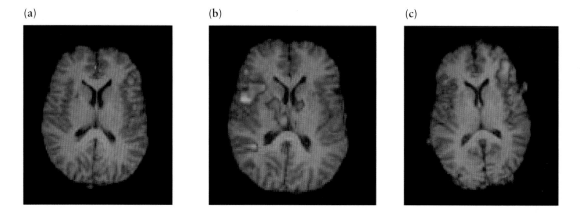

Fig. 1.11 The invasive Wada test is used to evaluate the lateralization of language and memory function in patients with temporal lobe epilepsy prior to possible surgery in order to minimize any potential for disability from the temporal lobe excision. There has been considerable interest in developing a non-invasive, fMRI-based method for lateralising language and memory functions. Here relative shifts in lateralization of brain activations in a verbal fluency task are illustrated. Each subject was presented with a visual letter cue and asked to recall as many words beginning with that letter during the active block of the fMRI paradigm. (a) A right-handed subject with right temporal lobe epilepsy demonstrates the pattern found in most healthy right- and left-handed controls showing almost entirely left-sided lateralization at this level of the brain, which includes Broca's area. (b) In contrast, a left-handed patient with left temporal lobe epilepsy demonstrates an almost complete shift in lateralization of activation to the right hemisphere. Here there is a more widely distributed pattern of activation at the same level, suggesting increased activation in more widely distributed nodes of the language network. (c) A right-handed patient with left temporal lobe epilepsy shows a bi-hemispheric pattern, suggesting that right hemispheric nodes in the putative language network become more active with damage to the left temporal lobe. (Images courtesy of Dr Jane Adcock, University of Oxford.)

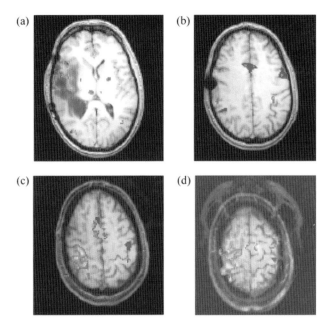

Fig. 1.12 Patterns of activation in patients with brain lesions may be useful in guiding neurosurgical excisions. This patient presented with a gliablastoma which was resected. With possible progression of the tumour the question of whether the excision margins could be extended arose. A concern was that the motor representation for movement of the contralateral (left) hand was too close to the excision margins to allow safe removal without subsequent disability. The patient then was studied using an FMRI paradigm involving simple movements of fingers of the left hand. The areas of significant activation are shown in blue. As can be seen particularly in images (b), (c) and (d), the patient (*blue*) shows predominantly ipsilateral cortical activation with movement of the hand. In contrast, healthy controls show predominantly contralateral sensorimotor cortex activation (*orange*). Panels (a) and (b) show loss of signal near the areas where the skull was interrupted by the craniotomy, a consequence of local magnetic susceptibility differences. (Images courtesy of Dr R. Pineiro, FMRIB Centre, Oxford.)

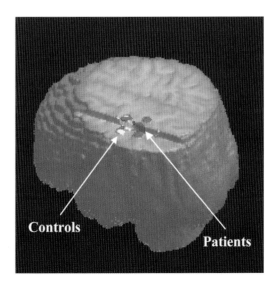

Fig. 1.13 Brain injury can lead to local adaptive changes in activation patterns from cortical 'plasticity' that can occur even in adults. This image illustrates a posterior shift in the centre of activation in the sensorimotor cortex for patients with established multiple sclerosis relative to a healthy control group. The yellow areas represent the mean centres of activation for a group of normal controls and the red areas shifted on average just under 1 cm more posterior) show similar centres of activation for a group of patients with established multiple sclerosis. Anatomically, this represents a shift in activation from the posterior wall of the pre-central gyrus in healthy controls to the anterior wall of the post-central gyrus in the patients. (Image courtesy of Drs H. Reddy and M. Lee, FMRIB Centre, Oxford.)

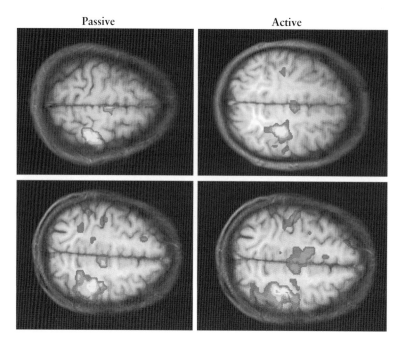

Passive   Active

Fig. 1.14 A major problem in studies of patients with disability from brain pathology is that of matching tasks between patients and controls to ensure that brain activation patterns represent responses to behaviourally comparable actions. One approach to the study of motor tasks may be to use the patterns of activation associated with passive movement of a limb. Because of the rich feedback from somatosensory and proprioceptive afferents to motor areas, activation patterns with passive movements generally recapitulate those accompanying active movement. Illustrated here are patterns of activation with either active (*upper panels*) or passive (*lower panels*) movements of a digit of the hand. (Images courtesy of Ms A. Floyer and Dr H. Reddy, FMRIB Centre Oxford.)

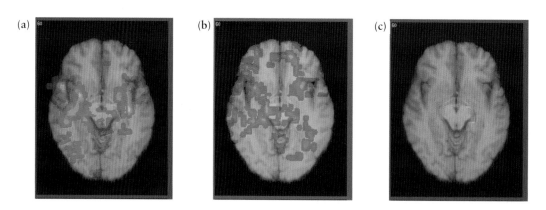

Fig. 1.15 One of the most exciting frontiers for fMRI is the objective description of subjective sensory experiences. A related area of excitement is the use of fMRI to assess the effects of pharmacological interventions. Here responses of the brain to a painful thermal stimulus are mapped using fMRI during intravenous infusion of a saline placebo (a). With infusion of 0.5 ng of the opiate analgesic remifentanil, there is small change in the pattern of activation, but the total volume of activation is little different from that with placebo and the subject reports little change in subjective pain perception (b). However, with infusion of 1 ng of remifentanil there is no subjective sensation of pain with the identical thermal stimulus. Associated with this is a loss of activation in this image slice, which includes the insula. (Images courtesy of Dr I. Tracey, FMRIB Centre, Oxford.)

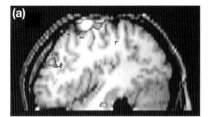 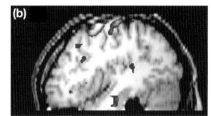

Fig. 4.9   PRESTO fMRI data, acquired with and without SENSE, overlaid on T1-weighted images acquired using the same resolution as the functional scan in order to demonstrate the spatial resolution of the functional sequence. The PRESTO parameters were TR = 24 ms, TE = 40 ms, θ = 9° and a voxel size of 3.5 × 3.5 × 3.5 mm³. Using a synergy coil consisting of two 20 cm surface coils placed on either side of the head both a two shot conventional PRESTO sequence: (a) matrix 64 × 48 × 30, 80 per cent rFOV, EPI Factor = 23, acquisition time = 2s, and a single shot PRESTO-SENSE sequence; (b) matrix 64 × 24 × 30, 40 per cent rFOV, EPI Factor 23, acquisition time = 1 s, SENSE factor = 2, were acquired. The coil sensitivities needed for the SENSE reconstruction were obtained by using the body coil to acquire an image with the same parameters. The fMRI paradigm consisted of finger-to-thumb opposition, with three activation periods interleaved with 3 resting periods, each of 20 s, leading to a total scan time of 2 min for both imaging sequences (60 or 120 dynamic scans respectively). All volumes were registered and spatially smoothed with a 6 mm Gaussian filter; *t* maps were then calculated and thresholded at p < 0.05. (Images courtesy of Xavier Golay, ETH, Zurich).

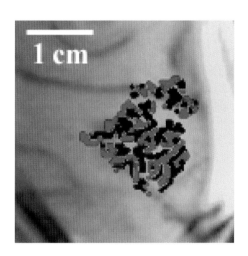

Fig. 7.1   Maps of ocular dominance along the medical bank of the right occipital cortex overlaid on structural MR images. Blue (red) represents image pixels whose fMRI response was greater in magnitude during left (right) eye stimulation. The image has been cropped for clarity. The back of the head is to the right of the image. In the calcarine sulcus, the map pixels of ocular dominance appear as stripes, consistent with the known columnar architecture of ocular dominance within the primary visual cortex. The functional image resolution in this case was 0.55 x 0.55 x 3mm³

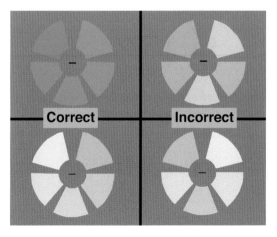

Fig. 10.2   Stimuli used by Beauchamp and colleagues in their colour discrimination task.

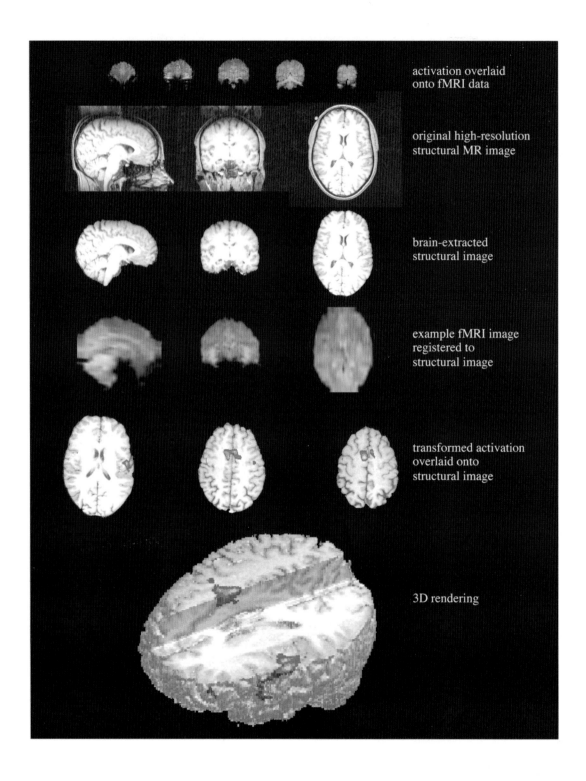

activation overlaid
onto fMRI data

original high-resolution
structural MR image

brain-extracted
structural image

example fMRI image
registered to
structural image

transformed activation
overlaid onto
structural image

3D rendering

Fig. 11.10   Various stages in the rendering of activation onto a high-resolution structural image.

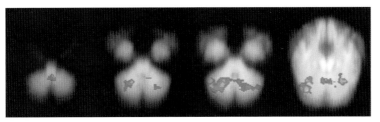

Fig. 11.12   Significant differences between the two subject groups in the pain-warm contrast.

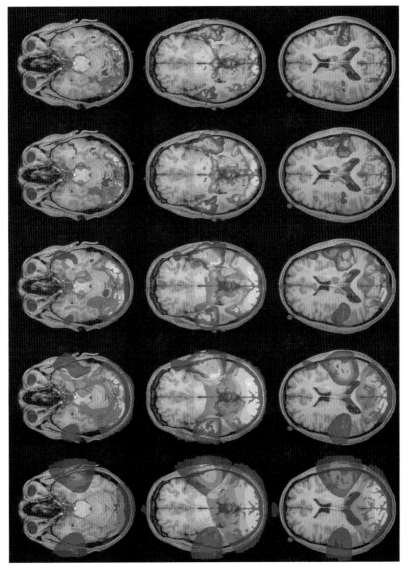

Fig. 12.5   Significant clusters of activation (Z > 2.3, P < 0.01) from an audiovisual experiment. The different rows were produced by processing with different spatial scales—filters of 0 (no filtering), 5, 10, 20, and 40 mm FWHM (from top row to bottom respectively). Red clusters show visual activation; blue clusters show auditory activation.

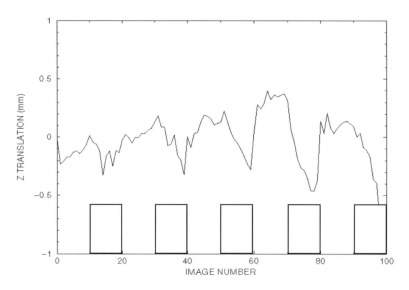

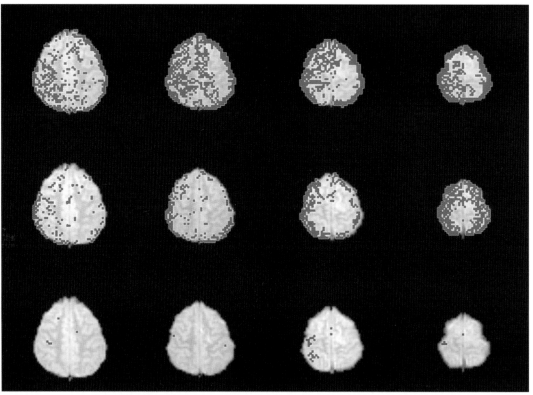

Fig. 13.1 Motion correction in a finger tapping experiment. Fig. 1(a) (*upper figure*) shows the motion component (z translation) exhibiting the strongest stimulus-correlated motion. The experimental 'on' periods are shown at the bottom of the figure. Fig. 1(b) (*lower figure*) shows a set of superior axial images with no correction (*top row*), after realignment only (*middle row*) and following full correction (*bottom row*).

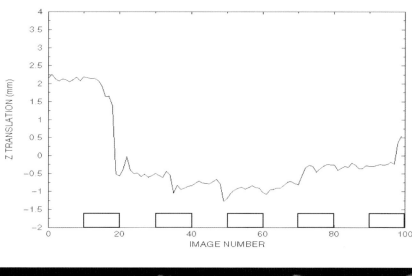

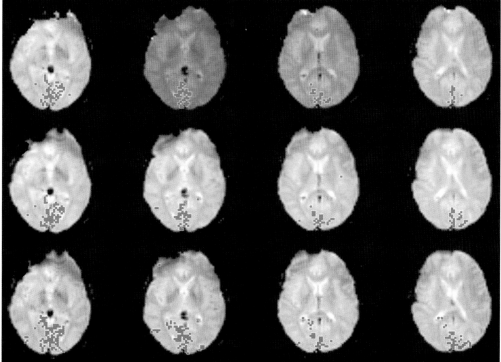

Fig. 13.2 Motion correction in a visual stimulation experiment. Fig. 2(a) (*upper figure*) shows the motion component (z translation) exhibiting the strongest stimulus-correlated motion. The experimental 'on' periods are shown at the bottom. Fig. 2(b) (*lower figure*) shows a set of superior axial images with no correction (*top row*), after realignment only (*middle row*) and following full correction (*bottom row*).

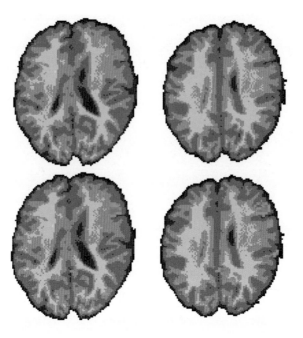

Fig. 13.3 Two slices from a group activation map (n = 6) in schizophrenic patients before (*upper row*) and after (*lower row*) group correction for subject motion.

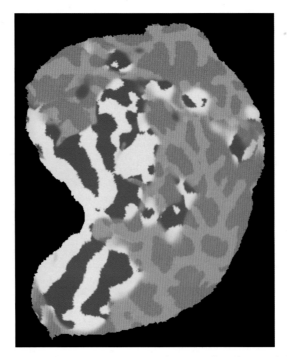

Fig. 15.18 An example of 'flattened activation' courtesy of R. Tootell and N. Hadjikhani. The different parts of the visual cortex are identified using phase-encoded visual stimulation.

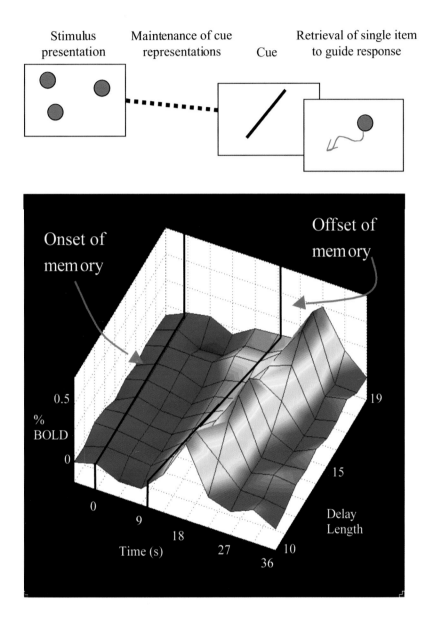

Fig. 17.3 Procedure and selected results adapted from Rowe *et al.* (2000). Subjects were required to memorize the positions of three dots presented on a screen (*top row*) and hold this information in memory for several seconds (see text). At the end of the delay period a line presented on the screen indicated to the subjects which of the three locations was to be recalled (but did not reveal its exact location, which was somewhere on that line). Subjects were then presented with a single dot and were required to move it to the required location. The data were modelled such that transient neuronal activations in the prefrontal cortex in response to selections from memory (*shown in lower part of figure*), could be reliably distinguished from sustained activation during the memory delay.

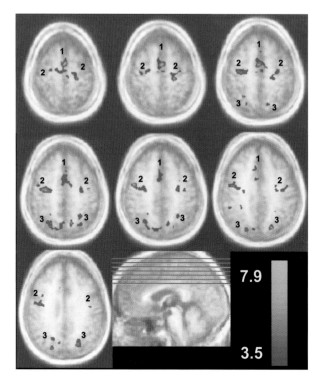

Fig. 18.1 Group activation map of a group (n=10) of adults performing the VGS paradigm (see p.332) analysed by a simple t-test (t threshold > 3.5) after excluding the 6 s transition periods. The supplementary eye fields (1), frontal eye fields (2) and intraparietal sulcus (3) are identified.

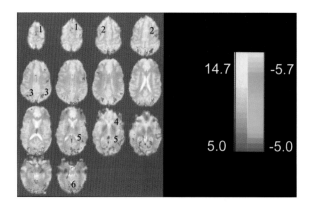

Fig. 18.2 Representative activation map of a normal adult performing the reading task paradigm (see p.333) analysed by a simple t-test (threshold > 5.0) after excluding the 6 second transition periods. In addition to the supplementary eye fields (1), frontal eye fields (2), and intraparietal sulcus (3), Broca's area (4) and Wernicke's area (5) and often the contralateral homologous areas are identified. Primary and association visual cortices (6) are identified.

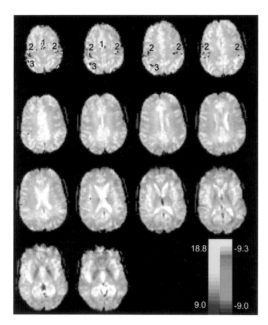

Fig. 18.3 Representative activation map of a normal adult performing the finger taping paradigm (see p. 334) analysed by a simple t-test (threshold > 9.0) after excluding the 6 s transition periods. The supplementary motor area (1), primary motor area (2) and primary somatosensory cortex (3) are identified.

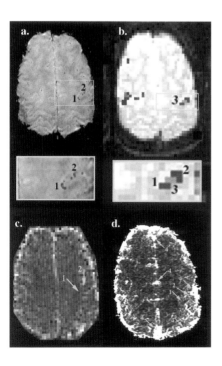

Fig. 18.5 Activation maps through the frontal eye fields from (a) high-resolution fMRI and (b) low-resolution using the VGS paradigm on the same subject. The gradient-echo echo planar imaging was performed with acquisition parameters: TR 3000 ms, TE 25 ms, with voxels dimensions of 0.8 x 1.6 x 3.0 mm, and 3.1 x 3.1 x 3.0 mm, respectively. Corresponding (c) apparent diffusion coefficient maps from diffusion weighted imaging and (d) high resolution venograms were obtained and used to localize tissue properties of the activation areas as shown in Table 18.1. The locations of the voxels with maximum t-value for the two clusters in the left frontal eye field on the high resolution map (1,2) are shown along with the voxel (3) at the center of the single equivalent cluster on low resolution image. These areas are projected onto the diffusion map and venogram. Areas (4) on the venogram represent veins.

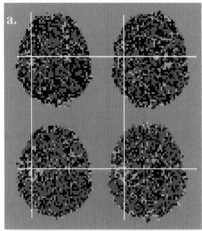

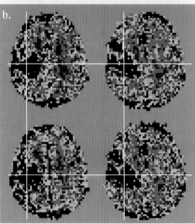

Fig. 18.8 (a) Selected adjacent slices from the TTT perfusion parametric map through the AVM (centre marked by crosshairs) for the pre-vasodilation (upper row) and post-vasodilation (lower row). The color scale graded in seconds is: black, 0–5 s; blue, 5–10 s; green, 10–15 s; pink, 15–20 s; red, 20–25 s; and yellow, >25 s. The displacement of blue voxels by green voxels is clearly evident, indicating vasodilation with concomitant longer transition times in all areas including the AVM. Thus perfusion reserve appears to be maintained. (b) Selected adjacent slices from the rCBV perfusion parametric map through the AVM (centre marked by crosshairs) for the pre-vasodilation (upper row) and post-vasodilation (lower row). The color scale is a relative scale of: blue, 1–50; green, 50–100; pink, 100–150; red, 150–200; yellow, 200–250 s and black, >200. The trend from low blood volumes (blue and green colors) to higher blood volumes (pink, yellow and black colors) is evident up to the edge of the AVM, indicating a relative haemodynamic reserve in all areas despite the AVM.

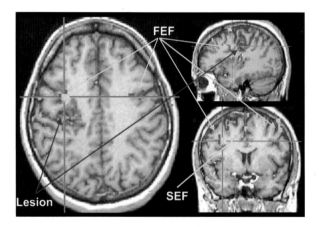

Fig. 18.9 Axial, sagittal and coronal activation maps through the right frontal eye field (FEF) showing the relative positions of the FEF and supplementary eye fields (SEF) to the AVM (lesion, red arrows) of Case 1. The t-statistic (threshold of 3.5) is displayed as a color scale: yellow > red > 3.5. The green lines show the relative location of each mapping plane. This presentation was derived from AFNI software.

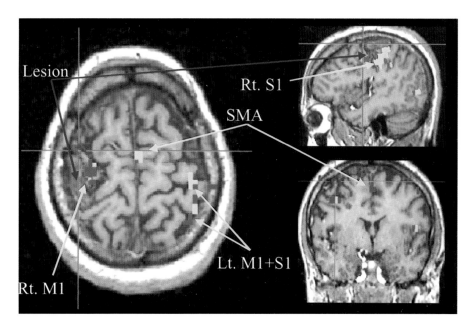

Fig. 18.10 Axial, sagittal and coronal activation maps through the right motor cortex (M1) showing the relative positions of M1 and supplementary motor area (SMA) to the AVM (lesion, red arrows) of Case 1. The t-threshold was set at 3.5 and is displayed as a color scale: yellow > red > 3.5. The green lines show the relative locations of each plane. The SMA is posterior to SEF shown in Fig. 18.9. M1 is posterior to FEF but anterior to the lesion. The left M1 and S1 were also strongly activated whereas this only weakly occurs in normal subjects. The right S1 (shown on the sagittal map) identified on a more inferior axial slice is posterior to the AVM.

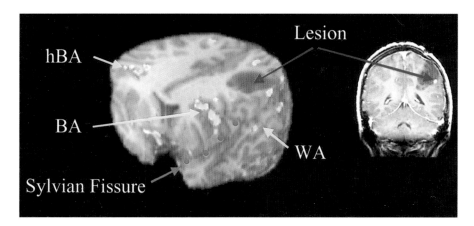

Fig. 18.13 Three-dimensional (3D) rendering of the activation map for Case 2. The exposed axial, coronal and sagittal planes through the AVM (lesion, red arrows) show the lesion's relative position to Wernicke's area (WA, posterior left superior temporal gyrus), Broca's area (BA, left inferior frontal lobe) and homologous Broca's area (hBA, right frontal lobe) and the Sylvian fissure (green dots). The t-threshold was set at 3.5 and is displayed as a color scale: yellow > red > 3.5. The coronal contrast enhanced image to the right shows the gadolinium contrast-enhancing nodule medial and superior to WA. This 3D presentation is an alternative presentation to three planes of Figures 18-9 and 18-10 and is also derived from AFNI software.

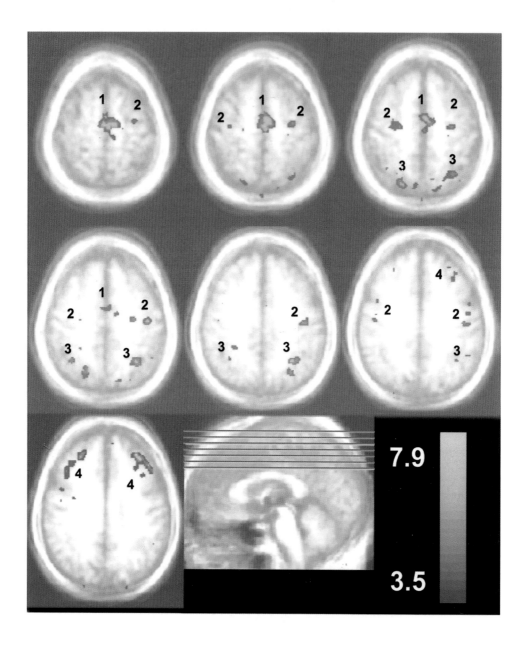

Fig. 18.14 Group activation map for a group of patients with Alzheimer's disease in which the group averages of the activation and the structural studies are superimposed. Such a group analysis is readily performed with AFNI software.

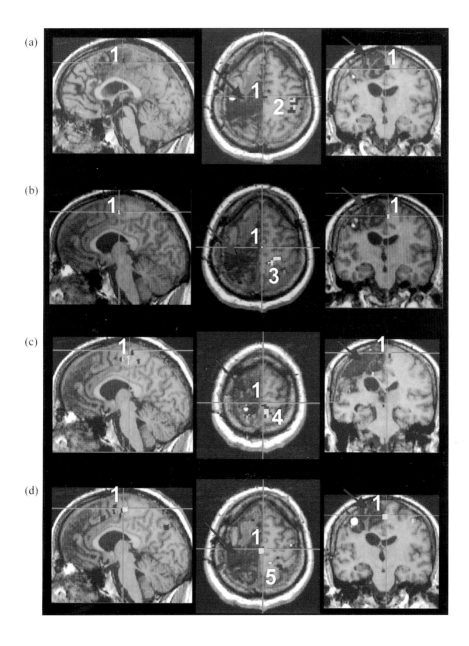

Fig. 18.16 Sagittal, axial and coronal activation maps for Case 3 through the supplementary motor cortex (1, SMA) and primary motor and somatosensory cortex of the left hemisphere in response to movement of the right upper (2), left upper (3), right lower (4) and left lower (5) extremities. The green lines show the relative locations of the three planes. This mapping shows robust activation elicited by movement of the left extremities in the left hemisphere adjacent to areas activated by the right extremities. The strokectomy (red arrows) clearly shows that the right motor cortex was resected. The patient was able to walk with a cane at 4 weeks following strokectomy suggesting that recovery was supported by redistribution of the cognitive workload to the left hemisphere.

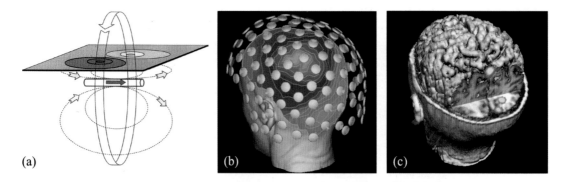

Fig. 19.1 Neural electromagnetic source localization. (a) Neuronal transmembrane currents give rise to longitudinal intracellular currents and extracellular volume return currents. A detectable magnetic field is associated with the intracellular current; extracellular currents tend to cancel in a spherical conducting volume. The extrema of the observed magnetic field distribution straddle and are orthogonal to the source current element. Extrema in the potential distribution are aligned with the current. (b) An array of electrodes or SQUID-based magnetic field detectors are positioned on or over the surface of the head. Potential and field distributions consistent with one or more simple dipole-like sources are often observed. (c) A source model based on a time-varying set of equivalent current dipoles is fit to the observed field distribution. In this figure, the uncertainty of source localization due to noise was estimated using Monte Carlo techniques and a 3D histogram of ECD location was constructed.

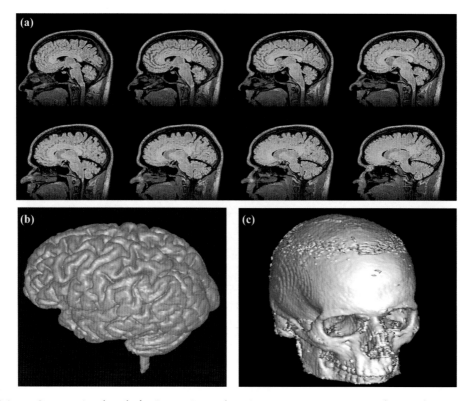

Fig. 19.2 Computational tools for interactive and semi-automatic segmentation of cortical anatomy allow extraction of computational geometries. (a) Region growing algorithms with adaptive criteria perform segmentation of white matter, and identification of grey matter by dilation. (b) 3D rendering of the cortical surface identified by an automatic algorithm. (c) Rendering of the skull segmented by region growing techniques from 3D MRI data.

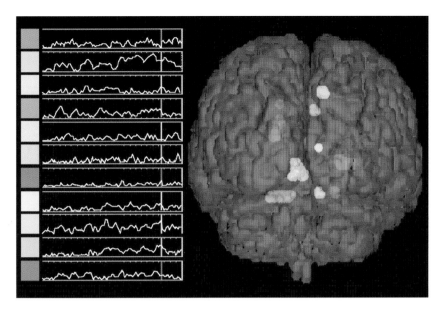

Fig. 19.4 Time courses of fMRI equivalent sources estimated from MEG data. FMRI visual data were acquired using blocked steady state stimulation, using the same video display as in a previous MEG experiment. Currents were assumed to vary within the source according to the distribution of FMRI activation. Currents were constrained to lie normal to cortex as indicated by anatomical MRI. Topographies were derived for each of the assumed sources, and used as basis functions for a linear decomposition of the time-varying field maps. Estimated time courses for 11 areas are coded in colour.

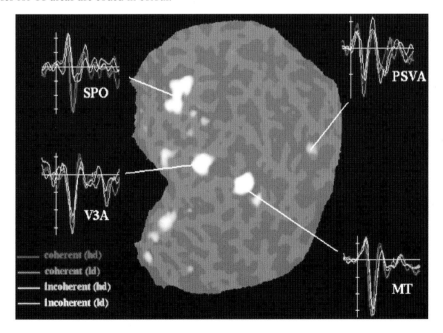

Fig. 19.5 MEG timecourses of fMRI sources using a weighted minimum norm procedure. Areas of activation from a visual fMRI experiment (involving visual motion) are shown on an unfolded cortex. A 0.9:0.1 weighted pseudoinverse procedure was applied to field maps at each time point. Estimated timecourses for activation in four identified visual areas are illustrated. Differences as a function of stimulus type are coded in color. (Data courtesy of Anders Dale and colleagues, Massachusetts General Hospital NMR Centre, Boston).

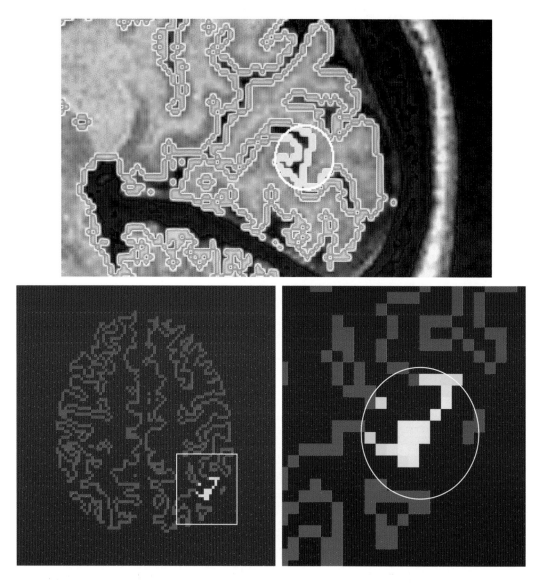

Fig. 19.7 Extended parametric source model used for Bayesian inference. A source defined by the intersection of cortex with a sphere centred on cortex. Note that adjacent sides of a sulcus or gyrus are often labeled together for extended sources. A source defined by a patch grown on the cortical surface. A location on cortex is seeded and adjacent bands of voxels are labeled in a series of dilation operations.

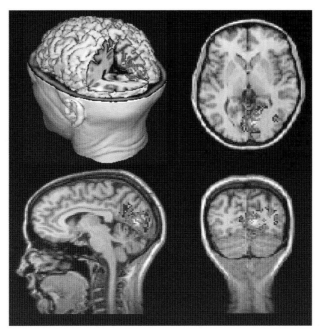

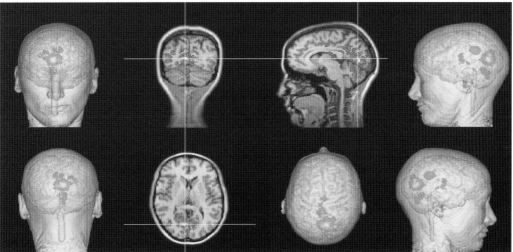

Fig. 19.8 Source probability maps estimated for visual evoked response data. Four views of a region found to contain activity at a 95 per cent probability level. This example is for left visual field stimulation. For right field stimulation, the most probable source is lateralized to the left hemisphere calcarine. Interactive visualization of spatial-temporal source probability maps co-registered with anatomical MRI for the same subject. The anatomical data set was used in the Bayesian inference procedure to constrain sources to lie in cortex.

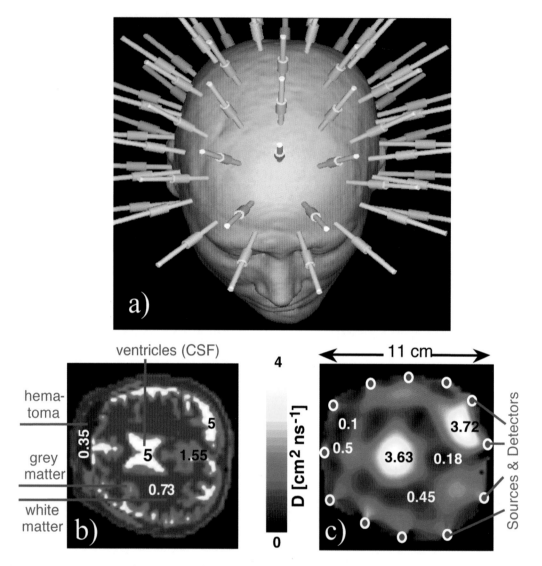

Fig. 19.12 Noninvasive dynamic optical imaging and time-resolved optical tomography. (a) Fiber optics in an array over the surface of the head are used as sources and detectors. Time resolved illumination and detection methods allow tomographic reconstruction or quantitative spectroscopy. Continuous wave methods (i.e. steady illumination and continuous detection) allow dynamic topographic imaging of haemodynamics and fast intrinsic neural signals. (b–c) Path length resolved optical techniques (time-resolved or frequency domain) can be employed for tomographic reconstruction. This reconstruction example used simulated data based on a MRI image (b) containing a haematoma as well as clear cerebral spinal fluid. The simulated optical data consisted of one source and eleven detectors for each of 12 source locations. Reconstructed data (c) captures the major features of the simulated medium although at low resolution.

In addition to the arterial side, larger draining veins that may be up to several centimetres away from the site of neural activity may also contribute to the measured BOLD fMRI signal (Lai *et al.* 1993; Menon *et al.* 1993; Segebarth *et al.* 1994; Lee *et al.* 1995). The problem arises because as the hyperoxygenated blood leaves the capillaries it drains into venules and veins whose volume can be a significant fraction of the volume in a voxel. Voxels with larger volume fractions are more easily detected by the statistical tests used in fMRI, even though there is usually dilution from the blood coming from other nonactivated areas. This effect can extend quite far, with the sagittal sinus often appearing 'activated' in fMRI experiements. This source of signal change is clearly not desired (Jueptner and Weiller 1995). The localization problem is further compounded by the statistics of detection. For example, the comparison of maps of brain function obtained using perfusion-based fMRI techniques with those obtained using BOLD fMRI has demonstrated that large BOLD signal changes are often associated with large draining veins, while tissue areas have low BOLD signal changes (Kim *et al.* 1997*a*). Hence, when high spatial resolution is employed, the resulting drop in signal-to-noise ratio (SNR) and contrast-to-noise ratio (CNR) means that only pixels exhibiting a large percentage change in signal will be detectable, and hence large vessels will dominate BOLD maps of brain function.

Optical imaging of intrinsic signals (OIS) has demonstrated that subsequent to the onset of neural activity, there is actually a transient increase in the tissue concentration of deoxyhaemoglobin caused by an increase in local oxygen consumption which precedes any commensurate change in blood flow or volume, resulting in a brief hypo-oxic state (Malonek and Grinvald 1996). (See also Chapter 8 for a discussion of this 'initial dip'). Several seconds later, in response to the increased metabolic demand, there is a vasodilation of the arterioles which results in a large fractional increase in cerebral blood flow (CBF). This CBF increase overcompensates for the increase in local oxygen consumption and leads to blood hyperoxygenation and the standard positive BOLD response. This temporal signature of initial dip in signal followed by positive BOLD increase is thought to correspond to that seen in fMRI studies of the visual system at very high magnetic fields (Menon *et al.* 1995; Hu *et al.*

1997). Thus, the haemodynamic response to neural activity is actually biphasic, an early hypo-oxic phase, termed the 'initial dip' (Menon *et al.* 1995; Malonek and Grinvald 1996; Hu *et al.* 1997), followed by a more pronounced hyperoxic phase. It is argued that the 'initial dip' is more spatially specific to the source of neuronal activity than the hyperoxic phase because while metabolic changes that give rise to the increased oxygen consumption are well co-localized with the neural activity, the spatial distribution of the resulting vascular flow response is not tightly coupled to neural activity. The 'initial dip' is very small and extremely difficult to map by MRI, even at 4 Tesla (~10 per cent of the amplitude of the familiar positive BOLD signal). Thus, for most experiments it is the latter phase that is used to make maps of human brain function in fMRI studies. However, careful studies have demonstrated that the 'initial dip' *is* resolvable within human visual cortex if sufficient signal averaging is performed (Hu *et al.* 1997; Yacoub and Hu 1999). More recently, fMRI studies at high magnetic field strengths of 4.7 and 9.4 Tesla have demonstrated that the 'initial dip' is detectable within cat visual cortex and can be used to resolve iso-orientation columns on a spatial scale of 100–200 μm (Duong *et al.* 2000; Kim *et al.* 2000).

Several studies commenting on the poor functional resolution capabilities of fMRI using the hyperoxic phase have employed stimuli of at least 10 s in duration to increase CNR (Engel *et al.* 1997; Kim *et al.* 2000), leading to a saturation of the hyperoxic response. When the hyperoxic phase of the haemodynamic response to neural activity reaches a plateau at 5 to 8 s after the onset of stimulation (Liu *et al.* 2000), the measured fMRI signal extends to areas well beyond the site of the excited neural tissue, making functional resolution at a submillimetre scale unlikely (however, see Cheng *et al.* 1999). If stimulation is brief (less than 4 s), the locus of neural activity may still be resolvable, at least from adjacent areas that are activated under an orthogonal stimulus condition. The use of short duration stimuli prevents the BOLD response from saturating and permits the use of peak fMRI signal magnitude as a measure of the amount of neural activity within a voxel (Boynton *et al.* 1996). The potential of short duration stimuli for submillimetre resolution studies has been shown in previous work demonstrating the temporal progression of functional maps obtained by optical imaging of intrinsic signals

(Grinvald *et al.* 1986; Frostig *et al.* 1990) and fMRI (Hu *et al.* 1997).

7.2.3 Spatial resolution of BOLD fMRI techniques

In a very elegant series of experiments characterizing the modulation transfer function in the visual system, Engel *et al.* (1997) showed that the fMRI signal could be localized to within 1.1 mm at 1.5 Tesla. As they also point out, this limit depends on the signal-to-noise ratio of the measurement and that there is no theoretical limit why it cannot be extended. There are a number of techniques that can be employed to increase CNR and minimize unwanted contributions to the BOLD fMRI signal. With regard to minimizing the contribution of large draining veins, these techniques involve modifications to the pulse sequence, as described in Chapter 6. The contribution of the 'inflow' of fresh blood into the imaging plane can be eliminated by pulsing slowly relative to the T1 recovery time after RF excitation. Additionally, inversion recovery-based fMRI techniques have shown that careful adjustment of the inversion recovery time can produce functional maps that are dominated by tissue areas rather than large vessels (Kim and Tsekos 1997). Alternatively, spin echo-based techniques can be used instead of conventional gradient-recalled echo-based techniques to refocus signal from stationary tissue at the time of the spin echo, while spins of fast flowing components dephase and are not refocused. One way to minimize macrovascular contributions is to use bipolar (flow crushing) gradients. However, it has been demonstrated that at a magnetic field strength of 1.5 Tesla, the use of bipolar gradients eliminates either all or the majority of the BOLD fMRI response, suggesting that macrovascular components are the dominant contributor to BOLD fMRI signals at this magnetic field strength (Boxerman *et al.* 1995). At high magnetic field strength (e.g. 4 Tesla), however, BOLD signal changes persist in the presence of flow crushing gradients, suggesting that extravascular and intravascular components coexist at high fields (Menon *et al.* 1994). The dependence of BOLD fMRI contrast on magnetic field strength has been studied in some detail (Gati *et al.* 1997), suggesting that in order to increase microvascular contributions to the BOLD signal a high static magnetic field strength (at least 3 or 4 Tesla)

should be used. Thus, the microvascular sensitivity that is associated with very high field scanners will likely be necessary to map at the columnar level. In addition to using high static magnetic field strength, BOLD fMRI contrast at submillimetre resolution can be enhanced through a number of other technical implementations. Quadrature surface coils (Lin *et al.* 1998) provide considerable SNR gains over head volume coils for cortical regions near the skull. However, since image signal decays rapidly with distance from a surface coil, head motion correction is difficult to implement due to gross differences in intensity throughout the image. Motion correction algorithms are beginning to address this problem (Nestares and Heeger 2000).

To increase CNR, physiological noise suppression schemes are necessary to remove fluctuations of image intensity caused by respiration and cardiac pulsation that mask the task-induced BOLD response and introduce spatial and temporal correlations in the data (Hu and Kim 1994; Le and Hu 1996; Glover *et al.* 2000).

Another consideration is the time it takes to collect high-resolution data. If all data necessary to reconstruct one high resolution image were collected after one RF excitation, as is the case with low resolution snap-shot EPI, there would be considerable blurring in the image due to signal decay over the time to collect the data (commonly referred to as T2* blurring). Hence, multi-shot EPI is favorable for collecting high resolution images in order to minimize this intrinsic blur (Menon *et al.* 1997; Menon and Goodyear 1999). Using these techniques, the spatial resolution capabilities of fMRI can be greatly enhanced. Ultimately, it is expected that the lateral connections in the horizontal layers of the cortex, as well as the vascular density (Zheng *et al.* 1991), will set the limiting resolution in fMRI, and these can vary in different areas of the brain.

7.2.4 Resolving ocular dominance columns within human visual cortex

An example of current high spatial resolution capabilities at 4 Tesla is shown in Fig. 7.1. This midline sagittal fMRI map and image of the right bank of the occipital pole of a normal volunteer shows ocular dominance stripes, corresponding to left and right eye inputs, that look very much like those seen in optical imaging (Grinvald *et al.* 1986; Frostig *et al.* 1990) and

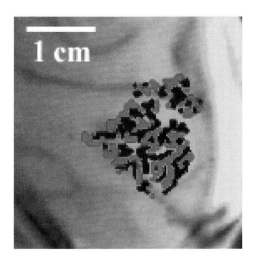

Fig. 7.1 Maps of ocular dominance along the medial bank of the right occipital cortex overlaid on structural MR images. Blue (red) represents image pixels whose fMRI response was greater in magnitude during right (left) eye stimulation than during left (right) eye stimulation. The image has been cropped for clarity. The back of the head is to the right of the image. In the calcarine sulcus, the map pixels of ocular dominance appear as stripes, consistent with the known columnar architecture of ocular dominance within the primary visual cortex. The functional image resolution in this case was $0.55 \times 0.55 \times 3$ mm^3. (See also colour plate section.)

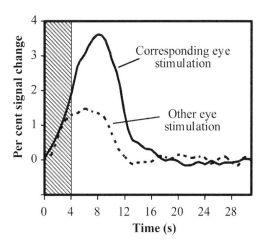

Fig. 7.2 Average time course of MR signal over one trial (expressed as a percentage change from baseline) within ocular dominant image pixels for one subject, as in Fig. 7.1. Corresponding (other) eye stimulation refers to blue (red) pixels during right eye stimulation and to red (blue) pixels during left eye stimulation. The hashed region indicates the duration of the visual stimulus (4 s).

post mortem studies (Horton *et al.* 1990). Figure 7.2 shows the time course of the fMRI signal from pixels within the ocular dominance map (as in Fig. 7.1) averaged over all stimulation trials. The stimulus duration in this case was 4 s. Notice that the magnitude of the fMRI response using a 4-s stimulus does not reach a plateau. The temporal resolution of the image time course (1 s) was insufficient to detect the 'initial dip'. The peak magnitude of the fMRI response when the eye corresponding to the pixel designation was stimulated (i.e. a red pixel during left eye stimulation and a blue pixel during right eye stimulation) is nearly three times the peak magnitude of the fMRI response within the same pixel when the fellow eye was stimulated (i.e. a red pixel during right eye stimulation and a blue pixel during left eye stimulation). We term the ratio of these responses as the 'fMRI response ratio'. A possible explanation for the non-zero signal within adjacent (other eye) image pixels in Fig. 7.2 is that even though the locus of the haemodynamic response may be within an ocular dominance column corresponding to

the eye being stimulated, there is a spill-over of the haemodynamic response into adjacent cortex corresponding to the other eye. If the duration of the stimulus is increased, this spill-over increases, as suggested in Fig. 7.3. As the duration of the stimulus increases, the fMRI response ratio approaches a value of approximately 1.96, as predicted by a randomly generated set of data simulating the fMRI response magnitude. Only for a stimulus duration of 2 or 4 s is the fMRI response ratio significantly greater ($p < 0.05$) than the ratio for a random data set. In fact, the stimulus duration at which the fMRI response ratio becomes the same as that predicted by random data closely corresponds to the time at which the hyperoxic phase of the haemodynamic response saturates, at which point functional resolution at submillimetre resolution becomes unachievable (however, see Cheng *et al.* 1999; Dechent and Frahm 2000).

It is important to stress that these results do not suggest that the hyperoxic phase of the haemodynamic response is as spatially specific as the initial hypo-oxic phase. Rather, a non-saturated hyperoxic response is capable of resolving adjacent and functionally different areas of neural activity with relatively high precision. Using the 'initial dip' is most likely to be better suited

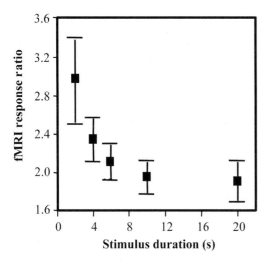

Fig. 7.3 The ratio of the average magnitude of the fMRI response within a blue (red) pixel during right (left) eye stimulation to the average magnitude of the fMRI response within the same pixel during left (right) eye stimulation (termed the 'fMRI response ratio') as a function of stimulus duration. Error bars indicate the standard error of the mean for all pixels in each functional map.

to accurate localization of the boundaries of a functional unit (i.e. determining where a functional unit is and where it is not). This is because the relative difference between the magnitude of signal in the active vs. non-active state is much higher and is independent of stimulus duration (see for example, Grinvald *et al.* 1986). However, it is suggested that using differential hyperoxic BOLD imaging techniques to resolve adjacent functional units may result in label reversal (Duong *et al.* 2000). This is a consequence of the complex dependence of the BOLD response on $CMRO_2$ changes, potentially causing the point spread function of the BOLD susceptibility effect to result in a larger BOLD response in inactive tissue rather than in active tissue. This remains to be confirmed by simultaneously measuring the BOLD and CBF responses. With further hardware improvements (e.g. higher gradient switching speed and more stable ultra-high static fields), it should become possible to make a direct comparison of maps created using the 'initial dip', the unsaturated BOLD response, and CBF response. Nonetheless, the fMRI technique is quickly becoming a feasible tool for non-invasively investigating the submillimetre functional organization of the human brain.

7.3 Limits to temporal resolution in fMRI

7.3.1 Overview of the temporal dynamics of human brain function

The temporal dynamics of human brain function have historically been embodied in a concept known as mental chronometry (Posner 1978). There is no particular temporal division for what is considered 'fast' or 'slow' in the brain. For example, many low level vision processes occur in the range 15–150 ms, while many higher order reasoning processes, or those that require action, take place over ranges that may extend from 250 ms to many seconds. As a point of reference, the fastest that a subject can press a button in response to a simple visual cue is about 250 ms. Tasks that probe the temporal dynamics of brain processing have been used extensively in cognitive neuroscience to elucidate mechanisms underlying cognitive processing, often using reaction times (RT) or other psychophysical measures to assess processing load. Such studies are not confined to 'higher order' functions. For example, low level vision has been studied using very clever masking paradigms to learn about visual cortical processing on the order of tens of milliseconds (Enns and Di Lollo 2000). While such psychophysical measurements yield considerable information by inference, they do not reveal directly the neural substrates or pathways involved in the processing of the stimulus. In the past few decades, neuroscientists have turned to a variety of neuroimaging techniques to fulfil this role and it is in this capacity that fMRI has been so successful. While fMRI has proved a tremendous tool to neuroscientists, it has been used primarily in the role of noninvasive mapping of human brain areas responsible for sensory and cognitive tasks, what some may consider 'mental cartography'. But what about mental chronometry? Because images required for BOLD sensitivity can be acquired on a time scale of tens of milliseconds with EPI, one of the tantalizing opportunities offered by fMRI is the chance to follow the temporal aspects of human brain function.

In the literature, the temporal properties of fMRI have been taken to include a confusing number of aspects related to the presentation of events as well as the timing between different areas. A number of investigators have examined the ability of fMRI to follow closely spaced events in time, these studies being motivated by the desire to understand the linearity of the fMRI response in order to deconvolve rapidly acquired single-trial fMRI data. Such studies are described in Chapter 9. Within the temporal context of the current chapter, we will examine the ability of fMRI to provide information regarding the temporal aspects of brain activation, such as the onset of neural activity and the duration of neural activity in a brain area, as well as the order of activations across different brain areas. Several recent papers review the topic in detail, emphasizing behavioural aspects (Menon and Kim 1999) or the deconvolution and timing issues (Miezin *et al.* 2000). At the time of writing, such studies have generally been performed as single-trials with repetition times on the order of 30 s in order that the fMRI response completely recovers to baseline prior to the next trial.

7.3.2 What does fMRI measure?

In order to explore the factors that may limit the application of BOLD-based fMRI in the study of mental chronometry, a few salient points about the BOLD signal are worth reviewing here, although they have been discussed extensively in earlier chapters. The BOLD signal reflects a delayed haemodynamic response to neural activity, though the exact mechanism of the coupling between the brain's activity and the vascular response is not well understood. This is an important issue, because it sets a limit on how consistent the vascular response might be between different brain areas (Miezin *et al.* 2000). For example, if the neuro-vascular coupling is brought about by the diffusion of a signaling molecule from the neurone to the blood vessel, then areas such as primary visual cortex (V1) which have high neural and vascular densities (Zheng *et al.* 1991) may show a BOLD response that is faster than areas where the distance between the neurone and the vascular regulation site (probably the arterioles) is greater. However, if the coupling mechanism is more direct, for example through membrane potentials on astrocytes that are in contact with both neurones and capillaries, then the BOLD response is likely to be more consistent between different areas. Because of the difficulty in evoking well timed neural responses in anything other than sensory cortex, where the stimulus can be easily controlled, the existing

imaging data cannot rule out either of these two possibilities.

Even the nature of brain 'activity' remains something of a mystery. It is thought that fMRI signals reflect metabolic activity in the brain. However, of the two main cell types in the brain, the neurones are in a significant minority with respect to the glia. It is known that the glia play an important role in neurotransmitter recovery and in maintaining homeostasis (Magistretti *et al.* 1999). Thus, any discussion of brain metabolic demand and its effect on blood flow should consider the presence of glial cells, although this is usually not done. The prevailing view is that it is the metabolic activity (presumably of neurones *and* glia) associated with synaptic firing which drives the vascular response, though the relative contribution to the BOLD response of spiking versus sub-threshold activity is unknown. Since sub-threshold potentials are also metabolically demanding, they must be reflected in the BOLD signal in some way. However, the time scale of sub-threshold activity is generally slower than spiking activity, so it is important to understand how each of these processes is reflected in the BOLD signal. Such measurements have yet to be done. A similar situation occurs in differentiating inhibitory from excitatory metabolic activity using the BOLD response. A recent report (Waldvogel *et al.* 2000) suggested that BOLD signal changes corresponding to inhibitory activity are not likely to be seen, since there is one inhibitory synapse for every five to six excitatory synapses. Furthermore, they argue that inhibitory signals are also more metabolically efficient since the inhibitory synapses are located on or near the soma of the pyramidal cells. Studies of somewhat similar go/no-go paradigms at 4 Tesla indicate otherwise (Richter *et al.* 1997), suggesting this issue is far from being resolved.

Single-unit recording is the 'gold standard' for studying neural coding, because it reflects both threshold and sub-threshold activity of individual neurones and, with some fortitude, can be used to obtain population averages as well. However, it is precluded in non-invasive human studies. The closest non-invasive analogues of single-unit electrophysiology are magneto-encephalography (MEG) and electro-encephalography (EEG), but even they suffer from subtle timing issues and major localization problems. Latencies observed in MEG and EEG are already displaced compared to single-unit recordings, perhaps not surprising given what is known about the sources of these electromagnetic signals. Similarly, MEG and EEG reflect bulk activity of neurones, which can only be spatially localized within certain constraints. Thus, while MEG, EEG and fMRI are good ways of measuring local population averages, many of the features of the individual neurones will be lost. There is no particular reason to believe that all the neurones are firing synchronously within the volume of interrogation, so if the neural code depends on the phase of the firing neurones, this information will likely be lost. This is certainly the case in some signaling pathways. Nonetheless, researchers are beginning to synthesize the temporal capabilities of EEG or MEG with the spatial resolution of fMRI (Ahlfors *et al.* 1999) to make 'brain movies'.

Given that a single voxel in a typical fMRI experiment may contain 10^7 neurones or more, is all hope lost for using fMRI to study the timing relationships of neurones in the brain? Perhaps not, at least on the scale where these temporal relationships govern behaviour. In many cognitive tasks, neural processing lasts from a few hundred milliseconds to a few s and in this domain of applicability, a number of recent papers suggest that fMRI may be used to examine both the sequence and the duration of neural activity in the brain.

7.3.3 Linking behaviour and fMRI

As mentioned earlier, psychologists have used sophisticated measurements of behaviour for years (known as psychophysics) to infer neural processing strategies. Except for what can be deduced from models fitted to the psychophysical data (e.g. Graham 1989; Wandell 1995), these techniques do not tell us where in the brain processing occurs, so these clever psychophysical techniques have been paralleled by electrophysiological recording studies in laboratory animals, and by neurological examination of human patients who have cortical lesions that impair neural processing, such as spatial, colour or form vision. While one cannot noninvasively examine the response of single neurones in human cortex, a number of investigators examining the visual cortex (Churchland and Sejnowski 1988; Britten *et al.* 1996; Lennie 1998; Boynton *et al.* 1999) have argued that behaviourally or perceptually significant activity occurs not at the level of single cells, but in large pools of neurones, not all of which need be driven optimally to elicit a behaviourally relevant deci

sion (Shadlen *et al.* 1996). It is a consequence of this circumstance that suggests a means for the use of neuroimaging techniques such as fMRI in the study of human behaviour.

However, there are several underlying assumptions implicit in any assertion that fMRI reflects behaviourally relevant neural responses. First, one must assume that the fMRI response from a selected region of cortex is proportional to the spatial average of individual neurones' metabolic activity integrated over some time. Neural responses to a stimulus are typically measured as impulses per second and one might think that the fMRI signal from any given voxel reflects this impulse rate multiplied by the number of units responding to that stimulus (Jueptner and Weiller 1995; Boynton *et al.* 1996). Second, one must assume that psychophysical judgements are governed by pooled neuronal activity as discussed above (as opposed to being determined by one or a small number of stimulus-specific neurones, such as the so-called 'grandmother cell'). A number of models support the assumption of population weighted or pooled neural activity as a determinant of psychophysical performance. See, for example, Shadlen *et al.* (1996) for results obtained in the visual cortex, and Platt and Glimcher (1999) for additional factors beyond the visual cortex. Further data has been obtained on contrast sensitivity in normals and amblyopes (Goodyear *et al.* 2000). The data of Boynton *et al.* (1999) and Rees *et al.* (2000) lend further support to this assertion. Third, we assume that a criterion threshold response can be defined in fMRI analogous to those used in single unit recording or psychophysical measurements (Bradley *et al.* 1987). This last assumption implies that the fMRI response in a given area of brain must reach a certain level for a behaviour to be initiated. The electrophysiological analogy is that a certain number of neurones must spike above a threshold mean rate in order for behaviour to occur. Whether fMRI has the sensitivity to show brain activity in the absence of behaviour is yet to be determined.

7.3.4 The temporal features of the fMRI response

In attempting to understand which aspects of the BOLD response might be useful in extracting the temporal order between neural substrates, it is useful

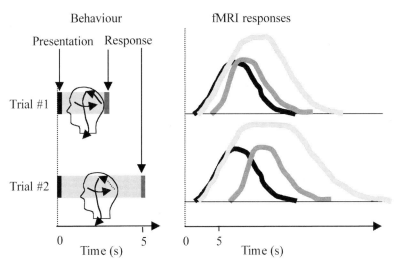

Fig. 7.4 A schematic representation of the BOLD responses to three stages of a typical paradigm, presentation (black), processing (light grey), and response (dark grey.)

to examine some features of the fMRI signal. With reference to Fig. 7.4, several features can be used to characterize the temporal aspects of the fMRI-measured haemodynamic response. As mentioned in Section 7.1.2, the 'initial dip' is small in magnitude, and it is not readily seen in humans. The figure demonstrates the well known haemodynamic delay of the positive-going BOLD signal which does not start to deviate from baseline for just over 2 s after the onset of the stimulus (black lines) or response (dark grey lines). The time to peak varies in part depending on how far the BOLD signal is rising, and is in general not a good measure of latency unless the fMRI task ensures consistent neural activity between trials. This is shown in the figure, where the light grey line peaks at a later time than the black line, despite the fact that the corresponding neural activity begins at approximately the same time. The light grey box and line denote a mental process and its corresponding BOLD response. The time to peak typically can vary from 1 s for a very short stimulus such as a flash of light, to 8 s for a continuing robust stimulus such as the typical 8 Hz blue-yellow flickering checkerboard used in many experiments. The curves also show that the total vascular response takes a considerable amount of time to return to zero and stabilize after the stimulus is turned off. The duration of this recovery phase places limits on how fast the stimulus can be repeated when

accurate timing derived from the BOLD response is required. For a stimulus duration of up to about 4 s, the time-to-peak depends on the duration and other parameters of the stimulus. Beyond 4 s, the neural (and hence BOLD) responses saturate (light grey line), and further increases in stimulus duration are manifested solely in the width of the peak, with some as yet poorly understood variations. It has been determined that the inflection point from baseline can be used as a measure of relative stimulus onset (Savoy *et al.* 1995; Kim *et al.* 1997*b*; Menon *et al.* 1998), while the width of the response can be used as a measure of stimulus processing time (Richter *et al.* 1997). These two aspects are illustrated later in this chapter.

If fMRI responses in all regions were identical and not signal-to-noise limited, it would be straightforward to compare temporal characteristics between regions using the width or inflection points of the fMRI response. Using the assumption of identical responses, averaged event-related fMRI has been used to determine sequential neural processing by timelocking the average fMRI response to the presentation of the visual cue (Buckner *et al.* 1996; Menon *et al.* 1998). However, if time-dependent modulation occurs (such as learning, alterations in strategy and errors, and habituation, all of which are common in cognition), averaging loses unique information associated with each individual execution of the task, information that could be used in powerful regression models with other parameters such as reaction time for in-depth analysis of the data. While the ability to image individual trials is a requirement for many studies, there remains much to be learned from averaged data. Of more concern is the fact that the intrinsic neurovascular coupling and the resultant BOLD responses among regions may differ. Under such conditions, it is not possible to conclude anything about the absolute temporal sequence of neural activity between different regions from the averaged time courses unless the a priori responses of each area can be characterized or calibrated. This is not easily done, because it is impossible to activate individual areas in isolation outside of a few select regions in sensory cortex.

7.3.5 Time-resolved event-related fMRI

One approach to separating intrinsic haemodynamic differences from neural activity differences is to use a time-resolved event-related fMRI technique (Rosen *et al.* 1998). Since it is difficult to calibrate the haemodynamic delays in different areas of the brain we manipulate some aspect of the timing of the stimulus presentation or task performance in order to cause variations of the fMRI signal that are neural in origin. By regressing one or more of the fMRI signal characteristics we have just discussed with a behavioural correlate, such as time to recognize an object or delay between storing and recalling a word list, one can then separate those components of the fMRI signal that are constants of the task from those that vary with the temporal regressor. This might seem onerous, but at very high magnetic fields such as 4 Tesla, there is often enough sensitivity to monitor fMRI signal with little or no averaging. Signal averaging can be performed using a behavioural correlate such as task performance (e.g. correct or incorrect) or response criteria (e.g. reaction time) to align the fMRI data prior to averaging. Subsequently, temporal characteristics such as onset time or width of the fMRI responses can be correlated with behavioural data such as response time. In this way, differences in the underlying temporal behaviour of neuronal activity can be distinguished from haemodynamic response time variations between subjects and brain areas, since the haemodynamic responses are constant while the delays of neural origin will increase or decrease.

7.3.6 Estimation of neural processing time from BOLD response onset

We have already suggested that the inflection point from baseline might be one way of characterizing the onset latency between different neural substrates, or at least of isolating the role of these substrates in neural processing. In Fig. 7.5, we demonstrate the use of onset time as an indicator of where the processing delays associated with a target tracking task may reside. In this task (Menon *et al.* 1998) 10 trials were presented in which a subject used a joystick to move a cursor from a start box to a target box as rapidly and accurately as possible. The BOLD responses for each trial were aligned to the onset of activity in V1, in order to try to compensate for the potential variation in haemodynamic response between trials and subjects. In this simple task, akin to a similar set of experiments on monkeys, the reaction time (RT) delay could originate in the planning of the movement or in the execution of the movement, and we wished to isolate the origin. We note that the spread in reaction time in the figure arises primarily from differences in task performance between subjects and that there is little time-dependent modulation of function in this very well practiced task. Surprisingly, the data demonstrate that in subjects of similar age, the relative haemodynamic delays scale consistently between subjects, and so RT between subjects can be used as a correlate in certain cases. In this particular experiment, it was shown that the subject-to-subject variation in RT arises from a delay somewhere between visual area V1 and the supplementary motor area (SMA), and not between the SMA and motor area M1. In other words, once the SMA is activated, the motor execution time is a predictable constant. It seems to be the planning of the trajectory that requires the processing delay and is the primary origin of the RT difference between subjects.

7.3.7 Estimation of neural processing time from BOLD response width

A second example is that of the well known comparison of photographs of two rotated objects. Shepard and Metzler (1971) demonstrated that the time to decide whether two rotated block-like objects were the same depended linearly on the rotation angle of one object relative to the other. Subjects indicated whether

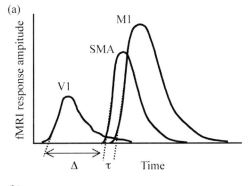

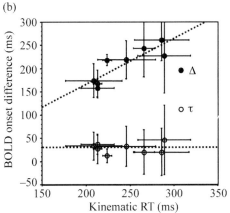

Fig. 7.5 (a) Stereotypical BOLD responses from three different areas of the cortex during a target tracking task, V1 (primary visual cortex), SMA (supplementary motor area), M1 (primary motor cortex). (b) The onset delays Δ and τ as a function of RT (reaction time) between subjects. The onset of the V1 activity was always referenced as 0 s, regardless of its absolute delay.

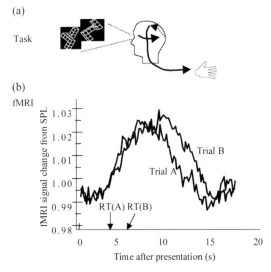

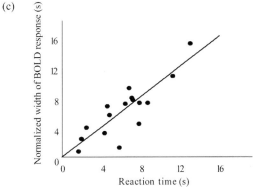

Fig. 7.6 (a) Showing the mental rotation task, including some of the salient brain areas involved. The dashed arrow denotes the pathway between primary visual cortex and the motor areas. (b) The BOLD response from the superior parietal lobule (SPL) for two different rotation angles of the block pair (Trial B > Trial A). (c) The width of the BOLD responses shown in (b) as a function of reaction time for a single subject.

the two objects were the same or different by pressing a button. If the task varied from trial to trial (because of the presentation of different rotation angles) the RT should also vary proportionally with rotation angle. One might then expect a component of the task whose width scales with duration of the mental rotation (computational component) and another component of the task whose onset varies with RT (response component). This is shown schematically in Fig. 7.6. It was found that the width of the fMRI response in the superior parietal area was well correlated with the RT, and that the onset time of that region remained constant. This suggests that the superior parietal lobule (SPL) is intimately involved in the mental rota-

tion process, not just as a constant of the task, but as a substrate involved in the actual rotation processing. Conversely, it would be expected that the onset of activity in the motor area correlated with the RT for a button press indicating the objects were the same or different, because the button press involves a well practiced stereotyped movement whose duration probably does vary significantly from trial to trial.

7.4 How might higher fMRI resolutions be achieved?

These developments open up the possibility of studying the temporal processing in the brain on the second and sub-second time scale. However, there are many impediments to pushing the temporal resolution further. Primary among these is the limited signal-to-noise ratio of the image (particularly as one images faster) as well as noise sources intrinsic to the measurement process. Cortical signal changes in fMRI of common stimulation tasks are small even at very high magnetic field strengths (< 3 per cent). Although the instrumental noise in modern MRI instruments can be well below 1 per cent peak-to-peak in a gel phantom, the signal fluctuation observed in the brain can be much larger. Even when motion is minimized by restraining the head, there are still signal fluctuations of physiological origin amongst which cardiac and respiratory induced components are the most dominant ones. With the best fast imaging techniques that can make an image in ~50 ms, effectively freezing some types of motion, the image-to-image signal fluctuation can exceed several percent. When physiological monitoring signals are collected during MRI measurements, some retrospective signal correction can remove the signal fluctuation induced by cardiac and respiration to a useful degree. When MRI image acquisition is carried out at double (or more) the highest frequency of interest, the physiological fluctuations can be visualized in the power spectrum of the time series data (Thomas and Menon 1998). Such physiological oscillations present in the time series can be filtered out in the post processing. Even if these issues can be conquered, there remains a host of biological variables. It is likely that the neural-haemodynamic coupling constant varies between brain areas and between people.

Correlations of the type described in this chapter may allow relative timing between areas to be determined, but the absolute timing currently seems out of reach using the temporal aspects of the BOLD response. However, an intriguing report that has just appeared suggests that the amplitude of the BOLD response can also be used to extract timing information about processing in the brain (Ogawa *et al.* 2000). Using paradigms more akin to masking or transcranial magnetic stimulation (TMS) studies, these researchers have shown that the amplitude modulation of the BOLD response as the timing between two events is varied (over the range of 100 ms) can be used to identify the direction and time of travel of electrical signals between hemispheres in the rat brain. These results are correlated with actual brain activity using EEG electrodes. While such studies do not allow acquisition of all the timing information for a task in a single trial, they do allow manipulation of stimulus parameters in such a manner as to discern interactions between neural substrates on the order of tens of milliseconds.

References

Ahlfors, S.P., Simpson, G.V., Dale, A.M., Belliveau, J.W., Liu, A.K., Korvenoja, A., Virtanen, J., Huotilainen, M., Tootell, R.B., Aronen, H.J., and Ilmoniemi, R.J. (1999). Spatio-temporal activity of a cortical network for processing visual motion revealed by MEG and fMRI. *Journal of Neurophysiology*, **82**, 2545–55.

Boxerman, J.L., Bandettini, P.A., Kwong, K.K., Baker, J.R., Davis, T.L., Rosen, B.R., and Weisskoff, R.M. (1995). The intravascular contribution to fMRI signal change: Monte Carlo modeling and diffusion-weighted studies *in vivo*. *Magnetic Resonance in Medicine*, **34**, 4–10.

Boynton, G.M., Engel, S.A., Glover, G.H., and Heeger, D.J. (1996). Linear systems analysis of functional magnetic resonance imaging in human V1. *Journal of Neuroscience*, **16**, 4207–21.

Boynton, G.M., Demb, J.B., Glover, G.H., and Heeger, D.J. (1999). Neuronal basis of contrast discrimination, *Vision Research*, **39**, 257–69.

Bradley, A., Skottun, B.C., Ohzawa, I., Sclar, G., and Freeman, R.D. (1987). Visual orientation and spatial frequency discrimination: A comparison of single neurones and behavior. *Journal of Neurophysiology*, **57**, 755–72.

Britten, K.H., Newsome, W.T., Shadlen, M.N., Celebrini, S., and Movshon, J.A. (1996). A relationship between behavioral choice and the visual responses of neurones in macaque MT. *Visual Neuroscience*, **13**, 87–100.

Buckner, R.L., Bandettini, P.A., O'Craven, K.M., Savoy, R.L., Petersen, S.E., Raichle, M.E., and Rosen, B.R. (1996). Detection of cortical activation during averaged single trials of a cognitive task using functional magnetic resonance imaging. *Proceedings of the National Academy of Sciences (USA)*, **93**, 14878–83.

Cheng, K. *et al.* (1999). Patterns of human ocular dominance columns as revealed by high-field (4T) functional magnetic resonance imaging (fMRI). *Society for Neuroscience Abstract*, 572.3.

Churchland, P.S. and Sejnowski, T.J. (1988). Perspectives on cognitive neuroscience. *Science*, **242**, 741–5.

Das, A. and Gilbert, C.D. (1995). Long-range horizontal connections and their role in cortical reorganization revealed by optical recording of cat visual cortex. *Nature*, **375**, 780–4.

Dechent, P. and Frahm, J. (2000). Direct mapping of ocular dominance columns in human primary visual cortex. *NeuroReport*, **11**, 3247–9.

DeYoe, E.A., Carman, G.J., Bandettini, P., Glickman, S., Wieser, J., Cox, R., Miller, D., and Neitz, J. (1996). Mapping striate and extrastriate visual areas in human cerebral cortex. *Proceedings of the National Academy of Sciences (USA)*, **93**, 2382–6.

Duong, T.Q., Kim, D.S., Ugurbil, K., and Kim, S.G. (2000). Spatiotemporal dynamics of BOLD fMRI signals: toward mapping submillimeter cortical columns using the early negative response. *Magnetic Resonance in Medicine*, **44**, 231–42.

Duyn, J.H., Moonen, C.T., van Yperen, G.H., de Boer, R.W., and Luyten, P.R. (1994). Inflow versus deoxyhemoglobin effects in BOLD functional MRI using gradient echoes at, 1.5 T. *NMR in Biomedicine*, **7**, 83–8.

Engel, S.A., Glover, G.H., and Wandell, B.A. (1997). Retinotopic organization in human visual cortex and the spatial precision of functional MRI. *Cerebral Cortex*, **7**, 181–92.

Enns, J.T. and Di Lollo, V. (2000). What's new in visual masking? *Trends in Cognitive Sciences*, **4**, 345–52.

Frahm, J., Merboldt, K.D., Hanicke, W., Kleinschmidt, A., and Boecker, H. (1994). Brain or vein-oxygenation or flow? On signal physiology in functional MRI of human brain activation. *NMR in Biomedicine*, **7**, 45–53.

Friston, K.J. (1997). Imaging cognitive anatomy. *Trends in Cognitive Science*, **1**, 21–7.

Frostig, R.D., Lieke, E.E., Ts'o DY, and Grinvald, A. (1990). Cortical functional architecture and local coupling between neuronal activity and the microcirculation revealed by *in vivo* high-resolution optical imaging of intrinsic signals. *Proceedings of the National Academy of Science (USA)*, **87**, 6082–6.

Gati, J.S., Menon, R.S., Ugurbil, K., and Rutt, B.K. (1997). Experimental determination of the BOLD field strength dependence in vessels and tissue. *Magnetic Resonance in Medicine*, **38**, 296–302.

Glover, G.H., Li, T.Q., and Ress, D. (2000). Image-based method for retrospective correction of physiological motion effects in fMRI: RETROICOR. *Magnetic Resonance in Medicine*, **44**, 162–7.

Goodyear, B.G., Nicolle, D.A., Humphrey, G.K., and Menon, R.S. (2000). BOLD fMRI response of early visual areas to perceived contrast in human amblyopia. *Journal of Neurophysiology*, **84**, 1907–13.

Graham, N. (1989). *Visual pattern analysers*. Oxford University Press, New York.

Grinvald, A., Lieke, E., Frostig, R.D., Gilbert, C.D., and Wiesel, T.N. (1986). Functional architecture of cortex revealed by optical imaging of intrinsic signals. *Nature*, **324**, 361–4.

Horton, J.C., Dagi, L.R., McCrane, E.P., and de Monasterio, F.M. (1990). Arrangement of ocular dominance columns in human visual cortex. *Archives of Ophthalmology*, **108**, 1025–31.

Hu, X. and Kim, S-G. (1994). Reduction of signal fluctuation in functional MRI using navigator echoes. *Magnetic Resonance in Medicine*, **31**, 495–503.

Hu, X., Le, T.H., and Ugurbil, K. (1997) Evaluation of the early response in fMRI in individual subjects using short stimulus duration. *Magnetic Resonance in Medicine*, **37**, 877–84.

Jueptner, M. and Weiller, C. (1995). Does measurement of regional cerebral blood flow reflect synaptic activity?—implication for PET and fMRI. *NeuroImage*, **2**, 148–56.

Kim, S.G., Hendrich, K., Hu, X., Merkle, H., and Ugurbil, K. (1994). Potential pitfalls of functional MRI using conventional gradient-recalled echo techniques. *NMR in Biomedicine*, **7**, 69–74.

Kim, S.G., Tsekos, N.V., and Ashe, J. (1997a). Multi-slice perfusion-based functional MRI using the FAIR technique: Comparison of CBF and BOLD effects. *NMR in Biomedicine*, **10**, 191–6.

Kim, S.G., Richter, W., and Ugurbil, K. (1997b). Limitations of temporal resolution in functional MRI. *Magnetic Resonance in Medicine*, **37**, 631–6.

Kim, D.S., Duong, T.Q., and Kim, S.G. (2000). High resolution mapping of iso-orientation columns by fMRI. *Nat. Neuroscience*, **3**, 164–9.

Kim, S-G. and Tsekos, N.V. (1997). Perfusion imaging by a flow-sensitive alternating inversion recovery (FAIR) technique: Application to functional mapping. *Magnetic Resonance in Medicine*, **37**, 425–35.

Lai, S., Hopkins, A.L., Haacke, E.M., Li, D., Wasserman, B.A., Buckley, P., Friedman, L., Meltzer, H., Hedera, P., and Friedland, R. (1993). Indentification of vascular structures as a major source of signal contrast in high resolution 2D and 3D functional activation imaging of the motor cortex at, 1.5 T: preliminary results. *Magnetic Resonance in Medicine*, **30**, 387–92.

Le, T.H. and Hu, X. (1996). Retrospective estimation and correction of physiological artifacts in fMRI by direct extraction of physiological activity from MR data. *Magnetic Resonance in Medicine*, **35**, 290–8.

Lee, A.T., Glover, G.H., and Meyer, C.H. (1995). Discrimination of large venous vessels in time-course spiral blood-oxygen-level-dependent magnetic resonance functional neuroimaging. *Magnetic Resonance in Medicine*, **33**, 745–54.

Lennie, P. (1998). Single units and visual cortical organization. *Perception*, **27**, 889–935.

Lin, C.S., Rajan, S.S., and Gold, J. (1998). A novel multi-segment surface coil for neuro-functional magnetic resonance imaging. *Magnetic Resonance in Medicine*, **39**, 164–8.

Liu, H.L., Pu, Y., Nickerson, L.D., Liu, Y., Fox, P.T., and Gao, J.H. (2000). Comparison of the temporal response in perfusion and BOLD-based event-related functional MRI. *Magnetic Resonance in Medicine*, **43**, 768–72.

Magistretti, P.J., Pellerin, L., Rothman, D.L., and Shulman, R.G. (1999). Energy on demand. *Science*, **283**, 496–7.

Malonek, D. and Grinvald, A. (1996). Interactions between electrical activity and cortical microcirculation revealed by imaging spectroscopy: implications for functional brain mapping. *Science*, **272**, 551–4.

Menon, R.S. and Kim, S-G. (1999). Spatial and temporal limits in cognitive neuroimaging with fMRI. *Trends in Cognitive Sciences*, **3**, 207–16.

Menon, R.S. and Goodyear, B.G. (1999). Submillimeter functional localization in human striate cortex using BOLD contrast at 4 Tesla: implications for the vascular point-spread function. *Magnetic Resonance in Medicine*, 41, 230–5.

Menon, R.S., Ogawa, S., Tank, D.W., and Ugurbil, K. (1993). 4 Tesla gradient recalled echo characteristics of photic stimulation-induced signal changes in the human primary visual cortex. *Magnetic Resonance in Medicine*, 30, 380–6.

Menon, R.S., Hu, X., Adriany, G., Andersen, P., Ogawa, S., and Ugurbil, K. (1994). Comparison of spin-echo EPI, asymmetric spin-echo EPI, and conventional EPI applied to functional neuroimaging: The effect of flow crushing gradients on the BOLD signal. *Proceedings of the Society of Magnetic Resonance*, 2, 622.

Menon, R.S., Ogawa, S., Hu, X., Strupp, J.P., Anderson, P., and Ugurbil, K. (1995). BOLD based functional MRI at 4 Tesla includes a capillary bed contribution: echo-planar imaging correlates with previous optical imaging using intrinsic signals. *Magnetic Resonance in Medicine*, 33, 453–9.

Menon, R.S., Thomas, C.G., and Gati, J.S. (1997). Investigation of BOLD contrast in fMRI using multi-shot EPI. *NMR in Biomedicine*, 10, 179–82.

Menon, R.S., Luknowsky, D.C., and Gati, J.S. (1998). Mental chronometry using latency-resolved functional magnetic resonance imaging. *Proceedings of the National Academy of Science (USA)*, 95, 10902–7.

Miezin, F.M., Maccotta, L., Ollinger, J.M., Petersen, S.E., and Buckner, R.L. (2000). Characterizing the hemodynamic response: effects of presentation rate, sampling procedure, and the possibility of ordering brain activity based on relative timing. *NeuroImage*, 11, 735–59.

Nestares, O. and Heeger, D.J. (2000). Robust multiresolution alignment of MRI brain volumes. *Magnetic Resonance in Medicine*, 43, 705–15.

Ogawa, S., Lee, T.M., Stepnoski, R., Chen, W., Zhu, X.H., and Ugurbil, K. (2000). An approach to probe some neural systems interaction by functional MRI at neural time scale down to milliseconds. *Proceedings of the National Academy of Science (USA)*, 97, 11026–31.

Platt, M.L. and Glimcher, P.W. (1999). Neural correlates of decision variables in parietal cortex. *Nature*, 400, 233–8.

Posner, M.I. (1978). *Chronometric explorations of mind.* Oxford University Press, New York.

Ress, D., Backus, B.T., and Heeger, D.J. (2000). Activity in primary visual cortex predicts performance in a visual detection task. *Nature Neuroscience*, 3, 940–5.

Richter, W., Andersen, P.M., Georgopoulos, A.P., and Kim, S.G. (1997). Sequential activity in human motor areas during a delayed cued finger movement task studied by time-resolved fMRI. *Neuroreport*, 8, 1257–61.

Rosen, B.R., Buckner, R.L., and Dale, A.M. (1998). Event-related functional MRI: Past, present and future. *Proceedings of the National Academy of Science (USA)*, 95, 773–80.

Savoy, R.L., Bandettini, P.A., O'Craven, K.M., Kwong, K.K., Davis, T.L., Baker, J.R., Weisskoff, R.M., and Rosen, B.R. (1995). Pushing the temporal resolution of fMRI: Studies of very brief visual stimuli, onset variability and asynchrony, and stimulus-correlated changes in noise. *Proceedings of the Society of Magnetic Resonance Abstracts*, 1, 450.

Segebarth, C., Belle, V., Delon, C., Massarelli, R., Decety, J., Le Bas, J.F., Decorps, M., and Benabid, A.L. (1994). Functional MRI of the human brain. Predominance of signals from extracerebral veins. *Neuroreport*, 5, 813–16.

Sereno, M.I., Dale, A.M., Reppas, J.B., Kwong, K.K., Belliveau, J.W., Brady, T.J., Rosen, B.R., and Tootell, R.B. (1995). Borders of multiple visual areas in humans revealed by functional magnetic resonance imaging. *Science*, 268, 889–93.

Shadlen, M.N., Britten, K.H., Newsome, W.T., and Movshon, J.A. (1996). A computational analysis of the relationship between neuronal behavioral responses to visual motion. *Journal of Neuroscience*, 16, 1486–1510.

Shepard, R.N. and Metzler, J. (1971). Mental rotation of three-dimensional objects. *Science*, 171, 701–3.

Thomas, C.G. and Menon, R.S. (1998). Amplitude response and stimulus presentation frequency response of human primary visual cortex using BOLD EPI at 4 T. *Magnetic Resonance in Medicine*, 40, 203–9.

Tootell, R.B.H., Dale, A.M., Sereno, M.I., and Malach, R. (1996). New images from human visual cortex. *Trends in Neuroscience*, 19, 481–9.

Tootell, R.B.H., Hadjikhani, N.K., Mendola, J.D., Marrett, S., and Dale, A.M. (1998). From retinotopy to recognition: fMRI in human visual cortex. *Trends in Cognitive Science*, 2, 174–83.

Waldvogel, D., van Gelderen, P., Muellbacher, W., Ziemann, U., Immisch, I., and Hallett, M. (2000). The relative metabolic demand of inhibition and excitation. *Nature*, 406, 995–8.

Wandell BA (1995). *Foundations of vision.* Sinauer Associates, Sunderland, MA.

Yacoub, E. and Hu, X. (1999). Detection of the early negative response in fMRI at, 1.5 Tesla. *Magnetic Resonance in Medicine*, 41, 1088–92.

Zheng, D., LaMantia, A.S. and Purves, D. (1991). Specialized vascularization of the primate visual cortex. *Journal of Neuroscience*, 11, 2622–9.

8 | *Quantitative measurement using fMRI*

Richard D. Hoge and G. Bruce Pike

8.1 *Introduction*

Recent developments have permitted the extension of magnetic resonance imaging into the realm of quantitative physiological monitoring. Previously, non-invasive quantitative measurement of physiological processes in internal structures such as the brain was almost the exclusive domain of techniques requiring the introduction of radioactive tracers via injection or inhalation, such as positron emission tomography (PET) and single photon emission computed tomography (SPECT). Currently, radioisotope-based methods retain the advantage of offering *absolute* quantitation of many variables in physical units (e.g. ml/100g/min for blood flow) compared with MRI-based techniques that offer only *relative* quantitation of most physiological parameters. That is, current MRI-based methods provide only the fractional or per cent change in a parameter (with the exception of blood flow). Nevertheless, MRI offers several extremely attractive strengths, which ensure it will play an important role in the study of brain physiology as well as clinical practice. These advantages include:

- The capability of continuously monitoring physiological processes and observing their dynamics throughout the brain with high time resolution.
- The ability to monitor several physiological processes, such as blood flow and oxygen utilization, at the same time.
- The ability to enhance the signal-to-noise ratio in individual subjects through extensive signal averaging without health risks due to ionizing radiation exposure.

While the above attributes constitute significant advances in our ability to probe brain function, it is not likely that functional MRI will fully replace PET. Indeed, the capabilities of the two methods are quite complementary. As noted above, PET provides absolute quantitation but with poor temporal resolution whereas fMRI offers excellent time resolution but in general may only provide relative quantitation. Another complementary aspect of the two techniques is that PET can measure cerebral blood flow changes with very high sensitivity while PET-based measurements of the cerebral metabolic rate of oxygen consumption ($CMRO_2$) are hampered by a fairly low signal-to-noise ratio (SNR). With MRI, this situation is reversed and changes in tissue oxygenation can be detected with relatively high sensitivity and it is flow monitoring that suffers in this respect. Translation of MRI observations into a quantitative measure of evoked oxygen consumption requires both flow and blood oxygenation information, however, so the low SNR of the flow signal propagates into $CMRO_2$ estimates. Nonetheless, we will see that flow-BOLD coupling relationships are highly sensitive to flow-metabolism regulation.

In this chapter we review the various features of the physiological response that can be monitored using fMRI, then discuss quantitative models linking physiology and MRI-visible physical parameters. Finally we show how these models can be used, in conjunction with suitable measurement techniques, to estimate changes in tissue energy utilization rates during stimulation.

8.2 *Features of the haemodynamic response*

As discussed in Chapter 2, focal increases in cerebral neuronal activity generally lead to co-localized increases in blood flow. It has long been believed that this acceleration of perfusion serves to sustain increased energy requirements at the site of activation, and recently introduced MRI-based techniques for physiological monitoring are playing an important role in establishing and refining this hypothesis.

One of the central aims of current physiological studies of brain activation is to determine quantitative relationships between blood flow, metabolism, and electrical activity in the brain under different conditions. Such quantitative models are important both for advancing our understanding of the basic biology of brain function, as well as for the interpretation of activation studies performed using PET-CBF, and blood oxygenation level dependent (BOLD) fMRI.

Before examining haemodynamic response models at a quantitative level, we give here a brief and qualitative overview of the main events generally observed during MR imaging of focal brain activation. The aim here is to describe the putative biological and physical origins of the various signal features, and identify those that are amenable to quantitative measurement.

In order to do this it is helpful to schematically divide the typical fMRI BOLD response into three epochs, as shown in Fig. 8.1. First, immediately after electrical activity commences there may be a brief period of approximately 0.5–1 s during which the MRI signal decreases slightly below baseline (~0.5 per cent). This is a very subtle effect and is often not seen at conventional 1.5 Tesla magnetic field strengths. This first epoch has become known as the 'initial dip'. Subsequently, the BOLD response increases, yielding a robust 'positive BOLD response' which peaks 5–8 s

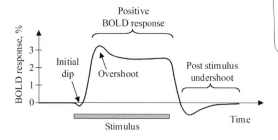

Fig. 8.1 Schematic representation of the common features of the fMRI BOLD response to a period of neuronal stimulation. During the first epoch a small negative 'initial dip' may be observed. Subsequently, a more robust 'positive BOLD response' is observed. Following cessation of the stimulus a return to baseline accompanied by a 'post-stimulus undershoot' is often seen.

after the stimulus commences. It is this positive BOLD response (2–3 per cent signal change at 1.5 Tesla) that is used by most fMRI researchers. Finally, upon cessation of the stimulus, there is a return of the BOLD response to baseline, often accompanied by a 'post-stimulus undershoot', during which the response passes through baseline and remains negative for several tens of seconds. Eventually, the response returns to baseline. All these features are shown schematically in Fig. 8.1. The figure also shows an 'overshoot' period during the early positive BOLD response, which is another common feature observed in fMRI experiments.

8.2.1 The positive BOLD response

From PET measurements it is known that when an individual is lying passively in the imager under quiet, visually neutral conditions, the baseline rate of blood flow through a typical 100 gramme sample of cortical tissue in the brain is in the neighbourhood of 50 ml/min (Matthew *et al.* 1993). Initiation of intense stimulation, such as rapid flashing of high contrast visual patterns, can increase perfusion rates in affected brain areas by 50–70 per cent (at locations that process visual input, in this case) (Fox *et al.* 1986). These flow increases elevate capillary blood oxygenation, accelerating the delivery of oxygen across the capillary wall and lowering venous deoxyhaemoglobin (dHb) levels. Since deoxyhaemoglobin decreases the MR signal in T2*-weighted images, activation-induced reductions in the tissue concentration of this compound lead to positive signal changes, which are usually around 2–3 per cent of the baseline signal level (at 1.5 Tesla). These blood oxygenation level dependent, or BOLD, signal changes are the basis for most MRI-based functional brain mapping.

While the magnitude of the blood flow response to a given stimulus is a basic physiological property of brain tissue, the size of the BOLD response depends on both the biological response and on the physics of the magnetic resonance imaging process. One of the objectives of this chapter is to identify physical factors influencing the BOLD signal, and then to use this insight to establish the physiological implications of characteristically observed response amplitudes.

It is worth remembering that, although functional MRI based on T2*-weighted image contrast is almost

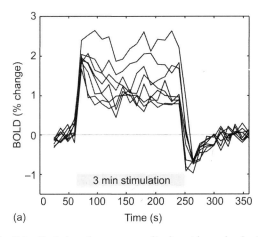
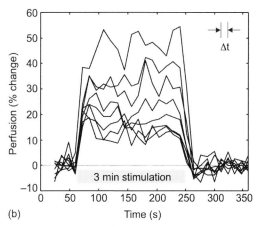

Fig. 8.2 Variation of response amplitudes with psychophysical contrast. All signals were recorded from the same portion of primary visual cortex (in multiple subjects; $n = 12$) and averaged. (a) BOLD response waveforms evoked by three min stimulation using a visual pattern with different luminance modulation amplitudes; (b) corresponding flow response waveforms. For both BOLD and flow, smaller modulation amplitudes produced smaller responses. Note that the shape of the step response seen in (a) changes with the intensity of stimulation.

universally referred to as blood oxygenation level dependent (BOLD) fMRI, there is really no direct sensitivity to the amount of oxygen in the blood. Only *deoxy*haemoglobin can affect the MR signal, and it is the assumed complementarity between oxy- and deoxyhaemoglobin which lets us view fMRI as a means of monitoring blood oxygenation. Under normal physiological conditions this is a valid assumption, but in certain abnormal states it could be quite wrong. Carbon monoxide poisoning is one example, as a victim's blood could be quite poorly oxygenated, with many of the haemoglobin O_2 binding sites occupied by CO molecules. Irreversible conversion of dHb into HbCO at the lung would reduce tissue dHb levels, enhancing the MR signal in spite of dangerously low tissue oxygenation.

In the following sections we will see that the BOLD response has a dynamic structure which, while often not exceedingly complex, must be taken into account when interpreting quantitative amplitude information.

8.2.2 BOLD overshoot and undershoot

MRI-based methods for measuring blood flow and oxygenation permit monitoring of these physiological variables on a relatively short time scale, so it becomes meaningful to talk in terms of *response waveforms* for the two parameters to a step or impulse input. In general, both the amplitude and the shape of the response waveform can vary. Obviously, the amplitude of the response will be zero in regions of the brain that are not affected by a particular stimulus. Also, response amplitudes (for both flow and oxygenation) may be diminished when the behavioural or psychophysical contrast between the baseline state and the activation condition of interest is reduced (Fig. 8.2).

Although short, impulsive stimuli have been found to produce response waveforms in both flow and BOLD with a relatively invariant form (well modelled as a gamma function (Burock *et al.* 1998)), the shape of the response waveforms to a step input (onset of sustained stimulation) is somewhat variable (Hoge *et al.* 1999*b*). The positive phase of the BOLD response waveforms often start with an overshoot phase, followed by an exponential decay to a lower (but still above baseline) steady-state level, with a post-stimulus negative undershoot upon cessation of stimulation that concludes in an exponential rise back to the pre-stimulation baseline level (Figs 8.1 and 8.3).

Although a pronounced positive response overshoot is often accompanied by a similarly large post-stimulus undershoot, the size of such transient signal features relative to the steady-state segment is highly variable and in some cases there is no discernible overshoot (or undershoot). Both extremes (pronounced or no overshoot) may be observed in a single cortical location

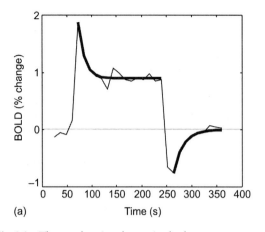 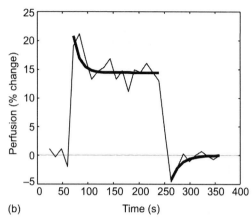

(a)   Time (s)   (b)   Time (s)

Fig. 8.3   The overshoot/steady-state/undershoot response pattern. (a) BOLD waveform. (b) Flow waveform. The heavier lines overlaid on the plots are fitted functions depicting the exponential decay to a new steady-state. The BOLD response waveform seen in (a) is often observed in fMRI experiments, but other shapes have also been reported.

during different types of stimulation, and there is no general correlation between overall response magnitude and the presence or absence of overshoot.

When present, the positive response overshoot appears to be much more pronounced in the BOLD signal than in the flow response waveforms. This observation suggests that some physical mechanism is probably amplifying the sensitivity of the BOLD signal to blood flow transients in the early phases following changes in stimulation state. One candidate for this amplifying influence, observed by Mandeville *et al.* during forepaw stimulation in rats, is the slow adjustment of cerebral blood volume (CBV, which weights the amount of deoxyhaemoglobin in the tissues) during changes in stimulation state (Mandeville *et al.* 1999). The elevated CBV levels associated with sustained stimulation may take up to a minute to evolve (Fig. 8.4), leading to a reduction in BOLD signal that is only significant in the late, steady-state phase. The reverse occurs upon stimulus cessation, when the elevated CBV levels (and accompanying BOLD signal reduction) persist briefly even as blood flow falls dramatically, contributing to a negative post-stimulus undershoot in the signal. Although this experiment has not yet been performed in humans or for multiple brain areas and stimuli, the time constant associated with CBV evolution in the rat (~20s) is similar to that of BOLD over/undershoot in many human studies (the method used to make these CBV measurements will be discussed below).

Positive response overshoot and negative post-stimulus undershoot are commonly, but not universally, observed features of the step-response function to sustained sensory or behavioural input. The main quantifiable parameters of this fMRI step-response function are the overshoot and undershoot amplitudes, their time-constants, and the steady-state signal level. If sensory or behavioural states are switched before recovery from previously sustained conditions is complete, then non-linear interactions between consecutive responses may occur. This can complicate generalization of response amplitude information, as the observed values then depend not only on the applied stimulus but also on the particular timing used in the experiment. It should also be noted that other temporal structures, more complex than the over/undershoot pattern, have been observed in some systems (Harms *et al.* 1999).

8.2.3   BOLD initial negative dip

A more subtle feature of the BOLD signal, observed more often at magnetic field values of 3 Tesla and above, is a small (~0.5 per cent), negative dip in the BOLD signal (Menon *et al.* 1993) lasting around one second following the onset of stimulation (prior to the much larger and universally observed positive signal change). This event, reported in both human and animal fMRI studies, corresponds to an apparent surge

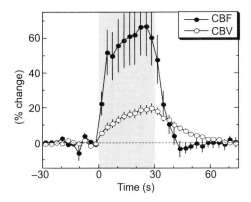

Fig. 8.4 Blood flow and volume signals. Blood flow exhibits an abrupt jump to its elevated level during stimulation, while blood volume adjusts gradually. Upon cessation of stimulation, blood volume returns slowly to its baseline value (adapted from Mandeville *et al.* 1996).

in tissue deoxyhaemoglobin (dHb) levels, occurring immediately following onset of stimulation, that has been observed using near-infrared spectroscopic (NIRS) reflectance imaging in cat visual cortex (Malonek and Grinvald 1996). This dHb surge has been attributed to an immediate, stimulus-driven increase in oxygen consumption accompanied by a slight latency in the circulatory response.

Observations of the initial dip have played an important role in reversing the previously prevalent view that stimulation of cortical tissue evokes little or no change in oxygen consumption (see Barinaga, 1997, for a review). It has also been suggested that BOLD functional MRI based solely on detection of the initial negative dip may offer more precise spatial localization of neuronal electrical activity (than detection of the larger positive response). This prediction is based on the hypothesis that the perfusion response is regulated on a more coarse spatial scale than oxygen utilization (see Chapter 7).

While the size of the initial negative dip is probably proportional to the evoked increase in $CMRO_2$, its exact amplitude depends on complex dynamic interactions between blood flow, blood volume, and tissue metabolism. There are currently no detailed models available for translation of initial dip amplitude into quantitative physiological parameters.

8.2.4 Metabolic attenuation of the positive BOLD response

The observations, described above, of a negative signal dip in the first second of stimulation illustrate the effect of a BOLD signal reduction caused by an increase in $CMRO_2$. While this negative dip is rapidly obliterated by the closely trailing CBF response, it is likely that $CMRO_2$ continues to increase during at least the first ten seconds of stimulation. This would suggest that the late-phase positive BOLD response is subject to considerable attenuation due to increased oxygen consumption by activated tissues. By comparing BOLD signals observed during elevation of perfusion rates to specific levels with either neural stimulation or CO_2-induced vasodilation, it is possible to isolate the effect of metabolic deoxyhaemoglobin production, providing a relatively direct demonstration of increased steady-state oxygen consumption by activated neurones.

Hypercapnia (increased blood CO_2) is a useful model for causing blood flow increases without causing an increase in the metabolic demand of oxygen. By calibrating the CBF increase caused by hypercapnia to be the same as the CBF increase caused by a neuronal stimulation paradigm it is possible to analyse the corresponding BOLD signal changes in order to deduce the BOLD contribution due to the increased metabolic demand of the stimulus. This requires the ability to independently measure CBF and BOLD signal responses. Figure 8.5(a) shows perfusion signals recorded in a region of human visual cortex at four levels of hypercapnia, superimposed with signals recorded from the same region of cortex at four levels of visual stimulation (with luminance contrast levels in the stimulus adjusted to match the hypercapnically induced flow increases). The corresponding BOLD signals (shown in Fig. 8.5(b)) reveal significant attenuation of the visually evoked BOLD responses (grey curves) compared with those produced by hypercapnia (thin black curves). This result shows that increased aerobic metabolism during neuronal activation does indeed exert a significant attenuating effect on the positive BOLD fMRI response, reducing the evoked response amplitude to approximately 50 per cent of the level that would be observed if oxygen consumption remained at baseline during activation. The amount of attenuation increases with perfusion, indicating that

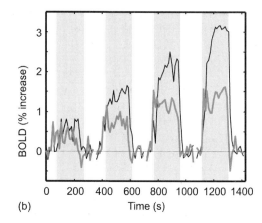

Fig. 8.5   Perfusion and BOLD signals as a function of time during graded hypercapnia and visual stimulation ($n = 12$; stimulation intervals indicated by grey background). (a) Flow signal during graded hypercapnia (thin black curve) and graded visual stimulation (grey curve) with contrast levels adjusted to match hypercapnia-induced flow increases. (b) BOLD signals during the perfusion increases shown on the left. BOLD signals during visual stimulation are significantly lower than those observed during hypercapnia at matched perfusion levels, revealing graded increases in oxygen consumption.

perfusion and oxygen consumption undergo coupled increases.

8.3   Quantitative measurement

In this section we will cover the basic physical principles involved in magnetic resonance imaging of cerebral blood flow (CBF), cerebral blood volume (CBV) and cerebral blood oxygenation. We will then show how these measurements can be incorporated into biophysical models that, in conjunction with physiological calibration procedures, can be used to estimate relative changes in the oxygen utilization rate of brain tissue. These techniques can also be used for comparing values of physiological parameters across different brain regions.

8.3.1   MRI measurement of cerebral blood flow

In the context of brain imaging, blood flow is usually defined as the volume of blood passing, per unit time, through the capillary bed in a given mass of tissue. The usual units for absolute measurement are ml/100g/min. As stated above, a typical baseline value for human cortex is 50 ml/100g/min and intense stimulation can increase local blood flow rates by up to 50–70 per cent.

There are many variants of MR-based flow imaging, and many technical details which must be considered in order to achieve accurate results. Much of this information is elsewhere in this book, so we focus here on those issues that impact on the quantitative accuracy of these methods. The basic concepts involved in measuring cerebral blood flow with magnetic resonance imaging are closely related to radiotracer methods, which have historically played an important role in quantitative physiological imaging. We therefore introduce these concepts by means of a brief overview of PET.

In PET CBF imaging, radioactively labelled water is introduced into the arterial blood, which carries the compound to the brain where it diffuses across the capillary wall and accumulates in tissue. The total number of radioactive decay events (the physical quantity imaged in PET) observed in an image voxel depends both on the rate of delivery of the tracer to the tissue and on the rate at which it is cleared from the volume by radioactive decay and venous outflow. This highly simplified description, known as the *two compartment model*, leads to a relatively straightforward set of differential equations predicting an approximately linear relationship between blood flow and tissue tracer concentration (Larson *et al.* 1987). While the existence of a linear relationship alone permits relative quantitation, knowledge of the amount of tracer in the inflowing blood, which can be obtained using arterial sampling, is required for calibration of the slope of this curve to provide an absolute measure of CBF.

Magnetic resonance imaging of cerebral blood flow is also based on the principles described above. Rather than injecting a radioactive tracer into the subject's blood, however, MRI-based methods utilize spatially selective spin inversion (or saturation) to label the water in the arterial blood that flows into the brain. Such techniques, known as arterial spin labelling (ASL) methods, achieve a sign-reversal in the magnetization vector associated with spins over a spatial band covering the arteries in the neck and lower brain. This negatively labelled magnetization, which assumes the role of a tracer in these methods, then flows into the brain where it contributes a flow-dependent component to the total tissue magnetization and hence to the MR image signal. As in PET, tracer clearance occurs by way of venous outflow and physical decay of the label (which in the case of MRI is longitudinal T1 relaxation).

A spatially selective inversion band can be established in approximately 10 ms by exciting the subject with a suitable pulse of radio frequency (RF) energy in conjunction with appropriately adjusted magnetic field gradients. It is then necessary to wait (on the order of 1–2 s) for the labelled blood to flow into the imaged region and diffuse into the tissue. Following this inversion time (commonly denoted TI), a conventional echo planar imaging sequence can be used to measure the distribution of tissue magnetization within the brain. This entire process can be carried out in under two seconds.

In order to isolate the flow-dependent component of tissue magnetization, the above process is repeated several seconds later without labelling the inflowing blood (various precautions must be observed to ensure that the two image acquisitions are otherwise identical). Subtracting the second image from the first eliminates the static tissue signal component, leaving only the flow-dependent contribution. In practice it is necessary to perform considerable signal averaging in order to achieve sufficient signal-to-noise ratio for measurements to be made.

Ideally, the ASL subtraction signal will be zero in regions with no blood supply and increase as a linear function of perfusion elsewhere. Unfortunately, a number of issues can lead to departures from this idealized behaviour (Buxton *et al.* 1998). The main complicating factors are arrival-time delay, finite bolus width, BOLD contamination, and macrovascular signal inclusion. To understand the first two effects it helps to remember that the spatially selective inversion process labels blood along a finite length of the arterial vessels falling within the inversion band, resulting in a plug-like volume or *bolus* of flowing blood destined for the image volume.

Arrival-time delay refers to the fact that some time is required for the leading edge of the bolus to travel between the inversion band and the image plane. The result of this is that the signal vs. flow function for regions with large arrival delays may have an intercept that is different from zero—that is, their ASL subtraction signal may be zero even though they are perfused. Arrival-time delays can be large when multi-slice imaging is performed and some slices are far from the labelling region.

Finite bolus width is a potential source of error because, at high flow rates, the trailing end of the bolus may pass through the image plane during the inversion time. When this happens, affected volume elements switch from a phase of net label accumulation to a period of net label elimination. As long as all the observations are made during either the period of net accumulation or of net elimination, then the ASL signal vs. flow function will be a linear function of flow. The problem, for a given inversion time, arises when flow increases or regional variations in transit time cause shifts between the two regimes. The bolus width may be particularly limited if the MRI system head RF coil is used to transmit inversion prepulses. By using the MRI system body coil to transmit inversion prepulses, however, a relatively large bolus width can be achieved. A large effective bolus width can also be attained using continuous labelling techniques (Wong *et al.* 1998*b*). More sophisticated pulsed labelling schemes, such as QUIPSS II (Wong *et al.* 1998*a*), manipulate the labelled magnetization to achieve a limited but consistent bolus duration and deliberately acquire images during the phase of label clearance. This permits accurate flow quantitation in multi-slice imaging without requiring a long bolus.

During ASL recording from tissues that are in a physiological steady-state, activation-related BOLD effects should be almost completely cancelled by the subtraction operation that is performed to isolate the flow-dependent signal component. This cancellation may not be effective during periods of physiological transition, however, particularly when gradient echo EPI readouts are preceded by a long echo time (TE). If there is a significant shift in tissue oxygenation between acquisition of two long-TE images used subsequently for ASL subtraction, there can be a considerable error in the apparent flow signal. One way to avoid this problem is to use only those flow values determined at a physiological steady-state. Inspection of Fig. 8.3a indicates that, in that experiment, flow data acquired during the first min after a change in stimulation state would be affected by BOLD drift associated with over/undershoot, and should (in this case) be disregarded. If depiction of flow dynamics is desired, then BOLD contamination errors can be minimized by using spin echo refocusing or, ideally, a single-shot fast spin echo readout with centric *k*-space ordering (Crelier *et al.* 1999). In all cases the shortest possible echo time should be used to minimize BOLD sensitivity (which will also boost the signal-to-noise ratio).

Since BOLD signal changes occur as a multiplicative effect applied to the baseline static tissue signal level, minimization of the static tissue signal will also reduce BOLD contamination of flow measurements. One way to achieve this is by selecting an inversion time which causes the recovering static tissue magnetization to be passing through zero when the echo planar images are acquired (note that the interaction between inversion time and bolus passage, discussed above, must always be considered).

A final potential source of error arises in image voxels in which a significant volume fraction is occupied by large, label-bearing vessels. The equations derived from the two compartment model are only accurate when labelled water is diluted by tissue water upon delivery. Inclusion of significant amounts of undiluted vascular blood water in the MR signal can lead to overestimation of blood flow in the region. This effect is particularly severe when very short inversion times (< 500ms) are used, as large arteries may receive labelled blood long before it arrives in the terminal capillary vessels where exchange occurs. The use of longer inversion times (≥800ms) and/or flow crusher gradients will minimize this problem.

In PET, measurements of accumulated tissue radioactivity can be translated into absolute blood flow values if the activity level of the arterial blood is known along with the decay time constant. Similarly, knowledge of the blood magnetization level and the longitudinal relaxation rate in tissue permit absolute quantitation of blood flow from MRI measurements according to the following equation (Calamante *et al.* 1999):

$$CBF = \frac{\Delta M \lambda}{2M_{ss}} \cdot \frac{T1}{a} \tag{8.1}$$

In the above formula, ΔM is the flow-related component of magnetization retained in the ASL subtraction signal, λ is a constant (the blood-brain partition coefficient, ~0.8) included to adjust for the difference in proton density between tissue and blood, M_{ss} is the steady-state equilibrium magnetization of the brain tissue ($2M_{ss}$ is therefore the maximum possible contrast achievable through inversion), T1 is the time constant for longitudinal relaxation (a clearance pathway for the label), and a is a factor which may be reduced from one to reflect incomplete inversion of inflowing spins.

Because of the requirement of additional measurements of fully relaxed magnetization and tissue T1 maps for absolute flow measurement with MRI, it is not uncommon to forgo these steps and accept only relative quantitation. Note, however, that regional variations in the above parameters, mainly T1, can affect the accuracy of relative flow measurements when comparing different spatial locations.

8.3.2 MRI measurement of cerebral blood volume

Cerebral blood volume is defined as the volume of blood present in a given quantity of brain tissue. It can be expressed either as a dimensionless volume fraction or in ml/g. Typical resting values in human cortex are around 2 per cent. Intense stimulation can increase CBV by up to approximately 30 per cent (Mandeville *et al.* 1999).

Mapping of cerebral blood volume was used to obtain the first human fMRI brain maps (Belliveau *et al.* 1991). Early experiments involved rapid imaging of the passage through the brain of a bolus of paramagnetic contrast agent (gadolinium-DTPA) using T2 or T2* weighted acquisitions (Rosen *et al.* 1990; Belliveau *et al.* 1991). The effect of the paramagnetic agent is to produce magnetic field inhomogeneities at the microvascular scale and thus to enhance the rate of decay of the transverse magnetization. Therefore, as the intravascular contrast agent passes through the brain a signal attenuation linearly proportional to the concentration of the contrast agent is observed (when plotted on log-linear axes). Integrating the area under such a concentration-time curve provides a measure of CBV. By repeating this experiment in baseline and activation conditions and subtracting the calculated CBV images, a functional activation map is produced. The major shortcomings of this fMRI technique are the poor temporal resolution and the requirement for an exogenous contrast agent, which limits the number of functional measurements that can be performed in humans.

Recently, intravascular contrast agents that can remain at stable concentrations in the blood for several hours have been developed, alleviating the requirement for bolus injection methods and greatly enhancing temporal resolution. One example is MION (monocrystalline iron oxide nanocolloid), which has been used in rats to provide a five-fold increase in SNR over BOLD contrast at 2 Tesla (Mandeville *et al.* 1998). While the MION concentrations used in these experiments are considerably higher than what is currently approved for humans, initial testing of other stable blood-pool contrast agents, such as ferumoxide, has begun in humans (Scheffler *et al.* 1999). The advantages of this approach are the potentially high SNR, temporal resolution, and physiologically quantitative nature of the measured signal (which is directly proportional to CBV). As with gadolinium-DTPA bolus methods, toxicity issues limit the number and frequency of studies that can be performed on an individual human subject.

There is also a third, indirect, avenue to estimation of relative cerebral blood volume changes that uses dynamic blood flow measurements. This indirect approach relies on earlier observations indicating that steady-state cerebral blood volume is highly correlated with steady-state perfusion level (Grubb *et al.* 1974; Mandeville *et al.* 1998). The actual relationship observed is usually a sub-linear (slightly less than square root) dependence of baseline-normalized CBV on baseline-normalized CBF:

$$\frac{CBV}{CBV_0} = \left(\frac{CBF}{CBF_0}\right)^\alpha \qquad (8.2)$$

where α is a constant with an approximate empirically derived value of 0.4 (Grubb *et al.* 1974) and the subscript '0' is used here and elsewhere in the text to refer to the baseline steady-state value of a variable. Relative CBV values can then be obtained implicitly from relative CBF values using this formula.

The above CBV–CBF coupling relationship has been found to hold in several species, including monkeys during modulation of CBF using hypercapnia (Grubb *et al.* 1974), and also in rats during both hypercapnia and electrical forepaw stimulation (Mandeville *et al.* 1996). It is also consistent with theoretical analyses of vascular response mechanics (van Zijl *et al.* 1998). It is important to note, however, that at the present time there are no data for awake human subjects providing independent measurements of CBF and CBV during physiological stimulation.

As we will see in the next section, knowledge of blood volume behaviour during stimulation is important for interpretation of BOLD signal changes. We need to know how much blood is present in tissues before we can estimate changes in dHb production rate based on changes in total tissue dHb levels.

8.3.3 MRI measurement of cerebral oxygen consumption

The cerebral metabolic rate of oxygen consumption, or $CMRO_2$, is a quantity that is of particular interest in brain mapping as it is tightly linked to tissue energy utilization rates and hence tissue information processing workload. $CMRO_2$ is usually defined as the number of moles of oxygen consumed, per unit time, by a given mass of tissue. A typical value for resting $CMRO_2$ in human cortex is 2 μmol/g/min (Mintun *et al.* 1984). Fractional increases in $CMRO_2$ during activation are generally smaller than changes in CBF, with maximal elevations of 30 per cent reported (Marrett and Gjedde 1997).

In the two previous sections we saw how the purely haemodynamic parameters of blood flow and volume could be estimated using MRI. In this section we will see how these methods can be combined with MRI acquisitions to estimate fractional changes in $CMRO_2$ during activation.

Sensitivity to blood oxygenation arises in T2*-weighted MR images of the brain because the local image intensity is generally subject to some degree of attenuation caused by deoxyhaemoglobin, a paramagnetic relaxation enhancer introduced into venous blood as tissues extract oxygen for aerobic metabolism. Increasing the perfusion rate in a tissue volume element generally leads to dilution of venous deoxyhaemoglobin (Haacke *et al.* 1997), reducing the tendency of the blood to decrease the magnetic resonance signal (i.e. leading to a signal increase). This increase in signal intensity, referred to as the BOLD response, can be detected in images and is often used as a surrogate marker for activation-induced increases in cerebral blood flow (Kwong *et al.* 1992; Ogawa *et al.* 1992).

Increases in blood flow also cause distension of the highly compliant venous vessels, however, and the resultant increase in the fraction of tissue volume occupied by blood (which will include paramagnetic deoxygenated blood) partially counteracts the diluting effect of the perfusion increase. Based on the assumption of a fixed relationship between CBF and CBV, application of mass conservation rules, and physical models of T2*-weighted signal dependence on tissue dHb concentration, a relatively simple relationship between fractional changes in CBF and BOLD signal is predicted for constant $CMRO_2$:

$$\frac{\Delta BOLD}{BOLD_0} = M\left(1 - \left(\frac{CBF}{CBF_0}\right)^{\alpha-\beta}\right). \quad (8.3)$$

M is the maximum possible BOLD signal change that would be observed upon complete elimination of all dHb from a tissue sample, α is the CBV-CBF coupling exponent from eqn (8.2), and β describes the attenuating power of deoxyhaemoglobin (range: $1 \leq \beta \leq 2$ (Boxerman *et al.* 1995)). The net exponent $\alpha-\beta$ is believed to be close to -1 under normal conditions, resulting in the relationship depicted graphically in Fig. 8.6(a) for a constant level of $CMRO_2$. The main characteristics of the predicted BOLD–CBF relationship are that there should be linear increases for moderate flow increases, but for larger CBF values the relationship becomes increasingly sublinear and the BOLD signal eventually plateaus to an asymptotic value of M.

If the rise in perfusion is due to heightened neuronal activity, then metabolic oxygen extraction may also increase, accelerating the production of deoxyhaemoglobin and counteracting the dilution effect. Extending eqn (8.3) to include variations in relative $CMRO_2$ results in the following expression:

$$\frac{\Delta BOLD}{BOLD_0} = M\left(1 - \left(\frac{CMRO_2}{CMRO_{2|0}}\right)^{\beta}\left(\frac{CBF}{CBF_0}\right)^{\alpha-\beta}\right) \quad (8.4)$$

Evaluating the above function at different levels of $CMRO_2$ results in a set of plots which can be viewed

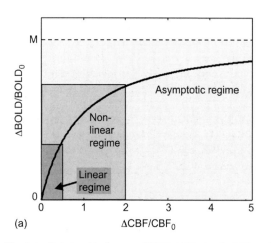

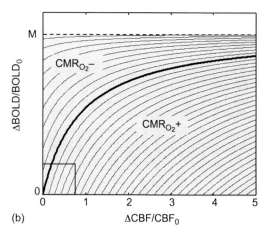

Fig. 8.6   Relationship between BOLD MRI signal, CBF, and $CMRO_2$ predicted at a) constant $CMRO_2$ (eqn (8.3)) and (b) different levels of $\Delta CMRO_2$ at 10 per cent interval (eqn (8.4)). Plots were calculated using parameter values $\alpha = 0.38$ and $\beta = 1.5$.

as iso-CMRO$_2$ contours on the BOLD-CBF plane, as shown in Fig. 8.6(b). It can be seen that increases in CMRO$_2$ pull the BOLD signal curves downward, reflecting signal attenuation due to increased dHb production.

The exact value of the parameter M depends both on the details of the pulse sequence used to monitor the BOLD signal and on the amount of deoxyhaemoglobin present in the tissue at baseline. In general this quantity is not known a priori. One way to estimate M is by mapping out the position of the baseline iso-CMRO$_2$ contour by driving flow increases, at a constant level of oxygen consumption, during simultaneous monitoring of relative BOLD and CBF signals. This can be done using graded hypercapnia to induce varying degrees of cerebral vasodilation. Ideally, flow would be increased until the BOLD signal reached the asymptotic limit, permitting direct observation of M. Comfortably tolerable levels of hypercapnia will not push a tissue sample beyond the linear regime of Fig. 8.6(a), but since the proportionality between the slope of the linear portion of the baseline iso-CMRO$_2$ contour and M is fixed by eqn (8.3), this is sufficient. Once M is determined (for a given subject, session, and tissue region), the vertical scaling of the iso-CMRO$_2$ plot is established and paired measurements of the fractional BOLD and CBF changes occuring during activation can then be translated into estimates of the fractional change in CMRO$_2$.

Experimental measurements of CBF and BOLD signal changes during graded hypercapnia at different levels of visual stimulation behave as predicted in Fig. 8.6(b). Figure 8.7(a) shows BOLD signal increases, as a function of flow increase, measured in a region of human visual cortex (averaged over multiple subjects) during graded hypercapnia at different levels of visual stimulation. The adjacent figure (Fig. 8.7(b)) shows data acquired in a separate experiment during graded hypercapnia and graded visual stimulation. It is clear that, with increasing neuronal activity (visual stimulation in this case), the BOLD-CBF response coordinates are driven across the iso-CMRO$_2$ contours into zones indicating increased metabolic activity. This behaviour is the foundation for CMRO$_2$ measurement using fMRI.

Equation (8.4) can be rearranged for computation of the fractional change in CMRO$_2$ as an explicit function of the fractional changes in BOLD and flow signal, provided that M is known for the tissue in question:

$$\frac{\text{CMRO}_2}{\text{CMRO}_{2|0}} = \left(1 - \frac{\Delta \text{BOLD}/\text{BOLD}_0}{M}\right)^{1/\beta} \left(\frac{\text{CBF}}{\text{CBF}_0}\right)^{1-\alpha/\beta}$$

$$(8.5)$$

Note that experimentally determined M values are likely to be specific to the conditions under which they were measured, including such factors as subject positioning in the magnet and their baseline physiological

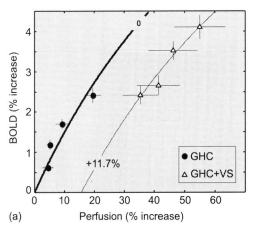

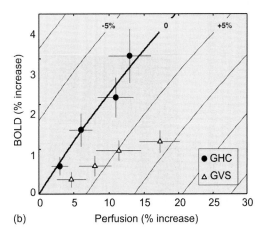

Fig. 8.7 Experimentally determined iso-CMRO$_2$ contours. a) Average BOLD and CBF responses during graded hypercapnia (GHC; black circles) and during graded hypercapnia plus a constant level of visual stimulation (GHC + VS; white triangles). The visual stimulus used was a low-contrast reversing checkerboard pattern. Iso-CMRO$_2$ contour lines were generated by fitting eqn (8.4) to the measured data, using the same model parameters listed in Fig. 8.6. (b) Average BOLD and CBF responses during graded hypercapnia (GHC; black circles) and during graded visual stimulation (GVS; white triangles) (Hoge *et al.* 1999a).

state and level of arousal. It is therefore preferable to perform the hypercapnic calibration procedure described above and all behavioural recording in a single session, with as little disturbance of the subject as possible. It is also preferable to record the BOLD and flow signals simultaneously, in order to maintain the closest possible matching of experimental conditions for the two measurements. This can be done using an interleaved imaging approach in which a BOLD acquisition is appended after each of the two inversion recovery scans required to produce a blood flow measurement (Fig. 8.8). The interleaving must be done in this fashion to ensure that the flow-sensitive and flow-insensitive phases of the ASL recording are iden-

tical. Although the echo-time may be shortened in the ASL acquisitions to reduce BOLD contamination, it is advisable to use identical EPI readout gradient waveforms for both the flow and BOLD phases. This will ensure that both measurements are spatially aligned, even in the presence of image distortions which can occur in EPI. Alternatively, image distortion correction should be performed to carefully realign BOLD and ASL images. Note also that the M parameter must be determined for each spatial location in the imaged volume.

There are two sets of issues affecting the accuracy of MRI-based $CMRO_2$ measurements. The first set involves possible inaccuracies in the measured values of

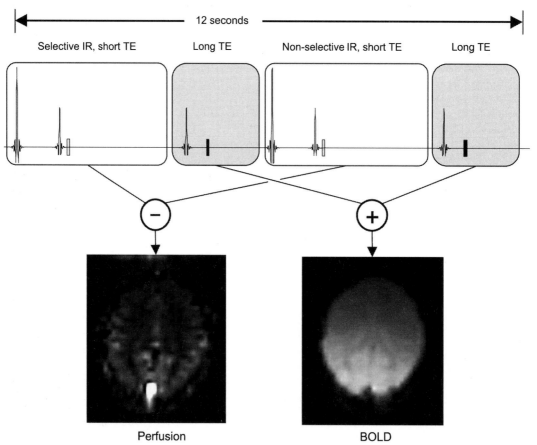

Fig. 8.8 Sample MRI pulse sequence for making interleaved measurements of flow and BOLD responses. The first and third sequence blocks (not shaded) comprise the flow-sensitive and flow-insensitive phases of an ASL acquisition. These EPI sub-sequences include an inversion prepulse and use a short echo time. The second and fourth blocks (shaded) use a longer echo time, providing sensitivity to BOLD signal changes. To produce flow and BOLD images that overlap in time, the inversion recovery scans are subtracted and the BOLD scans are added. (Adapted from Hoge *et al.* 1999*a*.)

CBF and BOLD signal changes, and the second involves the details of the BOLD signal model (eqn (8.4)) used to translate these measurements into $CMRO_2$ estimates.

Sources of error for flow measurements, described in detail above, include effects related to bolus passage, inclusion of macrovascular signal, and BOLD contamination. The inclusion of large vessel signals in BOLD images may also lead to minor errors in MRI-based $CMRO_2$ estimates, due to dependence of the model parameter β on vascular scale. Most of the tissue-dependent scaling of the model is lumped in the empirically determined parameter M, however, and the effect of realistic variations in β is likely to be small. Of greater concern is the possibility that the largest veins may exhibit strong BOLD signal changes at locations remote from the site of neuronal activation (i.e. the issue of 'draining veins').

Just as BOLD contamination can affect flow images, flow contamination is a potential source of error when BOLD images are used to estimate changes in the tissue dHb level. The same effects which lead to a flow-dependent signal component in ASL imaging can influence the intensity of BOLD images, especially if rapid imaging rates and high flip angles are used. If a short inter-scan (TR) interval must be used, it is important to consider the possible effects of inflow enhancement when interpreting BOLD response amplitudes.

A final factor affecting the scheme described above for MRI-based $CMRO_2$ measurement is that the relationship used to estimate CBV changes from flow increases may be invalid in the early stages of stimulation. The rat data of Mandeville *et al.* indicate that eqn (8.2) is only correct during the late, steady-state phases of stimulation (i.e. after any overshoot period).

8.3.4 Flow/metabolism coupling and the BOLD signal

The role and behaviour of oxidative metabolism during brain activation has been a central question in cerebral physiology (Barinaga 1997). Moreover, understanding the coupling between oxidative metabolism, blood flow, and the BOLD signal is of critical importance for the proper interpretation of cognitive neuroimaging data. The techniques described above provide a means for the mapping of regulatory relationships between cerebral blood flow and metabolism.

Figure 8.9(a) shows average steady-state increases in BOLD signal plotted as a function of perfusion increase in human primary visual cortex during presentation of a variety of different graded visual stimuli, as well as for graded hypercapnia. As described above, each combination of BOLD and perfusion values corresponds to a specific rate of oxygen consumption,

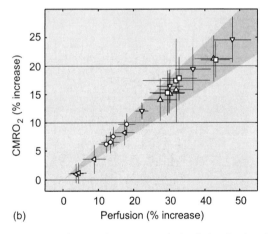

Fig. 8.9 Coupling relationships between CBF and $CMRO_2$ in primary visual cortex during neuronal stimulation. Regions in which the ratio between per cent changes in $CMRO_2$ and CBF is in the range 0.5 ± 0.1 are shaded in darker grey. (a) BOLD vs. perfusion data, including iso-$CMRO_2$ contours fit to graded hypercapnia data (black circles). Visual stimulation data, plotted using white markers, form a distinct linear cluster which progresses into regions indicating increased oxygen consumption. The different marker shapes denote different types of visual stimulation. (b) Relative $CMRO_2$ calculated from the data in (a) using eqn (8.5). The data reveal an invariant linear relationship between flow and metabolism.

with the hypercapnia data points tracing out a baseline iso-CMRO$_2$ contour. Non-baseline contours, plotted by fitting eqn (8.4) to the hypercapnia data, are shown at 10 per cent intervals. Figure 8.9(b) shows per cent changes in CMRO$_2$, computed by solving the fitted model function at measured BOLD and CBF values, plotted as a function of CBF. In this experiment, CMRO$_2$ and CBF responses exhibited a high degree of linear correlation with an average slope of 0.51 ± 0.02.

Figure 8.9(b) shows that, although a wide variety of stimulus-dependent response amplitudes may be observed in a given cortical location, the physiological coupling relationship between blood flow and oxygen consumption appears to be invariant. This consistent, linear relationship was observed in spite of the fact that different stimuli were designed to selectively excite populations of V1 neurones with varying levels of cytochrome oxidase.

The relationships depicted in Fig. 8.9(a-b) have an important implication for the interpretation of the BOLD signal. If the V1 BOLD responses are plotted against the corresponding CMRO$_2$ values, a highly linear relationship is revealed. This validates the BOLD fMRI mapping signal as an index of the information processing workload evoked by a particular stimulus.

It should be pointed out that all of the experimental CMRO$_2$ data shown above were obtained by pooling responses within V1, and then performing extensive multi-subject averaging. This is necessary because of the low signal-to-noise ratio of the MRI-based flow measurements required for estimation of CMRO$_2$. If reduced spatial resolution can be tolerated, then the required number of signal averages can be brought down to the point where images of CMRO$_2$ response patterns in single subjects can be produced.

Figure 8.10 shows quantitative images of various measured and computed physiological parameters acquired in an axial slice that passes through the visual cortex. The signal-to-noise ratio of these data was enhanced through extensive signal averaging in one subject combined with spatial low-pass filtering (12 mm FWHM). Figure 8.10(a) shows regional variations in the parameter M, which is related to the amount of deoxyhaemoglobin in the tissues at baseline. Clear grey-white matter contrast is seen, with grey matter showing higher resting levels of tissue dHb. Figure 8.10(b) shows the regional pattern of BOLD response produced by presentation of a visual stimulus, with intensity levels representing fractional change values. Figure 8.10c shows the corresponding pattern of increased blood flow, in units of percent signal change. Note that the spatial pattern of BOLD response appears to be determined by a weighting of the flow response pattern by the baseline distribution of tissue dHb. Figure 8.10(d) shows the pattern of increased oxygen consumption computed from the previous images. The boundaries of the CMRO$_2$ response pattern appear to match those of the flow response. The two dark bands at the front of the head in Fig. 8.10(d) are artefacts due to the low frontal SNR achieved with the occipital surface coil used in this study and would not be present in head-coil images. Responses in the posterior half of the brain are believed to be accurate to within the contour spacing.

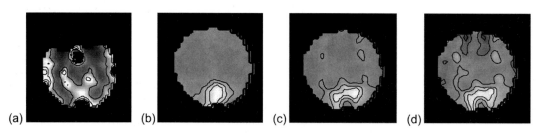

(a)   (b)   (c)   (d)

Fig. 8.10 Quantitative images of different physiological parameters. (a) Image of dHb-related MR signal attenuation at rest (M) based on combined BOLD and CBF responses to CO$_2$ inhalation. Grey-white matter contrast can be seen. Contour interval is 10 per cent; regions with no dHb appear black. (b) Image of the BOLD response pattern to visual stimulation. Contour interval is 0.5 per cent, regions with no change appear grey. (c) Image of CBF response pattern acquired simultaneously with BOLD data. Contour interval is 20 per cent, grey regions denote zero response. (d) Image of computed CMRO$_2$ response. Contour interval is 10 per cent, grey regions indicate zero response. Dark bands at front of head are artefacts due to non-uniform intensity of occipital surface coil.

8.4 Summary and conclusion

The previous sections describe techniques for monitoring physiological processes in the brain and show examples in which these methods have been combined to determine changes in metabolic activity in human visual cortex. While CBF and CBV changes have been measured in a number of experimental models, all of the $CMRO_2$ data shown above were acquired in human visual cortex. Additional work therefore needs to be done to investigate $CBF-CMRO_2$ coupling in multiple brain regions as well as in disease states. If the ~2:1 coupling between per cent changes in blood flow and oxygen consumption is observed throughout the brain, then the interpretation and predictive modelling of BOLD signal changes may be greatly simplified. If not, then regional idiosyncrasies in flow-metabolism coupling may yield insight into the physiological organization of the brain.

Refinement and validation of dynamic CBV monitoring approaches would strengthen confidence in MRI-based $CMRO_2$ measurements. The challenge of measuring dynamic CBV changes while retaining the ability to monitor BOLD signal levels and flow must also be overcome. Identification of a CBF–CBV coupling model that is accurate during the early phases of stimulation is one possible solution to this problem.

References

Barinaga, M. (1997). What makes brain neurones run? *Science*, **276**, 196–8.

Belliveau, J.W., Kennedy, D.N., McKinstry, R.C., Buchbinder, B.R., Weisskoff, R.M., Cohen, M.S., Vevea, J.M., Brady, T.J., and Rosen, B.R. (1991). Functional mapping of the human visual cortex by magnetic resonance imaging. *Science*, **254**, 716–9.

Boxerman, J.L., Bandettini, P.A., Kwong, K.K., Baker, J.R., Davis, T.L., Rosen, B.R., and Weisskoff, R.M. (1995). The intravascular contribution to fMRI signal change: Monte Carlo modeling and diffusion-weighted studies *in vivo*. *Magnetic Resonance in Medicine*, **34**, 4–10.

Burock, M.A., Buckner, R.L., Woldorff, M.G., Rosen, B.R., and Dale AM (1998). Randomized event-related experimental designs allow for extremely rapid presentation rates using functional MRI. *NeuroReport*, **19**, 3735–9.

Buxton, R.B., Frank, L.R. Wong, E.C. Siewart, B., Warach, S., and Edelman, R.R. (1998). A general kinetic model for quantitative perfusion imaging with arterial spin labeling. *Magnetic Resonance in Medicine*, **40**, 383–96.

Calamante, F., Thomas, D.L., Pell, G.S., Wiersma, J., and Turner, R. (1999). Measuring cerebral blood flow using magnetic resonance imaging techniques. *Journal of Cerebral Blood Flow and Metabolism*, **19**, 701–35.

Crelier, G.R., Hoge, R.D., Munger, P., and Pike, G.B. (1999). Perfusion-based functional magnetic resonance imaging with single-shot RARE and GRASE acquisitions. *Magnetic Resonance in Medicine*, **41**, 132–6.

Fox, P.T., Mintun, M.A., Raichle, M.E., Miezin, F.M., Allman, J.M., and Van Essen, D.C. (1986) Mapping human visual cortex with positron emission tomography. *Nature*, **323**, 806–9.

Grubb, R.L., Phelps, M.E., and Eichling, J.O. (1974). The effects of vascular changes in $PaCO_2$ on cerebral blood volume, blood flow and vascular mean transit time. *Stroke*, **5**, 630–9.

Haacke, E.M., Lai, S., Reichenbach, J.R., Kupusamy, K., Hoogenraad, F.G.C., Takeichi, H., and Lin, W. (1997). *In vivo* measurement of blood oxygen saturation using magnetic resonance imaging: a direct validation of the blood oxygen level-dependent concept in functional brain imaging. *Human Brain Mapping*, **5**, 341–6.

Harms, M.P. and Melcher, J.R. (1999). Understanding novel fMRI time courses to rapidly presented noise bursts. *NeuroImage*, **9**(2), 847.

Hoge, R.D., Atkinson, J., Gill, B., Crelier, G.R., Marrett, S., and Pike, G.B. (1999*a*). Investigation of BOLD signal dependence on CBF and $CMRO_2$: the deoxyhemoglobin dilution model. *Magnetic Resonance in Medicine*, **42**, 849–63.

Hoge, R.D., Atkinson, J., Gill, B., Crelier, G.R., Marrett, S., and Pike, G.B. (1999*b*). Stimulus-dependent BOLD and perfusion dynamics in human V1. *NeuroImage*, **9**, 573–85.

Kwong, K.K., Belliveau, J.W., Chesler, D.A., Goldberg, I.E., Weisskoff, R.M., Poncelet, B.P., Kennedy, D.N., Hoppel, B.E., Cohen, M.S., and Turner, R. (1992). Dynamic magnetic resonance imaging of human brain activity during primary sensory stimulation. *Proceedings of the National Academy of Sciences (USA)*, **89**, 5675–9.

Larson, K.B., Markham, J., and Raichle, M.E. (1987). Tracer-kinetic models for measuring cerebral blood flow using externally detected radiotracers. *Journal of Cerebral Blood Flow and Metabolism*, **7**, 443–63.

Malonek, D. and Grinvald, A. (1996). Interactions between electrical activity and cortical microcirculation revealed by imaging spectroscopy: implications for functional brain mapping. *Science* **272**, 551–4.

Mandeville, J.B., Marota, J., Keltner, J.R., Kosovsky, B., Burke, J., Hyman, S., and LaPointe, L. (1996). CBV functional imaging in rat brain using iron oxide agent at steady-state concentration, *Proceedings of the 4th International Society of Magnetic Resonance in Medicine*, p.292.

Mandeville, J.B., Marota, J.J.A., Kosofsky, B.E., Keltner, J.R., Weissleder, R., Rosen, B.R., and Weisskoff, R.M. (1998). Dynamic functional imaging of relative cerebral blood volume during rat forepaw stimulation. *Magnetic Resonance in Medicine*, **39**, 615–24.

Mandeville, J.B., Marota, J.J.A., Ayata, C., Moskowitz, M.A., and Weisskoff, R.M. (1999). MRI measurement of the temporal evolution of relative $CMRO_2$ during rat forepaw stimulation. *Magnetic Resonance in Medicine*, **42**, 944–51.

Marrett, S. and Gjedde, A. (1997). Changes of blood flow and oxygen consumption in visual cortex of living humans. *Advances in Experimental Medicine and Biology*, **413**, 205–8.

Matthew, E., Andreason, P., Carson, R.E., Herscovitch, P., Pettigrew, K., Cohen, R., King, C., Johanson, C.E., and Paul, S.M. (1993). Reproducibility of resting cerebral blood flow measurements with H2(15)O positron emission tomography in humans. *Journal of Cerebral Blood Flow and Metabolism*, **13**, 748–54.

Menon, R.S., Ogawa, S., Tank, D.W., and Ugurbil, K. (1993). 4 Tesla gradient recalled echo characteristics of photic stimulation-induced signal changes in the human primary visual cortex. *Magnetic Resonance in Medicine*, **30**, 380–6.

Mintun, M.A., Raichle, M.E., Martin, W.R., and Herscovitch, P. (1984). Brain oxygen utilization measured with ^{15}O radiotracers and positron emission tomography. *Journal of Nuclear Medicine*, **25**, 177–87.

Ogawa, S., Tank, D.W., Menon, R., Ellermann, J.M., Kim, S.G., Merkle, H., and Ugurbil, K. (1992). Intrinsic signal changes accompanying sensory stimulation: functional brain mapping with magnetic resonance imaging. *Proceedings of the National Academy of Sciences (USA)*, **89**, 5951–5.

Rosen, B.R., Belliveau, J.W., Vevea, J.M., and Brady, T.J. (1990). Perfusion imaging with NMR contrast agents. *Magnetic Resonance in Medicine*, **14**, 249–65.

Scheffler, K., Seifritz, E., Haselhorst, R., and Bilecen, D. (1999). Titration of the BOLD effect: separation and quantitation of blood volume and oxygenation changes in the human cerebral cortex during neuronal activation and ferumoxide infusion. *Magnetic Resonance in Medicine*, **42**, 829–36.

van Zijl, P.C.M., Eleff, S.M., Ulatowski, J.A., Oja, J.M.E., Ulug, A.M., Traystman, R.J., and Kauppinen, R.A. (1998). Quantitative assessment of blood flow, blood volume and blood oxygenation effects in functional magnetic resonance imaging. *Nature Medicine*, **4**, 159–67.

Wong, E.C., Buxton, R.B., and Frank, L.R. (1998a). Quantitative imaging of perfusion using a single subtraction (QUIPSS and QUIPSS II). *Magnetic Resonance in Medicine*, **39**, 702–8.

Wong, E.C., Buxton, R.B., and Frank, L.R. (1998b). A theoretical and experimental comparison of continuous and pulsed arterial spin labelling techniques for quantitative perfusion imaging. *Magnetic Resonance in Medicine*, **40**, 348–55.

III | Experimental design

9 | *Effective paradigm design*

David I. Donaldson and Randy L. Buckner

9.1 Introduction

Advances in functional magnetic resonance imaging (fMRI) are affording numerous new ways to design and analyse brain-imaging studies. A major driving force for these advances has been the widespread use of MRI scanners capable of ultra-fast imaging. For example, MRI scanners in many laboratories and clinical settings typically can acquire whole-brain images once every 2 s or even faster (see Chapter 4). However, the temporal resolution of fMRI is limited by the underlying physiological signals through which neuronal activity is indirectly measured (see Chapter 2). The optimal choice of an MRI experimental paradigm is determined by an interaction between methodological limitations and the properties of the physiology being measured. Extending the range of questions that can be addressed using the fMRI technique depends at least in part upon continued methodological advancement. This chapter aims first to review both key aspects of MRI technology and of the underlying physiology that constrain paradigm design for functional brain imaging.

Perhaps one of the most influential recent developments in terms of paradigm design has been the evolution and utilization of 'event-related' procedures. These procedures allow images to be formed of the transient neuronal changes associated with individual cognitive and sensory events, and even of the sub-processing stages within the events themselves. Event-related fMRI (ER-fMRI) allows experiments to depart solely from the use of 'blocked' procedures, introducing paradigms that isolate individual trial events separated by as little as a few seconds. A second aim of this chapter is to review issues related to the design of event-related experimental paradigms and how event-related procedures have extended the range of questions that can be asked. We will introduce the concept of mixed 'blocked *and* event-related' procedures. The development of such 'mixed' procedures widens the spectrum of task designs and analytical techniques that can be used, further extending the range of questions that can be addressed with fMRI.

Although aspects are discussed elsewhere in this book (Chapters 2 and 8), we first present a brief review of the underlying characteristics of the haemodynamic response, to provide a context for discussion event-related methods and their derivatives.

9.2 Origins of the signal

Haemodynamic techniques such as blood oxygenation level dependent (BOLD) fMRI and PET (positron emission tomography) index changes in blood properties (associated with relative oxygenation levels or blood flow respectively) that follow from changes in neural activity (as discussed in previous chapters). Haemodynamic techniques depend upon there being a close relation between neural activity and cerebral blood flow regulation within the brain—a coupling that is slow and that is affected by differences in regional vascular anatomy (cf. Lee *et al.* 1995; Robson *et al.* 1998; discussed in greater detail below). In fact, temporal evolution of the fMRI signal is an order of magnitude poorer than the evolution of the neural activity itself, at least when brief sensory events are considered. Thus, it is worthwhile reviewing the temporal properties of the signal, their limitations, and how certain forms of paradigm design can best exploit the temporal information provided by the signal.

9.2.1 The BOLD-contrast haemodynamic response

BOLD is the most commonly measured contrast mechanism used for fMRI (Ogawa *et al.* 1990; Kwong *et al.* 1992; Ogawa *et al.* 1992; see Chapters 1 and 2). At present the exact origin of the BOLD signal remains unclear. Nonetheless, even our present understanding of how the BOLD-contrast signal evolves in relation to neuronal activity (henceforth referred to as the 'haemodynamic response') provides important guides to effective MRI paradigm design. Thus, we briefly consider these findings here.

Perhaps the most relevant constraint of the haemo-dynamic response for issues related to paradigm design is that, as already noted, the response exhibits consid-erable temporal blurring in relation to the underlying neuronal activity. Although neural activity can occur very rapidly (in the order of milliseconds) in responses to a sensory event (Robinson and Rugg, 1988), changes in the haemodynamic response occur much more slowly (on the order of s). For example, even a brief period of sensory stimulation (as little as half a second) that presumably results in a proportionately brief period of neural activity, produces haemody-namic changes that do not begin for one to two s, and take place over a 10–12 s period (Blamire *et al.* 1992; Bandettini, 1993; Boynton *et al.* 1996; Konishi *et al.* 1996). Moreover, recent evidence suggests that, although the robust positive deflection of the haemo-dynamic response evolves over a 10–12 s time interval, there may be physiological effects that last consider-ably longer (e.g. the 'post-stimulus undershoot', see Buxton *et al.* 1998; Fransson *et al.* 1998, 1999). Thus, inherent to fMRI data is the fact that the changes are measured in time relative to the neural activity itself. As is discussed below, this is one of many factors that must be accounted for in the analysis procedures employed in event-related fMRI.

9.2.2 Reliability of the signal

The reliability of the BOLD signal as an indirect measure of neuronal activity has received support from a number of empirical observations. Most directly rele-vant to paradigm design is the finding that the response within a given subject and within a given region of cortex is extremely consistent from one set of measure-ments to the next (Dale and Buckner 1997; Menon *et al.* 1998; Miezin *et al.* 2000). Therefore, although the signal is temporally blurred, the lag of onset and time course of signal evolution are highly reproducible.

Reliable maps of brain activity further suggest that similar levels of BOLD-contrast can be generated reli-ably across the cerebral cortex. For example, Ojemann *et al.* (1998) (see also Clark *et al.* 1996; Casey *et al.*

1998), demonstrated reproducible patterns of activity associated with a speech production task in a compar-ison across studies produced in multiple laboratories employing both fMRI and PET. Several studies employing fMRI have demonstrated patterns of activity within striate and extrastriate cortex that could be predicted on the basis of the well-understood retinotopic organization of primary visual cortex (e.g. Sereno *et al.* 1995; DeYoe *et al.* 1996; Engel *et al.* 1997). Such evidence builds confidence that the BOLD response is tightly coupled to neuronal activity.

The studies discussed above demonstrate the stability and reliability of the signal provided by the haemodynamic response. Nonetheless, evidence sug-gests that there is some variability in the exact form of the response from one subject to the next and from one brain region to another. For example, Miezin *et al.* (2000) revealed differences in the timing and ampli-tude of the haemodynamic response from the primary visual cortex across subjects. More significant how-ever, is evidence that the haemodynamic response varies across brain regions within a given subject. This variability is exhibited in terms of the onset and shape of the response. Data from Buckner *et al.* (1998), for example, revealed the onset of the response in extras-triate cortex to be about 1 s earlier than the response in prefrontal cortex during a word generation task. A related finding was presented by Schacter *et al.* (1997) in the context of a memory study, revealing a differ-ence of several seconds between activity in anterior and dorsal prefrontal cortex. Even within visual cortex itself, Bandettini (1999) has shown variance in the timing of the response of 1–2 s across voxels. As these findings make clear, paradigm design and analysis must take into account the possibility of variance in the timing and shape of the haemodynamic response across regions.

9.3 Blocked paradigms

By far the most commonly used fMRI experimental paradigm is the 'blocked' task paradigm, whereby a series of trials in one condition is presented during a discrete epoch of time. The signal acquired during one blocked condition is then compared to other blocks involving different task conditions. In a typical study, task blocks will range in duration from 16 s to a minute and, in a single fMRI run (continuous period of data acquisition), multiple task blocks will be presented to allow the contrast of fMRI signals between task blocks. For example, to determine brain areas active during a language production task, task blocks in which subjects see words and produce a response to them could be contrasted with alternating task blocks in which subjects passively view words.

Reminiscent of earlier PET paradigms, blocked paradigms employ time-integrated averaging procedures. Not only were blocked paradigms the first approach to be employed in fMRI studies (Bandettini *et al.* 1992; Kwong *et al.* 1992; Ogawa *et al.* 1992), they were also the first targeted for the development of serious statistical analysis (e.g. Bandettini *et al.* 1993; Friston *et al.* 1994). Regions of activity change between one condition and another can be identified with considerable statistical power. Blocked procedures allow considerable experimental flexibility, for example allowing parametric designs and multi-factorial designs to be employed (Frackowiak and Friston 1995). The kinds of design possible with blocked paradigms have previously been reviewed extensively (for excellent reviews see Binder and Rao 1994; D'Esposito *et al.* 1999), and therefore, we will only touch upon one important conceptual consideration.

Because fMRI methods are limited to finding relative changes between task comparisons, a crucial question is how to best design task comparisons in a given study. One important question is how closely matched the different tasks should be. A useful distinction that can be made in this regard is between 'tight' and 'loose' task comparisons (cf. Buckner 1996; Buckner and Logan 2000). Tight comparisons aim at holding as many extraneous variables as possible constant across tasks. For example, consider a blocked design by Demb *et al.* (1995) that examined meaning-based decisions on visually presented words. They compared blocks involving a meaning-based semantic decision (deciding whether each item was abstract or concrete) relative to equivalent blocks of a nonsemantic decision (deciding whether each item was presented in upper or lower-case letters). To isolate differences related to processing word meaning, the two tasks were designed to differ in terms of the 'depth' of meaning based processing afforded to each item, whilst sharing other task demands, such as similar presentation of words, identical stimuli (when counter-

balanced across runs), and grossly similar response demands.

An alternative approach is possible however. That is, 'loose' comparisons between tasks that are not closely matched, employing a much broader comparison across task variables. For example, visual fixation could be used as a low-level task. Buckner and Koutstaal (1998) used just such a low-level visual fixation task in a study that also employed both the meaning-based semantic and nonsemantic tasks used by Demb *et al.* (1995). Buckner and Koutstaal were thus able to compare the two meaning-based task conditions to each other (tight comparisons), and either task condition to the 'fixation' task (loose comparisons). The resulting contrasts yielded brain areas active in common between the two word processing tasks *and* those that differed.

The use of 'loose' task comparisons described above may appear unnecessary. However, there are several clear merits in employing both loose and tight task comparisons simultaneously. First, the comparison between two closely matched tasks will only reveal regions that differ—any regions that are shared across the tasks will be subtracted out. It is often useful to see the entire set of regions that is activated during performance of a task, and not simply those regions that differ between two tasks, as a means of checking data quality and also as a means of identifying the entire network of brain regions active in a given task. For example, the two word processing tasks described above would, a priori, be expected to give rise to activity associated with viewing the stimuli and making a motor responses—excellent markers of whether the experiment has succeeded and of the overall quality of the data. These regions could only be examined using a 'loose' task comparison between each task and the low-level fixation condition. Moreover, several component processes may be shared between conditions being compared but nonetheless be important components of the high-level demands of a task. Shared regions of activation often only become apparent when multiple comparisons are made to low-level reference tasks (e.g. Buckner 1996). A final reason to employ reference to a low-level control is that the same reference task can serve for multiple conditions and even studies. As fMRI data provide information about relative signal change, interpretations across conditions and studies can be made easier if contrasts are made with respect to the same reference task.

This is not to imply that 'loose' comparisons (which come with their own interpretive problems, e.g. Shulman *et al.* 1997; Binder *et al.* 1999) are an alternative to the more closely matched 'tight' task comparisons. Nonetheless, it is often possible to include a variety of task comparisons within a study, building confidence in the quality of the data and answering theoretically driven questions—both loose and tight task comparisons should be considered.

9.4   Event-related paradigms

Event-related paradigms differ from blocked paradigms in that individual trial events (or even subcomponents of trial events) are measured, rather than a temporally-integrated signal. For example, in a typical event-related paradigm two separate trial types (e.g. words versus pictures) might be randomly intermixed in rapid succession. Then, the separate signal contributions of the two kinds of trial type are compared directly. Such a design may seem counterintuitive given the lag and temporally blurring inherent in the haemodynamic response. However, informative analysis of the complex signal is possible and affords considerable statistical power.

Several features of fMRI data proved to be critical in allowing event-related procedures to be developed. First, technological advances occurred in the speed with which fMRI data could be acquired. Second, the fact that even very brief periods of neural activity give rise to measurable signal changes—despite the delayed and prolonged nature of the time-course of the haemodynamic response. Third, the haemodynamic response has been shown to provide a highly consistent response that summates over sequential events in a roughly linear fashion. Each of these issues is considered in turn below.

9.4.1   Rapid data acquisition

Event-related procedures necessarily require that the signal of interest can be sampled frequently and repeatedly, allowing the data to be acquired over the time course of an individual event. Thus, it is an even more important feature of ER-MRI than of block designs

that signals can be acquired extremely rapidly (e.g. using echo planar or spiral imaging methods). If only a few slices through the brain are required, measurements can be repeated in less than 1 s. Generally, however, functional imaging studies require whole brain coverage and thus many slices must be acquired increasing the total acquisition time (sampling rate or repetition time, TR). Even so, for a scan that provides whole brain coverage, the total TR can be acquired in as little as 2 s on current commercial systems.

Whilst the actual sampling rate of fMRI measures is ultimately limited (due to factors such as saturation of spins in the brain and the speed with which the imaging gradients can be switched), it is possible to further reduce the *effective* sampling rate by appropriate paradigm design. By staggering the timing of stimulus presentation relative to the timing of image acquisition, reconstructed signals can be produced with a shorter effective sampling rate than is implied by the actual TR (cf. Josephs *et al.* 1997; Miezin *et al.* 2000). For example, consider the case whereby stimuli are presented every 5 s, and the signal is sampled (TR) every 3 s. The first sample is at zero seconds relative to the onset of the first stimuli, the second sample is at 3 s, the third sample is at one second relative to the onset of the second stimuli, etc. Thus, over the course of an experiment signals will, in effect, be acquired every second relative to the onset of the stimuli (Josephs *et al.* 1997). An even simpler example is shown in Fig. 9.1, whereby the effective sampling rate is doubled using an 'interleaved' procedure (Miezin *et al.* 2000). For a fixed TR of 2 s two data sets are acquired, providing odd and even sample points that contribute to a composite waveform with a 1 s sampling resolution.

Of course, for a given number of sampling points, such procedures result in less data being acquired, and therefore a poorer signal-to-noise ratio at each time point in the sample. Importantly, this *does not* imply a loss of power in the ability to detect the haemodynamic response signal over successive time points. In fact, in circumstances where fixed versus intermittent sampling procedures have been directly compared, the statistical power has been found to be either equivalent (Miezin *et al.* 2000) or better for intermittent sampling (Price *et al.* 1999).

In summary, it is clearly possible to increase the effective sampling rate beyond that of the TR, providing an increase in the temporal resolution of the

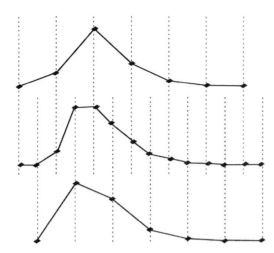

Fig. 9.1 Sampling the BOLD signal. The temporal resolution of the sampling of fMRI data can be increased beyond that of the basic sampling rate (TR) by simply varying the relationship between the onset of stimuli and the image acquisition. The figure demonstrates how staggering the point at which the signal is sampled can increase the temporal resolution. The averaged waveform (middle) is a composite of data from two separate sets of trials that sample sparsely, providing either odd (top) or even (bottom) data points. This method can be implemented by simply staggering the presentation of stimuli, presenting half the stimuli time-locked to the onset of the image acquisition (i.e. immediately) and the remaining stimuli half way between successive image acquisitions (i.e. delayed). Note that this method of improving the temporal resolution beyond the basic TR relies upon the averaging of data from different sets of stimuli and could not therefore be employed with single trial data.

data. Nonetheless, without such procedures, fairly rapid sampling procedures (~2 s per brain volume) are still achievable using currently available imaging systems, yielding a powerful means to estimate the haemodynamic response in event-related paradigms.

9.4.2 Sensitivity of the signal

The second feature of fMRI that was important in the development of event-related procedures is that the signal is highly sensitive, such that even a very brief period of neural activity elicits a measurable signal change. Transient increases in BOLD signal were initially demonstrated in sensory and motor cortex. For example, Blamire *et al.* (1992) presented subjects with visual stimuli lasting 2 s, intended to elicit corre-

spondingly brief periods of neuronal activity in visual cortex. As expected, transient increases in the BOLD signal were observed in response to each stimulus. Likewise, Bandettini (1993, 1999) observed the effects of brief versus prolonged motor activity, measuring signal changes in motor cortex while subjects made finger tapping movements lasting from 0.5–5 s in duration. Signal changes began around 2–3 s after finger tapping began, and continued for around 3–5 s, before returning to baseline. Increases in signal of around 2 per cent in magnitude were seen for even the briefest movements. Figure 11.2 shows an extreme example of the sensitivity of the BOLD signal, demonstrating that visual stimulation as brief as 34 ms in duration will elicit small, but clearly detectable, signal changes (cf. Savoy *et al.* 1995; and see Konishi *et al.* 1996).

Importantly, similar transient signal increases have also been demonstrated in cognitive task paradigms, even though the signal changes can be considerably lower in studies using sensory and motor tasks (i.e. with observed signal changes of less than 1 per cent). For example, Buckner *et al.* (1996) demonstrated that signal changes in visual and prefrontal brain areas can be detected during isolated trials of a word generation task. Similarly, Kim *et al.* (1997) defined haemodynamic responses in motor and visual cortex with tasks involving subject-initiated motor preparation. McCarthy *et al.* (1997) were able to measure transient responses in parietal cortex during infrequent presentation of target letter strings. Notably, all of these initial studies employed the constraint that trials were widely separated in time, allowing the haemodynamic response from one event to fully restore before the beginning of the next event.

Dale and Buckner (1997) extended the use of event-related procedures to circumstances in which different classes of stimuli were intermixed and presented close together in time. Dale and Buckner employed simple visual stimuli (flickering checkerboards), ensuring that relatively large and robust signal changes could be observed. In two experiments they showed that reliable signals could be detected in visual cortex when a single class of stimuli was presented *rapidly*—brief full-field flickering checkerboards, with as little as 2 s separation between successive stimulus presentations. Importantly, the response to these rapidly presented stimuli summed nearly linearly, so the individual responses to sequential events could be estimated. In

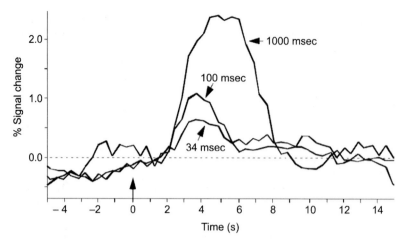

Fig. 9.2 Sensitivity of the BOLD signal. The fMRI BOLD signal change to visual stimulation. The stimuli varied in duration, lasting either 34, 100, or 1000 ms. Even the briefest period of stimulation gives rise to clear signal change. The signal change clearly increases in both amplitude and duration as the period of visual stimulation increases. Moreover, the signal is both delayed in onset and temporally blurred relative to the visual stimulation. Adapted from Savoy *et al.* (1995).

two further studies, Dale and Buckner demonstrated that reliable signals could be detected when two classes of stimuli were *intermixed* (stimuli were randomly presented to either left or right hemifield). Even though stimuli were randomly presented to left and right hemi-fields in too rapid a succession for the haemodynamic response to return to baseline, it was possible to extract the same lateralized patterns of visual cortex activity seen with much longer inter-stimulus intervals. Collectively, these observations made clear that fMRI can detect haemodynamic responses to extremely brief, rapidly presented and randomly intermixed neuronal events, making it possible to employ event-related signal-averaging procedures (for review see Rosen *et al.* 1998). The principles and specific procedures by which the haemodynamic response can be estimated in trains of rapidly presented stimuli will be discussed below.

9.4.3 Linearity of the signal

The study by Dale and Buckner (1997) discussed above and a seminal study by Boynton and colleagues (1996) highlight the third notable feature of fMRI data that proved crucial for the introduction of rapid presentation event-related procedures: namely that the shape of the BOLD haemodynamic response to a given period of stimulation is predictable and relatively

stable across events, even when there is an overlap in the responses to successive events.

Of particular interest is the finding that roughly the same response will be evoked even if the response to an initial event has not decayed, i.e. that the haemodynamic response summates in a roughly linear fashion (cf. Boynton *et al.* 1996; Dale and Buckner 1997; but see Friston *et al.* 1997; Vasquez and Noll 1998; Miezin *et al.* 2000). As can be seen in Fig. 9.3, fMRI signals evoked by a single event (1 s flickering checkerboard) exhibit the characteristic impulse-response function, with the haemodynamic responses to subsequently presented trials additively superimposing. Moreover, Fig. 9.3 shows that the estimated response to each successive trial closely matches that of the first trial with an onset around 2 s post-stimulus, a peak of between 4 s and 6 s, and a duration of around 12 s. This finding is important, because linear models of the haemodynamic response function underlie both the proper analysis of fMRI data, and the logic of certain forms of experimental designs such as rapid stimulus presentation and parametric manipulations (e.g. see Braver *et al.* 1997).

The even stronger claim of 'time-intensity separability' has been made in support of event-related procedures. This claim is that variations in the magnitude and duration of activity are essentially independent (Boynton, *et al.* 1996). This means that changes in the

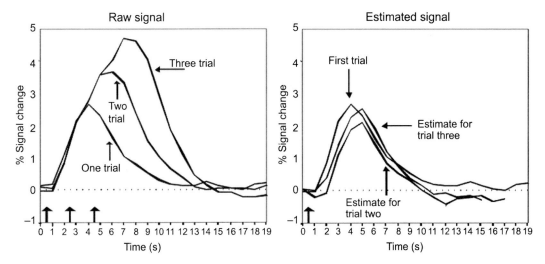

Fig. 9.3 Linear summation of the BOLD signal. Event-related fMRI data show approximately linear summation of the haemodynamic response in early visual cortex for closely spaced trials (2 s apart) of a 1 s visual checkerboard stimulus. Left. The raw fMRI signal intensity elicited by the presentation of one, two, or three trials. Note that the response is increased and prolonged by the addition of multiple trials, but does not saturate as successive trials overlap. Right. Estimates of the individual response to each of the three trials. Estimates were obtained by subtraction between the trial conditions (i.e. estimates for the second trial are the one trial condition subtracted from the two-trial condition, estimates for the third trial are the two-trial condition subtracted from the three-trial condition). Although subtle departures from linearity can be seen, the estimates are clearly very similar, supporting the assumption that the response to each stimulus summates linearly, at least under these specific conditions. Adapted from Dale and Buckner (1997).

intensity (strength) of neural activity result in equivalent changes in the intensity (magnitude) of the haemodynamic response, without any concomitant change in the duration of the response. In addition, a given change in the duration of neural activity results in an equivalent change in the duration of the haemodynamic response, without concomitant change in the magnitude of the activity.

Whilst the linearity and time-intensity separability assumptions may be valid working assumptions in many cases, it should be remembered that evidence suggests that there are limits to these assumptions. In particular, it seems possible that certain changes in the intensity of experimental stimulation are likely to break the linearity assumption—indeed even some of the earliest investigations of the BOLD signal showed some non-linear behaviours. In fact, all studies showing roughly linear summation properties have also revealed evidence for subtle (or not-so-subtle) nonlinearities. For example, Bandettini (1993) varied the rate at which subjects made finger-tapping movements, demonstrating that the magnitude of the signal

change in motor cortex did not vary in a monotonic fashion, i.e. it was not linearly related to the frequency of finger tapping.

One difficulty in resolving questions about how the haemodynamic signal summates over time is the fact that in many situations it is not known whether the underlying neuronal activity is itself linearly additive across time and trials. Thus, it is unclear whether departures from linearity reflect an intrinsic non-linear property of the haemodynamic response or of the underlying neuronal activity. For example, auditory word stimuli have been shown to exhibit roughly linear responses when stimuli were presented as frequently as one per 2 s or slower, but robust non-linearities in the response are observed at higher stimulus presentation rates (Friston *et al.* 1997). It may be the case that the neuronal response to auditory words at such rapid rates is different to that of more widely spaced words; alternatively, the neuronal response to words may be constant across rates but the haemodynamic response may saturate.

A practical question to ask—which to some degree

is agnostic as to the underlying mechanism by which non-linearities might arise—is whether the same, or different estimates of the haemodynamic response would be obtained at different trial presentation rates. Would the same response estimate be obtained when trials are spaced widely apart as when trials are so closely spaced as to yield overlapping responses? This was one of the questions asked in a recent analysis presented in Miezin *et al.* (2000). The rate of trial presentation was varied from one trial every 5 s (on average) to one trial every 20 s. Similar response function estimates were obtained at all rates. However, an amplitude reduction of about 20 per cent was noted at the fastest trial presentation rates, again suggesting either modest non-linear summation in the haemodynamic response itself, or interactions between trials. Neither the time-to-onset of the response, nor time-to-peak of the response was affected by the rate of trial presentation. Moreover, because of the increased numbers of trial events at the fastest rate, the greatest statistical power was present for detecting a response. Thus, in practical terms, these findings suggest that the haemodynamic response adds in a sufficiently linear fashion to provide a statistically powerful means of estimating responses—the necessary foundation for rapid event-related paradigm procedures.

9.5 Paradigm design and analysis of event-related studies

Haemodynamic imaging was originally limited to the use of 'blocked' recording procedures. As Raichle (2000) points out in an historical review of neuroimaging, the use of blocked procedures was a compromise, and the introduction of event-related procedures represents a major advance. Why? Fundamentally, because it allows the same procedures to be employed that have been so successfully employed elsewhere in the cognitive neurosciences. Enthusiasm for the 'event-related' approach stems from the fact that cognitive neuroscientists have traditionally employed procedures that allow for measurements of individual trials, or even sub-components of trials. Consider reaction time data, for example. Typically, reaction times are measured for individual trials, and then averaged according to different response categories (based on the type of stimuli presented and subject responses),

rather than being averaged across the entire experimental session. Equivalent procedures can now be easily accomplished in fMRI studies.

9.5.1 Extracting the signal of interest

From a methodological viewpoint, event-related and blocked procedures differ in the means by which the signal of interest is extracted. Blocked paradigms integrate activity over extended periods of up to a min during which a whole series of experimental trials (or a continuous extended task) are presented. By contrast, event-related procedures achieve similar signal-to-noise improvements by averaging data according to stimulus trial types, revealing activity that is time-locked to the onset of individual trial events. In most common settings these two forms of analysis largely proceed independently and are used to resolve different forms of signal. As will be discussed below however, in certain situations a given experimental data set can be analysed both in a blocked fashion and as part of an event-related analysis.

In blocked paradigms the time-averaged signal from one group of sequential trials is contrast with the time-averaged signal from another group. The signal reflects an average response from all trials presented during the task block—the signal changes associated with individual trials or trial types are not estimated separately. Moreover, averaged signal may also reflect multiple sources of activity. For example, imagine a visual brain region that increases in activity when a subject is asked to make judgements on visual stimuli, and further increases in activity each time an individual visual stimulus occurs during the task. Two separate components of the signal would likely be present, differing in their temporal evolution: (1) a sustained signal change across the entire task block and (2) a transient signal change with onset in a fixed relation to each trial event. In a blocked paradigm in which activity is averaged over an extended period the sustained and transient signal changes would not be resolved.

Event-related analyses explore signal changes in relation to the onsets of individual trial events, taking advantage of the finding that the BOLD haemodynamic response produces a transient (if temporally blurred) response to isolated trial events. The strength of the approach is twofold. First, transient signal

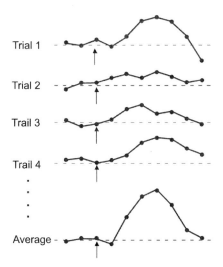

Trial 1

Trial 2

Trail 3

Trail 4

Average

Fig. 9.4 Event-related averaging. The figure shows how averaging can be used to reveal haemodynamic response that is consistently related to an event of interest. A series of trials is presented, involving the presentation of a stimulus on each trial, and haemodynamic changes are measured time-locked to the presentation of each stimulus. Individual trials are then averaged together to provide a representative average signal. Note that the signal on any given trial contains both the signal of interest and noise, and thus need not appear highly similar to the average signal. Nonetheless, assuming that noise is random across trials, the average signal reveals that part of the haemodynamic response that is systematically related to the event of interest.

changes that are not sustained across multiple trials can be detected. Second, because the transient signals are determined by individual trials, different kinds of trials can be randomly intermixed (or determined *post hoc*) for comparison. This allows the use of the kinds of paradigms that have been so well developed in other disciplines of cognitive neuroscience, such as for evoked potential studies. This allows the response to a specific event of interest to be defined. Note however, that a consequence of event-related procedures is that (as typically applied) they will likely miss activity that spans across successive trials—an issue that we will return to below in the section 'Introducing mixed "event-related and blocked" designs'. First, however, we provide a more extensive discussion of event-related procedures and their use in identifying transient signal events.

9.5.2 *Time-locked averaging*

As described above, event-related signal averaging most often requires the repetition of experimental trials, such that repeated time-locked epochs of data can be recorded and subsequently averaged together (cf. Buckner *et al.* 1996; Dale and Buckner 1997; Clark *et al.* 1998; Josephs *et al.* 1997; Zarahn *et al.* 1997; Friston *et al.* 1998*a*;). This, by definition, requires that an event is repeatable—or more commonly, that multiple instances of a class of event can be presented (such as old or new items in a memory test). The averaging procedure also requires that the data can be acquired in such a fashion that they can be aligned with the event of interest (i.e. averaged together based on a consistent reference point). As is illustrated in Fig. 9.4, in a typical event-related paradigm the presentation of each experimental stimuli is used as the temporal event to which the data is time-locked. However, this need not be the case. It is possible to time-lock to other events, such as the behavioral response made to each stimuli, and (at least in principle) to physiological measures such as heart rate. Moreover, in some circumstances it may be that one is interested in the pattern of neural activity leading up to an event, defining the event of interest as the end rather than the beginning of a trial.

In the most straightforward case the analysis of event-related trials reduces to simple selective averaging, i.e. calculating the mean and variance of the fMRI signal at each time point for each kind of trial event (e.g. Buckner *et al.* 1996; Dale and Buckner 1997). Inferential statistics can then be employed to ask questions about the presence or absence of differences between haemodynamic responses for each type of event (equivalent to the analysis of other physiological and behavioural data). Importantly, because of the temporal span of the haemodynamic response, it is necessary to consider the data across a range of time points. Whilst averaging procedures are typically performed off-line, alternative on-line procedures are currently being developed that allow real-time data processing and even statistical analyses (cf. Cox *et al.* 1995; Posse *et al.* 1998; Voyvodic 1999). Either way, given that the signal of interest is systematically associated with the time-locked event and invariant across trials, while background noise is random, the averaging procedure increases the signal-to-noise for signal changes that are time-locked to the experimental event. Clearly, the greater the number of trials that are averaged together the higher the signal-to-noise ratio becomes.

More recent approaches to the analysis of event-related fMRI data now involve a full implementation of the general linear model (GLM; cf. Friston *et al.* 1994; Worsley and Friston 1995; Josephs *et al.* 1997; Zarahn *et al.* 1997; Miezin *et al.* 2000). Analysis within the GLM is rooted in the simple assumption that the variance in the evolving fMRI BOLD-contrast signal that is systematically time-locked to the event *is* a direct measure of haemodynamic response. In practice, analysis of event-related data within the GLM requires that an explicit model is generated of the factors (i.e. effects) that are thought to contribute to variability in a data set. Effects can be modelled to account for the different kinds of trial events, as well as confounding effects such as a mean run intensity or slope that are theoretically uninteresting, but nonetheless present in the data.

For each voxel in a data set, estimates of the response to each effect are calculated by representing each time point in the data set by a linear equation. For each time point in the data set the linear equation represents the measured BOLD signal as the sum of the haemodynamic responses occurring at that point plus variance from noise (as illustrated in Fig. 9.5).

Because of overlap of successive haemodynamic responses to closely spaced trials, the ability to estimate the BOLD response is highly dependent upon the time between trials (cf. Burock *et al.* 1998). An important feature of the GLM approach is that the linear equations representing a data set can only be solved (i.e. estimates can only be derived) if there are as many equations as there are unknowns. When there is a fixed spacing between successive trials there is not enough information in the time-course data to arrive at a unique solution; there are more unknowns than equations, and the model is unsolvable. However, the introduction of 'jitter' (i.e. a variable temporal delay between successive trials) significantly increases the variance within the data set, providing more information from which to derive estimates of the BOLD response. The effects of introducing jitter on the available information is illustrated in Fig. 9.5.

The introduction of the GLM allows sophisticated approaches to data analysis to be employed, such as

interactions between response categories, time and performance measures (e.g. reaction time). Data can be selectively analysed for multiple independent factors (e.g. different response categories), extracting out that part of the on-going signal that is associated with each factor. Moreover, as will be discussed below, different factors that contribute to the ongoing waveform can be separated out using the GLM, allowing transient stimulus-related activity to be dissociated from more sustained state-related activity.

9.5.3 Trial ordering and jitter

When trials are spaced widely in time, the ordering of trial types has a marginal effect on the power of a paradigm. However, when trials are rapidly presented in succession, and must be linearly estimated, the trial ordering and/or temporal jittering between trials becomes a critical factor in designing a study. For example, Dale and Buckner (1997) provided a simple selective averaging procedure that allowed the separate contributions of different trial types to be estimated when they overlapped in time. It is important to stress that the power of the selective averaging procedures used by Dale and Buckner (1997) derived in part from the counterbalancing procedures employed. In their design, all trial types were made to follow each other equally often. That is, if a trial type 'A' was followed by a 'B' (yielding A–B), it was also followed by equally often an 'A' at another point in time (yielding A–A). When differences between event types were considered, the history of overlap simply, therefore, subtracted out.

The more general form of this counterbalancing technique is straightforward: trial orders are organized such that each type of trial is followed and preceded by every other trial type equally often. Because of the potential complexity of this, a computer program must be used to generate such trial sequences. The consequence of such counterbalancing is that when differences between trial types are considered the overlap between adjacent haemodynamic responses cancels out by simple subtraction. Within the context of the simple signal averaging procedure employed by Dale and Buckner (1997), without the use of this form of counterbalancing the overlapping haemodynamic responses to each successive stimuli are mixed together, making it difficult to assess the response for each type of stimuli.

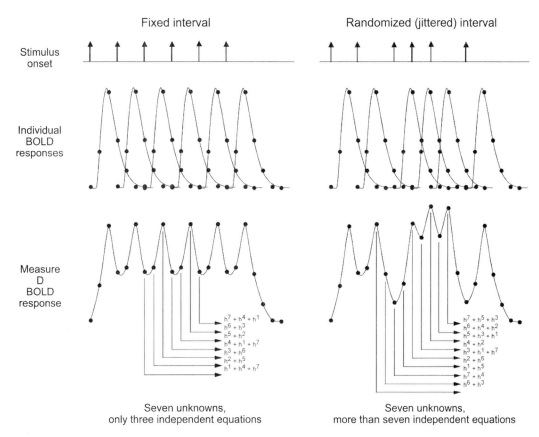

Fig. 9.5 The general linear model. The general linear model can only effectively estimate the separate contributions of the different trial types to the measured waveform when there are more equations than unknowns. The use of linear equations to estimate the haemodynamic response of overlapping events is consequently dependent upon the introduction of jitter between successive trial types. Each stimulus is associated with a transient signal change, evolving over several time points. The measured fMRI signal will be the linear summation of the signals to each stimulus—a complex waveform. The independent contributions of the different trials are unclear in the summated signal, however the contributions can be estimated using general linear equations. Left. When a fixed order of stimuli is employed in rapid event-related designs, with a fixed interval between successive trials, the resulting fMRI signal is repetitive. Analytically, the waveform is represented by fewer equations than unknowns, rendering the model unsolvable. Right. By introducing temporal jitter (variation) into the presentation rate of the trials the measured waveform becomes more complex. Consequently additional equations are required to represent the waveform, producing more equations than unknowns, making the general linear model tractable. Adapted from Miezin *et al.* (2000).

It is not always possible to counterbalance stimuli in this way, however, when interest lies in unpredictable responses to stimuli that may exhibit temporal dependencies or, by chance, yield sequences that are not counterbalanced. More generally, whenever trials are sorted *post hoc* according to subject performance it is unlikely that different trial types will be perfectly counterbalanced when only small numbers of trial events are considered. In such circumstances there are two

simple solutions. First, if a signal averaging procedure is used, then one solution is to change the experimental paradigm by spacing successive trials sufficiently far apart (i.e. around 10–12 s) for the haemodynamic response to return to baseline between trials (see Bandettini *et al.* 1998). This solution is probably not ideal as it will be of low power because relatively few trials can be presented in an acceptable time period. A second option is more appealing because it involves changing the analysis, rather than the paradigm. With this approach a more sophisticated analysis procedure is employed to obtain an overlap-corrected estimate of the haemodynamic response. Estimation within the GLM provides a powerful strategy. Although the GLM approach may provide a better estimate when stimuli are fully counterbalanced, it does not require the stringent counterbalancing procedures upon which the signal averaging technique is based. Power will increase to the degree that a variable amount of jitter between reoccurrence of the same trial type is presented, which is near its maximum in the design of Dale and Buckner (1997). However, a considerable amount of estimation power will exist so long as there is *sufficient* jitter between reoccurrence of the same event type.

The significance of introducing jitter between the representations of the same trial type is clear when one considers the difference between procedures that have a single trial type presented at fixed positions in time (i.e. without jitter) and those in which the trial is represented at varying intervals. When the interval between trials is fixed, very long intervals allow the haemodynamic response to return to baseline, producing some variance in the signal. By contrast, at very short intervals the response reaches a plateau because successive responses systematically overlap and never return to baseline, which reduces any variance in the signal. Put another way, the overlap cancels any modulation in signal; as the response increases for the next event, it will obscure the return to baseline of the earlier events. However, when the interval between trials fluctuates on any given trial there may be either a large or small amount of overlap between the haemodynamic response elicited on successive trials, depending on whether or not the trials were close together. Thus, as the presentation rate increases so does variability in the amount of overlap between trials, and hence variance in the signal will be larger (Burock *et al.* 1998). The greater this variance, the greater the information for deconvolution of individual time course.

The foregoing discussion should make clear that with rapidly presented stimuli it is necessary to introduce fluctuations in the interval between successive trials. Jitter increases the variance in the signal, and thereby increases the amount of information available, thus allowing the underlying haemodynamic response to be estimated for each class of trial. In practical terms

this feature of the event-related procedure is easy to incorporate into any given experimental design by simply introducing randomly inter-mixed 'null trials'—such as the presentation of a blank screen or fixation point during a visual experiment. From the subject's perspective, the gap between trials simply appears to vary slightly.

9.5.4 Detecting the response and constructing activation maps

A critical consideration when examining the signal using event-related procedures lies in estimating the time course of the signal, so that the averaged data includes the full evolution of a potential haemodynamic response, and then using that estimate to detect any haemodynamic response. The estimation procedures discussed above can be used without incorporating an explicit mathematical representation of the properties of the haemodynamic response. Linear estimation based on selective averaging or estimation within the GLM does not assume a specific response shape; only when statistical maps or quantitative variables must be derived are response shapes assumed.

Statistical map generation depends on the ability to detect those voxels in which a haemodynamic response is present. The most straightforward approach is to make no assumptions about the form (such as shape and temporal properties) of the haemodynamic response by examining for an effect over time (cf. Cohen *et al.* 1997). The disadvantage with this however, is that it is potentially less powerful than approaches that make use of the well-known characteristics of the haemodynamic impulse-response function. But in using a procedure that assumes a specific response shape and extracts activity that conforms to the particular properties of the haemodynamic response (e.g. using cross-correlation methods), the sensitivity will depend on what the shape of the haemodynamic response actually is, relative to what it is modelled to be.

While general characteristics of the response can be defined as described above, the specific shape of the response may vary in timing considerably between different regions of the cortex (Lee *et al.* 1995; Buckner *et al.* 1996; Schacter *et al.* 1997; Robson *et al.* 1998). Thus, when an idealized haemodynamic response is employed as the basis for analysis, it is important to employ a range (or set) of functions, to account for differences in the onset of the haemodynamic response across brain regions. Analysis that is restricted to a *single* function may systematically ignore activity that does not conform to the behavior of the chosen haemodynamic response (cf. Buckner *et al.* 1996; Schacter *et al.* 1997, discussed above). Fortunately, such variability can be relatively easily accounted for in practice. Multiple haemodynamic responses can be employed, using multiple delays, providing some robustness in detecting experimentally induced activity when a basic shape is assumed.

9.5.5 Some consequences of being event-related

Clearly, event-related averaging is a powerful technique for extracting the signal-of-interest. As with any method however, in addition to the inherent strengths, it has weaknesses. One clear caveat is that the averaged signal is not a direct measure of the response occurring on individual trials, and thus the averaged waveform could potentially show little relation to those of individual trials. The possibility of such distortion through averaging is important, because it leads to uncertainties in interpretation. For example, consider two averaged responses from different experimental conditions for a single brain region. If the magnitude of activity is greater in one case than the other this could be taken to reflect the presence of an underlying neural process that is graded, i.e. with greater processing in one case than the other. This need not necessarily be the case, however. The averaged responses also could reflect activity associated with an all-or-none neural process, with the difference between the two conditions lying in the proportion of trials in which the process is active.

Of course, this is not a problem specific to neuroimaging data—similar concerns arise in the interpretation of any dependent measure when averaged events are considered, whether behavioral or physiological. Nonetheless, such concerns reinforce the importance of studies examining single trial data (cf. Kim *et al.* 1997; Richter *et al.* 1997) or the distributions from many individual trials. Rapid event-related designs, in particular, are not easily modified to estimate the distribution of responses underlying the average. Estimation using parametric statistical methods such as the GLM implicitly ignores the possibility that

responses may not come from a single uni-modal distribution.

Notwithstanding concerns over the interpretation of differences between averaged event-related signals, it is clear that the introduction of event-related procedures has a major effect on the way fMRI data can be analysed. Perhaps the most significant effect of the event-related method is that it becomes possible to analyse data from different experimental trials according to either the type of stimuli presented, or subjects' responses to stimuli. Such approaches allow the neural correlates of performance on each experimental trial to be sorted *post hoc*. The advantages of this should be clear. For example, in studies of memory wherein the focus of interest lies in memory errors that are likely to occur relatively infrequently, the neural correlates of interest may only be visible using a trial based approach, where infrequently occurring memory errors can be cleanly isolated.

Studies of 'subsequent memory' effects highlight the utility of *post hoc* sorting. Wagner *et al.* (1998; also see Brewer *et al.* 1998) used event-related methods to study the neural correlates of memory encoding, by *post hoc* sorting haemodynamic response estimates according to whether subjects remembered each item during a later memory test. It was found that differences in the activation response associated with individual items at presentation were predictive of subjects' subsequent memory for those items. It is worth noting that the ability to sort data extends to other aspects of performance, such as reaction time (and in principal, to physiological measures such as heart rate). Thus, the use of event-related procedures allows one to ask questions concerning the covariation between neural activity and measurable aspects of behavior that are also likely to differ on a trial by trial basis.

Finally, the ability to sort trials *post hoc* also introduces the possibility of rejecting artifact-laden trials. It is clear that there are circumstances in which it is desirable to exclude responses to certain types of trial—for example, based on performance measures such as outlier responses (e.g. as measured by response times), incorrect responses, or when large movement artifacts are present. ER-fMRI procedures make this possible by allowing investigators to determine *post hoc* which trials contain artifacts and exclude them from further analysis. This kind of artifact rejection seems likely to be of particular use in studies involving difficult population groups, such as in experiments involving children (e.g. see Logan 1999; Thomas *et al.* 1999), or clinical patients (e.g. see Jezzard and Song 1996). Note that with blocked procedures this form of analysis is necessarily precluded because neural activity is averaged over a series of successive trials.

9.5.6 Issues related to experimental design

Not all of the effect of employing event-related procedures relates to data collection and analysis issues; the procedure also directly affects experimental design. The introduction of event-related procedures makes it more meaningful to inter-mix different types of stimuli. That is, randomized rather than blocked experimental designs can be employed. A study by McCarthy *et al.* (1997) highlights the way in which being able to employ randomized designs extends the range of questions that can be addressed using fMRI. The aim of the study was to examine the neural correlates of relatively infrequently occurring (rare) events, which occurred in amongst a series of frequently occurring (common) events. By averaging data in a time-locked manner dependent on each class of event, they were able to show that the infrequently occurring events elicited transient increases in activity in prefrontal and parietal cortex. This could not have been shown using blocked procedures however, because activity associated with each type of event could only have been separated had they been presented in separate blocks—making it difficult to have infrequent (rare) events.

Another clear example of the potential problems associated with this comes from studies of memory retrieval where old (studied) and new (unstudied) test items are presented in separate test blocks. After considering the first few trials in any block, subjects will be easily able to respond correctly to others in that block, without needing to consider whether the items are actually old or new. Employing a randomized experimental design can not only prevent subjects from suffering from fatigue and boredom, but also stop them from employing such strategies. However, it is worth stressing that the use of blocked designs in neuroimaging does not necessitate that trials of a certain type are grouped together. Indeed, researchers studying memory retrieval have purposely mixed old and new items at test, parametrically varying the proportions of each

trial type across blocks (e.g. see Rugg *et al.* 1996). The problem with this is that when the neural activity is measured across the block it is not possible to distinguish specifically the differences that occur between the different types of trials that are presented. This is only possible when event-related procedures are employed.

While the preceding discussion illustrates the potential problems of employing blocked data analysis procedures, it should not be taken to suggest that the displaying stimuli in blocks is undesirable *per se*. Indeed, in some circumstances a blocked experimental design is more appropriate. For example, requiring patients with frontal lobe damage to constantly alternate between tasks on a trial by trial basis may simply interfere with their ability to perform the tasks at all.

Unfortunately, it is not possible to simply produce an absolute index of which regions are involved in performing a given cognitive process—regardless of whether blocked or event-related procedures are employed. As with all neuroimaging techniques, information is provided by examining relative changes in activity—either in terms of differences between pairs (or a series) of tasks, or in correlations with behavioral measures.

9.6 *Introducing mixed 'event-related and blocked' designs*

A relatively subtle facet of paradigm design, and one that has been largely ignored to date, is the sensitivity of different kinds of paradigms to signal changes that evolve on distinct time scales. By definition, the event-related designs discussed above are sensitive to *transient* changes in activity that are time-locked to events of interest. Blocked paradigms are also sensitive to this form of signal change—but average over the events within the block. That is, a series of transient events will sum into a single extended signal change in standard blocked paradigms. However, as noted above, blocked paradigms are additionally sensitive to *sustained* changes in activity that exist across extended periods of time and that are not necessarily modulated on an event-by-event basis. In this regard, blocked and event-related procedures may be employed to investigate quite different questions.

The contrast between the use of event-related and blocked designs to investigate signal changes that develop over very different time scales is clear in two recent studies by Henson and colleagues that describe investigation of different aspects of memory retrieval. In one case (Henson *et al.* 1999*a*) event-related procedures were used because the focus of interest lay at the level of individual test items, i.e. in differences between *individual* recognition responses associated with trial-by-trial difference in experience. In a second study (Henson *et al.* 1999*b*) blocked procedures were employed because interest lay in defining any differ-

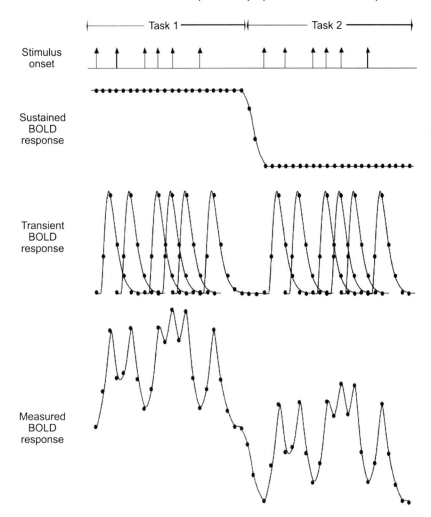

Fig. 9.6 Paradigm design for fMRI. A representation of the signal measured in a mixed 'blocked and event-related' paradigm. Stimuli are presented in two separate blocks (task 1 and task 2). Two distinct kinds of correlates of activity may occur, a sustained BOLD response that is modulated across the two tasks, and a transient BOLD response that is associated with the individual stimuli. The measured BOLD response will be a linear summation of these different signal changes. If blocked analyses were employed then a single aggregate measure of transient and sustained activity would be provided over each task period, confounding transient and sustained signal changes. By contrast, if event-related analyses were employed then only the transient signal changes would be examined. However, the general linear model can be used to provide independent estimates of (i) sustained activity associated with the different tasks, and (ii) transient signal changes associated with individual stimuli. This kind of paradigm design can be employed to distinguished between transient and sustained changes in activity, for example allowing different task states such as full versus divided attention or deep versus shallow encoding to be compared whilst holding the individual items constant.

ences that span across all test items. That is, differences between task blocks that differed in the retrieval instructions given to subjects—differences that might be expected to yield a sustained activity change reflecting the cognitive set (or mode) that a subject was engaged in.

The two experiments by Henson and colleges described above are interesting because they elucidate an important feature of experimental tasks; namely that performance on a task usually involves a combination of set-related processes and stimulus-related processes. Subjects are given an instructional set, and then use that set to dictate how they respond on each individual trial. A reasonable hypothesis is that certain components of the set-related responses are sustained while the set is maintained, while transient responses may modulate in response to the individual stimulus trials. That is, processes may exist that are elicited by the general situation or task setting (state), alongside processes that are elicited by the specific stimuli that are presented (item). Figure 9.6 provides an example of a paradigm in which both transient and sustained signal changes may be present.

As discussed above, blocked trial paradigms generally confound these two types of response (although for an interesting exception using Event-Related Potentials, see Duzel *et al.* 1999). In a typical blocked design fMRI experiment it is not possible to distinguish sustained changes in activity (effects that are tonic, lasting throughout a task period) from transient changes in activity (effects that are stimulus-specific and associated with current mental processes). Thus, any comparisons made between blocks will confound sustained and transient changes in activity, unless explicit attempts are made to control one or other type of response across blocks. By contrast, event-related paradigms are typically designed to be sensitive only to transient signal changes. Any sustained (tonic or task-related) activity that is present in *all* of the event-related responses during a task will therefore be subtracted out when comparisons are made between the responses to different conditions.

Of course, in many circumstances it may be that one is interested in neural activity associated with the processing of experimentally presented stimuli, and that sustained, ongoing set-related activity is essentially unwanted noise. However, in other settings, where one is explicitly manipulating the presentation

of individual stimuli and the context within which this is done, the distinction between sustained and transient effects can be crucial. For example, in studies of memory retrieval, neural activity associated with being in a 'retrieval mode' (related to the general requirement to perform a memory test) may be distinct from that associated with attempting or succeeding to retrieve information from memory (related to individual test items). Similarly, in the study of retrieval monitoring by Henson *et al.* (1999*b*) the effect of task states would ideally have been separated from the effects of the individual items presented during each task period. A thorough examination of the neural basis of performance thus necessitates investigations that allow a hybrid or combination of blocked and event-related procedures to be employed, allowing sustained or tonic neural effects to be distinguished from transient or item specific effects.

One of the exciting aspects of recent approaches to analysing fMRI data is that mixed 'event-related and blocked' analyses can be easily implemented. For example, the GLM approach allows multiple independent factors to be coded into the analytical model that is used to represent the experimental design. Thus, as long as an experiment is designed such that individual trials are separated into distinct blocks, transient (i.e. stimulus-related) and sustained (i.e. set-related) effects can be simultaneously incorporated into the GLM. Figure 9.6 provides one example of how an experiment can be designed to incorporate both blocked and event-related features.

When analysed using the GLM this kind of design allows sustained signal changes associated with the cognitive set to be estimated alongside independent estimates of the transient responses to individual stimuli. Moreover, with this type of paradigm design it should be possible to investigate the extent to which tonic or sustained neural activity contributes to, or interacts with, transient stimulus specific effects. For example, it may be that the pattern of transient activity associated with a given stimulus type is modulated (increased or decreased) dependent upon the subject's cognitive set. It is worth remembering however, that it is the introduction of event-related procedures that makes such a goal achievable. Thus, a detail that could be easily overlooked is that in a mixed blocked and event-related design, the trial types within the blocks must be jittered just as they would be in a purely event-related design. If that constraint is met, then solving for the independent sustained and transient components of the signal is simply the simultaneous solution to a set of effects that includes both the individual events and the blocks. Only with 'mixed' designs, however, is it possible to investigate the role of both transient and sustained activity in supporting cognitive processing, and any potential interplay between the two.

References

Aguirre, G.K., Zarahn, E., and D'Esposito, M. (1998). The variability of human BOLD hemodynamic responses. *NeuroImage*, 8, 360–9.

Bandettini, P.A. (1993). MRI studies of brain activation: dynamic characteristics. In: *Functional MRI of the Brain*, pp. 144–51, *Society of Magnetic Resonance in Medicine*, Berkeley.

Bandettini, P.A. (1999). The temporal resolution of MRI. In: *Functional MRI* (ed. C.T.W. Moonen and P. Bandettini), pp.205–20, *Springer-Verlag*, Mauer, Germany.

Bandettini, P.A., and Cox, R.W. (1998). In: *Contrast in single trial fMRI: Interstimulus interval dependency and comparison with blocked strategies*, 1, 161, Proceedings of the International Society for Magnetic Resonance in Imaging, 6th Meeting.

Bandettini, P.A., Wong, E.C., Hinks, R.S., Tikofsky, R.S., and Hyde, J.S., (1992). Time course of EPI of human brain function during task activation. *Magnetic Resonance in Medicine*, 25, 390–7.

Binder, J.R., and Rao, S.M. (1994). Human brain mapping with functional magnetic resonance imaging. In: *Localization and Neuroimaging in Neuropsychology* (ed. A. Kertesz), pp. 185–212, San Diego, Academic Press.

Binder, J.R., Frost, J.A., Hammeke, T.A., Bellgowan, P.S.F., Rao, S.M., and Cox, R.W. (1999). Conceptual processing during the conscious resting state. A functional MRI study. *Journal of Cognitive Neuroscience*, 11, 80–95.

Blamire, A.M., Ogawa, S., Ugurbil, K., Rothman, D., McCarthy, G., Ellerman, J.M., Hyder, F., Rattner, Z., and Shulman, R.G. (1992). Dynamic mapping of the human visual cortex by high-speed magnetic resonance imaging. *Proceedings of the National Academy of Sciences (USA)*, 89, 11069–73.

Boynton, G.M., Engel, S.A., Glover, G.H., and Heeger, D.J. (1996). Linear systems analysis of functional magnetic resonance imaging in human V1. *Journal of Neuroscience*, 16, 4207–21.

Braver, T.S., Cohen, J.D., Nystrom, L.E., Jonides, J., Smith, E.E., and Noll, D.C. (1997). A parametric study of prefrontal cortex involvement in human working memory. *NeuroImage*, 5, 49–62.

Brewer, J.B., Zhao, Z., Desmond, J.E., Glover, G.H., and Gabrieli, J.D. (1998). Making memories: brain activity that predicts how well visual experience will be remembered. *Science*, 281, 1185–7.

Buckner, R.L. (1996). Beyond HERA: Contributions of specific prefrontal brain areas to long-term memory retrieval. *Psychonomic Bulletin and Review*, 3, 149–58.

Buckner, R.L. and Koutstaal, W. (1998). Functional neuroimaging studies of encoding, priming, and explicit memory retrieval. *Proceedings of the National Academy of Science (USA)*, 95, 891–8.

Buckner, R.L. and Logan, J.M. (2001). Functional neuroimaging methods: PET and fMRI. In: *Functional Neuroimaging* (ed. R. Cabeza), pp. 27–48, Cambridge, MIT Press.

Buckner, R.L., Bandettini, P.A., O'Craven, K.M., Savoy, R.L., Petersen, S.E., Raichle, M.E., and Rosen, B.R. (1996). Detection of cortical activation during averaged single trials of a cognitive task using functional magnetic resonance imaging. *Proceedings of the National Academy of Science (USA)*, 93, 14878–83.

Buckner, R.I.., Koutstaal, W., Schacter, D.L., Dale, A.M., Rotte, M., and Rosen, B.R. (1998). Functional-anatomic study of episodic retrieval. II. Selective averaging of event-related fMRI trials to test the retrieval success hypothesis. *NeuroImage*, 7, 163–75.

Burock, M.A., Buckner, R.L., Woldorff, M.G., Rosen, B.R., and Dale, A.M. (1998). Randomized event-related experimental designs allow for extremely rapid presentation rates using functional MRI. *NeuroReport*, 9, 3735–9.

Buxton, R.B., Wong, E.C., and Frank, L.R. (1998). Dynamics of blood flow and oxygenation changes during brain activation: the balloon model. *Magnetic Resonance in Medicine*, 39, 855–64.

Carter, C.S., Braver, T.S., Barch, D.M., Botvinick, M.M., Noll, D.C., and Cohen, J.D. (1998). Anterior cingulate cortex, error detection, and the online monitoring of performance. *Science*, 280, 747–9.

Casey, B.J., Cohen, J.D., O'Craven, K., Davidson, R.J., Irwin, W., Nelson, C.A., Noll, D.C., Hu, X., Lowe, M.J., Rosen, B.R., Truwitt, C.L., and Turski, P.A. (1998). Reproducibility of fMRI results across four institutions using a spatial working memory task. *NeuroImage*, 8, 249–61.

Clark, V.P., Keil, K., Maisog, J.M., Courtney, S., Ungerleider, L.G., and Haxby, J.V. (1996). Functional magnetic resonance imaging of human visual cortex during face matching: A comparison with positron emission tomography. *NeuroImage*, 4, 1–15.

Clark, V.P., Maisog, J.M., and Haxby, J.V. (1998). fMRI study of face perception and memory using random stimulus sequences. *Journal of Neurophysiology*, 79, 3257–65.

Cohen, J.D., Perlstein, W.M., Braver, T.S., Nystrom, L.E., Noll, D.C., Jonides, J., and Smith, E.E. (1997). Temporal dynamics of brain activation during a working memory task. *Nature*, 386, 604–7.

Cox, R.W., Jesmanowicz A., and Hyde J. S. (1995). Real-time functional magnetic resonance imaging. *Magnetic Resonance in Medicine*, 33, 230–36.

Dale, A.M. and Buckner, R.L. (1997). Selective averaging of rapidly presented individual trials using fMRI. *Human Brain Mapping*, 5, 329–40.

Demb, J.B., Desmond, J.E., Wagner, A.D., Vaidya, C.J., Glover, G.H., and Gabrieli, J.D. (1995). Semantic encoding and retrieval in the left inferior prefrontal cortex: A functional MRI study of task difficulty and process specificity. *Journal of Neuroscience*, **15**, 5870–8.

D'Esposito, M., Zarahn, E., and Aguirre, G.K. (1999). Event-related functional MRI: Implications for cognitive psychology. *Psychological Bulletin*, **125**, 155–64.

DeYoe, E.A., Carman, G.J., Bandettini, P., Glickman, S., Wieser, J., Cox, R., Miller, D., and Neitz, J. (1996). Mapping striate and extrastriate visual areas in human cerebral cortex. *Proceedings of the National Academy of Sciences (USA)*, **93**, 2382–6.

Duzel, E., Cabeza, R., Picton, T.W., Yonelinas, A.P., Scheich, H., Heinze, H.J., and Tulving, E. (1999). Task-related and item-related brain processes of memory retrieval. *Proceedings of the National Academy of Sciences (USA)*, **96**, 1794–9.

Engel, S.A., Glover, G.H., and Wandell, B.A. (1997). Retinotopic organization in human visual cortex and the spatial precision of functional MRI. *Cerebral Cortex*, **7**, 181–92.

Frackowiak, R.S.J., and Friston, K.J. (1995). Methodology of activation paradigms. In: *Handbook of Neuropsychology*, Vol. 10. (ed. F. Boller and J. Grafman), pp.282–369, Elsevier, Amsterdam.

Fransson, P., Kruger, G., Merboldt, K.D., and Frahm, J. (1998). Physiologic aspects of event-related paradigms in magnetic resonance functional neuroimaging. *NeuroReport*, **9**, 2001–5.

Fransson, P., Kruger, G., Merboldt, K.D., and Frahm, J. (1999). Temporal and spatial MRI responses to subsecond visual activation. *Magnetic Resonance Imaging*, **17**, 1–7.

Friston, K.J., Jezzard, P., and Turner, R. (1994). The analysis of functional MRI time series. *Human Brain Mapping*, **1**, 153–71.

Friston, K.J., Buechel, C., Fink, G.R., Morris, J., Rolls, E., and Dolan, R.J. (1997). Psychophysiological and modulatory interactions in neuroimaging. *Neuroimage*, **6**, 218–29.

Friston K. J., Fletcher P., Josephs O., Holmes A., Rugg M. D., and Turner R. (1998*a*). Event-related fMRI: characterizing differential responses. *NeuroImage*, **7**, 30–40.

Friston, K.J., Josephs, O., Rees, G., and Turner, R. (1998*b*). Non-linear event-related responses in fMRI. *Magnetic Resonance in Medicine*, **39**, 41–52.

Henson R. N., Rugg M. D., Shallice T., Josephs O., and Dolan R. J. (1999*a*). Recollection and familiarity in recognition memory: an event-related functional magnetic resonance imaging study. *Journal of Neuroscience*, **15**, 3962–72.

Henson, R.N., Shallice, T., and Dolan, R.J. (1999*b*). Right prefrontal cortex and episodic memory retrieval: a functional MRI test of the monitoring hypothesis. *Brain*, **122**, 1367–81.

Jezzard, P., and Song, A.W. (1996). Technical foundations and pitfalls of clinical fMRI. *NeuroImage*, **4**, S63–75.

Josephs, O., Turner, R. and Friston, K. (1997). Event-related fMRI. *Human Brain Mapping*, **5**, 243–8.

Kim, S.G., Richter, W., and Ugurbil, K. (1997). Limitations of temporal resolution in functional MRI. *Magnetic Resonance in Medicine*, **37**, 631–6.

Konishi, S., Yoneyama, R., Itagaki, H., Uchida, I., Nakajima, K., Kato, H., Okajima, K., Koizumi, H., and Miyashita, Y. (1996). Transient brain activity used in magnetic resonance imaging to detect functional areas. *NeuroReport*, **8**, 19–23.

Kwong, K.K., Belliveau, J.W., Chesler, D.A., Goldberg, I.E., Weisskoff, R.M., Poncelet, B. P., Kennedy, D.N., Hoppel, B.E., Cohen, M.S., and Turner, R. (1992). Dynamic magnetic resonance imaging of human brain activity during primary sensory stimulation. *Proceedings of the National Academy of Sciences (USA)*, **89**, 5675–9.

Lee, A.T., Glover, G.H., and Meyer, C.H. (1995). Discrimination of large venous vessels in time-course spiral blood-oxygen-level-dependent magnetic-resonance functional neuroimaging. *Magnetic Resonance in Medicine*, **33**, 745–54.

Logan, W.J. (1999). Functional magnetic resonance imaging in children. *Seminars in Pediatric Neurology*, **6**, 78–86.

McCarthy, G., Luby, M., Gore, J., and Goldman-Rakic, P. (1997). Infrequent events transiently activate human prefrontal and parietal cortex as measured by functional MRI. *Journal of Neurophysiology*, **77**, 1630–4.

Menon, R.S., Gati, J.S., Goodyear, B.G., Luknowsky, D.C., and Thomas, C.G. (1998). Spatial and temporal resolution of functional magnetic resonance imaging. *Biochemistry and Cell Biology*, **76**, 560–71.

Miezin, F.M., Maccotta, L., Ollinger, J.M., Petersen, S.E., and Buckner, R.L. (2000). Characterizing the hemodynamic response: effects of presentation rate, sampling procedure, and the possibility of ordering brain activity based on relative timing. *NeuroImage*, **11**, 735–59.

Ogawa, S., Lee, T., Nayak, A., and Glynn, P. Oxygenation-sensitive contrast in magnetic resonance image of rodent brain at high magnetic fields. *Magnetic Resonance in Medicine*, **14**, 68–78.

Ogawa, S., Tank, D.W., Menon, R., Ellerman, J.M., Kim, S.G., Merkle, H., and Ugurbil, K. (1992). Intrinsic signal changes accompanying sensory stimulation: Functional brain mapping with magnetic resonance imaging. *Proceedings of the National Academy of Sciences (USA)*, **89**, 5951–5.

Ojemann, J.G., Buckner, R.L., Akbudak, E., Snyder, A.Z., Ollinger, J.M., McKinstry, R.C., Rosen, B.R., Petersen, S.E., Raichle, M.E., and Conturo, T.E. (1998). Functional MRI studies of word-stem completion: Reliability across laboratories and comparison to blood flow imaging with PET. *Human Brain Mapping*, **6**, 203–15.

Posse, S., Schor, S., Gembris, D., Muller, E., Peyerl., M., Krocker., R., Grosse-Ruken M. L., Elgghwaghi, B., and Taylor, J.G. (1998). Real-time fMRI on a clinical whole body scanner: Single-event detection of sensorimotor stimulation. *NeuroImage*, **7**, S567.

Price, C.J., Veltman, D.J., Ashburner, J., Josephs, O., and Friston, K.J. (1999). The critical relationship between the timing of stimulus presentation and data acquisition in blocked designs with fMRI. *NeuroImage*, **10**, 36–44.

Raichle, M.E. (2000). A brief history of functional brain imaging. In: *Brain mapping*: the systems (ed. A. Toga and J. Mazziotta), Academic Press, San Diego.

Richter, W., Georgopoulos, A. P., Ugurbil, K., and Kim, S.G. (1997). Detection of brain activity during mental rotation in a single trial by fMRI. *NeuroImage*, **5**, S49.

Robinson, D.L. and Rugg, M.D. (1988). Latencies of visually responsive neurons in various regions of the rhesus monkey brain and their relation to human visual responses. *Biological Psychology*, **26**, 111–6.

Robson, M.D., Dorosz, J.L., and Gore, J.C. (1998). Measurements of the temporal fMRI response of the human auditory cortex to trains of tones. *NeuroImage*, **7**, 185–98.

Rosen, B.R., Buckner, R.L., and Dale, A.M. (1998). Event-related fMRI: past, present, and future. *Proceedings of the National Academy of Sciences (USA)*, **95**, 773–80.

Rugg, M.D., Fletcher, P.C., Frith, C.D., Frackowiak, R.S., and Dolan, R.J. (1996). Differential activation of the prefrontal cortex in successful and unsuccessful memory retrieval. *Brain*, **119**, 2073–83.

Savoy, R.L., Bandettini, P.A., O'Craven, K.M., Kwong, K.K., Davis, T.L., Baker, J.R., Weiskoff, R.M., and Rosen, B.R. (1995). Pushing the temporal resolution of fMRI: Studies of very brief visual stimuli, onset variability and asynchrony, and stimulus-correlated changes in noise, 2, 450, *Proceedings of the Society of Magnetic Resonance* Third Scientific Meeting and Exhibition.

Schacter, D.L., Buckner, R.L., Koutstaal, W., Dale, A.M., and Rosen, B.R. (1997). Late onset of anterior prefrontal activity during true and false recognition: an event-related fMRI study. *NeuroImage*, **6**, 259–69.

Sereno, M.I., Dale, A.M., Reppas, J.B., Kwong, K.K., Belliveau, J.W., Brady, T.J., Rosen, B.R., and Tootell, R.B. (1995). Borders of multiple visual areas in humans revealed by functional magnetic resonance imaging. *Science*, **268**, 889–93.

Shulman, G.L., Fiez, J.A., Corbetta, M., Buckner, R.L., Miezin, F.M., Raichle, M.E., and Petersen, S.E. (1997). Common blood flow changes across visual tasks: II. Decreases in cerebral cortex. *Journal of Cognitive Neuroscience*, **9**, 648–63.

Thomas, K.M., King, S.W., Franzen, P.L., Welsh, T.F., Berkowitz, A.L., Noll, D.C., Birmaher, V., and Casey, B.J. (1999). A developmental functional MRI study of spatial working memory. *NeuroImage*, **10**, 327–38.

Vasquez, A.L., and Noll, D.C. (1998). Non-linear aspects of the BOLD response in functional MRI. *NeuroImage*, **7**, 108–18.

Voyvodic, J.T. (1999). Real-time fMRI paradigm control, physiology, and behavior combined with near real-time statistical analysis. *NeuroImage*, **10**, 91–106.

Wagner, A.D., Schacter, D.L., Rotte, M., Koutstaal, W., Maril, A., Dale, A.M., Rosen, B.R., and Buckner, R. L. (1998). Building memories: Remembering and forgetting of verbal experiences as predicted by brain activity. *Science*, **281**, 1188–91.

Worsley, K.J., and Friston, K.J. (1995). Analysis of fMRI time-series revisited—again. *NeuroImage*, **2**, 173–81.

Zarahn, E., Aguirre, G., and D'Esposito, M. (1997). A trial-based experimental design for fMRI. *NeuroImage*, **6**, 122–38.

10 | *The scanner as a psychophysical laboratory*

Robert Savoy

10.1 *Introduction*

The use of magnetic resonance imaging (MRI) for mapping human brain function has naturally required the presentation of stimuli, and recording of behavioural and physiological responses in the challenging MRI environment. The earliest human studies used very simple visual stimulation systems, such as goggles with blinking light-emitting diodes (Belliveau *et al.* 1991), or depended on the brain activity needed for simple motor tasks that did not require any extra simulation or recording equipment (e.g. Bandettini *et al.* 1993). There has been steady progress, both in individual laboratories and in the development of integrated commercial systems, for the sophisticated control of stimulus presentation and response recording during MRI. Some of this progress (and the general considerations for anyone establishing a functional MRI research environment) is articulated in the present chapter.

10.1.1 Information resources

The author of the present chapter reviewed these issues previously (Savoy *et al.* 1999), with more attention to the basic psychophysical limitations imposed by the visual and auditory systems themselves. The present chapter, while covering some similar topics, will focus on the latest developments relevant to an investigator establishing their own psychophysical laboratory in the magnet. In addition to the technical problems of stimulus presentation and response recording, there will be a brief discussion of the general need to adapt the psychophysical tasks themselves to be more compatible with the MRI environment.

The development of tools to create flexible psychophysical laboratories in the MRI environment is proceeding rapidly in research laboratories and also as commercial products. This makes it difficult to give 'up-to-date' information in a book. However, the material presented here should enable the reader to define the major issues and search the substantial Internet resources available. Some specific web sites will be mentioned, but as with any Internet reference, these should only be considered as starting points. The reliability of the web sites (in terms of existence, as well as content) is always subject to change. Nonetheless, virtually all vendors and laboratories will have a web presence. A subset of current vendors will be mentioned by name in the body of the chapter with contact information included in an Appendix at the end of the chapter.

10.1.2 Creating a psychophysical laboratory in the scanner

Without the constraints of having to operate within the MRI environment, the requirements for a general-purpose psychophysical laboratory are relatively straightforward. Computers are used to control stimulus presentation and behavioural response recording. Presentation of basic visual and auditory stimulation is routine (though calibration and quantitative control always require considerable care). Tactile, olfactory, gustatory, proprioceptive, pain, and other forms of stimulation can also be studied using relatively routine procedures in a psychophysical laboratory, albeit typically requiring human intervention or non-standard equipment. For example, the presentation of acupuncture stimulation (Hui *et al.* 2000) is not something that has yet been automated in any context.

The special enterprise of functional MRI adds many challenges. The first kind of challenge is the requirement for all equipment to function properly in the electromagnetically hostile MRI environment without distorting the images collected. The presence of a strong static magnetic field, large, rapidly varying gradient fields, and intense radiofrequency electromagnetic fields precludes the use of most standard psychophysical equipment both because they might pose safety hazards, and because they might not function properly. Moreover, such devices can interfere with the normal functioning of the MRI equipment, causing distortion or noise in the images. Because the signal modulations used in *functional* MRI are small fractions of the basic NMR signal modulations used in conventional (*structural*) MRI, even small amounts of distortion or noise can be a serious problem.

The presentation of auditory stimulation is a particular challenge because the pulse sequences commonly used for brain activation imaging (especially echo planar imaging (EPI) sequences), generate a great deal of acoustic noise. This noise poses both safety concerns and psychophysical challenges.

Beyond the measurement of traditional psychophysical and behavioural response parameters, it is sometimes desirable or necessary to obtain more general physiological activity measurements. These measures may be essential for safety or for scientific reasons, or they may be desirable as an approach to accounting for physiological noise not relevant to the brain activations of interest.

The challenge of physiological measurement is dealt with by commercial vendors because there are often clinical reasons (outside the context of brain activation MRI studies) for being able to monitor physiological conditions in a subject or patient during MRI. In the context of brain activation studies, it has been argued that information from monitoring of physiological parameters such as breathing, oxygenation level of the blood, blood pressure, heart beat, carbon dioxide concentration of the blood, etc., might allow corrections for 'physiological noise', and increase the effective signal-to-noise ratio of the measured brain activation response. While at least one published study has demonstrated some improvement (Hu *et al.* 1995), the increase was arguably modest relative to what would be needed to justify the expense of the equipment and the extra effort involved in using it with every subject. Nonetheless, some studies require the use of such equipment for both safety or scientific reasons (e.g. Breiter *et al.* 1977; Gollub *et al.* 1998), and it is likely that such physiological measures will eventually help us to better understand the physio-

logical noise components in functional brain activation studies.

Finally, subject movement during the imaging session is one of the most persistent challenges in fMRI. In a normal psychophysical laboratory, small movements of the subject's body or head are usually irrelevant. In the special cases where head movement must be controlled, a bite bar apparatus is simple, safe, inexpensive, and effective in reducing head movement to a level that is acceptable. Controlling movement in the context of brain activation MRI is much more difficult, and much more important. Head movement continues to be the single most serious cause of unusable data in fMRI.

The remainder of this chapter will be organized as follows: the general need to adapt tasks to the MRI environment; stimulus presentation, subdivided by modality (visual, auditory, tactile, etc.); voluntary response recording, including eye movements; physiological response recording; head movement, and related safety issues; and finally, a discussion of the tradeoffs between commercial systems, custom designed systems, and the goal of a completely integrated psychophysiological laboratory in the MRI environment.

10.2 Case studies in adapting tasks to functional MRI

In addition to the technical problems of making equipment work in the magnet while not interfering with the quality of the collected images, it is often impossible or impractical to use standard behavioural procedures in their normal manner. While there is no general solution to the problems involved, two specific examples are given below, as indications of the considerations necessary. The first example is a straightforward, but clever, adaptation of a standard procedure for assessing colour vision to the magnet environment. The second example addresses a more common problem in designing fMRI studies: the need for overt speech responses from subjects.

10.2.1 Quantifying colour vision

Developed in the 1940s, the 'Farnsworth-Munsell 100 Hue Test' (Farnsworth 1957) is the standard laboratory and clinical tool for assessing colour vision. While there are simpler, more quickly administered tests to detect dichromacy (defects in colour vision due to the absence of one class of cones), the 100 hue test is the most general tool. It also measures the ability of subjects to make fine colour discriminations—even people with normal trichromatic colour vision vary in their ability to detect small colour differences reliably. Because the procedure incorporates a difficult colour discrimination task, it is ideally suited for activating colour-processing areas of visual cortex.

The standard test is administered by presenting the subject with a row of 21 plastic caps, each of which has a coloured chip on the top, with two 'anchor' colours fixed at each end. The subject moves the caps until they form a sequence in which the colour changes continuously from one anchor to the other. This is repeated four times, for four different sets of colours. The chips are illuminated with a special lamp to control the colour temperature of the illumination. The test is designed so that the chips are of equal brightness, so that hue alone can serve as the cue for making the discrimination (see Fig. 10.1). (Note: it was the desire to make the differences in colours roughly equal in psychophysical terms that reduced the original 100 hues to the actual 84 in the test.)

Beauchamp and colleagues wished to take advantage of this procedure in an fMRI-based study of cortical visual areas (Beauchamp *et al.* 1999). However, they recognized that several modifications

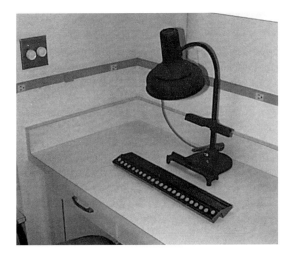

Fig. 10.1   The Farnsworth-Munsell 100 hue test.

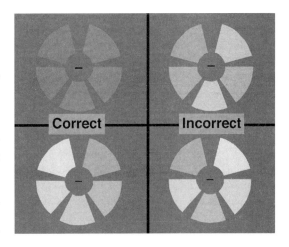

Fig. 10.2   Stimuli used by Beauchamp and colleagues in their colour discrimination task. (See also colour plate section.)

of the standard testing would be necessary. While the plastic chips would probably be MR-compatible, the special lamp would not have been. Moreover, there were several other reasons (beyond magnet compatibility) to alter the test for use in fMRI. For instance, if subjects viewed a collection of 21 'virtual' chips on a screen and had to use a cursor-controlling device to move these chips around until they were lined up in a computer version of the standard test, a wide array of cognitive systems would be activated that had little to do with the desired activations. In addition to the colour processing and colour discrimination tasks, there would be many eye and hand movements. Controlling for the consequences of taking different amounts of time to do different parts of the test would also be difficult with brain imaging.

Beauchamp and colleagues therefore tried to capture the essence of the colour discriminations needed, while keeping required eye movements and physical responses to a minimum. They used arrays of five coloured chips, arranged in a circle, as shown in Fig. 10.2. In the colour condition (mimicking the 100 hue test), the colours were either in correct sequence or not, and the subject had to respond accordingly (see upper half of Fig. 10.2). Brain responses during this task were contrasted with those during an achromatic condition in which five greys of different lightness were arranged in correct or incorrect sequence, and the subjects had to respond similarly (see lower half of

Fig. 10.2). The achromatic condition controlled for attention, fine perceptual discrimination, and motor output, but all in a context with no hue. Subjects were asked to perform these tasks while fixating a central point in the target, thus minimizing eye movements. Moreover, the experimenter could control the timing and duration of the stimulus presentations in a way that would not be possible in the traditional test.

10.2.2 Overt speech in functional MRI

Many classic psycholinguistic experiments and many functional imaging studies (e.g. Petersen *et al.* 1988) use overt speech as part of the experimental design. There are two major technical problems presented by overt speech in the context of fMRI. First, the movement of the subject's mouth is likely to be coupled to head movements. While head restraints can reduce this, and some subjects can speak while creating minimal head movement, overt speech is likely to cause head movement. The second problem is that when the subject speaks, the amount of air in the mouth is increased. This changes the local distortion of the magnetic field around, and within, the head (because the magnetic susceptibility of air is different from that of the brain itself). As discussed elsewhere in this book, this so-called 'susceptibility artifact' is more pronounced at higher magnetic fields (e.g. in 3 or 4 Tesla MRI systems).

One common solution to these problems is to adapt the tasks in such a way as to remove the need for overt speech. In the simplest cases, this consists of replacing an overt verbal response (such as 'yes' or 'no') with a motor response (pressing one of two keys to indicate 'yes' or 'no'). Such a solution is not always possible. For example, in the 1988 Petersen study mentioned above, the subjects had to generate and report a novel word, and it would not be easy to avoid overt speech in such a case. Recent work (Birn *et al.* 1999) has suggested an alternative approach, which permits overt speech in functional MRI experiments. This work exploits properties of the lag in the haemodynamic response (which is normally considered a limitation of fMRI). The kinds of motion and field distortion that overt speech produces occur on a very rapid time-scale, relative to the generation of the haemodynamically driven functional MRI signals of interest. When a subject says 'yes', gross head move-

ment is likely and, within the head, mouth movements create changes in the air pocket that distorts the MR images. These artifacts are introduced into the images that are collected *at the time* of the speech. For a single word, this rarely lasts longer than a second. But the images with the relevant changes based on neural activity coupled to the haemodynamic response will not be collected until several seconds later (starting at least 2 s later and continuing for 4–8 s). Thus, as long as the head and mouth return to their pre-speaking positions in a short time, the images contaminated by motion can be removed from the data analysis. (This type of experiment may be helped by use of a bite bar.) While no system of head restraint is perfect, one of the good features of bite bars is that they can serve as a physical cue for returning the head to a fixed position after speaking or inadvertent motion.

10.2.3 Every case is special

The preceding examples were presented to encourage careful thought about these kinds of issues *before* imaging begins. Simplifying a standard behavioural task to take into consideration ancillary brain activations accompanying the standard task (such as Beauchamp and colleagues did with the 100 hue test), or taking advantage of the differing time scales of MR imaging and the haemodynamic response to get good fMRI data despite physical movement by the subject (such as Birn and colleagues did for overt speech) are just two examples of what can be pulled out of an experimentalist's bag of tricks. However, just as there is no general algorithm for experimental design in psychology, so there is no general algorithm for deciding how best to adapt a behavioural task to the context of functional MRI.

10.3 Stimulus presentation

As stated in the introduction, the presentation below will be based on the perspective of someone planning to set up a new psychophysical laboratory in the MRI environment today. If you wish to see a more detailed discussion of the underlying issues, a reasonable place to start is the chapter mentioned previously (Savoy *et al.* 1999).

10.3.1 Visual stimulation

There is now a selection of different systems available for visual stimulus presentations. For general research, there are two primary considerations: cost and convenience. 'Cost', as it will be used here, refers specifically to the purchase price of equipment. Bear in mind, though, that there is another 'cost'—the time and effort needed to make a customized system work properly. This will be mentioned at various times and discussed more fully in the final section of this chapter. 'Convenience' refers both to ease of set-up for subjects (especially for more difficult subjects such as patients, elderly subjects, and children) and also to the commercial support for installation and technical problem solving.

The least costly visual display system is generally a computer projector with a custom lens, designed to project a small image onto a rear-projection screen. Mirror(s) (mounted on the radiofrequency coil or bite bar or other equipment) or prism(s) (typically worn as glasses by the subject) are required for enabling the subject to view the screen. For some specialized investigations (e.g. mapping multiple visual areas using retinotopy, or studying stereoscopic vision), there are special needs (such as maximizing the field of view of the stimulus display system, or presenting different stimuli to the two eyes, respectively). Several vendors offer workable systems for almost all standard situations. Some even include special features (like stereoscopic presentation, or high spatial resolution).

From the perspective of cost, the original systems that early labs have used (computer projector, screen and optics) are still the least expensive. They also can be reasonably easy to use, but demand local investment of time and resources in appropriately configuring them. From the perspective of convenience, commercial systems have some potential advantages, particularly in ease of set-up. Specific strengths and weaknesses of different types of systems are summarized below.

Spatial resolution

An advantage of projection systems is that, as the projection technology improves, it is straightforward to upgrade the projector with higher resolution versions. Early systems used NTSC video resolution, which is poor. The next generation systems used 640 × 480 pixel resolution, and now 800 × 600 or even 1024 × 768 is common. At the time of writing it would be inadvisable to use a projector with less than 800 × 600 pixels of spatial resolution for fMRI-based research. Each projector needs a special lens (e.g., from Bahl Optical) to cast a small image on the viewing screen.

Commercially available systems now allow viewing of the image through eyepieces via optical fibre cables. These also have a liquid crystal display (LCD) display as part of their optics, which, in theory, could be upgraded in a similar manner. In practice, however, the user has to wait for the system vender to choose to do that, and the associated costs are virtually guaranteed to be higher than for doing a simple swap of a projection system. Moreover, if the system uses fiber optic cable, increased spatial resolution of the projector may require increased fiber optic density to take advantage of the increased resolution of the source, which would add significant cost. In practice resolution also can be degraded in these systems by wear and tear on the optical fibre cables via progressive misalignment or fracture of individual fibers.

One approach that is not commonly used, but has obvious virtues in terms of cost and (after initial set up) simplicity, is to mount a conventional cathode ray tube (CRT) monitor in the MR room, far from the subject and bore of the magnet. Obviously, great care must be taken to assure that the monitor never comes near to the magnet. Subject then uses a system of mirrors, prisms and/or binoculars to see the CRT screen. Aside from the physical complexity and safety issues (as well as the optics) of the initial set up, the upgrade path is the least costly and the image quality can be excellent. Newer flat-screen technology can be made compatible with the high field environment to allow mounting of the screen at the end of the bore.

Temporal resolution

Virtually all modern visual presentation systems (both commercial and simple computer projection) have a temporal resolution of 20 or 17 ms (corresponding to the 50 or 60 Hz refresh rate of the projector or LCD screen). This is sufficient for most purposes, but not all. For example, if a task requires the tachistoscopic presentation of a stimulus for 5 ms, computer projectors are not sufficiently fast. Solutions include rapid shutters for the projected images (including traditional shutters used with a slide projector). Shutters normally need to go outside the MR scanner (and probably outside the MRI room) if they are controlled by solenoids, which can introduce RF-noise into the MRI system. In some traditional tachistoscopic devices the shutters go near the eyes, but this probably is not practical in the context of MRI.

There is another technology for projecting computer displays, known as Digital Light Processing (DLP). A commercial introduction can be found at http://www.ti.com/dlp/technology/. According to this, some 500 000 individual mirrors can be switched at 5000 Hz. In theory, this suggests that imaging presentation rates could be much faster than those described above. On the other hand, it appears that existing DLP products use the more modest 60–72 Hz that is similar to LCD and CRT systems. DLP products have various advantages (light and portable, possibly faster temporal resolution, allegedly excellent linearity across the three colours) but also have some disadvantages (spatial gradients away from the centre, e.g. non-uniform intensity of a nominally 'uniform' field). An informal discussion of these issues can be found at http://www.visionscience.com/mail/cvnet/1998/0172.html

Colour/intensity resolution

Colour and intensity *resolution* are not particular problems. Virtually all the technologies give a reasonable range (256-cubed, i.e. about 16 000 000 colours). Calibration is always challenging, however, especially in the context of the magnet. A telephotometer, which can measure intensities on a screen from a substantial distance (metres) away, can be helpful in calibrating visual projection systems.

Field of view

Virtually all current systems have a field of view that is at least a 20° wide by 10° high. This is more than adequate for most cognitive studies, although it is marginal for mapping cortical visual areas. Most commercial suppliers do not state the spatial extent of their systems in all their brochures, but this information can be requested directly. In the case of systems made 'in-house', the actual field of view will depend upon the size of the mirror that is put near the subject's face and the size of the screen and how close all of these can be to the subject's eyes. The bore of the magnet (and sometimes the size of the subject's chest or abdomen!) all limit the spatial extent of the visual display in such systems. In contrast, with systems that present the stimulus via fiber optics (e.g. Avotec) or via direct viewing of an LCD display (e.g. Psychology Software Tools and Resonance Technologies) the spatial extent is fixed.

Quality of the image

Direct viewing of a CRT or an active matrix LCD screen in the MR room probably yields the best image quality. Each of the other available systems is subject to various forms of degradation. Viewing an LCD through fiber optics is subject to defects caused by breaks in individual fiber optic cables. Some vendors have found new ways to minimize this problem. DLP displays, as noted above, have serious spatial non-uniformities (the centre of the screen is much brighter than the edges). The least expensive approach—projection on to a screen—typically has image quality in the middle of this range. Degradation in this case can come from the screen (which is imperfect to begin with and can be easily scratched in practice) or in the mirrors or lenses used to view the screen. For example, an inexpensive plastic mirror of the type often used for this application is usually a rear-surface mirror (i.e. the reflective coating is at the back of the object relative to the viewers' eyes). As a result, the image is contaminated by the surface (specular) reflection of the plastic. Front surface mirrors eliminate this problem, but they are more expensive and much more susceptible to scratches from mis-handling.

Having given a general impression of the overall issues in image quality, two things should be noted. First, these comments are qualitative, based on the author's observations (a published, quantitative comparison of visual display systems for fMRI is not presently known to the author). Second, despite the limitations listed above, virtually all the systems in current use give images of quality high enough to be used for all but the most demanding visual and cognitive experiments.

Ease of use

One of the 'selling points' of some of the commercial systems is the claim that it is easier to set up the system for use with each individual subject. Understandably, this is a significant concern for users. Early non-commercial visual display systems were often cumbersome and time-consuming to set up. Screens, lenses, and other optical apparatus had to be positioned painstakingly for the subject to see the stimuli properly. However, this issue has largely been addressed (both for systems made 'in-house' and in commercial systems). Set-up time for visual displays now should be only a minute or two.

There are other issues associated with ease of use. For instance, some display systems are easily portable from scanner to scanner, while others are specific to a given type of scanner or manufacturer. In general, it is in the interest of the manufacturers of commercial systems to make them adaptable to a broad range of scanners. In contrast, the systems made 'in-house' (typically consisting of some kind of mirrors for the subject, with a screen, a computer projector and a custom projection lens) are often specific to the particular scanner and room in which they are normally used. In particular, the projection lens must be customized for a specific (small) range of distances, and use of that system in a larger or smaller scanner room might be difficult. If a system is going to be used in a single scanner room, however, this is not an issue. Moreover, if the scanner is eventually changed, the cost for a new lens (a few thousand dollars, at most) is not likely to be a significant portion of the budget for the new scanner!

Cost

Commercial systems are much more expensive than the cost of constructing a visual stimulus presentation system 'in-house'. However, this comparison is not completely fair. There is a good deal of time and effort needed to figure out how to specify the required lens, and how to attach the mirrors and screens for use in the magnet with the projection system. The cost of commercial systems includes the cost of this engineering design, and these systems can have other features. For example, the system from Avotec includes the option of purchasing an integral eye-tracker with the visual display device (at a substantial additional cost, of course). Other vendors include response devices (buttons or cursor controllers) with their visual display systems (e.g. Resonance Technologies and Psychology Software Tools).

10.3.2 Auditory stimulation

Auditory stimulation is either straightforward, or nearly impossible, depending upon experimental needs. One annoyance is the ambient noise in the room (such as that caused by the continuous operation of the pumps used to help cool the liquid helium needed for the superconducting main magnet). But a much greater problem is the high level of acoustic stimulation generated by the gradient switching. This may be particularly severe at very high static field strengths. For simple auditory presentations (e.g. to cue the subject) there are a wide variety of solutions.

All clinical scanners have some version of auditory communication built in. That is, the operator can speak with the patient/subject through existing systems that come with the scanner. In some cases, the experimenter can tap directly into these systems (which have speakers built into the bore of the magnet). Thus, auditory output from computer stimulation packages can be connected to the scanner's own systems. Simple air-pressure driven systems (e.g. with a speaker outside the scanner room connected to long hollow plastic tubes running to a set of headphones) can be built 'in-house' or purchased. However, if one is attempting to do state-of-the-art auditory psychophysics in the scanner, a more specialized (and expensive) system may be needed, such as electro-static headphones. Air-pressure systems have a limited frequency response range and variable phase delays (e.g. Savoy *et al.* 1999).

10.3.3 Somatosensory, olfactory, gustatory, pain, and proprioceptive stimulation

The vast majority of experiments—especially cognitive experiments—rely on visual or auditory stimuli. Therefore, the greatest effort has gone into developing such systems, both in individual research laboratories and in the companies. Work on somatosensory, olfactory, gustatory, pain and proprioceptive stimulation is in progress, and there will, no doubt, soon be commercial systems available. Descriptions of some of the systems that have been used can be found in research reports.

Somatosensory

There are no standardized systems yet available, but there are a number under development. Until commercial systems are available, researchers are obligated to develop their own. Somatosensory fMRI experiments have been conducted using stimulation via air puffs, via piezo-electrically controlled physical manipulators (Harrington *et al.* 1998), and via direct human interaction (Hui *et al.* 2000).

Olfactory and gustatory

There have been a few studies using these modalities. In general, users have developed their own systems. Because the means of presentation generally involve plastic tubing coming into the scanner room (and to the subject) from outside, the MR-compatibility issues are not too difficult. Quantitative control of the stimuli is, of course, challenging, but not significantly more so than in a traditional psychophysical setting.

Proprioceptive and painful stimulation

While proprioceptive stimulation is, in principle, possible to make mechanically driven, in practice it is still most commonly applied directly by a person in the scan room. However, at least one electronically-controlled system has been reported using heat or cold (Davis *et al.* 1998). Painful stimuli based on transcutaneous electrical nerve stimulation were delivered via a commercial device previously used in a positron emission tomography study (Downs *et al.* (1998). The development of pneumatic stimulation for somatosensory experiments could, presumably, be adapted to applying painful stimulation or even mechanical movement of limbs and appendages for proprioceptive stimulation.

10.4 Recording voluntary responses

There is almost always a need to monitor behavioural responses in fMRI experiments. Various types of responses are considered below. In all cases, of course, it is important to use devices with little or no ferromagnetic material. The goal should always be to reduce such material to zero, though in practice it is possible for some devices to function properly and safely, if the amount of material is very small and as far from the imaging area as possible.

10.4.1 Buttons

Probably the most common type of response is a choice indicated by pressing one of several buttons. Ideally, the buttons should have no metal parts and should communicate the choice optically or pneumatically, to minimize interference with the images being collected by the MRI scanner. Several vendors (e.g. Psychology Software Tools, and others) offer such devices. In practice, the use of simple electrical switches at the hand (i.e. at a substantial distance from the head) introduces little radiofrequency noise, particularly if appropriate radiofrequency filters are used in the line. These signals (whether from a source that is originally optical or electronic) can be used to drive a special purpose interface board (e.g. from National Instruments), or can be used to simulate a button press on the keyboard (e.g. Savoy *et al.* 1999; http://pywacket.rowland.org/RURB).

10.4.2 Cursor controllers

Controlling a computer cursor (i.e. what would ordinarily be done with a mouse, trackball, joystick, or touch pad) can be more challenging. In contrast to a simple switch, there is much greater likelihood that significant radiofrequency interference will be generated. A simple switch only has to generate an electrical signal when a contact is made or broken; whereas cursor-controlling devices are generating many signals per second. Because of these issues, it is more desirable to use an optically based, rather than electrically based, device.

10.4.3 Continuous movements

Direct measurement of continuously moving body parts (hands in a tracking task, for instance) is probably most simply accomplished using digital video cameras in the MRI room, but far enough away from the scanner to be safe. Systems for processing such information would be the same as those used in conventional experiments. With appropriate radiofrequency filters, surface electromyography (EMG) is possible in the magnet. Similar strategies may be taken to address with safety concerns as described below for electroencephalography in the magnet (see also Lemieux *et al.* 1997).

10.4.4 Speech

As indicated in the example by Birn *et al.* (1999) earlier in this chapter, there are special challenges to recording MR images during overt speech. That example focused on the artifacts induced by movement and changes in air pockets in the head due to overt speech. Another challenge is simply hearing or recording the speech responses in the presence of the loud acoustic interference generated by the high speed imaging sequences (such as echo planar imaging). Most MRI systems have a built in microphone for patient communication, but it is far from the patient's mouth. An MR-compatible microphone nearer to the subject's mouth would help, and some vendors supply these as part of headphones or bite bar systems.

10.4.5 Eye movements

Eye movements are one of the most important variables in many cognitive experiments—from studies of motion perception to scanning the printed line in normal reading and reading disabilities. Consequently, there have been significant efforts by commercial vendors to make eye trackers outside the magnet, and some of these have been adapted for work within the magnet. In contrast to the visual display systems mentioned earlier, 'in-house' versions of this technology are rare or non-existent. Commercial eye tracking devices typically use a CCD-camera that monitors visible or, more commonly, infrared light. The light source may be outside the magnet (directed by mirrors and optics), or it may be from a small source mounted near the eye, or it may be part of the visual display equipment. Tracking itself is either based on multiple reflections from the eye (such as from the front of the cornea and back of the lens), or by following the outline of the iris or pupil. There are several vendors who supply MR compatible eye

trackers. A partial list includes: Cambridge Research Systems (Rochester, Kent, England); Applied Science Laboratories (Bedford, Massachusetts); and Sensor-Motoric Instruments, which can be purchased in an integrated package with the Avotec visual display system.

10.5 Recording physiological responses

In addition to the responses made voluntarily by the subject, there are many other behavioural or physiological responses that might be important for interpreting neuroimaging data. Some are useful for removing confounds in the fMRI data (e.g. movement of the brain induced by cardio-respiratory pressure changes). Others are the sorts of data that might be critical for future improvements to functional brain imaging, such as the integration of higher temporal resolution signals (e.g. from EEG) with fMRI (Halgren and Dale 1999). In addition, work with patients or in pharmacological studies may require the active monitoring of physiological signals for safety reasons.

10.5.1 Electrical signals

Although special considerations for safety must be made when recording electroencephalography and related electrical signals (ECG, EOG, EMG) in the MR environment, these are technically possible and clearly useful (Ives *et al.* 1993; Huang-Hellinger *et al.* 1995; Warach *et al.* 1996).

10.5.2 Other physiological signals

The chapter referred to previously(Savoy *et al.* 1999) includes a more detailed discussion of physiological monitoring. The following summary (based largely on a physiological monitoring system assembled, or being developed, by Dr Randy Gollub and colleagues at the MGH NMR Center in Charlestown, Massachusetts) gives an indication of the kinds of measurements that are possible with more-or-less standard commercial systems.

Complete, magnet compatible, clinically approved physiologic monitoring systems are available for both 1.5 Tesla and 3.0 Tesla MRI scanners. Monitoring systems (built and installed, for example, by InVivo Research, and with some equipment available from ADInstruments) allow continuous visual display of 4-lead electrocardiogram (ECG), non-invasive blood pressure (NIBP-measured mean, calculated systolic and diastolic pressures), pulse oximetry (SaO_2 and heart rate), and capnographic end tidal CO_2 ($ETCO_2$ and respiratory rate). The systems include alarms for notification of possible subject distress. They can be fully integrated with the scanner; and the output can be used for e.g. cardiac gating. The systems can be modified to allow access to the stream of ASCII character data fed to the monitoring screen that updates the clinical measures once per second. These data can be interfaced to a computer via the serial port, and analogue data (e.g. from the ECG leads) can be monitored via an analogue-to-digital interface card (e.g. hardware and LabView software from National Instruments). Several groups (at MGH) are developing additional physiological measurement capabilities for use in the scanners. New measures will include electrodermal skin resistance (also known as Electrodermal Activity (EDA) and, in older literature, as Galvanic Skin Response (GSR), skin temperature, pulse pressure (to get heart rate from a fingertip), invasive blood pressure, dual belt respiratory rate, spirometry, expired O_2 and CO_2 concentrations. The work at MGH is not unique, and other centres have developed analogous systems. The strategy at MGH has been to get as much as possible from the commercial systems, and to do further needed modifications in house.

10.6   Minimizing head movement

Discussion of head stabilization in fMRI is one of the topics that causes heated disagreement among practitioners. For example, some investigators swear *by* bite bars; others swear *at* them! The reason for such contention is that in attempting to minimize the head motion of subjects and patients, one has, in reality, much less control than one would like.

Head movement is perhaps the single most significant problem in the collection of high quality fMRI data. Given that each scanning session results in the collection of hundreds or even thousands of images of the brain, the standard method for dealing with the detection of head motion is the use of sophisticated computational algorithms using the image data itself. These same images and related algorithms can be used to attempt to compensate for the motion after it has been detected. However, the algorithms (see Chapter 13) have limitations. Therefore, the first line of defence against the problem of head movement must be to minimize it during the scanning session.

Objective studies of the efficacy of specific head stabilization techniques are starting to appear (Menon *et al.* 1997; Edward *et al.* 2000). These studies compare the target technique with a minimal head stabilization technique (such as foam padding). However, objective studies comparing different techniques against each other still are hard to find.

10.6.1   Behavioural feedback

One clever idea was to put a motion-detecting device on the head of a child, and let the *device* control the disappearance of a videotaped television programme that the child was watching. When head movement was below a certain threshold, the television stayed on. If movements stayed below threshold for a sustained period, the threshold was decreased. The training provided with this approach led to a degree of stability that allowed the imaging procedure to proceed without the need for a sedative (Slifer *et al.* 1993). However, this procedure was tested only for use with conventional structural scans, which last a few min and are not as sensitive to head movements as fMRI scans. Nonetheless, the use of behavioural feedback for behavioural control of head position is an idea worthy of exploration, and has been pursued in the context of adult fMRI experiments (Thulborn, 1999).

There are several common approaches to head stabilization, of which three of the most commonly used are foam padding, thermoplastic masks, and bite bars. All of these are non-invasive (the surgical alternative of installing screws in the skull to affix to an external frame is not justified for functional MRI with patients or volunteers!). None of these methods is totally effective. Subject motivation and ability is always important. Furthermore, even if the skull were fully stabilized, researchers would still need to contend with the small movements of the brain within the skull due to heartbeat. Various techniques can be used to take heartbeat into account (e.g. Guimaraes *et al.* 1998), but the motion detection and motion correction algorithms based on the brain images themselves are still needed (see Chapter 13).

10.6.2 Foam padding

In standard structural MRI scans it is also important for subjects to keep their heads still. The usual way to encourage this is to wrap the back and sides of the head in a comfortable pillow, and wedge foam between the pillow and the inside edges of the head receiver coil. Sometimes a chin strap or forehead strap are added to encourage subjects to be aware of when they begin to rotate their head about the x-axis (the axis from ear-to-ear). This direction of motion is usually the most difficult to control. Nonetheless, for a typical 20–30 min structural MRI session, pillow, foam, straps and encouragement to remain still are generally sufficient. Furthermore, virtually all subjects tolerate this procedure with no problems (except that it may be so comfortable and quiet as to encourage falling asleep). The pillow also introduces a measure of sound attenuation, which is good, though earplugs are still recommended or required in most EPI scanning sessions.

For normal, well-motivated adult subjects foam padding is often adequate for the longer functional imaging sessions as well. This is particularly true for the individual 2–6 min runs of functional data collection. It tends to be less true for the overall stability of head position across many runs of a 1–2 h functional imaging session.

10.6.3 Thermoplastic masks

There are several forms of mask that can be moulded to the shape of the subject's face and then bolted into position to help minimize head movements. Masks can be made from a mesh or a solid sheet of plastic. In both cases, the material is warmed to make it malleable so that it can be formed over the face, and so that holes can be cut out as needed for the eyes, nose, and mouth. This is the only form of head restraint that involves contact and some pressure over the whole face, and some subjects do not tolerate this well. Descriptions of these systems can be found at http://www.ccf.org/cc/radonc/spec_prog/rad_surg.html and http://www.oandp.com/organiza/aaop/jpo/63/6379.htm (Pilipuf and Berry 1994).

10.6.4 Plaster head cast

Another approach that has recently been tested is the creation of a plaster cast for the head (Edward *et al.* 2000). Some earlier attempts required that the head cast be removable simply by lifting the device off the head. This necessarily permitted some freedom of movement while in the cast. In the more recent report, the cast is created over most of the skull, and then split in half. The two halves can be bolted together later, thus yielding a tighter fit than would be possible with a 'pull-off' cast. Quantitative assessment of movement indicates that this approach is effective.

10.6.5 Bite bars

Bite bars (e.g. Menon *et al.* 1997; and Psychology Software Tools) are one of the most effective systems for minimizing head movements. An individualized mould of the subject's teeth is made using dental impression material, and the mould is affixed to some rigid structure attached to the patient table in the MRI scanner or the receiver coil. In comparison with the strategies mentioned above, bite bars have the advantage of coupling directly to the skull (through the upper teeth) rather than the scalp, which can move significant distances over the surface of the skull. They also are easy for the subject to use to recover a previous position (e.g. if they move slightly or talk or sneeze). However, bite bars have some special problems. Some subjects simply do not tolerate them. Much shorter bite bars (e.g. which couple only to the front four upper teeth and four lower teeth, instead of going further back in the mouth) may be more easily tolerated, but these also are less effective in minimizing motion. Finally, there are some safety concerns with bite bars that do not apply to the previous systems. For example, it is critically important that the dental impression material not be brittle, because the subject is lying in the magnet (rather than sitting upright, as in a normal psychophysical experiment), and if the bite bar shattered, the pieces would represent a choking hazard. These and related safety issues are addressed more fully in the previously mentioned chapter (Savoy *et al.* 1999).

At a practical level, one of the most significant advantages of bite bars is apparent when using an experienced subject for many experiments. The bite bar is made once, and set-up time for the subject is subsequently minimal. For subjects who are comfortable with bite bars they can be the fastest and easiest way to support the subjects' attempts to stay still.

10.7 Safety

There are a number of issues related to safety in the context of general MRI, and a few special considerations in the context of functional MRI. The standard safety reference remains Shellock and Kanal's book (Shellock and Kanal, 1996). Everyone who engages in MRI-based research should be familiar with the issues discussed in that book. Each of the sources of possible danger are discussed in turn: the dangers associated with lying in a magnet (the main one being flying ferromagnetic objects); the dangers associated with systemic heating of body tissues by radio frequency (RF) energy; the dangers associated with nerve or cardiac effects from the rapidly switching gradients; the dangers associated with bio-mechanical and bio-electrical implanted devices; and acoustic noise (McJury *et al.* 1994; Shellock *et al.* 1994; McJury 1995; Cho *et al.* 1997; Counter *et al.* 1997; Hedeen and Edelstein 1997; Shellock *et al.* 1998). Shellock and Kanal also have a web site devoted to the topic of MR safety at: http://kanal.arad.upmc.edu/MR_Safety/. As indicated previously, there are some special safety concerns associated with head stabilization and bite bars, and with electrical monitoring devices for EEG, EOG, and EMG.

10.8 Integrating the psycho-physiological laboratory with MRI for brain activation studies

When contemplating the creation of a psychophysiological laboratory to be associated with functional MRI work, there are at least two general themes that must be considered. The first is whether (or to what extent) to work 'in-house' to make special systems for stimulus presentation and response recording or to purchase commercially available systems. The second is how tightly the psychophysiological laboratory is going to be integrated with the functioning of the MR scanner.

10.8.1 Commercial systems versus 'in-house' construction

In the early days of any scientific enterprise, there is no choice—the investigator must build, rather than buy, the tools needed. Therefore, in the early days of fMRI-based research, each laboratory worked hard to develop its own systems for head stabilization, visual stimulus display, response recording, etc. Today, however, there are commercial systems for many of these tasks.

Some of the tradeoffs involved are obvious: in terms of cost of equipment, the commercial systems will be more expensive; in terms of time, effort, and ongoing obligation to maintain systems, systems developed 'in-house' will be more 'expensive'. Moreover, a great deal of 'reinventing-the-wheel' goes on when creating systems 'in-house' and in the case of 'reinventing' procedures for RF-noise insulation and control, the issues can be much trickier than for wheels! In theory, commercial systems have worked out many of the problems that would be new headaches for the local developer. On the other hand, if an adaptation or improvement to a system is needed immediately, it is often difficult or expensive to get rapid help from a vendor. Of course, it also is difficult to do it oneself, but the issues of communication, delay, and costs are very different.

There are a few points that can be summarized from the earlier contents of this chapter. It is probably better to purchase, rather than design and build physiological monitoring equipment 'in-house'. It is not just that this will be easier, but that there may also be medico-legal issues associated with using some of these devices because of implications for subject health and safety. (Those are non-trivial issues, so it is probably wiser to use equipment that has already been certified.) In contrast, 'in-house' construction may be ideal for other equipment. There is no perfect visual display system, but all are likely to work adequately for basic cognitive studies. There is no gold standard for head stabilization systems and it may be advantageous to try a variety of them.

Other considerations include the number of available staff for designing, implementing, and maintaining custom-designed systems and any special needs of individual investigators. An illustrative case study is the ongoing renovation of the MRI imaging suites at the MGH-NMR Center based in Charlestown, Massachusetts. Because MGH was one of the earliest fMRI-based research centres, many of the pieces of testing equipment in its existing psychophysiological laboratories had been developed 'on-the-fly' and were both outdated and not well integrated with each other. Thus, the renovation created a natural opportunity for implementing new psychophysiological laboratories. This case is unusual in that there is a particularly large group of researchers involved—in a smaller research setting, some of the options and choices would have been different. But in the MGH context, extensive discussion among practitioners led to the clear conclusion that no one approach would suffice. Individual investigators needed specific features that were not typically available in a general commercial system. To address both the needs of the general user and also the needs of individual researchers, many people agreed to contribute a non-trivial fraction of their time to equipment design and development because the group needed the unique features such development would provide. Finally, because the MGH-NMR Center would need to duplicate these systems for several MRI machines across laboratory and hospital settings, the investment of time would have broader benefit functionally, as well as financially. If we had decided to purchase an integrated system for many MRI suites, the cost would have been considerable (though still a small fraction of the cost for the scanner and its room). Having made the effort to design and implement one system, it was much easier to duplicate that system for a number of MR suites.

Consider an alternative extreme case: a small laboratory with available funding for a single fMRI suite. One of the options for such a group is to purchase an integrated, reasonably extensive collection of stimulus presentation, response recording, head stabilization, scanner synchronizing, and data analysis tools in a package from one company (e.g. Psychology Software Tools' Integrated Functional Imaging System, IFIS), or various components from a collection of companies (e.g. Avotec, Resonance Technology, etc). In either of the above cases, the issue of integration with the scanner and the integration with experimental design and analysis software needs to be explored, as indicated below.

10.8.2 Integration of psychophysiological laboratory and MR scanner

While simple in concept, integration of all the psychophysiological laboratory hardware with both the software that is used for experimental design and presentation and with the pulse sequences of the imaging scanner itself can be complex in practice. Standard software for the presentation of stimuli often needs to be modified for use in functional MRI experiments. The most common problem is timing. In most behavioural studies it is sufficient to have precise timing during a single trial—if there is a 100 ms uncertainty in timing *between* trials, it is not of any practical importance. However, in the context of functional MRI, when a single imaging run might entail hundreds of stimulus presentations, small errors in timing accumulate. This can be disastrous for data analysis, as it is the known correspondence between stimulus presentation and MR image that governs almost all approaches to analysis (with the primary exception being 'principle component analysis' and its relatives). Experimental designs using single trial presentation or rapid-single-trial presentations (Buckner *et al.* 1996; Dale and Buckner 1997; Rosen *et al.* 1998) require even more accurate correspondence than do the older block designs.

New software packages for stimulus presentation have been developed that have the necessary timing accuracy, and older packages have been suitably modified. It is critically important that the user understand how important this issue can be and that the timing for any experiment is checked beforehand.

A related issue is synchronizing events in the experimental paradigm with image acquisition. With the exception of triggering the scanner at specific points in the cardiac cycle (to minimize the variance introduced into the MR data by the pulsatility of blood flow (Guimaraes *et al.* 1998)), it is rare that the scanner's operation itself is triggered by the experimenter's protocol. More commonly, the scanner operates at a fixed regular rate, and the stimuli are hopefully being presented in a suitably coordinated manner. At the very least, it is desirable to have a record of when the MR images were *actually* collected, relative to the stimulus presentation. Better would be the control of either the scanner or the stimulus presentation software so that correspondence in time is maintained throughout the imaging run. It should be noted that some scanner manufacturers have in the past generated timing information in their output files that were only specified to an accuracy of about 1 s. In many situations in functional MRI, greater temporal precision is important. Rewriting pulse sequences is not always within the technical competence of an imaging centre, and waiting for MR manufacturers to address these problems can sometimes be frustrating.

Again, there are both commercial and 'in-house' approaches to these issues. At least one vendor (Psychology Software Tools, 'IFIS') makes a concerted effort to integrate all of these aspects, including the clever use of an RF-detector (so that the hardware/software combination is somewhat independent of the particular scanner being used, thus obviating the need to modify or control pulse sequences), and a sophisticated experimental control programme in which behavioural responses are integrated with this image acquisition information. An alternative approach is to build relatively simple electronics so that the signal supplied by the scanner whenever an imaging sequence begins is output directly for purposes of software recording and/or synchronization. There are relatively convenient interface tools for supplying such a signal to modern computers that use the 'USB' interface for peripheral devices.

It should be understood that neither of the above approaches actually controls the scanner. To do that would require much greater sophistication, but is possible with research (rather than clinical) scanners. In some applications there can be advantages in the tight coupling of modifiable pulse sequences based on imaging and/or behavioural data as an imaging run or experimental session progresses.

10.9 Conclusion

There are substantial challenges in adapting standard psychological, psychophysical, and physiological measurement techniques to the MR environment. Nonetheless, it is possible to perform versions of virtually all standard psychophysical tasks in the magnet. Presentation of visual, tactile, olfactory, gustatory, pain, and other stimuli is reasonably straightforward. Presentation of auditory stimuli is problematic because of the acoustic noise generated by the scanner,

but is otherwise straightforward. Recording voluntary responses is easy for simple responses such as button presses or brief overt speech. Responses that involve movement of larger body parts remain a potentially difficult (and largely unexplored) challenge for the MR environment. Recording physiological responses, including such challenging responses as eye movements, is well served by available commercial hardware.

The key question for investigators establishing new fMRI-based laboratories is: 'How much of the technology for a psychophysical laboratory should I buy "off-the-shelf", and how much should I design and implement 'in-house'? While there is no absolute answer to this question, the present chapter has highlighted considerations that should be kept in mind.

Acknowledgments

The author wishes to thank the many people who have helped develop the psychophysical laboratory at the MGH-NMR Center. The NMR Center is currently in the process of revamping its psychophysical systems, and the author is grateful for many helpful discussions with people involved in this work. This includes, among others, Russell Poldrack, Sean Marrett, Rick Hoge, Roger Tootell, and Randy Gollub. Early work by Terry Campbell and Mark S. Cohen set the stage for many additions. Thanks also go to Don Rogers, Winfield Hill, and Robert Newton at the Rowland Institute for Science for work on optical, mechanical, and electronic devices. Specific thanks are due to Michael Ravicz for helpful discussions regarding the issues of auditory stimulus presentation and management of acoustic noise. Additionally, Randy Gollub of MGH helped in the description of the current and future implementations of physiological monitoring systems. In addition, we wish to thank the various vendors (including Paul Bullwinkel of Avotec, Walter Schneider of Psychology Software Tools, Sol Aisenberg of International Technology Group, Virginia Salem of Applied Science Laboratories) who have come to the MGH-NMR Center's Visiting Fellowship Program in Functional MRI to demonstrate their equipment. Finally, thanks to Michael Beauchamp for supplying the two figures used in this chapter.

Appendix: list of existing vendors

The following list is not exhaustive, and is given for illustrative purposes and as a basis to start searches. The list is in alphabetical order:

ADInstruments
Clinical monitoring systems, some of which are MR compatible
Mountain View, California
http://www.adinstruments.com

Applied Science Laboratoris
Bedford, Massachusetts
http://www.a-s-l.com

Avotec, Inc. [vendor]
MR-compatible visual and auditory stimulus presentation; integration with SMI Eye Tracker
Jensen Beach, Florida
http://www.avotec.org

Buhl Optical
Pittsburgh, Pennsylvania
http://www.buhloptical.com

Cambridge Research Systems
Visual Stimulus Generators; MR/MEG/PET—compatible eye tracker
Rochester, Kent, England
http://www.crsltd.com

InVivo Research
MR-compatible clinical monitoring equipment
Orlando, Florida
http://www.invivoresearch.com

National Instruments
LabView software and D->A and A->D boards for computers
Austin, Texas
http://www.ni.com/

Psychology Software Tools, Inc. (PST)
IFIS (Integrated Functional Imaging System); E-Prime (Software for Stimulus Presentation and Response Recording).
Pittsburgh, Pennsylvania
http://www.pstnet.com/

Resonance Technology, Inc.
MR-compatible visual and auditory stimulus presentation, response recording
Northridge, California
http://www.mrivideo.com

SensoriMotoric Instruments, Inc. (SMI)
MR-compatible Eye-Tracker; can be integrated with Avotec display system

Needham, Massachusetts
http://www.smiusa.com

References

Bandettini, P.A., Wong, E.D., Hinks, R.S., Tikofsky, R.S., and Hyde, J.S. (1993). Time course EPI of human brain function during task activation. *Magnetic Resonance in Medicine*, 25, 390–7.

Beauchamp, M.S., Haxby, J.V., Jennings, J.E., and De Yoe, E.A. (1999). An fMRI version of the Farnsworth-Munsell 100-hue test reveals multiple color-selective areas in human ventral occipitotemporal cortex. *Cerebral Cortex*, 9, 257–63.

Belliveau, J.W., Kennedy, D.N. Jr., McKinstry, R.C., Buchbinder, B.R., Weisskoff, R.M., Cohen, M.S., Vevea, J.M., Brady, T.J., and Rosen, B.R. (1991). Functional mapping of the human visual cortex by magnetic resonance imaging. *Science*, 254, 716–19.

Birn, R.M., Bandettini, P.A., Cox, R.W., and Shaker, R. (1999). Event-related fMRI of tasks involving brief motion. *Human Brain Mapping*, 7(2), 106–14.

Breiter, H.C., Gollub, R.L., Weisskoff, R.M., Kennedy, D.N., Makris, N., Berke, J.D., Goodman, J.M., Kantor, H.I., Gastfriend, D.R., Riorden, J.P., Mathew, R.T., Rosen, B.R., and Hyman, S.E. (1997). Acute effects of cocaine on human brain activity and emotion. *Neuron*, 19(9), 591–611.

Buckner, R.L., Bandettini, P.A., O'Craven, K.M., Savoy, R.L., Petersen, S.E., Raichle, M.E., and Rosen, B.R. (1996). Detection of cortical activation during averaged single trials of a cognitive task using functional magnetic resonance imaging. *Proceedings of the National Academy of Sciences (USA)*, 93, 1478–83.

Cho, Z.H., Park, S.H., Kim, J.H., Chung, S.C., Chung, S.T., Chung, J.Y., Moon, C.W., Yi, J.H., Sin, C.H., and Wong, E.K. (1997). Analysis of acoustic noise in MRI. *Magnetic Resonance Imaging*, 15, 815–22.

Counter, S.A., Olofsson, A., Grahn, H.F., and Berg, E. (1997). MRI acoustic noise: sound pressure and frequency analysis. *Journal of Magnetic Resonance Imaging*, 7, 606–11.

Dale, A.M. and Buckner, R.L. (1997). Selective averaging of rapidly presented individual trials using fMRI. *Human Brain Mapping*, 5, 329–40.

Davis, K.D., Kwan, C.L., Crawley, A.P., and Mikulis, D.J. (1998). fMRI of the anterior cingulate cortex during painful thermal and motor tasks in individual subjects. *NeuroImage*. 7(4): (abstract) S426.

Downs, J.H.I., Crawford, H.J., Plantec, M.B., Horton, J.E., Vendemia, J.M.C., Harrington, G.C., Yung, S., and Shamro, C. (1998). Attention to painful somatosensory TENS Stimuli: an fMRI study. *NeuroImage*, 7(4): (abstract) S432.

Edward, V., Windischberger, C., Cunnington, R., Erdler, M., Lanzenberger, R., Mayer, D., Endl, W., and Beisteiner, R. (2000). Quantification of fMRI artifact reduction by a novel plaster cast head holder. *Human Brain Mapping*, 3, 207–13.

Farnsworth, D. (1957). *The Farnsworth-Munsell 100-hue test for the examination of color vision*. Munsell Color Company, Balitmore.

Gollub, R.L., Breiter, H.C., Kantor, H., Kennedy, D., Gastfriend, D., Mathew, R.T., Makris, N., Guimarhes, A., Riorden, J., Campbell, T., Foley, M., Hyman, S.E., Rosen, B., and Weisskoff, R. (1998). Cocaine decreases cortical cerebral blood flow but does not obscure regional activation in functional magnetic resonance imaging in human subjects. *Journal of Cerebral Blood Flow and Metabolism*, **18**, 724–34.

Guimaraes, A.R., Melcher, J.R., Talavage, T.M., Baker, J.R., Ledden, P., Rosen, B.R., Kiang, N.Y.S., Fullerton, B.C., and Weisskoff, R.M. (1998). Imaging subcortical auditory activity in humans. *Human Brain Mapping*, **6**, 33–41.

Halgren, E. and Dale, A.M. (1999). Combining electromagnetic and hemodynamic signals to derive spatiotemporal brain acivation patterns: theory and results. *Biomedizinishe Technik (Biomedical Engineering)*, **44**(2), 53–60.

Harrington, G.S., Raman, M.P., Kassell, N.F., Down, J.H., III (1998). Somatosensory response to vibrotactile stimuli in fMRI. *NeuroImage*, 7(4): (abstract) S401.

Hedeen, R.A. and Edelstein, W.A. (1997). Characterization and prediction of gradient acoustic noise in MR Imgages. *Magnetic Resonance in Medicine*, 37, 7–10.

Hu, X., Le, T.H., Paris, T., and Erhard, P. (1995). Retrospective estimation and compensation of physiological fluctuation in functional MRI. *Magnetic Resonance in Medicine*, **34**(2), 201–12.

Huang-Hellinger, F.R., Breiter, H.C., McCormack, G.I., Cohen, M.S., Kwong, K.K., Sutton, J.P., Davis, T.L., Savoy, R.I., Weisskoff, R.M., Belliveau, J.W., and Rosen, B.R. (1995). Simultaneous functional magnetic resonance imaging and electrophysiological recording. *Human Brain Mapping*, 3(1), 13–23.

Hui, K.K.S., Liu, J. *et al.* (2000). Acupuncture modulates the limbic system and subcortical gray structures of the human brain: evidence from fMRI studies in normal subjects. *Human Brain Mapping*, 9, 13–25.

Ives, J.R., Warach, S., Schmitt, F., Edelman, R.R., and Schomer, D.L. (1993). Monitoring the patient's EEG during echo planar MRI. *Electroencephalography and Clinical Neurophysiology*, 87(6), 417–20.

Lemieux, L., Allen, P.J., Franconi, F., Symms, M.R., and Fish, D.R. (1997). Recording of EEG during fMRI experiments: patient safety. *Magnetic Resonance in Medicine*, 38(6), 943–52.

McJury, M.J. (1995). Acoustic noise levels generated during high field MR imaging. *Clinical Radiology*, 50, 331–4.

McJury, M., Blug, A., Joerger, C., Condon, B., and Wyper, D. (1994). Short communication: acoustic noise levels during magnetic resonance imaging scanning at 1.5 T *British Journal of Radiology*, 67(796), 413–15.

Menon, V., Lim, K.O., *et al.* (1997). Design and efficacy of a head-coil bite bar for reducing movement-related artifacts during functional MRI scanning. *Behavior Research Methods, Instruments and Computers*, 29(4), 589–94.

Petersen, S.E., Fox, P.T., Posner, M.I., and Raichle, M.E. (1988). Positron emission tomographic studies of the cortical anatomy of single-word processing. *Nature*, 331(6157), 585–9.

Pilipuf, M.N., Berry, J.M. *et al.* (1994). Prosthetic and orthotic lab applications in medical imaging head immobilization. *Journal of Prosthetics and Orthotics*, 6(3), 79–82.

Rosen, B.R., Buckner, R.L., and Dale, A.M. (1998). Event-related functional MRI: past, present, and future. *Proceedings of the National Academy of Sciences (USA)*, 95(3), 773–80.

Savoy, R.L., Ravicz, M.E., and Gollub, R. (1999). The psychophysiological laboratory in the magnet: stimulus delivery, response recording, and safety. In: *Functional MRI*, (ed. C.T.W. Moonen and P.A. Bandettini), pp. 347–65, Springer-Verlag, Berlin.

Shellock, F.G. and Kanal, E. (1996). *Magnetic resonance: bioeffects, safety, and patient management*, 2nd edn, New York, Lippincott-Raven.

Shellock, F.G., Morisoli, S.M., and Ziarati, M. (1994). Measurement of acoustic noise during MR imaging: evaluation of six 'worst-case' pulse sequences. *Radiology*, 191, 91–3.

Shellock, F.G., Ziarati, M., Atkinson, D., and Chen, D.Y. (1998). Determination of gradient magnetic field-induced acoustic noise associated with the use of echo planar and three-dimensional, fast spin echo techniques. *Journal of Magnetic Resonance Imaging*, 8(5), 54–7.

Slifer, K.J., Cataldo, M.F., Cataldo, M.D., Connor, R.T., and Zerhouni, E.A. (1993). Behavior analysis of motion control for pediatric neuroimaging. *Journal of Applied Behavioral Analysis*, 26(4), 469–70.

Thulborn, K.R. (1999). Visual feedback to stabilize head position for fMRI. *Magnetic Resonance in Medicine*, 41, 1039–43.

Warach, S., Ives, J.R., Schlaug, G., Patel, M.R., Darby, D.G., Thangeraj, V., Edelman, R.R., and Schoner, D.L. (1996). EEG-triggered echo planar functional MRI in epilepsy. *Neurology*, 47(1), 89–93.

IV | *Analysis of functional imaging data*

11 | *Overview of fMRI analysis*

Stephen M. Smith

11.1 Introduction

After an fMRI experiment has been designed and carried out, the resulting data must be passed through various analysis steps before the experimenter can get answers to questions about experimentally-related activations at the individual or multi-subject level. This chapter gives a brief overview of the various analysis steps, whilst Chapters 12–16 cover these areas in greater detail.

11.2 fMRI data

In a typical fMRI session a low-resolution functional volume is acquired every few seconds. (MR volumes are often also referred to as 'images' or 'scans'). Over the course of the experiment, 100 volumes or more are typically recorded. In the simplest possible experiment, some images will be taken whilst stimulation[1] is applied, and some will be taken with the subject at rest. Because the images are taken using an MR sequence which is sensitive to changes in local blood oxygenation level (BOLD imaging; see Chapters 2 and 3), parts of the images taken during stimulation should show increased intensity, compared with those taken whilst at rest. The parts of these images which show increased intensity should correspond to the brain areas which are activated by the stimulation.

The goal of fMRI analysis is to detect, in a robust, sensitive, and valid way, those parts of the brain which show increased intensity at the points in time that stimulation was applied.

A single volume is made up of individual cuboid elements called voxels—see Fig. 11.1. An fMRI data set from a single session can either be thought of as t volumes, one taken every few seconds, or as v voxels,

each with an associated time series of t time points. It is important to be able to conceptualize both of these representations, as some analysis steps make more sense when thinking of the data in one way, and others make more sense the other way.

An example time-series from a single voxel is shown in Fig. 11.2. Image intensity is shown on the y axis, and time (in scans) on the x axis. As described above, for some of the time points, stimulation was applied, (the higher intensity periods), and at some time points the subject was at rest. As well as the effect of the stimulation being clear, the high frequency noise is also apparent. The aim of fMRI analysis is to identify in which voxels' time-series the signal of interest is significantly greater than the noise level.

11.3 Preparing fMRI data for statistical analysis

Initially, a 4D data set is pre-processed, i.e. prepared for statistical analysis. (Chapters 12 and 13 describe the pre-processing steps in more detail.) Once data has been acquired by the MR scanner, the pre-processing starts by reconstructing the raw 'k-space' data into images that actually look like brains. Very often, the next step applied is slice-timing correction; because each slice in each volume is acquired at slightly different times, it necessary to adjust the data so that it appears that all voxels within one volume had been acquired at exactly the same time (all subsequent processing is far simpler if this is done). Each volume is now transformed (using rotation and translation) so that the image of the brain within each volume is aligned with that in every other volume; this is known as motion correction.

Most researchers now blur each volume spatially,

---

[1] For the remainder of this chapter, reference to 'stimulation' should be taken to include also the carrying out of physical or cognitive activity.

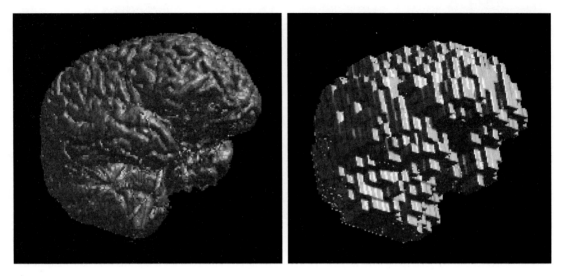

Fig. 11.1 What are voxels? Shown here are surface renderings of 3D brain images. On the left is a high-resolution image, with small ($1 \times 1 \times 1.5$mm) voxels; the voxels are too small to see. On the right is a low-resolution image of the same brain, with large ($7 \times 7 \times 10$mm) voxels, clearly showing the voxels making up the image.

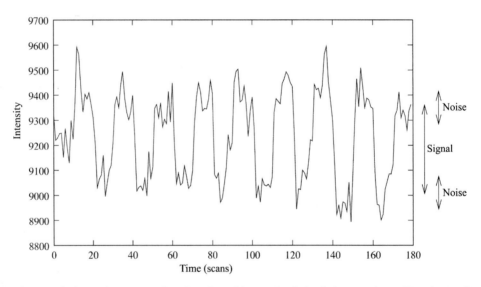

Fig. 11.2 An example time series at a strongly activated voxel from a visual stimulation experiment. Here the signal is significantly larger than the noise level. Periods of stimulation are alternated with periods of rest–a complete stimulation-rest cycle lasts 20 scans.

principally to reduce noise, hopefully without significantly affecting the activation signal. After this, each volume's overall intensity level is adjusted so that all volumes have the same mean intensity—this intensity normalization can help reduce the effect of global changes in intensity over time. Reduction in low and high frequency noise is normally desired as a final step; each voxel's time series is filtered by linear or non-linear tools in order to achieve this.

The purpose of the preprocessing is to remove various kinds of artefacts in the data, and to condition the data, in order to maximize the sensitivity of later statistical analysis, and also, in some situations, to increase the statistical validity.

11.4 Statistical analysis of activation images

In this section can be found a very brief overview of different approaches to obtaining activation maps, followed by a slightly more detailed introduction to analysis via the general linear model (GLM—currently the most popular statistical approach) and also various methods of thresholding the resulting statistics maps. (Note that Chapter 14 covers these areas in much more detail.)

After the pre-processing steps, statistical analysis is carried out to determine which voxels are activated by the stimulation. This can be simple correlation analysis or more advanced modelling of the expected haemodynamic response to the stimulation. Various possible statistical corrections can be included, such as correction for smoothness of the measured time series at each voxel. The main output from this step is a statistical map which indicates those points in the image where the brain has activated in response to the stimulus.

It is most common to analyse each voxel's time series independently ('univariate analysis'). For example, standard general linear model (GLM) analysis is univariate (although cluster-based thresholding, commonly used at the final inference stage, does use spatial neighbourhood information and is therefore not univariate). However, there are also 'multivariate' methods (e.g. Friston *et al.* 1996) which process all the data together; these methods make more use of spatial relationships within the data than univariate analysis.

Note that most model-free methods (see the following paragraph) are also multivariate.

There is also a distinction between model-based and model-free methods. In a model-based method (e.g. Friston *et al.* 1995), a model of the expected response is generated and compared with the data. In a model-free method, (e.g. McKeown *et al.* 1998), effects or components of interest in the data are found on the basis of some specific criterion (for example, the spatial or temporal components should be statistically independent of each other). This allows for 'surprise' in the data, and also the analysis of data where it is difficult to generate a good model. There are also a few methods which lie between model-based and model-free, for example (Clare *et al.* 1999), where the only 'model' information given is the time of the beginning of each simulation period (the actual time-course within each period is not pre-specified). A statistic map is generating by comparing the variance within periods with the variance across periods.

11.4.1 General Linear Model—overview

General linear modelling (more correctly, just 'linear modelling') sets up a model (i.e. a general pattern which you expect to see in the data) and fits it to the data. If the model is derived from the timing of the stimulation that was applied to the subject in the MRI scanner, then a good fit between the model and the data means that the data was probably caused by the stimulation.

As the GLM is normally used in a univariate way, the rest of this section considers one voxel only, and the fitting of models to a single voxel's time-course. Thus consider that the data of interest comprises a single 1D vector of intensity values.

A very simple example of linear modelling is

$$y(t) = \beta * x(t) + c + e(t), \tag{11.1}$$

where $y(t)$ is the data, and is a 1D vector of intensity values—one for each time point, i.e. is a function of time. $x(t)$ is the model, and is also a 1D vector with one value for each time point. In the case of a square-wave block design, $x(t)$ might be a series of 1s and 0s—for example, 0 0 0 0 0 1 1 1 1 1 0 0 0 0 0 etc. β is the parameter estimate for $x(t)$, i.e. the value that the square wave (of height 1) must be multiplied by to fit the square wave component in the data. c is a constant, and in this example, would correspond to the baseline (rest) intensity value in the data. e is the error in the model fitting. Thus the model fitting involves adjusting the baseline level and the height of the square wave, to best fit the data; the error term accounts for the residual error between the fitted model and the data.

If there are two types of stimulus, the model would be

$$y = \beta_1 * x_1 + \beta_2 * x_2 + c + e. \qquad (11.2)$$

Thus there are now two different model waveforms corresponding to the two stimulus time-courses. There are also two interesting parameters to estimate, β_1 and β_2. Thus if a particular voxel responds strongly to model x_1 the model-fitting will find a large value for β_1; if the data instead looks more like the second model time-course, x_2, then the model-fitting will give β_2 a large value. Different model waveforms within a complex model are often referred to as explanatory variables (EVs), as they explain different processes in the data.

In order to get the best possible fit of the model to the data, the 'stimulus function' (which is often a sharp on/off waveform) is convolved with the haemodynamic response function (HRF). This process mimics the effect that the brain's neuro-physiology has on the input function (the stimulation). The brain's haemodynamic response is a delayed and blurred version of the input time-series, so a mathematical operation is applied to the stimulus function to take the square wave input and create a delayed and blurred version, which will better fit the data. For example, see Fig.

11.3, showing the raw stimulation timing waveform and the HRF-convolved model—$x(t)$— which will be used in the model fitting.

The GLM is often formulated in matrix notation. Thus all of the parameters are grouped together into a vector $\boldsymbol{\beta}$, and all of the model time-courses are grouped together into a matrix X, often referred to as the design matrix. Figure 11.4 shows an example design matrix with two such model time-courses. Each column is a different part of the model. For example, in a particular experiment, both visual and auditory stimulations are applied, but with different timings; the left column (x_1 or EV 1) models the visual stimulation, and the right column (EV 2 or x_2) models the auditory stimulation.

As described above, when the model is fit separately to the data at each voxel, there will be found an estimate of the 'goodness of fit', of each column in the model, to that voxel's time-course. In the example visual/auditory experiment, the first column will generate a high first parameter estimate in the visual cortex. However, the second column will generate a low second parameter estimate, as this part of the model will not fit the voxel's time-course well.

To convert a parameter estimate (PE, i.e. the estimated β value) into a useful statistic, its value is compared with the uncertainty in its estimation (resulting in what is known as a T value; $T = PE/$ standard error (PE)). If the PE is low relative to its estimated uncertainty, the fit is not significant and vice versa. Thus T is a good measure of whether the estimate of the PE value is significantly different from zero, i.e. whether there is believable activation. (Remember, all of this is carried out separately for each

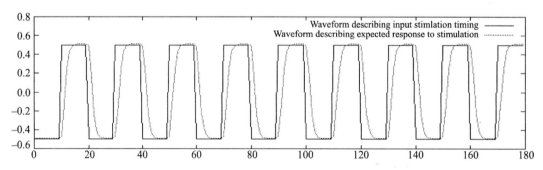

Fig. 11.3   Model waveform formation: the square waveform describes the input stimulation timing; the smoothed waveform results from convolving the first with the haemodynamic response function, a transformation which leaves the model looking much more like the measured data.

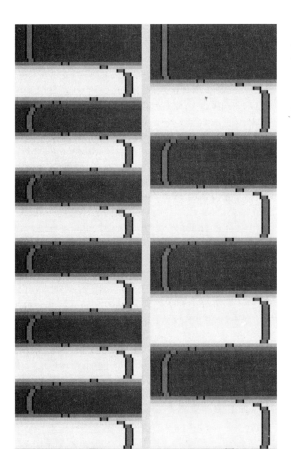

Fig. 11.4 Example design matrix with two explanatory variables; two different stimulations are being applied. Because they have different timings, they are modelled separately—see eqn (11.2). Time is on the *y* axis, pointing downwards. Note that a column has two representations of the model's value at each point in time: the underlying intensity encodes the model's value at a particular time point, and so does the line graph.

voxel.) To convert a *T* value into a *P* (probability) or *Z* statistic[2] requires standard statistical transformations; however, *T*, *P*, and *Z* all contain the same information—they describe how significantly the data is related to a particular part of the model (x_1 or x_2).

As well as producing images of *Z* values which describe how strongly each voxel is related to each EV

(one image per EV), parameter estimates can be compared to test directly whether one EV is more 'relevant' to the data than another. To do this, one *PE* is subtracted from another, the standard error for this new value is calculated, and a new *T* image is created. All of the above is controlled by setting up 'contrasts'. To compare two EVs (for example, to subtract one stimulus type—EV 1—from another type—EV 2), set EV 1's contrast value to −1 and EV 2's to 1. This is often written as a contrast of [−1 1], as the contrasted parameter estimate equals $-1 \times \beta_1 + 1 \times \beta_2$. A *T* statistic image will then be generated according to this request, answering the question 'where is the response to stimulus 2 significantly greater than the response to stimulus 1?'

It is possible that the response to two different stimuli, when applied simultaneously, is greater than that predicted by adding up the responses to the stimuli when applied separately. If this is the case, then such 'non-linear interactions' need to be allowed for in the model. The simplest way of doing this is to setup the two originals EVs, and then add an interaction EV, which will only be 'up' when both of the original EVs are 'up', and 'down' otherwise. In Fig. 11.5, EV 1 could represent the application of a drug, and EV 2 could represent visual stimulation. EV 3 will model the extent to which the response to drug + visual is greater than the sum of drug-only and visual-only. A contrast of [0 0 1] will show this measure, whilst a contrast of [0 0 −1] shows where negative interaction is occurring.

Ideally, all of the EVs should be independent of each other. If any EV is close to being a sum (or weighted sum) of other EVs in the design, then the fitting of the model to the data does not work properly (the design matrix is not of 'full rank'). A common mistake of this type is to model both rest and activation waveforms, making one an upside-down version of the other; in this case EV 2 is −1 times EV 1, and therefore linearly dependent on it. It is only necessary to model the activation waveform.

With 'parametric designs', there are typically several different levels of stimulation, and it is common to estimate the response to each level separately. This requires a separate EV for each stimulation level. The

---

[2] *Z* is a 'Gaussianised *T*'; if the noise in the data is Gaussian, then *T* can be simply converted (taking into account the number of time points) into *Z*. When there is no activation, *Z* follows a Gaussian distribution, with zero mean and unit variance.

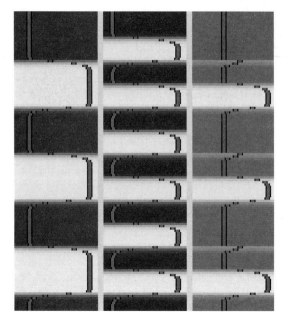

Fig. 11.5 Example of modelling a nonlinear interaction between stimuli. The first two EVs model the separate stimuli, whilst the third models the interaction, i.e. accounts for the 'extra' response when both stimuli are applied together.

different contrasts ask different questions about these responses: For example, for an experiment with 3 stimulation levels, [1 0 0] shows the response to stimulation level 1 versus rest (likewise [0 1 0] for level 2 vs rest and [0 0 1] for level 3). [−1 1 0] shows where the response to level 2 is greater than that for level 1. [−1 0 1] shows the general linear increase across all three levels. [1 −2 1] shows where the level dependence deviates, in an upwardly-curving way, from being linear.

11.4.2 Inference ('Thresholding')

Thus we now have a statistic map (for example, T or Z). The next step is to threshold this, in order to decide, at a given level of significance, which parts of the brain were activated. There are a variety of ways of carrying out thresholding. These are now briefly outlined.

The simplest method of thresholding is to select a significance (P) threshold and apply this to every voxel in the statistic map (it is straightforward to convert a P level to a suitable threshold for the map type, e.g. a T threshold). A problem with this is that there are many tests being carried out, because there are so many voxels in the brain. If 20 000 voxels are tested for at a significance of $P < 0.01$ then it is expected that 200 will activate by chance, even if no stimulation is applied. It is not ideal to blindly accept these as being activated! This 'multiple-comparison problem' means that it is not valid to accept all activations reported by this method of thresholding; a correction is necessary to reduce the number of false positives. Typically a Bonferroni correction is used, where the significance level at each voxel is divided by the number of voxels; this corrects for the number of comparisons being made. However, this results in very stringent thresholding (i.e. in the case given above, the resulting P threshold is $0.01/20000 = 0.0000005$).

A refinement of the above voxel-wise thresholding is to use Gaussian random field (GRF) theory to threshold the image. The main difference is that this method takes into account the spatial smoothness of the statistic map (i.e. estimates the number of statistically independent voxels, which is smaller than the original number). This method is less 'over-conservative' than simple voxel-wise thresholding with Bonferroni correction; typically the correction to P values is reduced (compared with Bonferroni correction) by a factor of 2–20.

Finally, it is possible, again using GRF theory, to take into account spatial extent (i.e. size) of clusters of activations, before estimating significance. Thus instead of assigning a P-value to each voxel, clusters of voxels are created on the basis of an initial thresholding, and then each cluster is assigned a P-value, which may or may not pass the final significance test. It is often the case that this method is more sensitive to activation than the voxel-based methods. A limitation is the arbitrary nature of the initial thresholding, used to create the clusters.

11.5 Multi-subject statistics

Although so far we have only discussed single-session analyses, it is common to run an experiment several times, either on the same subject, or with several different subjects, or both. This can both increase the sensitivity of the overall experiment (as more data can lead to increased sensitivity to an effect) or allow the generalisation of any conclusions to the whole population.

In order to combine statistics across different sessions or subjects, the first necessary step is to align the brain images from all sessions into some common space. This is done using generic registration tools (for more detail see Chapter 15) and can be carried out either on the raw data (i.e. before the single-session, or 'first-level', analyses) or on the statistic maps created by the first-level analyses.

Once all the data is aligned, there are a variety of statistical methods for combining results across sessions or subjects, to either create a single result for a group of subjects, or to compare different groups of subjects (for example, placebo group versus drug treatment group). These methods include 'fixed-effects' and 'random-effects' analyses. Fixed-effects assumes that all subjects within a group activate equally, and is only interested in within-session errors. Random-effects analysis additionally takes into account between-session errors, and therefore makes less assumptions about the data; its results are therefore valid for the whole population from which the group of subjects is drawn (whereas fixed-effects results are not). However, the random-effects analysis tends to give more 'conservative' results.

How many subjects are required, in order for multi-subject statistics to be sensitive and robust? The answer is not simple, as it depends on many factors including the level of response to the stimulation, between-subject variability and scanner characteristics. (Furthermore, all things being equal, a smaller number of subjects is generally required for a fixed-effects group analysis than for a random-effects analysis.) However, it is generally accepted that groups containing less than about 10 subjects are suboptimal. For more detail see (Friston *et al.* 1999).

11.6 Registration, brain atlases and cortical flattening

As described above, registration (aligning different brain images) is often used when combining fMRI data from different sessions or subjects. It can also be used to align the low-resolution fMRI images to a high-resolution structural image, so that the activations can be viewed in the context of a good quality brain image; this aids in the interpretation of the activations.

A related issue is the use of templates and brain atlases. These consist of data which is transformed into some 'standard brain space', for example the co-ordinate system specified by (Talairach and Tournoux, 1988). A template is typically an average of many brains, all registered into any given common co-ordinate system. An example is the MNI 305 average (Collins *et al.* 1994). An atlas is also based in a common co-ordinate system, but contains more sophisticated information about the brain at each voxel, for example, information about tissue type, local brain structure, or functional area. Atlases can inform interpretation of fMRI experiments in a variety of ways, helping the experimenter gain the maximum value from the data.

Finally, another related issue is that of cortical flattening. Here a high-resolution structural image is used to estimate the convoluted cortical surface (this can be considered to be the simple 2D surface, consisting of all cortical grey matter, which has been 'crumpled' into the skull). Because cortical activation should only lie on this surface, new statistical constraints and preprocessing methodologies can be developed which use this spatial information, in order to improve on the simple 3D processing most commonly used. Also, it can be of value to 'project' estimated activations onto a flattened version of the surface, enabling interesting interpretation of the relative placements of different activations. For more detail on the structural analysis issues described in this section, see Chapter 15.

11.7 Extracting brain connectivity

So far, we have only discussed the estimation of sites of activation and their relationship to stimulation or cognitive activity. No mention has been made of the relationships *between* different sites in the brain. Connectivity analysis attempts to try to estimate such networks, in order to build up a more sophisticated picture of the functioning of the brain.

Connectivity analysis is carried out on the basis of either similarities in time-courses or relationships between final activation levels between different brain regions. This exciting new area of research is described in Chapter 16.

11.8 Appendix—GLM-based analysis example

This appendix describes briefly the practical and numerical details involved in the analysis of a particular fMRI experiment. Most of the analysis concepts referred to within this section are explained more fully in the following chapters.

The experiment attempted to compare the response to thermal stimulation between two groups of subjects. One group comprised 10 clinical patients and the second was a control group of eight subjects. Within each session, brief periods of warm or hot thermal stimulation were applied briefly to the back of the subject's hand. For each session, 250 volumes were acquired, one every 3 s. A question of interest was how the relative response to hot and warm stimulation differed between the two groups. All analysis was carried out within the fMRI analysis package FEAT (FMRI Expert Analysis Tool) (Smith *et al.* 2001).

11.8.1 First-level analysis

Each individual subject's session was processed independently, using the following analysis: head motion correction was carried out using MCFLIRT (Bannister and Jenkinson 2001), a tool which corrects for rigid-body (rotation and translation) motion, using an accurate and robust multi-scale optimization strategy. Figure 11.6 shows the estimated rotation and translation parameters used to correct for the head motion. MCFLIRT is fully automated, i.e. requires no user-interaction.

Spatial filtering was carried out on every volume using a Gaussian profile filter of full-width–half-maximum 5 mm. Example slices from an example volume, before and after spatial filtering, are shown in Fig. 11.7. Each session's data set was intensity normalized to have a mean within-brain intensity of 10 000 units. No volume-by-volume intensity normalization was carried out.

Nonlinear (Gaussian-weighted running line detrending) high-pass filtering was applied, with FWHM 50 s. The high-pass cutoff was this low because this is a single-event design, which allows more aggressive high-pass filtering than block-design experiments. No low-pass filtering was applied, due to the nature of the later GLM procedure; as pre-whitening of each voxel's time series was used, low-pass filtering is inappropriate. An example time-course from a single (activated) voxel is shown in Fig. 11.8, before and after high-pass filtering.

Next, GLM analysis was carried out on each subject's pre-processed data using FILM (Woolrich *et al.*, 2000): Generalized least-squares multiple regression was used; the model was initially fit to the data and fitted activation subtracted from the data. The resulting first-pass residuals were then pre-whitened by estimating the autocorrelation structure (calculating the autocorrelation coefficients, then using Tukey tapering and within-tissue-type spatial regularisation to improve estimation accuracy and robustness). The model was then refit to the pre-whitened data to give maximum efficiency estimation.

The model used is shown in Fig. 11.9 (and an example fit of the model to one voxel's timecourse is shown in Figure 11.8). EV 1 models the periods of painful heat, EV 3 models 'pain conditioning' (a light of a certain colour was shown just before the painful heat), EV 5 models warm thermal stimulation and EV 7 models 'warm conditioning' (using a different coloured light). The even numbered EVs are simply the temporal derivatives of the odd numbered EVs. These are included because they can correct for slight overall temporal shifts between the model and the data.[3]

As the single-subject statistics were then to be fed into a multi-subject second-level analysis, thresholding was not in general carried out on the first-level results. However, an example single-session activation map was created by thresholding one contrast (pain-warm, i.e. a contrast of [1 0 0 0 −1 0 0 0]) from one subject's data with cluster-based thresholding; clusters were formed by thresholding at $Z > 2.3$, and then each cluster was tested for significance at $P < 0.01$. Also, as an example of using a single-subject's structural image to render activation onto, one subject's fMRI data was registered onto that subject's high-resolution image: first, the structural was brain-extracted (i.e. non-brain matter removed) using BET (Smith, 2000). Then the fMRI image was registered to the brain-extracted high-

---

[3] Adding, to an original signal, a small amount of the temporal derivative of that signal, is equivalent to shifting the original signal slightly in time.

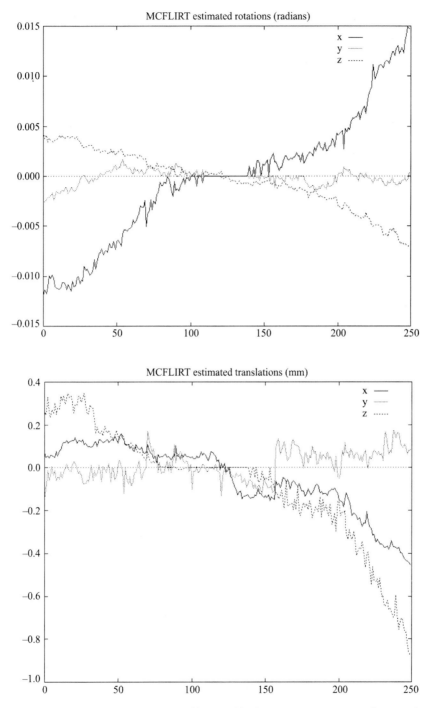

Fig. 11.6 Rotation and translation parameters estimated by a rigid-body motion correction procedure, as a function of scan number.

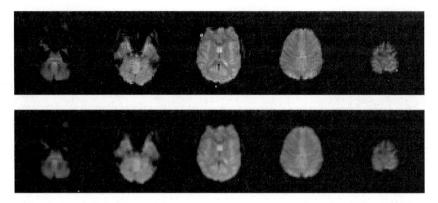

Fig. 11.7 Example slices from an example fMRI volume, before and after spatial filtering of 5 mm FWHM.

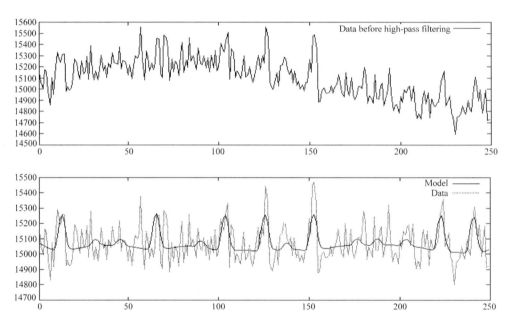

Fig. 11.8 An example time-course from a single (activated) voxel: *Top*: time-course before high-pass filtering. *Bottom*: after filtering, and plotted against the fitted model.

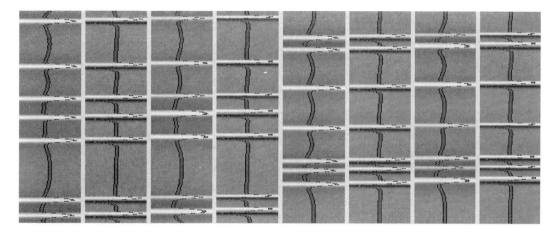

Fig. 11.9 The model, or design matrix, used in the GLM analysis of the heat-warm experiment. EVs 1 and 5 model pain and warm, EVs 3 and 7 model conditioning to pain and warm, and the even numbered EVs are simply the temporal derivatives of the odd numbers; these allow phase shifts in the fitting.

resolution image using FLIRT (Jenkinson and Smith, 2001), and this transform was applied to the thresholded activation map. The various stages involved can be seen in Fig. 11.10.

11.8.2 Second-level analysis

Second-level analysis was carried out to test for differences in the pain-warm contrast between the two subject groups. The single-session data sets were registered into standard space using FLIRT in a two-step process. First the low-resolution fMRI data from each subject was registered to that subject's (brain-extracted) high-resolution structural MRI using a 7 degrees-of-freedom (DOF) linear fit (see Chapter 15). Then the high-resolution image was registered to a Talairach-space standard brain image (the MNI 152 image) using a 12 DOF linear fit. The average image from all 18 subjects is compared with the standard space target image in Fig. 11.11. Then, for each subject, the two transforms were combined mathematically to give a single transform taking the fMRI data into standard space; this was applied to the first-level statistic maps (activation parameter estimates and variance estimates) to take them into standard space. Thus all subjects' statistical data are now in alignment.

Second-level fixed-effects and random-effects analyses were then carried out on the first-level statistic maps to test for differences in activation between the

two subject groups. The resulting statistic maps were thresholded as above, i.e. using clusters formed by $Z > 2.3$ and then tested with $P < 0.01$. These results can be seen in Fig. 11.12. These final results are in Talairach co-ordinate space, so meaningful co-ordinates can be given for the centres of activation. Thus the only remaining process is the final interpretation of this group comparison.

References

Bannister, P. and Jenkinson, M. (2001). *Robust affine motion correction in fMRI time series*. Seventh International Conference on Functional Mapping of the Human Brain.

Clare, S., Humberstone, M., Hykin, J., Blumhardt, L., Bowtell, R., and Morris, P. (1999). Detecting activations in event-related fMRI using analysis of variance. *Magnetic Resonance in Medicine*, **42**, 1117–22.

Collins, D., Neelin, P., Peters, T., and Evans, A. (1994). Automatic 3D intersubject registration of MR volumetric data in standardized Talairach space. *Journal of Computer Assisted Tomography*, **18**(2), 192–205.

Friston, K., Holmes, A., and Worsley, K. (1999). How many subjects constitute a study? *NeuroImage*, **10**(1), 1–5.

Friston, K., Holmes, A., Worsley, K., Poline, J.-B., Frith, C., and Frackowiak, R. (1995). Statistical parametric maps in functional imaging: A general linear approach. *Human Brain Mapping*, **2**, 189–210.

Friston, K., Poline, J.-B., Holmes, A., Frith, C., and Frackowiak, R. (1996). A multivariate analysis of PET activation studies. *Human Brain Mapping*, **4**, 140–51.

Jenkinson, M. and Smith, S. (2001). Global optimisation for

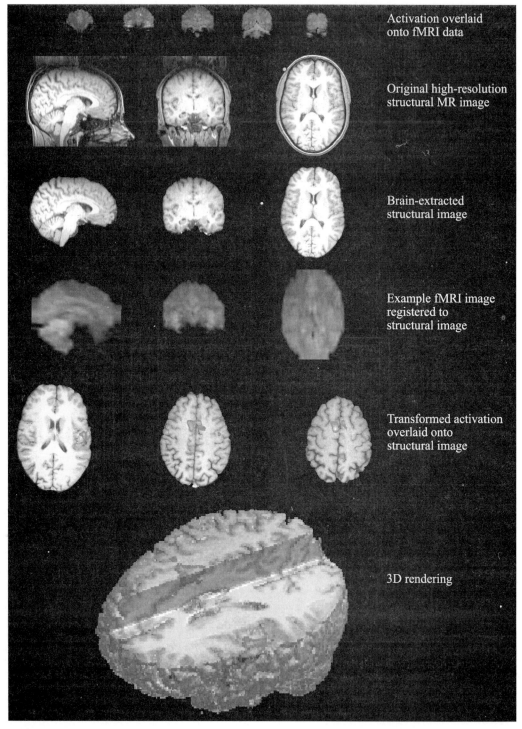

Activation overlaid
onto fMRI data

Original high-resolution
structural MR image

Brain-extracted
structural image

Example fMRI image
registered to
structural image

Transformed activation
overlaid onto
structural image

3D rendering

Fig. 11.10 Various stages in the rendering of activation onto a high-resolution structural image. (See also colour plate section.)

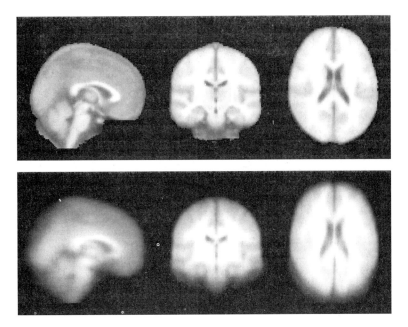

Fig. 11.11 Comparison of the standard space MNI 152 image (*top*) and the mean of the 18 subjects' high-resolution structural images after transformation into standard space (*bottom*). The mean of the subjects' MR 'high-resolution' images is fairly blurred, due to the relatively low resolution of most of the structural scans taken for this study.

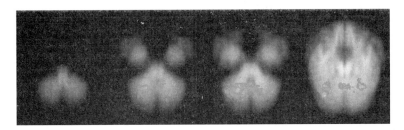

Fig. 11.12 Significant differences between the two subject groups in the pain-warm contrast. (see also colour plate section)

robust affine registration of brain images. *Medical Image Analysis.* **5**(2), 143–156.

McKeown, M.J., Makeig, S., Brown, G.G., Jung, T.P., Kindermann, S.S., Bell, A.J., and Sejnowski, T.J. (1998). Analysis of fMRI data by blind separation into independent spatial components. *Human Brain Mapping*, **6**(3), 160–88.

Smith, S. (2000). *Robust automated brain extraction.* Sixth International Conference on Functional Mapping of the Human Brain, p. 625.

Smith, S., Bannister, P., Beckmann, C., Brady, M., Clare, S., Flitney, D., Hansen, P., Jenkinson, M., Leibovici, D., Ripley, B., Woolrich, M., and Zhang, Y. (2001). *FSL: new tools for functional and structural brain image analysis.* Seventh International Conference on Functional Mapping of the Human Brain.

Talairach, J. and Tournoux, P. (1988). *Co-planar Stereotaxic Atlas of the Human Brain.* Thieme Medical Publisher Inc., New York.

Woolrich, M., Ripley, B., Brady, M., and Smith, S. (2000). *Nonparametric estimation of temporal autocorrelation in FMRI.* Sixth International Conference on Functional Mapping of the Human Brain, p. 610.

12 | *Preparing fMRI data for statistical analysis*

Stephen M. Smith

12.1 Introduction

This chapter (along with Chapter 13) describes the various pre-processing steps necessary to take raw data from the scanner and prepare it for the 'heart' of fMRI analysis, namely statistical analysis (estimating where significant activation occurred, described in Chapter 14). These pre-processing steps take the raw MR data, convert it into images that actually look like brains, then reduce unwanted noise of various types, and precondition the data, in order to aid the later statistics. Later statistical analysis is often seen as the most 'important' part of fMRI analysis; however, without the pre-processing steps, the statistical analysis is, at best, greatly reduced in power, and at worst, rendered invalid.

Having stated the importance of data pre-processing, it should however be noted that, from the researcher's point-of-view, it is much easier to 'automate' the pre-processing steps than the statistical analysis. This is because optimal tuning of pre-processing algorithms is less dependent on details of any particular experiment than is the case with later statistics.

12.2 Reconstruction from raw k-space data

As described in Chapter 3, the raw MR signal is obtained by digitising the demodulated RF signal that is detected by the receiver coil. The raw data that is thus generated does not resemble a real image, but instead is 'k-space' data, that is, a spatial frequency transformation of real-space. (The principles of k-space are described in Chapter 3). Fig. 12.1 shows an example slice of k-space data.

In order to reconstruct the k-space data into real-space so that the image may be viewed and analysed, a Fourier transform is generally required. This may be run in 2D or 3D, depending on the MR sequence used; it is normally 2D for fMRI data, i.e. each slice is processed separately.

Additional reconstruction steps are also often necessary in order to correct for various artefacts in the data, or to otherwise improve the quality of the resulting image. A particular case in point is the additional processing steps that are necessary for echo planar imaging (EPI). The most significant artefact suffered by EPI data is the so-called 'Nyquist ghost' that causes a lower intensity replication of the main image, shifted by half the field-of-view with respect to the main image (at least for snapshot EPI). Generally some additional phase information is collected with the fMRI data that enables a 'ghost correction' to be applied to the data. This typically reduces the intensity of the ghost image to less than 5 per cent of the intensity of the main image. A detailed treatment of the data correction steps that are applied to EPI data can be found in (Schmitt *et al.* 1998).

Note that some researchers (e.g. Wowk *et al.* 1997; Hu *et al.* 1995) carry out additional pre-processing steps on the raw (k-space) data *before* reconstruction into real-space, for example, in order to apply a phase and amplitude correction to the data in an attempt to correct for physiological noise effects. Although this is not a very common approach, it does have some computational and conceptual advantages over the more common approach of working in real-space. Another good example is certain image registration procedures (Eddy *et al.* 1996); translation is achieved in real-space by applying a first order phase-shift in k-space, before reconstruction.

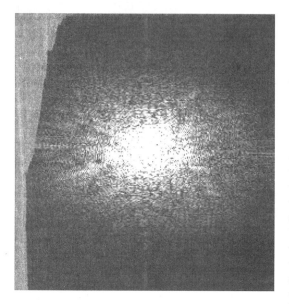

Fig. 12.1 Example single-slice FID data, where different pixels represent a different point in *k*-space (spatial frequency space).

12.3 Slice timing correction

Functional volumes are normally formed one slice at a time; the capture of these slices is spread out in time over the few seconds that the total volume capture takes. A problem with this is that later fMRI analysis assumes that all slices were captured at the same time (and, moreover, instantaneously). For example, fitting a model to each voxel's time series normally assumes that the data for each time point was taken at the beginning of the corresponding volume's scan time. However, because different points in the volume were scanned at slightly different times, the model fitting is not optimal. The fitting will be improved if each voxel's time series is adjusted so that it really does appear as if all voxels were scanned at the same time.

This adjusting of time series is normally referred to as slice timing correction (the same correction is applied to each voxel within any given slice), and is achieved by phase shifting the time series of values at each voxel. Phase shifting means sliding the 1D time plot forwards or backwards; because the correction is small, (less than the time between consecutive volumes) a very small amount of 'sliding' is required. This is normally achieved by Fourier transforming each voxel's time series into a frequency representation, applying a phase shift to this data, and then applying the reverse Fourier transformation to recover the corrected time series. (Note that it is not possible to carry out this phase shift on the original raw *k*-space data, as this raw data is in 'Fourier space' only in the spatial dimension, and not in time.)

There is a complication to the above solution to the slice timing problem. If there is much head motion during the capture of a functional volume, then the whole image is distorted, as well as containing timing variation between slices. Thus ideal pre-processing would combine slice timing correction and geometric correction, as these different corrections cannot really be separated. (Geometric correction includes functional image unwarping—see Chapter 15, within-volume movement-related distortion correction, and correction for movement 'between' volumes.) However, to date, very little research of this sophistication has been carried out.

12.4 Motion correction

If a subject moves their head during an fMRI session, the position of the brain within the functional images will vary over time. This means that any particular voxel's time series does not (over time) refer to the same point in the brain. Correcting for such head motion is a large topic, and is the subject of the following chapter; it is therefore not discussed further here.

12.5 Spatial filtering

The next stage of fMRI analysis is the spatial filtering ('blurring') of each volume. There are two reasons for applying spatial filtering as a pre-processing step; first, blurring can increase signal-to-noise ratio in the data, and second, certain later statistical steps, in order to be valid, may require the functional images to be spatially smooth.

12.5.1 Reasons for spatial filtering

The 'signal-to-noise ratio' is a measure of how big the signal of interest is, compared with the noise level. The signal of interest, in this case, is the change in image intensity which arises as a result of application of stimulation. The noise is the unavoidable random variations in image intensity which are present even when no stimulation is applied. Typically, the change in intensity due to stimulation is between 0.5 per cent and 5 per cent of the average intensity, and the noise level is between 0.5 per cent and 1 per cent.

The main point of spatial filtering of the fMRI data is to reduce the noise level whilst retaining the underlying signal. It is obvious why noise is reduced; the blurring function is effectively a local averaging, so the 'noise' values in the local neighbourhood will tend to cancel each other out. In order for the underlying signal to not be reduced along with the noise, it is required that the extent of the blurring is not larger than the size of the activated region; if very small activation regions are expected then spatial filtering should not be carried out.

The secondary reason for spatial filtering is that certain statistical theory which may be used in later processing requires the data to be spatially smooth for the assumptions underlying the statistical theory to be valid (Friston *et al.* 1994*b*). However, the amount of smoothing required for this is generally quite small (a 4 mm width blurring function is generally adequate).

Whilst the approach of 'tuning' the extent of the spatial blurring to the expected extent of activation is a simple strategy in spatial filtering, a related, more sophisticated approach is to involve a number of spatial scales. Such 'scale-space' methods analyse the effect of a wide range of spatial filtering extents on final activation (Poline and Mazoyer 1994; Worsley *et al.* 1996). A range of results can be obtained, each having resulted from a different amount of spatial blurring, and these can be searched for activations of interest. Clearly this can increase the chance of false positives unless statistical corrections are made, but such problems can be avoided, for example by choosing an appropriate spatial scale on the basis of one fMRI data set, and then applying this amount of smoothing to a second data set.

Some researchers have recently started looking at ways of combining spatial information that are more sophisticated than simple blurring (Descombes *et al.* 1998). Using non-linear filtering (or, in general, any neighbourhood information fusion method such as Markov random fields) it is possible to spread information spatially without necessarily blurring the signal of interest. In other words, voxels can 'use' information from their neighbours selectively, and thus reduce noise in an intelligent way. This should result in clearer fine detail within activation clusters. As such develop-

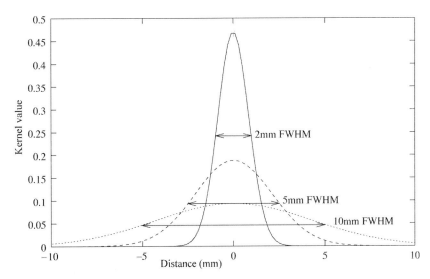

Fig. 12.2 Three example Gaussian profile convolution kernels. Note that the wider the kernel, the greater the smoothing effect. Note also that the wider the kernel, the smaller the central value. This is so that the area under the kernel is always 1; thus overall image intensity is unchanged by the filtering process, regardless of the width.

ments mature, the use of simple spatial filtering may become obsolete.

12.5.2 Implementation of spatial filtering

The commonest method of carrying out spatial filtering is to convolve each volume with a Gaussian profile filter (see Appendix for a brief explanation of convolution). The width of this filter (usually expressed in mm) determines the extent of the blurring that takes place. It is common to use a width of between 3 and 10 mm full-width–half-maximum (FWHM) for fMRI images. The term FWHM refers to the full width of the kernel

at the points which have half of the central maximum value. In Fig. 12.2 three example 1D Gaussian kernels are shown, with full widths 2, 5, and 10 mm.

Figure 12.3 shows an example image and the effect that a 10 mm FWHM smoothing filter has on this. Both the images themselves and the example intensity profiles through the images clearly show the effect of the blurring.

A Gaussian profile is a continuous mathematical curve, whereas a digitized version of this profile is required in order to be able to convolve the filter with the digitized data. Thus the Gaussian profile is sampled at intervals corresponding to the data voxel dimen-

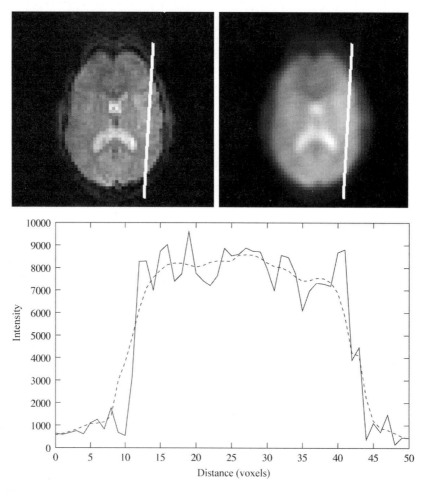

Fig. 12.3 Effect of spatial filtering. *Upper left*: single slice from original image with source of 1D profile (plotted as solid line) shown. *Upper right*: single slice from filtered image (FWHM = 10 mm) with source of 1D profile (plotted as dashed line) shown.

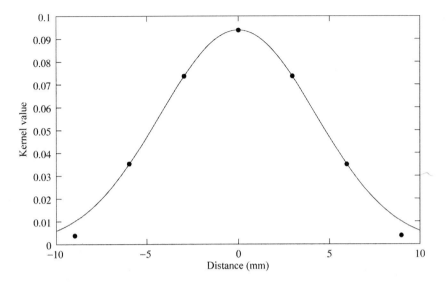

Fig. 12.4 Example Gaussian profile filter showing discrete sampling (dots) of the original continuous function. The distance between samples corresponds to the voxel size—in this case 3 mm. The end samples have been reduced from the theoretical value by a 'windowing' function.

sions (see Fig. 12.4). Note that the original Gaussian profile never quite falls to zero, so the the digitized filter needs to be 'truncated' (i.e. the tails are chopped off) at some point. It may be desirable to ameliorate the effects of this truncation by 'rolling off' the kernel values at the ends of the digitized filter.

The 2D equivalent of the 1D convolution filters shown in Figs 12.2 and 12.4 can be thought of as a 'hat' function. The 3D convolution filter can be visualized as a blurred sphere. However, in practice, a 3D filter is rarely implemented. Instead, it is far more computationally efficient to implement 3D Gaussian filtering as three separate 1D filters (in *x*, *y*, and *z*), each passed in turn over the data. This is mathematically equivalent to a single-pass 3D filter.

12.5.3 Example results

An example of the effect of different amounts of spatial filtering is given in Fig. 12.5. Both auditory and visual stimulation was applied, but with different paradigm frequencies, enabling activation due to the different stimuli to be found separately. The following pre-statistics processing was applied; simple 3D motion correction; a variety of spatial filtering extents (none, 5, 10, 20, 40 mm FWHM); non-linear high-pass

temporal filtering (Gaussian-weighted LSF straight line fitting, with sigma = 67.5 s). Statistical analysis was carried out using FILM (FMRIB's Improved Linear Model) with local autocorrelation correction (Woolrich *et al.* 2000). Z (Gaussianised T) statistic images were thresholded using clusters determined by Z > 2.3 and a cluster significance threshold of *p* = 0.01. Registration of fMRI images to a T1-weighted structural was carried out using FLIRT (FMRIB's Linear Image Registration Tool) (Jenkinson and Smith 2001).

The results clearly show the blurring of activation areas as spatial filtering extent increases, even causing 'activation' outside of the brain. In general, little appears to have been gained in these results by increased smoothing.

12.6 *Intensity normalization*

Intensity normalization refers to the rescaling of all intensities in an fMRI volume by the same amount, i.e. a general change in overall brightness. This process is applied separately to each functional volume, normally so that each ends up having the same mean intensity.

Historically, this process was a necessary step in PET pre-processing, as there were expected to be

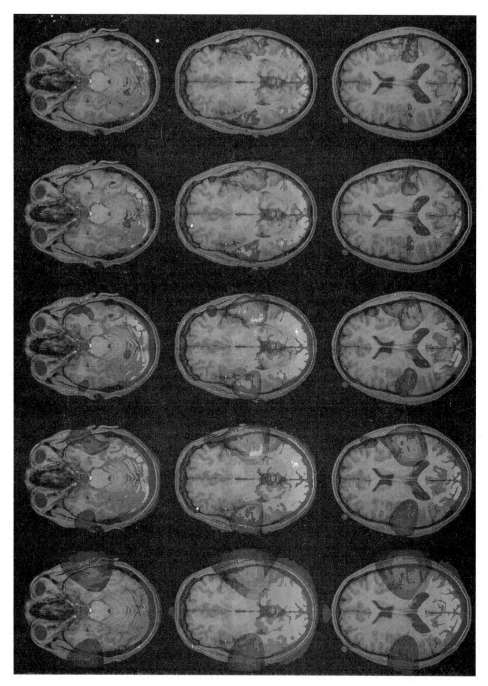

Fig. 12.5 Significant clusters of activation ($Z > 2.3$, $P < 0.01$) from an audiovisual experiment. The different rows were produced by processing with different spatial scales—filters of 0 (no filtering), 5, 10, 20, and 40 mm FWHM (from top row to bottom respectively). Red clusters show visual activation; blue clusters show auditory activation. (See also colour plate section.)

global (i.e. volume-wide) changes in intensity from one volume to the next, due to the radioactive decay of the agent injected to give the PET signal. In fMRI, there is less of a likelihood of much change in overall intensity, but it is still enough of an issue for an intensity normalization step to be normal practice. One possible cause of changes in overall intensity over time is the scanner itself, where electrical or temperature effects may occur (although any such effects which change slowly over time would be removed by high-pass temporal filtering—see next section).

In fMRI, intensity normalization is commonly carried out by finding, for each volume separately, the mean intensity across all voxels which have an intensity above a predetermined threshold[1]; then all intensity values (within the volume) are rescaled by a constant value, so that the new mean intensity becomes a preset value—for example, 10 000. A common alternative procedure is to take the mean intensity value for each volume, and include this set of values in later statistical analyses (as a 'confound variable'); statistical modelling can then fit each voxel's time series to both the mean intensity values and the expected response to stimulus at the same time.

There is, however, a widely recognized problem with such methods of intensity normalization. This is that if strong activation occurs, then the activation itself will increase the mean intensity; a volume which contains strong activation will have an artificially high mean intensity. Thus after normalization the 'non-activated' parts of the volume will be negatively correlated with the stimulation, and will show up as 'deactivation' in the final statistical image. This is clearly to be avoided; see, for example (Aguirre *et al.* 1998). Similarly, some experiments directly alter mean intensity level, for example, if overall oxygenation is being modulated during the session; in this case, again, mean-based intensity normalization is too simple an approach.

There are two possible solutions to this problem. The easy solution is simply not to carry out intensity normalization—it is arguably unnecessary for normal fMRI data. A more sophisticated approach, if one believes intensity normalization to be necessary, is to use a more robust estimation of 'global intensity'—one

that is not sensitive to strong local activation. For example, a median intensity, instead of a mean, might be expected to be appropriate, as it is relatively insensitive to 'outliers' in data. A second approach is to carry out statistical analysis, and then go back to the original data and carry out intensity normalization whilst ignoring activated areas. The resulting data is then re-analysed (see Andersson 1997). However, to date, no general robust solution is in wide use.

Figure 12.6 shows example results from analyses of the experiment described in Section 12.5.3, with different normalization methods used. The 'mean-in-GLM' method uses the time series of global mean intensity values as a confound in the general linear model. Each plot shows the histogram of values in the Z statistic image; this image effectively shows the extent of (positive or negative) correlation between each voxel's time series and the time series model created from the stimulation timing. Thus strongly activated voxels will have high Z—the figure shows this as a raised tail at the far right end of the plots. Non-activated voxels show up as noise in the Z image, and should form a Gaussian distribution which is zero-centred and of unit variance. Because mean-based intensity normalization causes all non-activated voxels to become negatively correlated with the model, (or less strongly positively correlated if they were initially positively correlated), there is a clear negative shift in the peak of the mean-based normalization plot. The median-based and mean-in-GLM normalization methods also show such a shift, albeit less marked. Only the un-normalized method gives a zero-centred Z histogram. Images of significant activation clusters show noticeably less activation in the cases where normalization was used, compared with the un-normalized case. Thus, overall, it is clear that if normalization is to be applied, a more sophisticated approach (than those tested here) is required.

Note that if intensity normalization is not carried out, there can be a problem with second-level (e.g. multi-subject) analyses. For example, if one session (i.e. 4D data set) has twice the mean intensity than another, the fitted activation parameter estimates would also be double (given the same activation). A random-effects group analysis would then see this, incorrectly, as between-session variability in response. The simple

---

[1] This could be defined, for example, as 10 per cent of the maximum volume intensity. The reason for thresholding is that one is only interested in the mean intensity of 'brain' voxels, and not background.

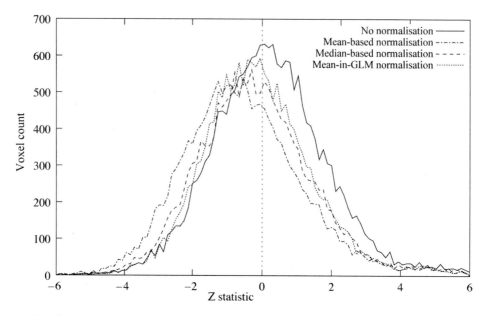

Fig. 12.6 Plots of Z statistic histograms, produced using four different analyses of visual activation. The four cases differ only with respect to the kind of global intensity normalization applied. Only the results produced using no normalization show a correctly zero-centred plot. Note the raised tail at the extreme positive end of all plots, due to the activation voxels.

way of avoiding this problem, if intensity normalization is not carried out, is to scale each 4D (single-session) data set to have a preset mean intensity. This is sometimes referred to as 'grand mean' normalization, and has the effect of causing all single-session data sets to have the same overall mean intensity.

12.7 *Temporal filtering*

Temporal filtering, instead of working on each (spatial) volume separately, as with spatial filtering and global intensity normalization, works on each voxel's time series separately. Because most basic statistical analyses also operate directly on voxel time series, it makes sense to carry out this step after all the previously described pre-processing stages, as each voxel's time series should then be optimally conditioned.

The main point of temporal filtering is to remove unwanted components of a time series, without, of course, damaging the signal of interest. For example, if a stimulation is applied for 30 s, followed by 30 s rest, and this pattern is repeated many times, the signal of interest will be close to a square wave of period 60 s.

Temporal filtering will normally attempt to remove components in the time series which are more slowly varying than this 60 s periodic signal (high-pass filtering or drift removal) and also remove components which are more quickly varying (low-pass filtering, or noise reduction). Figure 12.7 shows an example time series, decomposed into the different frequency components.

12.7.1 High-pass

High-pass filtering attempts to remove all slowly varying unwanted signals in each voxel's time series. Such confounds could be physiological effects like heartbeat or breathing, or scanner-related drifts. Note that although the physiological effects may primarily occur at higher frequencies than the (stimulus-related) signal of interest, the temporal sampling (taking one volume every few seconds) can interact with the original frequency to give an apparent signal at a much lower frequency. This is known as aliasing, and is equivalent to watching wagon wheels appear to turn slowly when viewed on television. (Note that some researchers—e.g. Hu *et al.* 1995—have attempted to remove physiological artefacts in a more sophisticated

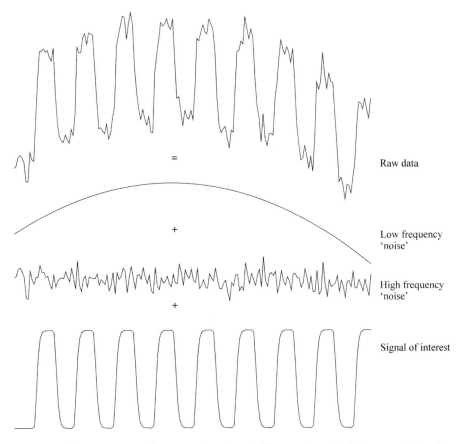

Fig. 12.7 An example unfiltered time series from an activated voxel. The raw time series is decomposed into three components: low frequency artefact (or drift), high frequency artefact (or noise) and the expected signal of interest, caused by the stimulation.

way than simple high-pass filtering, including feeding measurement of the cardiac and respiratory cycles into the algorithm, but this kind of approach is not yet in common use.)

If slowly varying signals are not removed from a voxel's time series then the apparent noise in the later statistical analysis will be higher than necessary. (This noise is also often referred to as residuals in the model fitting process.) If one supposes that low frequency signals do not relate to the stimulation, it is therefore worthwhile removing them. This will result in better fitting of the stimulation-derived model to the data, and more significant activation.

Of course, it is important that the high-pass filtering does not corrupt the stimulus-related signal. If the cutoff period of the filter is too low (i.e. cutoff frequency too high), the signal of interest will be reduced or even eliminated. (This is particularly important in block-design experiments; the danger is much reduced in the case of event-related designs.) Thus it is normal to set the cutoff period at 1.5 times the period of the stimulation. For example, if the stimulation is 10 volumes off, 10 volumes on, repeated many times, then a cutoff period of $1.5 \times (10 + 10) = 30$ volumes is safe. The selection of an appropriate cutoff period when complex block-design experiments are to be analysed requires careful thought. For example, take an ABA-CABAC . . . design, where A is the rest (or control) condition, and B and C are different types of stimulation; all blocks (A, B, and C) consist of 10 volumes. If the response to B is to be compared with the response to C, the cutoff period should be at least $1.5 \times 4 \times 10$;

anything smaller would result in a loss of sensitivity to this contrast.

High-pass filtering is often achieved by finite impulse response (i.e. convolution-based—see Appendix) linear filters, with designs such as the Butterworth filter; as well as choosing the cutoff period, this allows one to choose the sharpness of the cutoff itself. Although this kind of filtering is simple and in common use, it has an unfortunate side-effect; it can induce negative auto-correlations into the signal (i.e. an oscillatory component), which can confound later measurements of intrinsic temporal smoothness (see the following section for more on this).

Alternatively, a method which is fairly similar in effect is to model low frequencies within later statistics instead of removing them at this stage; they are thus treated as confounds within the modelling and so effectively 'ignored'. This is commonly achieved by placing a series of low frequency cosine waves at a range of frequencies in the model—a linear combination of these then fits the actual drift in the data. This solution does not suffer from the problem of inducing negative auto-correlations in the data.

As an alternative to linear filtering, non-linear high-pass filtering can be relatively robust to certain types of outliers in the data, and does not need to introduce negative autocorrelations. A simple non-linear filter is

achieved by fitting a straight line through a fixed number of time points either side of any given time point, and recording the central fitted value. After this has been carried out for each time point, the central fitted value at each point is subtracted from the original value—this has the effect of removing slow trends.

Figure 12.8 shows the effect of three different filters on a range of sinusoidal input frequencies; a Butterworth linear filter, a flat-weighted non-linear filter (where the weighting along the straight-line fit is constant) and a Gaussian-weighted non-linear filter (where the weighting along the straight-line fit is larger close to the central point, giving better stability to the fit). The x axis shows the period of the input signal, in time points, i.e. the number of time points required for a complete cycle in the input sine wave. (Note that period is 1/frequency—thus the highest frequencies are at the leftmost end of the plot.) The y axis shows the relative signal strength after filtering—the smaller the value, the greater the suppression of a given frequency by a filter. All filters suppress the lowest frequencies (largest periods) in the input data. The plots show a typical cutoff period of about 12 time points. Note that the Butterworth linear filter gives the sharpest suppression at periods greater than the cutoff period; note also the rather strange response of the flat-weighted non-linear filter.

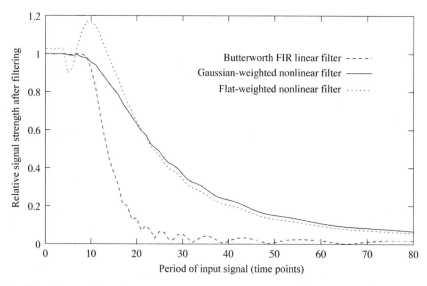

Fig. 12.8 The effect of three different high-pass temporal filters on a range of sinusoidal input frequencies, with the cutoff period set at approximately 12 time points.

12.7.2 Low-pass

Low-pass filtering attempts to reduce high frequency noise in each voxel's time series, without affecting the signal of interest. As with the high-pass filtering, it is important to choose a filter that removes noise without corrupting the underlying stimulus-related signal.

It is common to carry out low-pass filtering via a simple linear convolution with a Gaussian kernel. This can be thought of as a 'blurring' function, and is identical in theory to the Gaussian spatial filtering described earlier. Because it is normal to use a fairly narrow Gaussian, i.e. carry out relatively little blurring, this does not do much more than replace each time point with the original value plus a small fraction of the immediate neighbours (in time).

One obvious danger with low-pass filtering can appear with event-related experiments which often contain signals of interest which are rapidly changing. For example, very brief stimulation may give rise to narrow peaks in the resulting time series. Low-pass filtering may suppress these signals, thus reducing the power of later statistical analysis.

Another danger arises because of the increases in smoothness of the time series due to low-pass filtering. ('Smoothness'—sometimes referred to as positive auto-correlation—means that the intensity at any given time point is likely to be closer to its neigbours' values than values elsewhere in the time series.) Smooth data contains less 'effective' (i.e. truly independent) time points than the actual number of points. Later analysis needs to correct for this smoothness, otherwise reported significances may be overestimated, resulting in false positives. Related to this, certain statistical approaches *rely* on low-pass filtering, in order for later calculations of smoothness to be well-conditioned (see Chapter 14 and Friston *et al.* 1994a; Friston *et al.* 1995 for more details).

It has recently been shown (Woolrich *et al.* 2000) that if one is able to robustly and accurately characterize the nature of the smoothness of the fMRI data, then the most efficient approach is to carry out no smoothing at all, and instead 'prewhiten' the data within the statistical analysis (see Chapter 14). Thus, with this method, no low-pass filtering is applied.

Other researchers have looked at more sophisticated low-pass filtering, including wavelet filtering, Markov random fields, local enforced monotonicity and local neighbourhood smoothing (Kruggel *et al.* 1999). It has not yet been conclusively shown that such approaches are of general benefit; however, whilst many researchers still regularly use linear low-pass filtering of fMRI data, the interest in more sophisticated non-linear methods (or, as discussed above, no low-pass filtering at all) is increasing.

12.8 Appendix—Convolution

Convolution is a standard image and signal processing operation, often used in fMRI analysis. For example, convolution is regularly used to carry out linear spatial filtering and linear high-pass and low-pass temporal filtering. This section gives a brief description of how convolution works.

Convolution involves taking two signals or images and combining them to give a single output. For example, a long 1D time series might be convolved with a short 1D time series; the short time series is normally known as the convolution kernel or filter. Thus the kernel is used to act on the main input time series, for example, to shift it forwards or backwards in time, or blur it, or remove low frequency components from it.

Convolution does not have to act in 1D; the input data and the kernel can be 2D or 3D, although in practice these would often be carried out as separate 1D convolutions for reasons of computational efficiency.

The convolution kernel can be thought of as existing within a 'window' that is slid across the input signal. The window is centred around each point in the input signal, and an output value is formed, which is a weighted sum of all of the points in the input signal which fall within the window. The weights in the sum are given by the shape of the kernel. Thus if the kernel is Gaussian-shaped, the furthest points (in the input signal) from the current central point contribute less to the weighted sum than the closest points.

In Fig. 12.9, an example kernel is shown. In this case, it is a low-pass or smoothing kernel. The 'lag' is half of the window size, and determines the extent by which the input signal will be shifted in time. The full-width–half-maximum of the kernel determines the extent to which the input signal will be blurred. To carry out the convolution at any point in time, a mirror-image of the kernel is taken, and point-wise

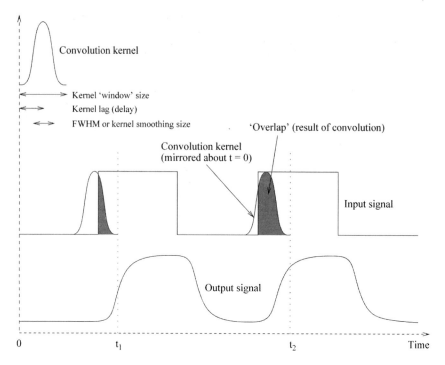

Fig. 12.9 Example convolution of an input square wave and a low-pass filter. The resulting output is both blurred and delayed. This is a typical operation when converting the stimulation waveform into the expected haemodynamic response to this input. If the convolution were simply blurring the data without introducing a delay, the kernel would be centred on $t = 0$ instead.

multiplied by the original signal—the two example shaded areas show the results of two such multiplications—in this case the overlap area between the input signal and the kernel gives the result of the convolution, and determines the height of the output signal at that point in time.

Mathematically, if the input 1D signal is $i(t)$ and the kernel is $k(t)$, where t is, for example, time, then the output of the convolution, $o(t)$, is given by:

$$o(t) = \int_{-U}^{U} i(t + u) * k(-u)\, du \qquad (12.1)$$

for continuous signals, and

$$o(t) = \sum_{-U}^{U} i(t + u) * k(-u) \qquad (12.2)$$

for discrete signals. (Continuous signals have a value at *every* point in time, whereas discrete signals have a fixed number of values, for example, a sample taken

every 3 s. All signals of interest in this chapter are discrete.) The extent of the kernel's window is given by $\pm U$.

References

Aguirre, G., Zarahn, E., and D'Esposito, M. (1998). The inferential impact of global signal covariates in functional neuroimaging analyses. *NeuroImage*, **8**, 302–6.

Andersson, J. (1997). How to estimate global activity independent of changes in local activity. *NeuroImage*, **6**, 237–44.

Descombes, X., Kruggel, F., and von Cramon, D.Y. (1998). Spatio-temporal fMRI analysis using Markov random fields. *IEEE Transactions on Medical Imaging*, **17**(6), 1028–39.

Eddy, W., Fitzgerald, M., and Noll, D. (1996). Improved image registration by using Fourier interpolation. *Magnetic Resonance in Medicine*, **36**(6), 923–31.

Friston, K., Jezzard, P., and Turner, R. (1994a). Analysis of Functional MRI time-series. *Human Brain Mapping*, **1**, 153–71.

Friston, K., Worsley, K., Frackowiak, R., Mazziotta, J., and Evans, A. (1994b). Assessing the significance of focal activations using their spatial extent. *Human Brain Mapping*, **1**, 214–20.

Friston, K., Holmes, A., Poline, J.-B., Grasby, P., Williams, S., Frackowiak, R., and Turner, R. (1995). Analysis of fMRI time series revisited. *NeuroImage*, **2**, 45–53.

Hu, X., Le, T., Parrish, T., and Erhard, P. (1995). Retrospective estimation and correction of physiological fluctutaion in functional MRI. *Magnetic Resonance in Medicine*, **34**(2), 201–12.

Jenkinson, M. and Smith, S. (2001). Global optimization for robust affine registration of brain images. *Medical Image Analysis*. 5(2) 143–156.

Kruggel, F., von Cramon, D., and Descombes, X. (1999). Comparison of filtering methods of fMRI datasets. *NeuroImage*, **10**, 530–43.

Poline, J.-B. and Mazoyer, B. (1994). Enhanced detection in brain activation maps using a multi-filtering approach. *Journal of Cerebral Blood Flow and Metabolism*, **14**, 639–42.

Schmitt, F., Stehling, M., and Turner, R., editors (1998). *Echo-Planar Imaging: Theory, Technique, and Application*. Springer-Verlag, Berlin.

Woolrich, M., Ripley, B., Brady, J., and Smith, S. (2000). *Nonparametric estimation of temporal autocorrelation in FMRI*. Sixth International Conference on Functional Mapping of the Human Brain, p.610.

Worsley, K., Marrett, S., Neelin, P., and Evans, A. (1996). Searching scale space for activation in PET images. *Human Brain Mapping*, **4**, 74–90.

Wowk, B., McIntyre, M., and Saunders, J. (1997). *k*-space detection and correction of physiological artifacts in fMRI. *Magnetic Resonance in Medicine*, **38**, 1029–34.

13 | Head motion and its correction

Mick J. Brammer

13.1 Introduction—the problem

The aim of fMRI data analysis is, in simple terms, to identify small, spatially localized changes in image intensity that accompany the performance of some experimental task. This is normally accomplished by collecting a series of images covering part or all of the brain at intervals of a few seconds and analysing the resulting time-series obtained at each voxel. The experimentally-associated intensity changes are frequently only a few per cent of the mean value at that spatial location and are embedded in a noisy signal contaminated by electronic and physiological effects. Head motion is one further and critically important confound. Very small movements of the head, on a scale of less than a millimetre, can be a major source of error in fMRI analysis if not identified and treated correctly—a problem drawn to the attention of workers in this area in 1994 by Hajnal *et al.* This problem can be particularly acute in areas lying close to a high-contrast boundary in the brain image, where movement-related changes in image intensity may be large. In analysing the image intensity at each voxel over a time series of brain volumes, we make the assumption that we are sampling an identical region of the brain at every point in an experiment. Head motion renders this assumption incorrect by moving samples of other, nearby, brain regions in and out of the voxel being studied. Two obvious possible effects of this process will be apparent. If the head moves in time with the experimental stimulus, the resulting changes in image intensity may be indistinguishable from a 'true' experimental response. Conversely, if head motion occurs with timing completely divorced from the experimental design, this will generally have the effect of producing changes in image intensity that will appear as an additional source of noise when the experimental effect is modelled, worsening the signal to noise ratio and making detection of a response more difficult. The purpose of this chapter is to illustrate some of these problems and to discuss some of the methods that have been developed to counter them.

13.2 Estimating head motion

The realization that head motion is a potentially serious confound in fMRI has led to the development of a number of strategies for dealing with this problem. These have ranged from simple inspection of the images to computationally expensive full 3-D realignment procedures. However, a significant number of centres still report studies with no attempt either to estimate or to correct head motion. A commonly used 'first pass' attempt to assess the extent of head motion involves viewing a video loop of one or more slices of data over the time-course of the experiment. Even sub-voxel head motion can be seen by this method as a variation in image intensity. In many cases, this approach is simply used to make a decision as to whether or not to reject a data set. However, as fMRI is an expensive process and the session may not be easily repeatable (a common problem when patients are involved), motion correction should be attempted when feasible.

The correction process begins with estimation of the extent of head motion. In order to simplify calculations and bring processing times down to acceptable levels, the assumption is often made that head motion is a rigid-body process, i.e. that the head changes its position and orientation but does not undergo shape change. Even if the shape of the head and brain should indeed remain constant, a complicating factor is that head motion within the time taken to collect a single brain volume will lead to *apparent* shape changes in the MRI data. However, independent motion of parts of the brain (e.g. pulsation in ventricular fluid spaces (see Enzmann *et al.* 1992; Dagli *et al.* 1999) not only can but does occur, leading to temporally varying shape changes which differ across brain structures. At present, these problems are often ignored but it is becoming possible to remove the rigid body assumption as computer processing power increases and higher resolution fMRI images are taken. With sufficient processing power, this would allow much higher-order warping algorithms to be employed. Such algorithms not only exist but are often used at present for warping data sets onto standard templates during spatial normalisation for multi-subject studies. Detailed discussion of these methods is outside the scope of this chapter; however for some ideas of methods and issues involved see Christensen *et al.* (1994); Davatzikos (1996); Ashburner *et al.* (1999). At present these methods are still prohibitively expensive in computational terms for routine correction of fMRI experiments involving the acquisition of hundreds of image volumes.

Returning to our assumption that a rigid body transformation is acceptable, the problem in estimating head motion can be formulated in terms of computing the image transformation (the set of translations in x, y, and z and rotations around the x, y, and z axes) that will match an image at time point t to some template or target image. Ideally, the required transformation should be computed rapidly and without operator intervention. The latter constraint has led to most of the algorithms used for within-experiment head motion correction in fMRI being based on automatically computed measures of image similarity rather than identification of landmarks. Automated 'image similarity' based methods operate by attempting to minimize or maximize some merit function used to assess similarity between the brain volume at time point t and some reference template used to act as a target for the realignment process. The reference template is commonly chosen to be the first image volume in the fMRI time series (see Friston *et al.* 1996) but an alternative strategy is to use the voxel-wise average volume computed across the whole time series (Bullmore *et al.* 1999).

The most widely used automatic, 'image-similarity' based motion correction algorithms for within-experiment fMRI motion at present are that of Friston *et al.* (1995, 1996) in the Statistical Parametric Mapping (SPM) package and that described by Woods *et al.* (1992, 1998) in the Automated Image Registration (AIR) package. Some of the issues involved in the use of these and similar algorithms will now be described.

If we make the assumption that only a small percentage of all intracerebral voxels will show experimentally-related changes in image intensity, that these changes will be small (in the order of a few per cent of the average image intensity at any voxel), and that there is no systematic change in global image intensity, we can state as a first approximation that all images will be identical in image intensity distribution but simply displaced in position and orientation. The set of rotations and translations required to minimize either the sum of absolute image intensity differences, or the squares of these differences over all voxels between the volume at time t and the reference volume can then be computed. The second of these alternatives is much the more commonly used and is often referred to as the least-squares or LS cost function. The first method can be described as the least absolute difference (LAD) cost function. In either case, the volume at time t is rotated and translated until it best overlaps the target volume.

Friston *et al.* (1996) compute the minimum of the LS function by linearizing the problem as a first-order Taylor approximation. Numerical approximations of the differentials of image intensity with respect to small rotations and translations are computed and used to compute the vector of rotations and translations required to minimize the sums of squares of image differences. This approach is quick to compute, non-iterative (although some workers have iterated it), and valid if the movements are small compared with the smoothness of the image. In the AIR 3.0 package (Woods *et al.* 1998), a similar cost function is used, but the best fit is found, in this case, with a choice of two iterative Newton-based minimisation algorithms, using first or first and second derivatives of the cost function with respect to the transformation parameters. Another approach (Bullmore *et al.* 1999) uses a multidimensional minimization algorithm (Powell–Davidon–Fletcher) to find the vector of rotations and translations that minimizes the LAD whilst allowing for a global rescaling of image intensity.

During the process of minimizing the LS or LAD cost function, the image at time point t is iteratively rotated and translated relative to the target image by successively smaller amounts as the best match is approached. For acceptable accuracy in an fMRI experiment, this will involve rotations and translations leading to motion on a sub-voxel level. Calculating the cost function under these circumstances will involve estimating the image intensity at different points *within* voxels (interpolation) during the process of finding the required set of transformation parameters. There are a number of types of interpolation of varying computational speed and accuracy (the two having an inverse relationship). They all use information on the intensity of a voxel and its neighbours to compute an estimate of sub-voxel image intensity distribution. All the image realignment methods described above principally use trilinear interpolation to estimate new voxel intensity values during realignment for reasons of computational speed. However, when the final realigned image is written out, following attainment of an acceptable value of the cost function, more complex interpolation algorithms are employed such as tricubic or sinc interpolation. The reason for this is that trilinear interpolation can lead to unacceptable amounts of image smoothing, which becomes worse as motion approaches half a voxel.

Before leaving this area, it should be mentioned that many other techniques can be used to improve speed and efficiency of realignment. For example, it is common practice to subsample the images during realignment. Thus, the cost function is calculated on the basis of a chosen subset of voxels in the images. This can lead to impressive increases in speed of minimisation with little loss of accuracy. The performance of some algorithms can also be improved slightly by image smoothing using Gaussian filters. These issues are discussed with clarity and in detail in Woods *et al.* (1998).

13.3 Residual effects of head motion following image realignment

At first sight, it may appear that realignment of all the image volumes collected during an fMRI experiment may provide a satisfactory solution to head motion, subject to the caveat, raised above, that the movement was that of a rigid body. It has however been pointed out that there is an additional potential complication arising for fMRI data. Friston *et al.* (1996) argued that the image intensity in a small volume of the brain, for example in a single voxel in an fMRI scan, can under certain circumstances be strongly dependent on its

position in the magnetic field. They point out that excitation of spins at the edge of a slice, during multi-slice acquisition, 'will be sensitive to small displacements in and out of that slice'.

If we accept that this is the case, realignment of images to a reference volume will not in itself be sufficient to remove motion related effects from those images. Additional processing steps will be required to remove these residual effects. The strategy suggested by Friston *et al.* (1996) was to model these effects using second order polynomial functions of the instantaneous and lagged displacements estimated during the realignment process. In other words, the position-related changes in image intensity at time *t* will be a simple quadratic function of how much movement had occurred at that time and during the previous image acquisition. The dependence of image intensity on the present and previous position of a brain volume has led to the use of the term spin-excitation history (see Friston *et al.* 1996). The correction strategy employed to remove these effects is quite simple. Once the realignment process has been completed, a vector of *x*, *y*, and *z* translations and rotations is available for the volume at each time point, describing the estimated motion at that time relative to the template image (see above). These values can be used to compute the estimated displacements of each voxel in *x*, *y*, and *z* relative to the template image. Using these displacements, their squares and the displacements, and their squares at the previous time point, it is possible to formulate a multiple regression model for the relationship between the displacement and the resulting change in image intensity. Carrying out this operation on each voxel's time series allows any movement-related intensity changes to be removed from that time series.

13.4 Stimulus-correlated motion and stimulus-uncorrelated motion

Bullmore *et al.* (1999) have discussed at some length the possible impact of various types of subject motion on fMRI activation mapping. Without entering into details regarding any particular method of image analysis, we can make the basic point that it is normal to compute a standardized statistic and then ascertain its probability of occurrence under a null hypothesis.

The larger the value of the statistic the more likely we are to accept a voxel as showing significant activation. If we represent the test statistic (S) as POW/ERR, POW is the power of the response correlated with the experimental paradigm and ERR is the standard error of POW. When subject motion is uncorrelated with the experimental paradigm, motion correction will reduce ERR but leave POW unchanged, increasing S and making activation analysis more sensitive. However, if motion is stimulus-correlated, motion correction (if it includes the previously described intensity adjustment) will reduce POW as the motion is similar to a true experimental effect and correcting the former will diminish the size of the latter. In this case, motion correction will reduce the apparent level of activation, a situation described by Friston *et al.* (1996) as 'throwing out the baby with the bath water'. Though this is clearly a potential problem a number of observations may be warranted. First, if stimulus-correlated motion is a serious problem in an experiment, it is clearly more desirable to make a very conservative activation map, than to produce output dominated by false activations. Second, recent advances in experimental design, such as the use of event-related approaches, in which responses to individual stimuli are studied, often permit better separation of true responses from motion artefacts than might be possible using 'blocked designs'. Third, approaches to correcting the problem are available at group level (see below).

13.5 *Practical implications of motion correction*

It will be appreciated from the description above that motion correction is a computationally expensive process and workers involved in fMRI might reasonably ask whether this processing load is justified. Unfortunately, much of the literature on image registration in fMRI is somewhat daunting for the less mathematically inclined and concentrates on questions such as choice of cost function, interpolation algorithm, and function minimisation strategy.

Detailed consideration of these questions is of course essential but most non-mathematicians involved in fMRI data analysis may be more interested in the apparently simple question, 'how much will it affect my activation maps?' The rest of this chapter is intended to give an indication of how different types of subject motion can affect activation maps when different motion correction methods are used. Figure 13.1 illustrates motion correction of an experiment involving finger tapping with the left hand. The experiment involved the acquisition of 14 axial slices of 7 mm thickness every three seconds for 5 min. Finger tapping occurred in 30 s blocks separated by 30 s periods of the rest. Figure 13.1(a) shows the estimated translation in the *z* axis (up and down movement of the head) throughout the experiment. It can be seen that there was gradual movement of the head but with a pronounced periodicity superimposed on this drift. This periodic change clearly occurs close to the experimental frequency—a good example of stimulus-correlated motion. Similar, though less pronounced movements were apparent in some of the other rotations and translations. Figure 13.1(b) shows the results of activation analysis using our own software (Bullmore *et al.* 1996) on four of the upper slices of the dataset, expected to include motor cortex activated in this experiment. The top row shows extraordinarily widespread artefactual activations, including classic 'ring' artefacts around the brain, characteristic of motion of the slices in and out of plane (*z* translation). Realignment of the image volumes (middle row) to an average template by minimizing the sum of absolute differences in image intensity (see above), resulted in a considerable reduction in the apparent level of activation but the map is still effectively uninterpretable. The final row shows the effect of including the regression step suggested by Friston *et al.* (1996) as implemented in our software (Bullmore *et al.* 1999). We can see a small area of activation close to the motor strip, which might have been expected in this experiment. Here the stimulus-correlation was not great enough to completely abolish activation in the expected area though we can presume that it was severely reduced.

Figure 13.2 shows a visual activation experiment in which the stimulus was a flashing checkerboard (8 Hz) presented for 30 s epochs with intervening periods of darkness (see above). All other image acquisition parameters were as described for Fig. 13.1. In Fig. 13.2(a) the largest movement is shown, again this is translation along the *z* axis, but this time the pattern is very different. There is a large downward movement of the

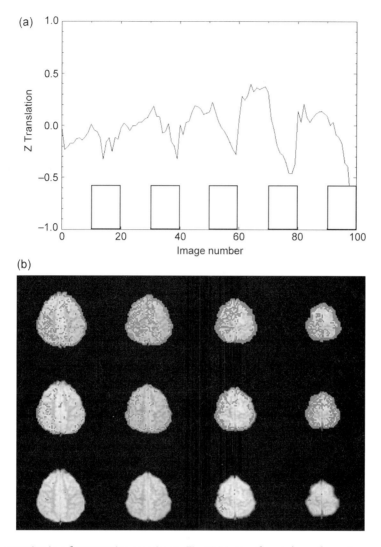

Fig. 13.1 Motion correction in a finger tapping experiment. Fig. 1(a) (*upper figure*) shows the motion component (z transla-tion) exhibiting the strongest stimulus-correlated motion. The experimental 'on' periods are shown at the bottom of the figure. Fig. 1(b) (*lower figure*) shows a set of superior axial images with no correction (*top row*), after realignment only (*middle row*) and following full correction (*bottom row*). (See also colour plate section.)

head of approximately 3 mm 1 min into the experi-ment and some small motion afterwards. However, the motion was not stimulus-correlated, this time leading to a small increase in the number of apparently acti-vated voxels in the visual cortex as can be seen in Fig. 13.2(b), in which the three rows represent the same image processing steps as those described for Fig. 13.1(b).

These two experiments show the actual impact of the theoretical ideas discussed above in real fMRI data. It is notable that the artefacts produced in experiment 1 were much more severe, even though the actual amplitude of the z translation was considerably smaller than in experiment 2, well below the voxel dimension along the z axis. The combined computa-tion load of realignment and subsequent correction by

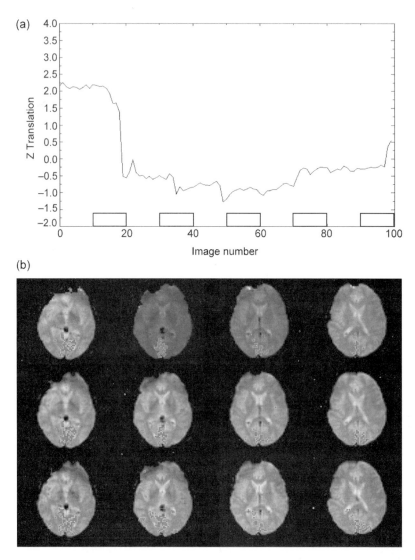

Fig. 13.2 Motion correction in a visual stimulation experiment. Fig. 2(a) (*upper figure*) shows the motion component (z translation) exhibiting the strongest stimulus-correlated motion. The experimental 'on' periods are shown at the bottom. Fig. 2(b) (*lower figure*) shows a set of superior axial images with no correction (*top row*), after realignment only (*middle row*) and following full correction (*bottom row*). (See also colour plate section.)

regression of movement-related intensity changes is considerable, accounting for 60–70 per cent of the time taken to produce a single-subject activation map from raw data using our algorithms. We firmly believe, however, that failure to compute and at least attempt to correct motion related artefacts in fMRI can result in very severe problems, particularly in the case of patients who often move considerably more in the scanner than healthy volunteer controls. Patients can be difficult and expensive to scan and all possible attempts should be made to obtain the best possible data in clinical studies where rescanning of subjects can be problematic.

13.6 Motion correction at the group level

There are a number of reasons for attempting to obtain images from a group of subjects. Some of these are statistical. Group data is required to form any assessment of population behaviour. We often need to know which brain regions are reliably activated across multiple subjects. Increasing subject numbers clearly gives us more power to detect inter-group differences. There is also some logic in making group maps to overcome motion-related problems in fMRI. It is likely (and has been found by examining a large number of scans in our unit) that subject motion in the scanner is highly idiosyncratic and computation of an average or median image across a group will produce a reliable view of task-related brain activation relatively free from motion artefacts as these will be different in different subjects and will not produce significant activations in a group. This is particularly the case if a median image is computed to minimize outlier effects (see Brammer *et al.* 1997). However, we still make a routine check for stimulus-correlated motion in all subjects by fitting the estimated *x*, *y*, and *z* translations and rotations to the experimental design and assessing

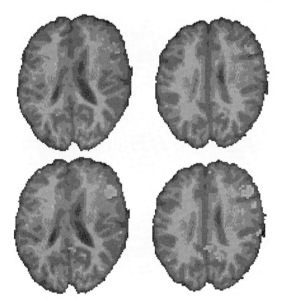

Fig. 13.3 Two slices from a group activation map (*n* = 6) in schizophrenic patients before (*upper row*) and after (*lower row*) group correction for subject motion. (See also colour plate section.)

the extent of the correlations. We have found occasions when, although exact type of motion differs from subject to subject in terms of its manifestation in different rotations and translations, there are consistent, high levels of stimulus-correlated motion across a whole subject (typically patient) group. We described one such example in detail in Bullmore *et al.* (1999). In this case, groups of control subjects and schizophrenic patients (five subjects in each group) were scanned whilst performing a verbal fluency task using a block A/B design similar to those described above. There was little evidence of stimulus-correlated motion in the control group but clear evidence in the schizophrenic subjects. Computation of median group images without attempting to correct this problem and subsequent statistical comparison of these images, revealed considerably more activation in the control group in several brain regions, including frontal and parietal cortices. This is important in view of the theory that schizophrenia is accompanied by hypo-activation of frontal cortical regions. Our uncorrected data would clearly have supported such a hypothesis but we had every reason to believe that at least part of the hypoactivity may have been due to loss of activation during motion correction. We have suggested a simple, regression-based approach to the correction of stimulus-correlated motion effects at the group level (see Bullmore *et al.* 1999). This involves computing our test statistic (*S*—see above) with and without motion correction, and evaluating the change in *S* due to motion correction (ΔS) at every voxel. Thus, following this operation, we have a standardized activation statistic and the effect of motion correction on this statistic, for every individual at every voxel. The values of *S* following motion correction and of ΔS are then transformed into standard space (Talairach and Tournoux 1988) to allow voxel-wise statistical operations at the group level. The median value of these operations is to produce a group activation map in which individual variations due to the motion correction process have been removed.

The results of these operations are shown in Fig. 13.3. The upper two images show activation across the group of schizophrenic subjects before correction for stimulus-correlated motion and the lower two images the same data after correction as described above. The most notable finding is the considerable enhancement of activation in the left prefrontal cortex (top right of the images) after the correction process. Failure to carry out this operation might have led to erroneous interpretations being drawn concerning the extent of 'hypofrontality' in the schizophrenic subjects.

13.7 Conclusions

Subject motion remains a potentially serious problem in fMRI. There are yet no complete solutions to the problem but a number of approaches to minimizing the effects of motion do exist. This chapter has described some of the available methodology and the practical impact of correction on activation mapping. Use of motion correction algorithms in fMRI is strongly advocated.

References

Ashburner, J., Andersson, J.L.R. and Friston, K.J. (1999). High dimensional; image registration using symmetric priors. *Neuroimage*, 9, 619–28.

Brammer, M.J., Bullmore, E.T., Simmons, A., Williams, S.C.R., Grasby, P.M., Howard, R.J., Woodruff, P.W.R., and Rabe-Hesketh, S. (1997). Generic brain activation mapping in fMRI: a nonparametrix approach. *Magnetic Resonance Imaging*, 15, 763–70.

Bullmore, E.T., Brammer, M.J., Rabe-Hesketh, S., Curtis, V.A., Morris, R.G., Williams, S.C.R., Sharma, T., and McGuire, P.K. (1999). Methods for diagnosis and treatment of stim-ulus-correlated motion in generic brain activation studies using fMRI. *Human Brain Mapping*, 7, 38–48.

Christiansen, G.E., Rabbit, R.D., and Miller, M.I. (1996). Deformable templates using large deformation kinematics. *IEEE Transactions of Image Processing*, 5, 1435–7.

Dagli, M.S., Inglehom, J.E., and Haxby, J.V. (1999) Localization of cardiac-induced signal change in fMRI. *Neuroimage*, 9, 407–15.

Davatzikos, C. (1996) Spatial normalization of 3D images using deformable models. *Journal of Computer-Assisted Tomography*, 20, 656–65.

Enzmann, D.R. and Pelc, N.J. (1992). Brain motion. Measurement with phase-contrast MR imaging. *Radiology*, 185, 653–60.

Friston, K.J., Ashburner, J., Frith, C.D., Poline, J.-B., Heather, J.D., and Frackowiak, R.S.J. (1995). Spatial registration and normalization of images. *Human Brain Mapping*, 2, 165–89.

Friston, K.J., Williams, S.C.R., Howard, R., Frackowiak, R.S.J., and Turner, R. (1996). Movement-related effects in fMRI time series. *Magnetic Resonance in Medicine*, 35, 346–55.

Hajnal, J.V., Myers, R., Oatridge, A., Schwieso, J.E., Young, I.R., and Bydder, G.M. (1994). Artefacts due to stimulus-correlated motion in functional images of the brain. *Magnetic Resonance in Medicine*, 31, 283–91.

Talairach, J. and Tournoux, P. (1988). *A co-planar stereotactic atlas of the human brain*. Thieme, Stuttgart.

Woods, R.P., Cherry, S.R., and Mazziotta, J.C. (1992). Rapid automated algorithm for aligning and reslicing PET images. *Journal of Computer Assisted Tomography*, 16, 620–33.

Wood, R.P., Grafton, S.T., Holmes, C.J., Cherry, S.R., and Mazziotta, J.C. (1998). Automated image registration: I. General methods and intrasubject, intramodality validation. *Journal of Computer Assisted Tomography*, 22, 139–52.

14 | Statistical analysis of activation images

K.J. Worsley

14.1 Introduction—Why do we need statistics?

Statistical analysis is concerned with making inference about underlying patterns in data that often contain a large amount of random error. This is certainly the case with fMRI data, where the effect of a stimulus may be as little as 1 per cent of the BOLD signal. However, by careful averaging of the data over time, such as averaging the BOLD response at the times when the stimulus is ON, and subtracting the average when the stimulus is OFF, we are often able to detect such a small signal in the presence of considerable background noise.

More complex experimental designs require more complex analysis. The type of analysis can be guided by constructing a *model* for the way in which the BOLD response depends on the stimulus. Such a model must include a component of random error which explains how the observations vary even if the experiment is repeated on the same subject under exactly the same conditions. Statistics can be used to best estimate the parameters in the model, including the variability of the errors. It is this random variability of the errors that can then be used to assess the random variability, or standard error, of the estimated parameters themselves. This key quantity allows the experimenter not only to say that the BOLD response is increased by say 20 units due to a particular stimulus, but also how accurate that estimate is, say ±8 units.

Finally, comparing the size of the increase to its standard error allows the experimenter to decide if any increase has really taken place; after all, the 20 unit increase could have occurred by chance alone when in fact the true increase (after a very large number of repetitions of the experiment) was very close to zero. However, the fact that the increase is 20/8 = 2.5 times larger than its standard error makes this extremely unlikely; in fact this would happen with a probability of less than 1 per cent (under certain reasonable assumptions) if in fact there really was no true increase. We usually report this as 'z = 2–5, P < 0.01' or we sometimes give the exact P-value, or probability of a more extreme value of z than that observed, which is 0.0062.

Motivated by the above discussion, our first step in this chapter is build up a model of the fMRI data, beginning with the haemodynamic response to the stimulus (Section 14.2), then the random error (Section 14.3). The remainder of the chapter then deals with estimating the parameters of these models, assessing their variability, and making decisions about whether the fMRI data shows any evidence of a BOLD response to the stimulus.

Theoretical statistics material in this chapter, that can be skipped by the non-technical reader, is marked *.

14.2 Modelling the response to the stimulus

In this section we model the way in which the BOLD response depends on an external stimulus. Time will be denoted by t and the external stimulus will be denoted by $s(t)$. For example, $s(t)$ could take the value 1 when the stimulus is ON and 0 when the stimulus is OFF (see Figure 14.1(a)). The BOLD response at a particular voxel, denoted by $x(t)$, usually occurs between 3 and 10 s after the stimulus, peaking at about 6 s. This delay and blurring is modelled by a haemodynamic response function (HRF) $h(t)$ (Figure 14.1(b)) which weights past stimulus values by a *convolution* as follows:

$$x(t) = \int_0^\infty h(u)\, s(t - u)\, \mathrm{d}u. \qquad (14.1)$$

The HRF can be modelled as a simple gamma function

(Lange and Zeger, 1997). Friston (1998a) proposes a difference of two gamma functions that captures the fact that there is a small dip after the HRF has returned to zero:

$$h(t) = \left(\frac{t}{d_1}\right)^{a_1} \exp\left(\frac{-(t - d_1)}{b_1}\right) -$$
$$c\left(\frac{t}{d_2}\right)^{a_2} \exp\left(\frac{-(t - d_2)}{b_2}\right) \qquad (14.2)$$

where $d_j = a_j b_j$ is the time to the peak, and $a_1 = 6$, $a_2 = 12$, $b_1 = b_2 = 0.9$ s, and $c = 0.35$ (Glover, 1999). This particular choice of HRF is shown in Figure 14.1(b). The resulting convolution of $h(t)$ with

$s(t)$ is shown in Figure 14.1(c). This is then sampled at the n FMRI volume acquisition times $t_1, \dots t_n$ to give the response $x_i = x(t_i)$ at volume i.

In many experiments several different stimuli are presented. In the experiment used to illustrate the methods in this chapter, a subject was given a painful heat stimulus (49°C) to the left forearm for 9 s, followed by a neutral stimulus for 9 s, interspersed with 9 s when no stimulus was presented. These two stimuli $s_1(t)$ and $s_2(t)$ are shown in Figure 14.1(a). We can denote their corresponding responses by $x_1(t)$ and $x_2(t)$ by convolution with $h(t)$ as in (14.1). We usually assume that the responses have different magnitudes, denoted by β_1 and β_2 and that they add together to

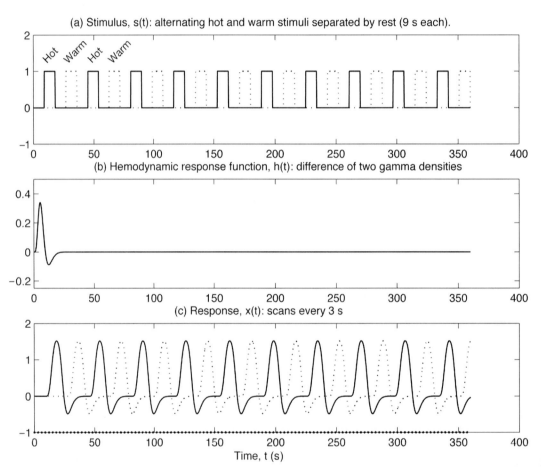

Fig. 14.1 (a) The hot and neutral stimuli $s(t)$, (b) the hemodynamic response function $h(t)$ and (c) its convolution with $s(t)$ to give the response $x(t)$. The time between volumes is $\Delta t = 3$s, so $x(t)$ is then subsampled at the $n = 118$ volume acquisition times $t_i = 3i$ to give the response $x_i = x(t_i)$ at time index $i = 1, \dots n$.

produce the final BOLD response. In general, the effect of m different responses in volume i, denoted by $x_{i1}, \ldots x_{im}$ is modelled as the linear model (Friston *et al.*, 1995)

$$x_{i1}\beta_1 + \ldots + x_{im}\beta_m. \qquad (14.3)$$

Many voxels in fMRI data also show a slow variation over time, known as drift. The removal of drift, or low frequency noise, was described in Chapter 12. Recall that drift can be removed either by high-pass filtering or by introducing low frequency drift terms, such as cosines, polynomials, or splines, into the linear model. However, drift also appears in this chapter, as the problem of drift interacts with model design; the presence of drift limits the type of stimulus design that can be used with fMRI experiments. Any stimulus that behaves like drift, such as a steadily increasing stimulus intensity, cannot be easily distinguished from drift and is either impossible or very difficult to estimate (i.e. estimable with very high error). This includes block designs with very long blocks, such as presenting a stimulus continually during the second half of an experiment. This type of design should be avoided. The best designs should try to present the stimulus fairly rapidly so that its effect can be assessed over a short period where the drift has little effect (see Section 14.8 for further discussion of optimal design).

14.3 Modelling the random error

Statistical models usually contain two parts: the fixed effects and the random error. The fixed effects are the parts of the model that do not vary if the experiment is repeated; they capture the underlying scientific 'truth' that we hope to discover. The random error is the part left over that varies every time new data is obtained. Random error is very important for two reasons: first, it tells us how to best estimate the effect of the stimulus, and second, and more importantly, it gives us a way of assessing the error in the effect. This then allows us to compare the effect with its random error, and select those voxels where the effect is much larger than its random error, that is, voxels with high signal-to-noise ratio.

The way to do this is to first combine the response and the drift terms, if high-pass temporal filtering has

not been applied, into a single linear model for the fixed effects as in (14.3). Then a random error ε_i is added to obtain the observed fMRI data, Y_i, at time index i:

$$Y_i = x_{i1}\beta_1 + \ldots + x_{im}\beta_m + \varepsilon_i. \qquad (14.4)$$

The observations tend to be correlated in time, particularly in cortical regions, with correlations up to 0.4 between time points 3 s apart (Fig. 14.2(a)). This effect is known as temporal autocorrelation (correlation of the errors separated by a fixed time lag) or smoothness; it can be caused, for example, by simply blurring the data in time, but is most likely due to some influence of the random error of the preceding time points on that of the current time point.

14.3.1 *Modelling the temporal correlation

Why is the temporal correlation structure important? The reason has to do not so much with how to estimate the signal strengths β_i, but with how to assess the standard errors of these estimates, and hence how to detect the presence of the signal. For this reason, we must take some care to model the correlation structure.

The simplest is the first order autoregressive model. This is generated by combining the error from the previous time point with a new error term to produce the error for the current time point:

$$\varepsilon_i = \rho\varepsilon_{i-1} + \chi_{i1},$$

where $|\rho| < 1$ and χ_{i1} is a 'white noise' sequence of independent and identically distributed normal random variables with mean 0 and standard deviation σ_1, written as $\chi_{i1} \sim N(0, \sigma_1^2)$. With such a model, the temporal correlation decays exponentially as the lag l increases:

$$\text{Cor}(\varepsilon_i, \varepsilon_{i-l}) = \rho^{|l|}.$$

More complex oscillatory behaviour as well as exponential decay can be obtained by adding more terms to give autoregressive models of order p, known as AR(p) models:

$$\varepsilon_i = \alpha_1\varepsilon_{i-1} + \ldots + \alpha_p\varepsilon_{i-p} + \chi_{i1},$$

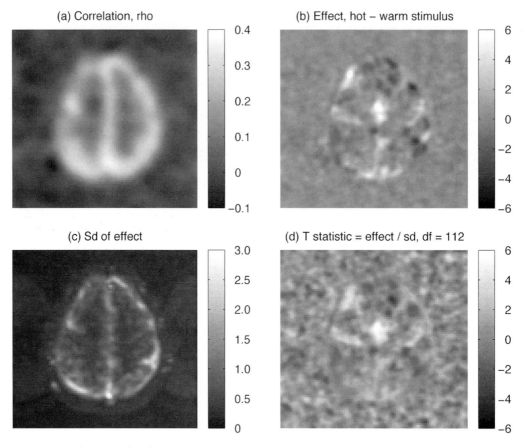

Fig. 14.2 Statistical analysis of the fMRI data. (a) The estimated AR(1) autocorrelation parameter ρ after bias correction and spatial smoothing with a 15mm FWHM Gaussian filter. Note that the correlation is high in cortical regions. (b) The effect of the hot stimulus minus the neutral stimulus, $c'\hat{\beta}$. (c) The estimated standard deviation of the effect $(\hat{Var}(c'\hat{\beta}))^{1/2}$. Note that it is much higher in cortical regions than elsewhere in the brain. (d) The T statistic T equal to (b) divided by (c), with $\theta = 112$ degrees of freedom.

To take into account white noise from the scanner, Purdon *et al.* (1998) has extended the AR(1) model as follows:

$$\eta_i = \rho\eta_{i-1} + \chi_{i1}, \tag{14.5}$$

$$\varepsilon_i = \eta_i + \chi_{i2}, \tag{14.6}$$

in which a second independent white noise term $\chi_{i2} \sim N(0,\sigma_2^2)$ is added to an AR(1) component. This extra component χ_{i2} accounts for the scanner white noise which is added to physiological 'coloured' (temporally correlated) noise η_i from the brain itself.

The correlation then becomes

$$\text{Cor}\,(\varepsilon_i, \varepsilon_{i-l}) = \frac{\rho^{|l|}}{1 + (1 - \rho^2)\sigma_2^2/\sigma_1^2},$$

if $l \neq 0$ and 1 if $l = 0$. In other words, there is a jump at zero lag, known in the geostatistics literature as a 'nugget effect'. Further autoregressive terms can be added. This is a special type of state space model (Caines 1988) in which (14.5) is the state equation, and (14.6) is the observation equation. State space models are extremely powerful at capturing complex dynamic relationships, including drift.

14.4 Estimating the response magnitudes

So far we have built a simple model for the BOLD response (Section 14.2) and the random error that is added to that response (Section 14.3). The magnitudes β_j of the responses are still unknown, and the purpose of this section is to find good estimates of them (Sections 14.5 and 14.9 look at how we estimate the noise). We present three methods: the 'best possible' (fully efficient, that is, most accurate) method, the potentially more robust SPM'99 method, and the Fourier space method. Finally we compare the three methods.

14.4.1 *Notation

To do the theoretical work in this section we shall need matrix notation:

$$Y = \begin{pmatrix} Y_1 \\ h \\ Y_n \end{pmatrix},$$

$$X = \begin{pmatrix} x_{11} & \cdots & x_{1m} \\ h & & h \\ x_{n1} & \cdots & x_{nm} \end{pmatrix},$$

$$\beta = \begin{pmatrix} \beta_1 \\ h \\ \beta_m \end{pmatrix}, \quad \varepsilon = \begin{pmatrix} \varepsilon_1 \\ h \\ \varepsilon_n \end{pmatrix}$$

As before, n is the number of time points (volumes) and m is the number of different stimuli or drift terms (explanatory variables) being modelled.

We will denote the variance of the vector of errors ε by the matrix $V\sigma^2$, where σ^2 is an unknown scalar, and the element of V in row i and column j, multiplied by σ^2, is the covariance between ε_i and ε_j. For the AR(1) model, for example,

$$V = \begin{pmatrix} 1 & \rho & \rho^2 & \cdots & \rho^{n-1} \\ \rho & 1 & \rho & \cdots & \rho^{n-2} \\ \rho^2 & \rho & 1 & \cdots & \rho^{n-3} \\ h & h & h & & h \\ \rho^{n-1} & \rho^{n-2} & \rho^{n-3} & \cdots & 1 \end{pmatrix}, \quad \sigma^2 = \frac{\sigma_1^2}{1 - \rho^2}$$

We further assume that the distribution of ε is multi-variate normal, so that we can write the entire linear model as:

$$Y = X\beta + \varepsilon, \quad \varepsilon \sim N_n(0, V\sigma^2). \tag{14.7}$$

A general unbiased estimator of β can be found by first multiplying (14.7) through by an $n \times n$ matrix A (various possible choices of A will be discussed below) to give:

$$\tilde{Y} = AY, \quad \tilde{X} = AX,$$

$$\tilde{Y} = X\beta + \tilde{\varepsilon} \quad \tilde{\varepsilon} = A\varepsilon \sim N_n(0, AVA'\sigma^2). \tag{14.8}$$

The least squares estimator of β is the value of β that minimizes the sum of squared errors in (14.8), that is,

$$\min \|\tilde{Y} - \tilde{X}\beta\|^2.$$

We shall adopt conventional statistical notation and denote estimators by ^ throughout. It can be shown that

$$\hat{\beta} = \tilde{X}^+ \tilde{Y},$$

where $^+$ denotes the Moore–Penrose pseudoinverse, the 'best possible' inverse that minimizes the error sum-of-squares. For any choice of A, $\hat{\beta}$ is unbiased and its variance matrix is given by:

$$E(\beta) = \hat{\beta}, \quad \text{Var}(\hat{\beta}) = \tilde{X}^+ AVA' \tilde{X}^{+'} \sigma^2.$$

Note that the estimation of β (by calculating the pseudoinverse of the design matrix and then using $\hat{\beta} = \tilde{X}^+ \tilde{Y}$) is what is referred to generally as fitting the model to the data.

14.4.2 *The fully efficient estimator

The fully efficient (most accurate, i.e. minimum variance) estimator of β is obtained by choosing A so that the variance of the errors is proportional to the identity matrix, equivalent to 'whitening' the errors, by the Gauss–Markov Theorem. This process removes any temporal smoothness in the data, whether caused by the intrinsic smoothness of the random errors, or by pre-filtering. This is accomplished by factoring V, for example by a Cholesky factorization, then inverting the transpose of the factor:

$$\mathbf{V} = \mathbf{H'H}, \quad \mathbf{A} = (\mathbf{H'})^{-1}, \quad \mathbf{AVA'} = \mathbf{I},$$

where $\mathbf{I}$ is the $n \times n$ identity matrix. Doing this in practice can be very time consuming if it is repeated at every voxel. Fortunately there are computationally efficient ways of finding $\mathbf{A}$ if the errors are generated by an AR(p) process or a state space model (using the Kalman filter). For the AR(1) model, for example,

$$\mathbf{A} = \begin{pmatrix} 1 & 0 & 0 & \ldots & 0 \\ -\rho R & R & 0 & \ldots & 0 \\ 0 & -\rho R & R & \mathtt{j} & \mathtt{h} \\ \mathtt{h} & \mathtt{j} & & \mathtt{j} & 0 \\ 0 & \ldots & 0 & -\rho R & R \end{pmatrix}$$

where $R = 1/\sqrt{(1 - \rho^2)}$, so that $\widetilde{\mathbf{Y}}_1 = \mathbf{Y}_1$ and $\widetilde{\mathbf{Y}}_i = (Y_i - \rho Y_{i-1})/\sqrt{(1 - \rho^2)}$, $i = 2, \ldots n$.

14.4.3 *The more robust estimator of SPM '99

An alternative, adopted by SPM '99, is to 'precolour', or smooth, the data (and the model). This yields an unbiased estimator of β, but with slightly increased variance. This small loss of efficiency is offset by a more robust estimator of the variance, that is, an estimator of β whose estimated variance is less sensitive to departures from the assumed form of $\mathbf{V}$. Rather than modelling the correlation structure of the original observations, SPM'99 adopts an AR(1) model for the smoothed data.

14.4.4 *Estimation in Fourier space

Still another possibility is to choose $\mathbf{A}$ so that the transformed observations $\widetilde{\mathbf{Y}}$ are independent though not necessarily equally variable (as for the fully efficient estimator). It is a remarkable fact that if the error process is stationary (the same correlation structure at any time) then this can be achieved by choosing the rows of $\mathbf{A}$ to be the Fourier transform sine and cosine basis functions (the reason is that these basis functions are almost eigenvectors of $\mathbf{V}$). This would be exactly so if the correlation structure were periodic; non-periodicity is less important if the sequence is long. Multiplying by $\mathbf{A}$ is then equivalent to taking the Fourier transform, a very rapid operation.

The advantage is that the resulting errors $\widetilde{\varepsilon}$ become almost independent, but with variances equal to the spectrum of the process (in engineering terms, the expected power of the process at each frequency). This simplifies the analysis; fitting the model (14.8) is then equivalent to weighted least squares, with weights inversely proportional to the spectrum. From this point of view, the SPM '99 method can be seen as weighted least squares with weights proportional to the spectrum of the haemodynamic response function, which gives more weight to the frequencies that are passed by the haemodynamic response, and less weight to those that are damped by the haemodynamic response.

An added advantage of working in Fourier space is that convolution of the stimulus with the haemodynamic response function (14.1) becomes simple multiplication of their Fourier transforms. We make use of this to estimate the haemodynamic response itself in Section 14.11.

14.4.5 Comparison of the methods

The fully efficient method, based on pre-whitening the data, produces the best estimators if the correlation structure is correctly modelled. The SPM method is more robust to biases in modeling and estimating the correlation structure, at the expensive of losing a little accuracy (again if the correlation structure is correctly modelled). It is not easy to choose between them, but fortunately both methods give very similar answers in most situations. The Fourier space method is simply a convenient way of implementing either the fully efficient or the SPM methods, particularly when the design is periodic.

It should be noted that parameter estimation for some types of experimental design is unaffected by the choice of $\mathbf{A}$. It can be shown that if the columns of $\mathbf{X}$ are linear combinations of p eigenvectors of $\mathbf{A'A}$, then the same estimator can be obtained by using least squares in model (14.4), i.e. ignoring multiplication by $\mathbf{A}$ altogether. For fully efficient estimation, $\mathbf{A'A} = \mathbf{V}^{-1}$, which has the same eigenvectors as $\mathbf{V}$. Now as remarked above, the eigenvectors of $\mathbf{V}$ are the Fourier sine and cosine functions, provided the error process is stationary.

This implies that stimuli whose intensity varies as a sine or cosine function can be estimated with full efficiency by ignoring $\mathbf{A}$. Furthermore, for the SPM '99 method, $\mathbf{A'A}$ is a Toeplitz matrix whose eigenvectors are almost the Fourier sines and cosines, so here again a design of this sort is estimated with full efficiency by the SPM '99 method. The reason should now be clear: for this design, the regressors are just 1 at a subset of p of the frequencies, and zero elsewhere. Data at only these m frequencies are used to estimate m parameters, so any weighting scheme yields the same parameter estimates.

Block designs are almost sine functions, so these are estimated with almost full efficiency by the SPM '99 method. Random event-related designs have a more complex spectrum so these are most affected by the choice of method; precolouring can result in a fairly inefficient analysis in the case of dense event-related designs.

14.5 *Estimating the variance

In this section we look at how to estimate the error variance σ^2, assuming for the moment that the error correlation structure $\mathbf{V}$ is known (we shall look at estimating $\mathbf{V}$ a little later in Section 14.9). The estimator is based on the residuals, defined as the difference between the data and the estimated fixed effects

$$\mathbf{r} = \tilde{\mathbf{Y}} - \tilde{\mathbf{X}}\hat{\beta} = \mathbf{R}\tilde{\mathbf{Y}},$$

where $\mathbf{R} = \mathbf{I} - \tilde{\mathbf{X}}\,\tilde{\mathbf{X}}^+$. The estimator of σ^2 is the sum of squares of the residuals divided by a constant chosen so that $\hat{\sigma}^2$ is unbiased:

$$\hat{\sigma}^2 = \mathbf{r'r}/\mathrm{tr}(\mathbf{RAVA'}).$$

Its effective degrees of freedom, based on matching second moments, is

$$\nu = \mathrm{tr}(\mathbf{RAVA'})^2/\mathrm{tr}((\mathbf{RAVA'})^2),$$

so that the distribution of $\nu\hat{\sigma}^2/\sigma^2$ is well approximated by a χ^2 distribution with ν degrees of freedom, known as the Satterthwaite approximation. If the estimation is fully efficient, so that $\mathbf{AVA'} = \mathbf{I}$, then the degrees of freedom becomes the usual $\nu = n - \tilde{m}$, where $\tilde{m}$ is the rank of $\tilde{\mathbf{X}}$, and the Satterthwaite approximation is exact.

For example, say we have $n = 118$ volumes, two parameters for the fMRI response, and four para-

meters for a polynomial drift of degree 3, giving $m = 6$ total parameters. If the fully efficient estimator is used (i.e. 'prewhitening'), the degrees of freedom is $\nu = 118 - 6 = 112$.

14.6 Detecting an effect

In the previous two sections we have given methods for estimating both the signal and noise parameters. Usually we are more interested in comparing signal parameters, such as whether the hot stimulus gives a bigger response than the neutral stimulus. In other words, we are interested in the difference between the hot stimulus and the neutral stimulus, $\beta_1 - \beta_2$. This is known as an effect (an effect could of course be just a single magnitude, say β_1). In this section we give estimates for an effect and its variance. We then turn to the crucial question of detecting an effect, that is, whether or not there is any evidence for an effect. In this way we can detect those voxels where there is evidence that the pain stimulus produces a BOLD response over and above that produced by the neutral stimulus.

14.6.1 *T*-tests

The particular differences of the parameters β that make up the effect are specified by a *contrast* vector $\mathbf{c}$, a vector of the same length as β, which specifies a linear combination of the parameters $\mathbf{c'}\beta$. First of all, this is estimated by the same linear combination of the estimated parameters $\mathbf{c'}\hat{\beta}$ (from now on we shall use the term effect to refer to the estimator as well as to the combination of parameters to be estimated).

The simplest contrast involves only one explanatory variable. For example, to test activation in the hot condition versus rest, the contrast vector is $\mathbf{c'} = (1\,0\,0\,0\,0\,0)$ (the first zero excludes the neutral condition from the contrast and the other four exclude the cubic drift). This means that the estimate of the effect is simply $\mathbf{c'}\hat{\beta} = \hat{\beta}_1$. If, however, we are interested in the difference between the hot stimulus (β_1) and the neutral stimulus (β_2), then the contrast vector is $\mathbf{c'} = (1\,-1\,0\,0\,0\,0)$. This means that the estimate of the effect is $\mathbf{c'}\hat{\beta} = \hat{\beta}_1 - \hat{\beta}_2$ (Figure 14.2(b)).

We have now defined the effect via the contrast vector, and given a natural estimator of it. As usual, we would also like to estimate the variance of the effect, which is given by

$$\hat{\mathrm{Var}}(\mathbf{c}'\hat{\beta}) = \mathbf{c}'\tilde{\mathbf{X}}^+\mathbf{AVA}'\tilde{\mathbf{X}}^{+'}\,\mathbf{c}\hat{\sigma}^2. \qquad (14.9)$$

An example of the estimated standard deviation (the square root of the estimated variance (14.9)) is shown in Figure 14.2(c). Note that it is much higher in cortical regions than elsewhere in the brain.

Finally we test whether or not there is any evidence for the effect, that is whether the effect differs from zero, using the ratio of the effect to its standard error, called the T statistic:

$$T = \frac{\mathbf{c}'\hat{\beta}}{\sqrt{\hat{\mathrm{Var}}(\mathbf{c}'\hat{\beta})}}$$

This has an approximate t distribution with ν degrees of freedom (exact if $\mathbf{AVA}' = \mathbf{I}$) when there is no effect, that is, $\mathbf{c}'\beta = 0$. An example is shown in Figure 14.2(d), where large values of T indicate evidence for an effect.

Note that T (or F) statistic images are often converted into Z statistic images, where the theoretical T (or F) null distribution (given the relevant degrees-of-freedom) is converted into a unit-variance Gaussian distribution (which does not depend on degrees-of-freedom). Thus Z statistic images are often referred to as 'Gaussianised T-statistics' etc. (Note however that the random field theory in Sections 14.12.1 and 14.12.2 does not apply to an image of Gaussianised statistics, and must be applied to the original non-Gaussianised images of T or F statistics.)

14.6.2 *F-tests for several contrasts*

Sometimes we may wish to make a simultaneous test of several contrasts at once. For example, we may wish to detect *any* difference between the hot and neutral stimuli and rest. This can be done by using a contrast matrix

$$\mathbf{c}' = \begin{pmatrix} 1 & 0 & 0 & 0 & 0 & 0 \\ 0 & 1 & 0 & 0 & 0 & 0 \end{pmatrix}.$$

The first row compares hot to rest, the second compares neutral to rest. To test $K > 1$ contrasts at the same time, that is, if $\mathbf{c}$ is a $K \times m$ matrix, the T statistic is replaced by an F statistic defined by

$$F = \frac{\hat{\beta}'\mathbf{c}(\hat{\mathrm{Var}}(\mathbf{c}'\hat{\beta}))^{-1}\mathbf{c}'\hat{\beta}}{K}$$

which has an approximate F distribution with K and ν degrees of freedom (exact if $\mathbf{AVA}' = \mathbf{I}$) when there is no effect, $\mathbf{c}'\beta = 0$. The effects are then detected simultaneously by large values of F. If $K = 1$, then $F = T^2$, so the F-test is equivalent to the T-test.

An alternative is to use the increase in error sum of squares when the model is restricted so that $\mathbf{c}'\beta = 0$. One way of doing this is to replace $\mathbf{X}$ with $\mathbf{X}(\mathbf{I} - \mathbf{cc}^+)$. If $\mathbf{R}_0$ is the equivalent of $\mathbf{R}$ under the restricted model, so that the restricted residuals are $\mathbf{r}_0 = \mathbf{R}_0\mathbf{Y}$, then the resulting F statistic is

$$\bar{F} = (\mathbf{r}_0'\mathbf{r}_0 - \mathbf{r}'\mathbf{r})/(\mathrm{tr}((\mathbf{R} - \mathbf{R}_0)\,\mathbf{AVA}')\hat{\sigma}^2)$$

which has an approximate F distribution with $\bar{K}$ and ν degrees of freedom, where

$$\bar{K} = \mathrm{tr}[(\mathbf{R} - \mathbf{R}_0)\mathbf{AVA}']^2/\mathrm{tr}\{[(\mathbf{R} - \mathbf{R}_0)\mathbf{AVA}']^2\}.$$

If the estimation is fully efficient ($\mathbf{AVA}' = \mathbf{I}$) then the two F-tests are identical ($\bar{F} = F$).

14.6.3 **When to use *F*-tests**

F-tests should only be used when we are interested in any linear combination of the contrasts. For example, an *F*-test would be appropriate for detecting regions with high polynomial drift, since we would be interested in either a linear, quadratic or cubic trend, or any linear combination of these. In this case we could use the contrast matrix

$$\mathbf{c}' = \begin{pmatrix} 0 & 0 & 0 & 1 & 0 & 0 \\ 0 & 0 & 0 & 0 & 1 & 0 \\ 0 & 0 & 0 & 0 & 0 & 1 \end{pmatrix}$$

Another good use of the *F*-test is for detecting effects when the haemodynamic response is modelled by a set of basis functions (see Section 14.11).

The *F*-test could also be used for detecting differences between a set of stimuli as in (14.10), but a significant result would simply say that there were *some* differences between the stimuli, without saying which ones were different. Researchers would probably be more interested in comparing each stimulus with a baseline, or paired comparisons between all pairs of stimuli, using a simple *T*-test. If desired, a Bonferroni correction could be used to correct for multiple *T*-tests, in which the *P* values are multiplied by the number of tests made. In other words, most scientific questions can be handled by a few well-chosen *T*-tests, rather than an *F*-test.

14.7 Setting up the model—an example

For the experimenter, specifying the the stimuli $s(t)$ and the contrasts **c** are the most difficult steps in the analysis, because these relate the design of the experiment to the scientific questions. A few examples should help clarify some important issues.

14.7.1 A linear intensity effect

Suppose a single stimulus is compared to a baseline, but the intensity of the stimulus varies. We are interested first in whether the stimulus was detected, and then whether the effect increases with stimulus intensity. Suppose the stimulus is presented sequentially in the first 10 blocks, with intensity values 0 (no stimulus), 1, 2, 3, 4, 5, and two stimulus functions (explanatory variables) $s_1(t)$ and $s_2(t)$ are set up to capture a linear intensity effect, as follows (recall that $x(t)$ is $s(t)$ convolved with $h(t)$):

Linear model, orthogonalized

Block	1	2	3	4	5	6	7	8	9	10
Intensity	0	1	0	2	0	3	0	4	0	5
$s_1(t)$	0	1	0	1	0	1	0	1	0	1
$s_2(t)$	0	—2	0	—1	0	0	0	1	0	2

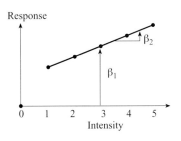

Each block might comprise say 3 volumes of 3 s each, and these 10 blocks might be repeated say 4 times in one run to give 120 volumes in all. Recall that the constant term, which models the baseline level (horizontal axis), would normally be included in the drift terms.

Note that the second stimulus model $s_2(t)$ has been centered by subtracting its mean. This allows us to look at two (nearly) orthogonal contrasts, that is, contrasts whose estimators are statistically independent: $\mathbf{c}' = (1\ 0)$ which tests for an overall effect of the stimulus compared to baseline (β_1), and $\mathbf{c}' = (0\ 1)$ which tests for a linear effect of stimulus intensity (β_2). These contrasts are not quite orthogonal because of the temporal correlation. Note that if $s_2(t)$ had been replaced by 0 1 0 2 0 3 0 4 0 5 as follows:

Linear model, not orthogonalized

Block	1	2	3	4	5	6	7	8	9	10
Intensity	0	1	0	2	0	3	0	4	0	5
$s_1(t)$	0	1	0	1	0	1	0	1	0	1
$s_2(t)$	0	1	0	2	0	3	0	4	0	5

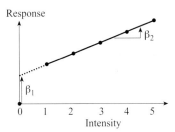

then the fit of the model would be identical, but the interpretation of the tests would be different. The second contrast $\mathbf{c}' = (0\ 1)$ would still test for a linear effect of stimulus intensity (β_2), but the first contrast $\mathbf{c}' = (1\ 0)$ would now test for the intercept of the intensity response (β_1), that is, whether zero intensity gives zero response. Replacing it with $\mathbf{c}' = (1\ 3)$, where 3 is the average of the non-zero intensities, would once again test for an overall effect of the stimulus as above.

14.7.2 A quadratic intensity effect

Sometimes the relationship of intensity to response may be non-linear. This can be captured by adding higher order terms, such as the quadratic term $s_3(t) = s_2(t)^2$:

Quadratic model

Block	1	2	3	4	5	6	7	8	9	10
Intensity	0	1	0	2	0	3	0	4	0	5
$s_1(t)$	0	1	0	1	0	1	0	1	0	1
$s_2(t)$	0	1	0	2	0	3	0	4	0	5
$s_3(t)$	0	1	0	4	0	9	0	16	0	25

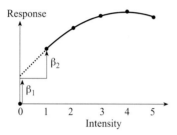

The contrast $\mathbf{c'} = (1\ 0\ 0)$ tests for whether zero intensity gives zero response, $\mathbf{c'} = (0\ 1\ 0)$ tests for whether the slope at the origin (β_2) is zero, and $\mathbf{c'} = (0\ 0\ 1)$ tests for a quadratic (non-linear) response. These terms can be orthogonalized (approximately) by replacing $s_2(t)$ with $0 -2\ 0\ -1\ 0\ 0\ 0\ 1\ 0\ 2$ and $s_3(t)$ with $0\ 2\ 0 -1\ 0 -2\ 0 -1\ 0\ 2$, in which case $\mathbf{c'} = (1\ 0\ 0)$ tests for an overall effect, $\mathbf{c'} = (0\ 1\ 0)$ tests for a linear effect, and $\mathbf{c'} = (0\ 0\ 1)$ tests for the same quadratic effect as before.

14.7.3 Intensity as a factor

The factor model assigns a separate parameter to each level of the intensity, allowing for an arbitrary relationship between stimulus intensity and response:

Factor model

Block	1	2	3	4	5	6	7	8	9	10
Intensity	0	1	0	2	0	3	0	4	0	5
$s_1(t)$	0	1	0	0	0	0	0	0	0	0
$s_2(t)$	0	0	0	1	0	0	0	0	0	0
$s_3(t)$	0	0	0	0	0	1	0	0	0	0
$s_4(t)$	0	0	0	0	0	0	0	1	0	0
$s_5(t)$	0	0	0	0	0	0	0	0	0	1

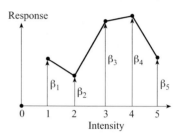

The coefficients $\beta_1, \beta_2, \beta_3, \beta_4, \beta_5$ are now the effects of each stimulus level relative to the baseline (0 stimulus). To test for an arbitrary unspecified non-linear effect, use an F-test with contrast matrix

$$\mathbf{c'} = \begin{pmatrix} 1 & 0 & 0 & 0 & 0 \\ 0 & 1 & 0 & 0 & 0 \\ 0 & 0 & 1 & 0 & 0 \\ 0 & 0 & 0 & 1 & 0 \\ 0 & 0 & 0 & 0 & 1 \end{pmatrix}$$

The factor model is identical to a fourth degree polynomial because a fourth degree polynomial can be fitted exactly through any five points. We can still test for polynomial effects using the factor model: to test for an overall effect, use $\mathbf{c'} = (1\ 1\ 1\ 1\ 1)$; to test for a linear effect, use $\mathbf{c'} = (-2\ -1\ 0\ 1\ 2)$; to test for a quadratic effect, use $\mathbf{c'} = (2\ -1\ -2\ -1\ 2)$.

What is the difference between testing for a linear effect using the contrast $\mathbf{c'} = (-2\ -1\ 0\ 1\ 2)$ in the factor model and the contrast $\mathbf{c'} = (0\ 1)$ in the linear model? The estimated effect is identical in both cases, but their standard deviations might be different. The reason is that the linear model only allows only for a linear effect, whereas the factor model allows for more polynomial effects.

If the effect is predominantly linear, then the F-test may fail to detect it, in other words, it has less sensitivity than a T-test with the contrast $\mathbf{c'} = (-2\ -1\ 0\ 1\ 2)$. This is the price paid for not knowing where to look; the F-test looks for all possible effects: overall, linear, quadratic, cubic and quartic, so naturally it has to sacrifice some sensitivity against a directed search for any one of them. The usual advice applies here: first look in the direction where you expect to see something (T-test), then look in all possible directions for the unanticipated (F-test).

14.7.4 The design

Two comments on the design of this experiment. First, the design could be improved by rearranging the temporal order of the intensity levels, because a linear intensity effect could be confounded with drift. The reason is that if an effect of interest looks like drift, then it will be partially removed by the drift terms in the linear model. A good choice might be to present the stimulus intensities in the order 4 1 3 5 2 which is orthogonal to a linear drift. Second, since the primary interest is probably detection of the stimulus, it has been alternated with the baseline, rather than say putting all the baselines together at one end. The next section, 14.8 on optimal design, gives a justification for this.

14.7.5 The baseline or rest condition

In the factor model there is no explicit indicator variable, such as 1 0 1 0 1 0 1 0 1 0 for the baseline or rest condition of no stimulus; the same is true for the hot/neutral example. What is special about this condition? What would happen if we simply had the five intensity levels, or the hot and neutral stimulus, with no rest or baseline in between? Which one would we treat as the baseline? The answer is that the baseline is the condition of the subject *before* volume acquisition commenced. In the varying intensity experiment, we are assuming that the condition of 0 stimulus persisted before scanning commenced, so this is the baseline and it is not modelled as a separate condition. In the hot/neutral experiment, the subject was at rest with no heat stimulus before scanning commenced, so this is the baseline.

If the hot/neutral experiment consisted of alternating hot and neutral stimuli applied at the start of the first volume, with no rest in between, then the hot and neutral conditions should still be modelled with a separate stimulus response, as in Figure 14.1 but without the gaps. The baseline or rest condition would appear in the first few volumes, carried over by the haemodynamic response function. The first coefficient β_1 would then measure the difference between the hot stimulus and this small amount of pre-scanning baseline; the same would be true for the neutral stimulus coefficient β_2. Obviously by themselves these coefficients would not be very informative (due to high

standard deviation; one explanatory variable is very nearly the inverse of the other, leading to poorly conditioned estimation of the individual parameters). However, the main interest is the difference between the hot and the neutral, and this would still be well estimated (low standard deviation) by the difference of the coefficients $\beta_1 - \beta_2$. If on the other hand the neutral stimulus was continuously applied preceding the first volume, then it would become the baseline and only the hot stimulus would be used; the coefficient β_1 of the hot stimulus would then measure the difference hot–neutral.

14.8 Optimal experimental design

The question arises of how to optimally design the experiment in order for the data to contain the maximum possible amount of extractable information. In other words, how should we choose the frequency and duration of the stimuli in order to have the greatest sensitivity in detecting the effects, and to estimate the effects as accurately as possible. If an on-off stimulus is presented too rapidly in short blocks then the haemodynamic response function will smooth the response to near-uniformity. On the other hand, a short stimulus presentation is desirable since it capitalises on the temporal correlation, which reduces the variance of the on minus the off volumes. Optimal designs have been investigated by Friston *et al.* (1999*b*).

The problem comes down to finding the stimulus that minimizes Var($\mathbf{c}'\hat{\beta}$) from (14.9). To simplify the discussion, assume that there is just one parameter, $c = 1$, no drift, $\sigma = 1$, and we use the fully efficient estimator so that $\mathbf{AVA}' = \mathbf{I}$. Then

$$\text{Var}\,(\hat{\beta}) = \frac{1}{\mathbf{X}'\mathbf{V}^{-1}\mathbf{X}} = \frac{1}{\sum_{j=0}^{n-1} |\tilde{s}_j|^2\,|\tilde{h}_j|^2/v_j},$$

where $\tilde{h}_j$ and $\tilde{s}_j$ are the Fourier transforms of the haemodynamic response function and the stimulus at frequency $2\pi j/n$, and v_j is the variance of the Fourier transform of the errors (spectrum) at that frequency, e.g. $v_j = 1/(1 - 2a_1 \cos(2\pi i j/n) + a_1^2)$ for a (periodic) AR(1) process. For fixed total stimulus sum of squares

$$\sum_{i=1}^{n} s(t_i)^2 = \sum_{j=0}^{n-1} |\tilde{s}_j|^2,$$

(14.11) is minimized by placing all of the weight of $|\tilde{s}_j|$ at the value of j that maximizes $|\tilde{h}_j|^2/v_j$, and zero elsewhere. In other words, the optimal design should be a sine wave with frequency that maximizes the spectrum of the haemodynamic response function divided by the spectrum of the noise. Interestingly enough, this is precisely the stimulus whose estimation is unaffected by the choice of $\mathbf{A}$.

The block design with equal on and off periods should be close to optimal since it closely matches a sine wave. For the haemodynamic response function (14.2) and an AR(1) process with $0 < \rho < 0.5$ at 3 s volume intervals, the optimal period of the block design is 21 to 16 s, or about 4 to 3 times the delay of the haemodynamic response. This optimal period is not changed greatly by drift removal, which mainly affects low frequency stimuli. For comparing the response between two stimuli the same result applies: the two stimuli should be presented alternatively in equal blocks with a period of 21 to 16 s.

For event-related designs, in which the stimulus duration is one volume or less, optimal design depends on the volume interval. For the example analysed here, the optimal design is one event every 5 to 4 volumes, or 15 to 12 s, as ρ varies between 0 and 0.5.

14.9 *Estimating the correlation structure*

Getting the correct correlation structure, specified by $\mathbf{V}$, is very important for three reasons: first, it guides us to the best estimator (see Section 14.4), second, it tells us how to best design the experiment, (see Section 14.8), but third, and most importantly, it leads to the correct estimator of the variance of the estimator, vital for getting the correct T or F statistic. In this section we look at how to estimate $\mathbf{V}$, which we have so far assumed is known.

Estimating $\mathbf{V}$, or the parameters such as ρ that make up $\mathbf{V}$, is not as straightforward as estimating β and σ^2. There are no simple methods that give best unbiased answers; the better methods all involve costly iterative calculations that are expensive to compute. One of the simplest methods is the Cochrane–Orcutt method that

first estimates β by least squares for the original unsmoothed data (14.7), that is with $\mathbf{A} = \mathbf{I}$. This estimator is always unbiased, though perhaps not the most accurate, but at least it ensures that the residuals $\mathbf{r}$ contain only error and no signal, due to the fact that the expectation of the residuals is zero, that is, averaged over all random instances of the errors. Moreover the correlation structure of the residuals is closely approximated by the matrix $\mathbf{V}$ that we wish to estimate.

The parameters of an AR(p) model are easily estimated from the autocorrelations of the residuals via the Yule–Walker equations, but $\mathbf{A} = \mathbf{V}^{-1/2}$ can be estimated directly from the autocorrelations (see Worsley *et al.* 2000). This is based only on an estimate of the first $(p + 1) \times (p + 1)$ elements of $\mathbf{V}$, given by the sample autocorrelation out to lag p:

$$\hat{\mathbf{V}} = \mathrm{Cor}\,(\varepsilon_i, \varepsilon_j) = \frac{\displaystyle\sum_{l=|i-j|+1}^{n} r_l r_{l-|i-j|}}{\displaystyle\sum_{l=1}^{n} r_l^2}$$

$$1 \leqslant i, j \leqslant p+1$$

A slight bias creeps into these estimators due to the correlation of the residuals induced by removing an estimated linear effect from the observations. Typically, they are about 0.05 lower than expected. Worsley *et al.* (2000) gives a simple method of correcting this. Using the estimated $\hat{\mathbf{A}}$, the parameters β can be re-estimated from (14.8) and the above procedure can be iterated to convergence, but in practice just one iteration seems to be enough.

The parameters of a state space model can be estimated by using a Kalman predictor to obtain the likelihood of the parameters. This must then be maximized by iterative methods to find maximum likelihood estimators. Purdon *et al.* (1998) avoided this by estimating the white noise variance from outside the brain, where the AR(1) contribution is assumed to be zero, then estimating the AR(1) component from voxels inside the brain, assuming the white noise variance is the same as outside.

Lange and Zeger (1997) took a non-parametric approach. Noting that the Fourier transform of a stationary error sequence diagonalizes $\mathbf{V}$ (that is, makes the variance matrix into a diagonal matrix), they assumed that the diagonal components (the spectrum) is a smooth function of the frequency. Instead of fitting a model to the spectrum, they simply smoothed it avoiding the frequencies which contained the signal. This works well for a periodic stimulus, since the signal is then confined to the frequency of the signal and its higher harmonics. Taking this further, other authors have proposed simply averaging the spectrum either side of the main harmonic, in effect using linear interpolation as a form of smoother (Marchini and Ripley 2000). These approaches are much more complicated to implement in the case of non-periodic stimuli.

14.10 Spatial smoothing

So far no information has been used from neighbouring voxels, and all our models have been fitted independently at each voxel. If it is felt that the signal extends over a certain predetermined region (region of interest, ROI) in space then it can be shown that signal detection is optimal if the data is simply averaged over all voxels in that region (the ROI approach).

Since we do not usually know the location of the ROI, a reasonable compromise is to smooth the data with a kernel whose shape matches the assumed spatial activation pattern. The most common choice is a Gaussian shaped kernel. For example, if it is felt that the signal covers a 10 mm region, then the data should be smoothed with a 10 mm wide kernel (see also Chapter 12). The ROI approach can be seen as a special case in which we smooth the data with a 'box' kernel whose shape matches the ROI.

14.10.1 Scale space

Smoothing the data has been criticised because it sacrifices resolvability for detectability. Moreover, we need to know in advance the width of the signal to be detected; smoothing with a 10 mm kernel will be optimal for 10 mm signals but less optimal for 5 or 20 mm signals. A way out of this was first proposed by Poline and Mazoyer (1994) in which a range of filter widths is used to create an extra scale dimension to the data, known as 'scale space'. To maintain constant resolution in scale space, filter widths should be chosen to be equally spaced on a log scale, e.g. 8, 12, 18, 27 mm. The data is now searched in location as well as

scale, though there is a small price to pay in terms of an increase in the critical threshold of the resulting T statistics (see the end of Section 14.12.1).

14.10.2 Spatial information

Solo *et al.* (2000) have proposed a novel approach to overcoming the problem of incorporating spatial information without smoothing the data. The idea is to estimate the signal parameters without smoothing, but to estimate the noise parameters by smoothing the likelihood, not the data. An information criterion is used to set the extent of the smoothing, producing an adaptive smoother. The result is that local information is used to estimate the variability of the signal, but not the signal itself.

Worsley *et al.* (2000) took a similar approach by advocating smoothing the parameters $\alpha_1, \dots \alpha_p$ of an AR(p) model for the noise, without smoothing the estimators of the signal β or the variance σ^2 (Figure 14.2).

SPM '99 takes this idea to the limit by averaging the AR parameters over all voxels, to produce a global estimate common to the whole brain. The robustness conferred by high frequency filtering offsets the bias in this estimator.

14.11 Estimating the haemodynamic response function

So far we have assumed a fixed parametric form for the haemodynamic response function. Although the parameters are usually reasonably well known, it is still worth estimating these parameters. For some types of experiment, the parameters themselves, such as the delay, are of intrinsic interest.

First we shall present some methods for estimating the haemodynamic response function parameters, then in Sections 14.11.1 and 14.11.2 we shall look at the cost of over and under estimating these parameters. Finally in Section 14.11.3 we shall look at non-linear alternatives to the basic convolution model (14.1).

The problem with estimating parameters of the haemodynamic response is that its parameters enter the model in a non-linear fashion, requiring time-consuming iterative estimation methods. Lange and Zeger (1997) take this route, estimating the parameters of a gamma model by non-linear regression techniques.

Rajapakse *et al.* (1999) instead modified the form of the haemodynamic response to make it easier to estimate. They chose a Gaussian function for the haemodynamic response, whose mean and variance parameters can then be estimated by least squares in the frequency domain. Even though the Gaussian is not a realistic model for the haemodynamic response, since its support includes negative lags, this method appears to give reasonable results.

Liao *et al.* (2001), inspired by SPM'99, have proposed linearizing the scale of the haemodynamic response by expanding $h(t)$ as a Taylor series in an unknown scale change δ:

$$e^{-\delta}h(te^{-\delta}) \approx h(t) + (-h - t\dot{h}(t))\delta,$$

where $\dot{h}(t) = \partial h(t)/\partial t$. We can then convolve the stimuli with $-h - t\dot{h}(t)$ and add these to the model, which allows for different scales for different types of stimuli. It is then possible to estimate δ from the ratio of the two coefficients to produce a 3D image of the delay of the haemodynamic response, and a 3D image of its standard error.

To give yet greater flexibility, SPM'99 proposes modeling the haemodynamic response function as a linear combination of a set of J basis functions $b_j(t)$, $j = 1, \ldots J$ that capture possible differential delays and dispersions:

$$h(t) = \sum_{j=1}^{J} \gamma_j b_j(t), \qquad (14.12)$$

where $\gamma_j, j = 1, \ldots J$ are unknown parameters to be estimated. One such set of basis functions is a set of gamma density functions with different delays and dispersions, or a single gamma density modulated by one period of a sine wave with different frequencies.

The advantage of this approach is that the response (14.4) is still linear in the unknown parameters:

$$x(t) = \int_0^\infty h(u)\, s(t - u)\, du$$

$$= \sum_{j=1}^{J} \gamma_j \left(\int_0^\infty b_j(u) s(t - u)\, du \right).$$

If we allow different parameters γ_j for different stimuli, then the resulting model (14.4) is still a linear model,

now in Jm instead of m parameters. This means that all the above methods can be used to rapidly estimate the parameters and test for activation.

Burock and Dale (2000) have taken this further by replacing the integral in (14.1) by a sum over the first few lags, then simply modeling the haemodynamic response by arbitrary coefficients. In effect, they propose modeling the haemodynamic response function by a linear combination of basis functions as above, with one basis function for each lag taking the value 1 at that lag and 0 elsewhere. This highly parameterized linear model is easy to estimate, but there is an attendant loss of sensitivity at detecting activation, relative to knowing the haemodynamic response exactly, which we shall discuss in the next section 14.11.1.

Finally, Genovese *et al.* (2000) have taken the most sophisticated approach. Each part of the haemodynamic response is modelled separately: the time to onset, the rate of increase, the duration of the response, the rate of decline, the undershoot, and the recovery. Priors are constructed for each of these parameters, and all the other signal and noise parameters, and the entire model is estimated by Bayesian methods using the Gibbs sampler. This makes it possible to generate the posterior distribution of any combination of parameters, though the time required for such an analysis is forbidding.

14.11.1 Over-specifying the haemodynamic response function

The reason for the loss of sensitivity when using a large number J of basis functions for the haemodynamic response is quite simple. The null model with no activation due to one stimulus has no effect of that stimulus and hence no convolution with a haemodynamic response function. It therefore has J less parameters than the model with activation, so we must use the F statistic with J and $\nu - J$ degrees of freedom to detect activation. The sensitivity of the F test decreases as J increases. It can be shown that this translates into having only about $n/J^{0.4}$ observations instead of n observations, for large n. In other words, the extra parameters dilute the effect of the activation, making it harder to detect.

However, it must be remembered that a haemodynamic response function with too few parameters may be biased, resulting also in a loss of sensitivity because it will fail to capture all of the response. Obviously one should try to strike a balance between too few parameters to adequately capture the response, and too many parameters that overfits the response.

The lesson is that the more flexibility allowed for the response, the more difficult it is to detect it. The best strategy is to try to model the haemodynamic response with a small number of well chosen basis functions, or preferably just one basis function. These comments apply equally well to the non-linear models in Section 14.11.3.

14.11.2 Misspecifying the haemodynamic response function

What is the cost of mis-specifying the haemodynamic response function? First, there is no effect at all on the validity of the analysis. *P*-values for detecting pure activation are still correct even if the haemodynamic response is wrong because they are based on the null model in which there is no activation and hence no haemodynamic response. However, it is still important to get the haemodynamic response correct when comparing activations, because now the null model does contain a haemodynamic response, equal for the conditions to be compared.

The main cost of misspecifying the haemodynamic response is a loss of sensitivity. This is more pronounced for event-related designs than for block designs, because the block stimulus with long blocks is less affected by convolution with the haemodynamic response function. In fact some stimuli are completely unaffected by convolution with the haemodynamic response function. One such is the sine wave stimulus with arbitrary amplitude and phase, that is, a linear combination of sine and cosine with the same known frequency ω:

$$s(t) = \beta_1 \sin(\omega t) + \beta_2 \cos(\omega t).$$

Convolution of $s(t)$ with any haemodynamic response function changes β_1 and β_2 but leaves the form of the model unchanged. This means that for this design, there is no cost to misspecifying the haemodynamic response—in fact it can be ignored altogether.

14.11.3 Non-linear haemodynamic response and stimulus non-additivity

The linearity of the haemodynamic response, and hence the additivity of signals closely separated in time, has been questioned by several authors. Is the response always a simple convolution of stimuli with a haemodynamic response function? Friston *et al.* (1998b) have addressed this by expanding the haemodynamic convolution itself as a set of Volterra kernels. The second-order model is:

$$x(t) = \int_0^\infty h_1(u_1)s(t - u_1)\,\mathrm{d}u_1 +$$

$$\int_0^\infty \int_0^\infty h_2(u_1, u_2)s(t - u_1)\,s(t - u_2)\,\mathrm{d}u_1\,\mathrm{d}u_2.$$

$$(14.13)$$

The first term is the simple convolution model (14.1) in which past stimuli have a linear effect on the current response. The second term is the second-order Volterra kernel in which past stimuli have a quadratic (including interactions) effect on the current response. (Note that without loss of generality h_2 is symmetric: $h_2(u_1, u_2) = h_2(u_2, u_1)$.) In other words, this model allows for the possibility that the effect of stimuli may not be purely additive; the response to two stimuli in close succession may be different from the sum of the separate responses if the two stimuli are far apart in time.

It might be possible to estimate the second-order kernel by extending the method of Burock and Dale (2000) (Section 14.11). The integrals in (14.13) could be replaced by summations over the first few lags, and the discrete kernels become arbitrary unknown parameters. The result is once again a large linear model including linear and quadratic terms in the first few lags of the stimulus. However, the large number of parameters to be estimated might make this method prohibitive.

A more practical suggestion, due to Friston *et al.* (1998b), is to model the first and second order kernels by a linear combination of a small number of basis functions $b_j(t)$, $j = 1, \ldots J$, extending (14.12):

$$h_1(u_1) = \sum_{j=1}^{J} \gamma_j b_j(u_1),$$

$$h_2(u_1, u_2) = \sum_{j=1}^{J} \sum_{k=1}^{J} \gamma_{jk} b_j(u_1) b_k(u_2)$$

where γ_j, γ_{jk}, $1 \leq j \leq k \leq J$ are unknown parameters to be estimated. The convolution of each basis function with the stimulus is $z_j(t) = \int_{-\infty}^{\infty} b_j(u)s(t-u)$, so that the response becomes:

$$x(t) = \sum_{j=1}^{J} \gamma_j z_j(t) + \sum_{j=1}^{J} \sum_{k=j}^{J} \gamma_{jk} z_j(t) z_k(t),$$

which is once again linear in the unknown parameters, so it can be fitted by the linear models methods above. Linearity of the haemodynamic response and stimulus additivity can now be tested by an F statistic for the bivariate terms γ_{jk}, $1 \leq j \leq k \leq J$ as in Section 14.6.

14.12 Detecting an effect at an unknown location

In this section we shall look at the question of detecting an effect $c'\beta$ or activation ($c'\beta > 0$) at an unknown spatial location, rather than at a known location as in Section 14.6. Very often we do not know in advance where to look for an effect, and we are interested in searching the whole brain, or part of it. This presents special statistical problems related to the problem of multiple comparisons, or multiple tests. Two methods have been proposed, the first based on the maximum of the T or F statistic, the second based on the spatial extent of the region where these statistics exceed some threshold value. Both involve results from random field theory (Adler 1981).

14.12.1 The maximum test statistic

An obvious method is to select those locations where a test statistic Z (which could alternatively be the T statistic or F statistic of Section 14.6) is large, that is, to threshold the image of Z at a height z. The problem is then to choose the threshold z to exclude false positives with a high probability, say 0.95. Setting z to the usual (uncorrected) $P = 0.05$ critical value of Z (1.64 in the Gaussian case) means that 5 per cent of the unactivated parts of the brain will show false positives. We need to raise z so that the probability of finding any activation in the non-activated regions is 0.05. This is a type of multiple comparison problem, since we are

testing the hypothesis of no activation at a very large number of voxels.

A simple solution is to apply a Bonferroni correction. The probability of detecting any activation in the unactivated locations is bounded by assuming that the unactivated locations cover the entire search region. By the Bonferroni inequality, the probability of detecting any activation is further bounded by

$$P(\max Z > z) \leq N\, P(Z > z), \qquad (14.14)$$

where the maximum is taken over all N voxels in the search region. For a $P = 0.05$ test of Gaussian statistics, critical thresholds of 4–5 are common. This procedure is conservative if the image is smooth, although for fMRI data it often gives very accurate thresholds.

Random field theory gives a less conservative (lower) P-value if the image is smooth. As with time series analysis, if the statistic image is smooth, then there are less truly independent voxels than the original voxel count. Thus the N used above should be reduced to the correct number of independent voxels, giving less conservative thresholding. The smoothness of the statistic image is estimated and a 'resel' size is derived, where a resel is larger than a voxel and represents the size of 'independent voxels'. The resulting thresholding is thus:

$$P(\max Z > z) \approx \sum_{d=0}^{D} \text{Resels}_d \text{EC}_d(z) \qquad (14.15)$$

where D is the number of dimensions of the search region, Resels_d is the number of d-dimensional resels (resolution elements) in the search region, and $\text{EC}_d(z)$ is the d-dimensional Euler characteristic density. The approximation (14.15) is based on the fact that the left hand side is the exact expectation of the Euler characteristic of the region above the threshold z. The Euler characteristic counts the number of clusters if the region has no holes, which is likely to be the case if z is large. Details can be found in Worsley *et al.* (1996a).

The approximation (14.15) is accurate for search regions of any size or shape, even a single point, but it is best for search regions that are not too concave. Sometimes it is better to surround a highly convoluted search region, such as the cortical surface, by a convex hull with slightly higher volume but less surface area, to get a lower and more accurate P-value.

For large search regions, the last term ($d = 3$) is the most important. The number of resels is

$$\text{Resels}_3 = V/\text{FWHM}^3,$$

where V is the volume of the search region and FWHM is the effective full width at half maximum of a Gaussian kernel used to smooth the data. The corresponding EC density for a T statistics image with ν degrees of freedom is

$$\text{EC}_3(z) =$$

$$\frac{(4 \log_e 2)^{3/2}}{(2\pi)^2} \left(\frac{\nu - 1}{\nu} z^2 - 1 \right) \left(1 + \frac{z^2}{\nu} \right)^{-(1/2)(\nu-1)}$$

For small search regions, the lower dimensional terms $d < 3$ become important. However, the P-value (14.15) is not very sensitive to the shape of the search region, so that assuming a spherical search region gives a very good approximation. In practice, it is better to take the minimum of the the the two P-values (14.14) and (14.15). Figure 14.3 shows the T statistic thresholded at the $P = 0.05$ value of $z = 4.86$, found by equating (14.15) to 0.05 and solving for z.

Extensions of the result (14.15) to scale space random fields are given in Worsley *et al.* (1996*b*). Here the search is over all spatial filter widths as well over location, so that the width of the signal is estimated as

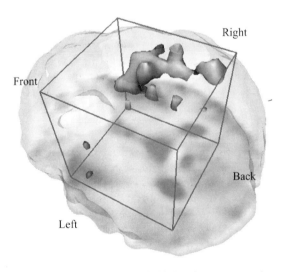

Fig. 14.3 The T statistic thresholded at the $P = 0.05$ value of 4.86.

well as its location. The price to pay is an increase in critical threshold of about 0.5.

14.12.2 The maximum spatial extent of the test statistic

An alternative test can be based on the spatial extent of clusters of connected components of supra threshold voxels where $Z > z$ (Friston *et al.*, 1994). Typically z is chosen to be about 3 for a Gaussian random field. Once again the image must be a smooth stationary random field. The idea is to approximate the shape of the image by a quadratic with a peak at the local maximum. For a Gaussian random field, it can be shown that the second spatial derivative of this quadratic is well approximated by $\ddot{Z} = -z\Lambda$, where $\Lambda = \text{Var}(\dot{Z})$, for large z. The spatial extent S is then approximated by the volume of the quadratic of height H above z:

$$S \approx cH^{D/2},$$

where

$$c = \frac{(2\pi/z)^{D/2}}{\det (\Lambda)^{1/2} \Gamma(D/2 + 1)}. \tag{14.16}$$

For large z, the upper tail probability of H is well approximated by

$$P(H > h) =$$

$$\frac{P(\max Z > z + h)}{P(\max Z > z)} \approx \exp(-zh), \tag{14.17}$$

from which we conclude that H has an approximate exponential distribution with mean $1/z$. From this we can find the approximate P-value of the spatial extent S of a single cluster:

$$P(S > s) \approx \exp(-z(s/c)^{2/D}). \tag{14.18}$$

The P-value for the largest spatial extent is obtained by a simple Bonferroni correction for the expected number of clusters N:

$$P(\max S > s) \approx E(N) \, P(S > s),$$

$$\text{where } E(N) \approx P(\max Z > z) \tag{14.19}$$

from (14.15).

We can substantially improve the value of the constant c by equating the expected total spatial extent, given by $V P(Z > z)$, to that obtained by summing up the spatial extents of all the clusters $S_1, \dots S_N$:

$$V P(Z > z) = E(S_1 + \dots + S_N) = E(N) E(S).$$

Using the fact that

$$E(S) \approx c\Gamma(D/2 + 1)/z^{D/2}$$

from (14.16), it follows that

$$c \approx \frac{\text{FWHM}^D z^{D/2} P(Z > z)}{\text{EC}_D(z) \Gamma(D/2 + 1)}$$

Cao (1999) has extended these results to T and F fields, but unfortunately there are no theoretical results for non-smooth fields such as raw fMRI data.

14.12.3 Searching in small regions

For small pre-specified search regions such as the cingulate, the P-values for the maximum test statistic are very well estimated by (14.15), but the results in section 14.12.2 only apply to large search regions. Friston (1997) has proposed a fascinating method that avoids the awkward problem of pre-specifying a small search region altogether. We threshold the image of test statistics at z, then simply pick the nearest peak to a point or region of interest. The clever part is this. Since we have identified this peak based only on its spatial location and not based on its height or extent, there is now no need to correct for searching over all peaks. Hence, the P-value for its spatial extent S is simply $P(S > s)$ from (14.18), and the P-value for its peak height H above z is simply $P(H > h)$ from (14.17).

14.13 Multiple runs, sessions, and subjects

fMRI experiments are often repeated for several runs in the same session, several sessions on the same subject, and for several subjects drawn from a population. We shall assume that all the images have been aligned to a common stereotactic space (see Chapter 15), so that anatomical variability is not a problem.

Nevertheless, there remains a very different sort of statistical problem.

It has long been recognized that a simple fixed effects analysis, in which we assume that the signal strength β is identical in all runs, sessions and subjects, is incorrect (Holmes and Friston, 1998). A random effects analysis seems the most appropriate, in which the error of the effect is calculated from independent repetitions, not from the noise error σ. Unfortunately this leads to an awkward practical problem: usually the number of repetitions (runs, sessions, subjects) is small, so the available degrees of freedom is small. For most purposes this would not be too serious, but in brain mapping we are often looking in the extreme tails of the distribution, where low degrees of freedom give very large critical thresholds for maximum test statistics, which substantially reduces the sensitivity of detecting any activation. Added to this is the problem of the Gaussian assumption for the errors; although the Central Limit Theorem assures good normality for test statistics, it is not clear that normality is maintained far into the tails of the distribution.

In PET data, degrees of freedom can be increased by spatially smoothing the random effects variance to produce a global estimate for the entire brain. Unfortunately this cannot be done for fMRI data because the variance is much too spatially structured. Instead, Worsley et al. (2000) assume that the ratio of random effects variance σ^2_{random} to fixed effects variance σ^2_{fixed} is locally constant. The degrees of freedom is increased by spatially smoothing this ratio with a $\omega_{\text{ratio}} = 15$ mm FWHM Gaussian kernel, then multiplying back by the unsmoothed fixed effects variance. The residual variance is then estimated by

$$\sigma^2_{\text{residual}} = \sigma^2_{\text{fixed}}\text{smooth}(\sigma^2_{\text{random}}/\sigma^2_{\text{fixed}}).$$

The result is a slightly biased but much less variable estimate of the variance of an effect, that comes midway between a random effects analysis (no smoothing, $\omega_{\text{ratio}} = 0$) and a fixed effects analysis (complete smoothing, $\omega_{\text{ratio}} = \infty$, to a global ratio of 1).

A simple formula, based on random field theory, gives the effective degrees of freedom of the variance ratio:

$$\nu_{\text{ratio}} = \nu_{\text{random}}(2(\omega_{\text{ratio}}/\omega_{\text{data}})^2 + 1)^{3/2},$$

where ν_{random} is the random effects degrees of freedom and ω_{data} is the FWHM of the fMRI signal, usually taken to be that of the raw data (typically 6 mm). The final effective degrees of freedom of the residuals, $\nu_{residual}$, is estimated by

$$1/\nu_{residual} = 1/\nu_{ratio} + 1/\nu_{fixed},$$

where ν_{fixed} is the fixed effects degrees of freedom. In practice we choose the amount of smoothing ω_{ratio} so that the final degrees of freedom $\nu_{residual}$ is at least 100, ensuring that errors in its estimation do not greatly affect the distribution of test statistics.

14.13.1 Conjunctions

An alternative method of dealing with multiple subjects is through conjunctions. A conjunction is simply the locations where all the subjects' test statistics exceed a fixed threshold (Friston *et al.*, 1999*a*). We are interested in the *P*-value of this event if in fact there is no activation for any of the subjects, which is equivalent to the *P*-value of the maximum (over location) of the minimum (over subjects) of the test statistic images. There is a neat formula for this based on random field theory (Worsley and Friston 2000).

It is useful to compare this with the above regularized random effects analysis. As it stands, conjunction analysis is still a fixed effects analysis, since the distribution of the test statistic is based on errors estimated within subjects, rather than between subjects. The random effects analysis assumes that there is an effect for each subject that is zero when averaged over all subjects. In other words, the random effects analysis is using a much weaker null hypothesis than the fixed effects analysis; the random effects analysis assumes that there is an effect, but this effect is randomly distributed about zero; the fixed effects analysis demands in addition that the variability of this random effect is zero, forcing the effect on each subject to be identically zero.

However, Friston *et al.* (1999*a*) turns the conjunction analysis into a neat test for a type of random effect. He asks the following question: suppose we say that a given subject shows an effect if it passes a usual $P = 0.05$ test based on a fixed effect; what is the probability that all subjects will show this type of effect in some small region (i.e. a conjunction), if in fact a

proportion γ do, and the rest do not? The paper then gives a lower bound for γ, based on the data, such that the true γ is larger than the lower bound with a probability of at least 0.95. In other words, we obtain a type of (conservative) confidence interval for the proportion of subjects that show a fixed effect.

14.14 Conclusion

This chapter has presented a review of methods for setting up a model for fMRI data, described how to estimate the parameters of this model, and how to assess the errors in these estimates. It obviously presupposes that the experimenter knows quite a lot about how and when the stimulus affects the BOLD response, but it does not suppose that we know which regions of the brain are affected. Thresholding and looking at cluster size of activated regions, will detect those regions that are affected above background noise.

There are other approaches that make far fewer assumptions about the time course of the expected BOLD response. Most of these are based on some sort of decomposition of the data into time courses and spatial patterns that are uncorrelated (singular value decomposition (SVD), principal components analysis (PCA)), or independent (independent components analysis (ICA)). These methods can be extremely useful at suggesting or generating hypotheses that can be captured and confirmed by the models presented in this chapter.

The idea of using a hypothesis test to detect activated regions does contain a fundamental flaw that all experimenters should be aware of. Think of it this way: if we had enough data, *T* statistics would increase (as the square root of the number of time points or subjects) until *all* voxels were 'activated'! In reality, *every* voxel must be affected by the stimulus, perhaps by a very tiny amount; it is impossible to believe that $\beta = 0.000000000$ exactly. So thresholding simply excludes those voxels where we do not yet have enough evidence to distinguish their effects from zero. If we had more evidence, perhaps with better scanners, or simply more time points, we would surely be able to do so. But then we would probably not want to detect activated regions. As for satellite images, the job for statisticians would then be signal *enhancement* rather than signal detection. The distinguishing feature of our fMRI data is that there is so little signal to enhance. Even with the advent of better scanners this is still likely to be the case, because neuroscientists will surely devise yet more subtle experiments that will push the signal to the limits of detectability.

References

Adler, R.J. (1981). *The geometry of random fields*. Wiley, New York.

Caines, P.E. (1988). *Linear stochastic systems*. Wiley, New York.

Cao, J. (1999). The size of the connected components of excursion sets of χ^2, t and F fields. *Advances in Applied Probability*, 31, 577–93.

Burock, M.A., and Dale, A.M. (2000). Estimation and detection of event-related fMRI signals with temporally correlated noise: a statistically efficient unbiased approach. *Human Brain Mapping*, 11(4), 249–60.

Friston, K.J. (1997). Testing for anatomically specified regional effects. *Human Brain Mapping*, 5, 133–6.

Friston, K.J., Worsley, K.J., Frackowiak, R.S.J., Mazziotta, J.C., and Evans, A.C. (1994). Assessing the significance of focal activations using their spatial extent. *Human Brain Mapping*, 1, 214–20.

Friston, K.J., Holmes, A.P., Worsley, K.J., Poline, J-B., Frith, C.D., and Frackowiak, R.S.J. (1995). Statistical parametric maps in functional imaging: a general linear approach. *Human Brain Mapping*, 2, 189–210.

Friston, K.J., Fletcher, P., Josephs, O., Holmes, A.P., Rugg, M.D., and Turner, R. (1998a). Event-related fMRI: Characterising differential responses. *NeuroImage*, 7, 30–40.

Friston, K.J., Josephs, O., Rees, G., and Turner, R. (1998b). Non-linear event-related responses in fMRI. *Magnetic Resonance in Medicine*, 39, 41–52.

Friston, K.J., Holmes, A.P., Price, C.J., Büchel, C., and Worsley, K.J. (1999a). Multi-subject fMRI studies and conjunction analyses. *NeuroImage*, 10, 385–96.

Friston, K.J., Zarahn, E., Josephs, O., Henson, R.N., and Dale, A.M. (1999b). Stochastic designs in event-related fMRI. *NeuroImage*, 10, 607–19.

Friston, K.J., Josephs, O., Zarahn, E., Holmes, A.P., Rouquette, S. and Poline, J.-B. (2000). To smooth or not to smooth: Bias and efficiency in fMRI time series analysis. *NeuroImage*, 12, 196–208.

Genovese, C.R. (2000). A Bayesian time-course model for functional magnetic resonance imaging data (with discussion). *Journal of the American Statistical Association*, 95, 691–719.

Glover, G.H. (1999). Deconvolution of impulse response in event-related BOLD fMRI. *NeuroImage*, 9, 416–29.

Holmes, A.P., and Friston, K.J. (1998). Generalizability, random effects, and population inference. *NeuroImage*, 7, S754.

Lange, N. and Zeger, S.L. (1997). Non-linear Fourier time series analysis for human brain mapping by functional magnetic resonance imaging (with discussion). *Applied Statistics*, 46, 1–29.

Liao, C., Worsley, K.J., Poline, J-B., Duncan, G.H., and Evans, A.C. (2001). Estimating the delay of the haemodynamic response of fMRI data. *NeuroImage*, 13, S185.

Marchini, J.L. and Ripley, B.D. (2000). A new statistical approach to detecting significant activation in functional MRI. *NeuroImage*, 12, 366–80.

Poline, J-B., and Mazoyer, B.M. (1994). Enhanced detection in activation maps using a multifiltering approach. *Journal of Cerebral Blood Flow and Metabolism* 14, 690–9.

Purdon, P.L., Solo, V., Brown, E., Buckner, R., Rotte, M., and Weisskoff, R.M. (1998). fMRI noise variability across subjects and trials: insights for noise estimation methods. *NeuroImage*, 7, S617.

Rajapakse, J.C., Kruggel, F., Maisog, J.M., and von Cramon, D.Y. (1998). Modeling haemodynamic response for analysis of functional MRI time-series. *Human Brain Mapping*, 6, 283–300.

Solo, V., Purdon, P., Brown, E., and Weisskoff, R. (2001). A signal estimation approach to functional MRI. *IEEE Transactions on Medical Imaging*, 20(1), 26–35.

Worsley, K.J., Marrett, S., Neelin, P., Vandal, A.C., Friston, K.J., and Evans, A.C. (1996a). A unified statistical approach for determining significant signals in images of cerebral activation. *Human Brain Mapping*, 4, 58–73.

Worsley, K.J., Marrett, S., Neelin, P., and Evans, A.C. (1996b). Searching scale space for activation in PET images. *Human Brain Mapping*, 4, 74–90.

Worsley, K.J., Liao, C., Grabove, M., Petre, V., Ha, B., and Evans, A.C. (2000). A general statistical analysis for fMRI data. *NeuroImage*, 11, S648.

15 | *Registration, atlases and cortical flattening*

Mark Jenkinson

15.1 Introduction

As we have seen in previous chapters, fMRI analysis involves taking a series of low resolution functional images and analysing these to produce a map of brain regions which are thought to have been significantly activated by experimental stimulation. As well as these (relatively low resolution) functional images, an fMRI experiment will also normally include a single high resolution structural MR scan. This can be used in a variety of ways to provide more advanced interpretation and analysis of the initial low resolution fMRI activation maps.

The main objectives in fMRI-related structural analysis are to interpret, relate, and compare spatial locations. For example, imagine that the location of an interesting activation is at voxel coordinate (23,31,7). The question that structural analysis aims to answer is: what does this mean physically? This may require determining whether the activation is within a particular area (say Broca's area) or where the corresponding location is in another individual or group.

Registration is the main tool in such structural analyses. The basic task of registration is to align two images. That is, to move or reshape one image to match the other by finding a relation between the voxel coordinates of one image and the other. This is particularly useful since it allows the information at corresponding physical locations to be compared, effectively combining the information contained in both. For example, the location of an activation can be compared to the anatomy by registering the functional volume to an anatomical scan of that individual. Another example is in the registering of fMRI results from one subject to those of other subjects for inter-subject statistical analysis.

In general then, registration is useful as it allows different sources of information to be combined (even

for simple repeat trials of the same experiment). An extension of the concept of combining information from just a few input images (via registration) is the use of atlases. Atlases are images which are a rich source of information such as anatomical structure, histological data, or functional response, and are therefore particularly useful for higher level analysis of fMRI data. Such atlases act as standard maps of the brain, just as pictures in an anatomy textbook do. In addition, atlases can also be used to specify a standard physical coordinate system which allows spatial locations to be reported and interpreted in a consistent way. An example of a standard coordinate system is the one proposed by Talairach and Tournoux (Talairach and Tournoux 1988).

Another component of structural analysis that will be discussed here is cortical flattening. This deforms the convoluted (3D) surface of the cortex into a flat (or spherical) surface. The resulting cortical map is helpful because in the flattened representation, areas which appear close are likely to be functionally 'close'; this is not the case in the original 3D image, where two regions that lie on either side of a sulcus are physically close, but are likely to be functionally 'distant' (being involved in relatively dissimilar tasks). In addition, cortical flattening enables the whole cortex to be viewed at once, which is not possible in three dimensions where the overall shape and individual folds obscure certain regions for any particular viewing angle.

In this chapter the details of structural analysis methods will be discussed, starting with a section devoted to some preliminary and related processing methods. Registration is covered next, including both manual and automatic registration, followed by sections on atlases and cortical flattening. The final sections look at some example applications.

15.2 Preliminaries

There are three useful preprocessing steps which are often beneficial for registration (and other related structural methods). The first is to reduce the amount of geometric distortion present, for example in EPI (echo planar imaging) fMRI images, by applying an unwarping map. The second is to remove non-brain structures such as the scalp and skull, and the third is to reduce large scale intensity inhomogeneities caused by bias fields. These steps are now described.

15.2.1 Unwarping geometric distortion

The acquisition of MR images is not perfect for a number of physical reasons, and so the resultant images are also imperfect. In particular, the magnetic field inside the head is usually inhomogeneous, even after careful shimming, and this results in geometric distortion of the image. The magnitude of the distortion depends upon the parameters of the imaging sequence used, where these parameters are chosen as a compromise between speed, contrast and other factors. Unfortunately, EPI sequences, which are commonly used to acquire fMRI time-series, are particularly susceptible to this form of geometric distortion. This is most

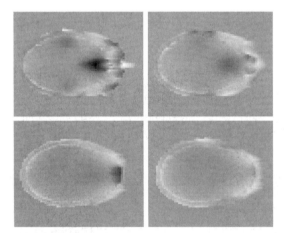

Fig. 15.1 Four slices from a single field map showing typical static magnetic field variations inside the brain. Dark areas represent fields less than the external field while bright areas represent fields higher than the external one. The total range corresponds to approximately ± 0.5 ppm.

notable near regions where there is a tissue/air interface such as sinuses, and so can have drastic effects on the frontal and temporal lobes (see Fig. 15.1).

Fortunately, there is a simple method available which reduces this geometric distortion to low levels (Jezzard and Balaban 1995). It involves acquiring a field map by appropriately combining additional EPI images taken with different gradient echo weightings. That is, an image is produced that shows the strength of the deviation in magnetic field at each voxel. This field deviation is proportional to the amount of distortion, which principally occurs along the phase encode direction for EPI data. Therefore, by calculating the magnitude of the distortion, the image can be transformed by 'warping' the distorted voxel positions to the non-distorted voxel positions.

The resulting images then contain minimal distortion and can be better aligned with images taken with other, less distorting, sequences (such as a T1-weighted structural image). This can be seen in Fig. 15.2, where the EPI image shown on the left (corresponding to the bottom left field map slice shown in Fig. 15.1) is transformed to that shown on the right. Note the large effect that this has on the frontal lobe.

15.2.2 Removing non-brain structures

For most analyses it is only areas within the brain that are of interest, and not surrounding tissue such as the scalp, skull or eyeballs. Moreover, these non-brain structures can vary significantly between individuals or between scans of the same individual. Therefore it is often helpful to remove these structures prior to further structural analysis. In fact, some registration programs, like AIR (Woods *et al.* 1993), specifically require that non-brain structures should be removed beforehand.

The simplest way to remove non-brain structures is to carry this out manually with an appropriate graphical software tool. However, as this takes a considerable amount of time, various semi-automated and fully automated methods have been developed. In general, these depend on the layer around the brain surface having an intensity which is significantly different than brain tissue. This change in intensity is then used as a barrier to constrain the brain surface estimate. For example, one approach is to start with a small spher-

Before unwarping   After unwarping

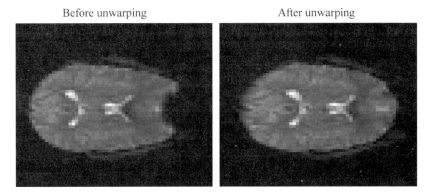

Fig. 15.2   An example application of the unwarping transformation to remove geometric distortion.

ical surface inside the brain and inflate it like a balloon until it reaches the barrier, so that in the end it models the whole brain surface, smoothing over any points where the barrier was absent or badly placed. This is the approach taken in (Dale *et al.* 1999; Smith 2000), as illustrated in Fig. 15.3. Less fully automated methods often rely on user-defined intensity thresholding resulting in a binary image; this image is then processed with morphology (shrinking and expanding operations) to isolate and identify the brain region.

Automated methods have the advantage that they are often much faster than manual methods, they are repeatable and they are more objective. However, it is often difficult to distinguish between the brain sur-face and various membranes, skull and fatty tissue, depending on the contrast and resolution of the images. Therefore, care must be taken to check that only non-brain structures have been removed and that no significant amount of non-brain structures remain. However, for the purposes of registration, small errors at this stage have little effect on registration results.

15.2.3 Bias field removal

As well as the geometric distortions (described above) which are often present in MR images, there are often intensity variations across the image, due primarily to radio frequency (RF) field inhomogeneity. These vari-

Original image   After brain extraction

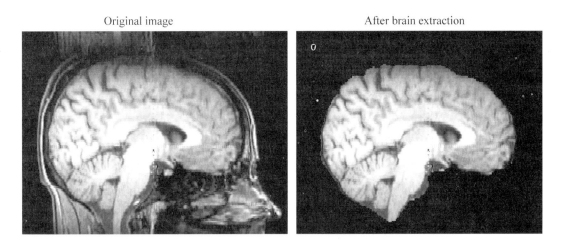

Fig. 15.3   An illustration of automatic removal of non-brain structures using BET (Smith, 2000).

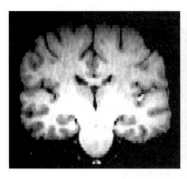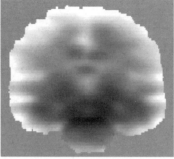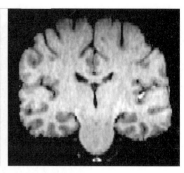

Fig. 15.4 An example of bias field removal; original image, estimated bias field and restored image (Zhang *et al.* 2001).

ations are sometimes known as *bias field*, and are seen as slowly varying changes in intensity across an image. Consequently the intensity corresponding to a given tissue type varies with position, which can be undesirable.

Various methods exist for removing bias field, since it has a very significant effect on automatic tissue segmentation procedures. With most modern scanners and volume coils, however, the bias field is small enough to be neglected when the only concern is whether bias field would damage registration quality. When this is not true and the effect is significant, one of the bias field removal methods should be applied prior to later structural analysis. For example images, see figure 15.4.

Existing methods either tend to integrate bias field estimation with tissue segmentation (Zhang *et al.* 2001) (where a correct segmentation directly gives the bias field and a correct bias field allows simple segmentation; therefore iterating the two processes ultimately

gives a good final solution for both problems) or attempt to find a bias field correction which maximizes some measure of 'sharpness' or entropy in the image (Sled *et al.* 1998).

15.3 Registration

15.3.1 Concepts

We start by giving a brief overview of the important concepts involved in registration in general, before describing manual and automatic registration in more detail.

Transformations

In the context of registration, a spatial transformation is applied to an image in order to change the position, orientation or shape of structures (such as the brain) in

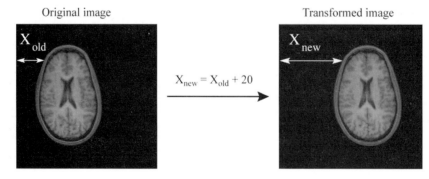

Fig. 15.5 An illustrative example showing a translation of 20 units to the right together with the corresponding equation relating the coordinates.

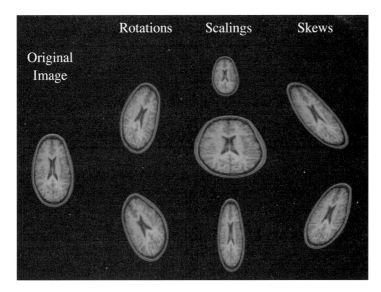

Fig. 15.6   Various examples of linear transformations of an original image (*left*). Note that, in general, these individual transformation types can be mixed in any order (e.g. scalings and rotations and skews).

the image. Mathematically it is expressed as a set of equations relating the old image positions (coordinates) to the new ones. For example, consider a translation of the image to the right. This is accomplished by moving all the positions to the right, represented by adding a constant value to the old coordinates to get the new coordinates (see Fig. 15.5).

Thus there are three different parameters (separate constants for x, y, and z) that define a translation. These 'separately selectable' parameters are known as degrees of freedom (DOF) and the number of DOF is a useful classification of the transformation type. In general, increasing the number of degrees of freedom gives greater flexibility to the registration process, in terms of the range of transformations that can be applied to make one image look like the other. The two commonest classes of transformation are linear transformations, which have 12 DOF or less, and non-linear transformations, or warps, which can have anything from tens to millions of DOF (or more). Each of these classes will now be discussed more fully.

Linear transformations

The simplest, but extremely useful, class of transformations is that of linear (also known as affine) transformations. In three dimensions they can have up to 12 DOF which include three translation, three rotation, three scaling and three skew parameters.[1] These are illustrated in Fig. 15.6.

Common sub-classes of linear transformations are:

- Rigid body (6 DOF)—translation and rotation only.
- Similarity (7 DOF)—translation, rotation and a single global scaling.
- Affine (12 DOF)—most general; includes translation, rotation, scalings and skews.

When registering an image of a particular subject's brain with another image of the same brain, a rigid body transformation would, in an ideal world, allow for a perfect registration; only translation and rotation should be necessary in order to give a good registration between the two images. In practice, various factors mean that to achieve optimal registration, the number

---

[1] Mathematical note: the use of the term 'linear' derives from the constraint that the change in each of the x, y, and z coordinates is a linear function of the original coordinates—no non-linear terms (e.g. values squared) are allowed.

of DOF often needs to be increased, usually to 12 DOF (full linear fit), or possibly even further, to non-linear warping. The factors that give rise to this necessity include geometric image distortion (as described in Section 15.2.1), changes in actual brain shape (as the brain is not a completely rigid body) and head motion during the scanning process.

In contrast, when registering one subject's brain to that of a different subject, or to an atlas (e.g. several brains averaged together), one would definitely *not* expect to achieve good results with only a rigid body transformation. At least a full linear (12 DOF) transformation should be used to achieve reasonable results.

At this point it may seem tempting to include more and more DOF in order to allow for more subtle changes in shape and scanner distortion. However, using linear transformations has several advantages. First, the fewer the DOF, the faster and more reliably the registration can be performed. This is because each additional DOF requires an additional parameter value to be found, requiring extra calculations. There is a balance between setting the DOF too low, giving a poor final fit, and setting the DOF too high, giving a slow fit, and a possibly invalid fit (physically). Second, the theory for linear transformations is simpler and so a wider variety of registration methods have been developed that use them. Third, it is possible to verify the accuracy of such transformations by comparing them to results obtained with stereotactic markers, which is much harder to do for transformations with many DOF.

Warps

Any transformation where the equations relating the coordinates of the images are non-linear can be described as a warp or warping transformation. They encompass a very wide range of transformations from the simplest, with few DOF, to the most general transformations which have three separate DOF for each voxel, giving well over a million DOF for typical images. In principle, these higher DOF transformations allow any geometric change between images to be modelled; in practice there are fewer implementations available at this end of the spectrum (especially for multi-modal registration), and these also tend to be very computationally expensive.

For general warps, with many DOF, it is usually necessary to impose an additional constraint. This constraint is that the final warp field be physically sensible—for example, that the topology of the image should be preserved. The topology of the image refers to how it is connected together, rather than its shape. Therefore, preserving topology implies that two structures which are joined in an image should remain joined after the transformation. In this way the integrity of brain structures is assured. Otherwise, without this constraint, the topology could be violated which could lead to structures such as the ventricles being split into fragments, which is undesirable. Examples of topology preserving and non-preserving warps are shown in Fig. 15.7

In general, warps are useful for higher resolution or higher contrast images where the changes are due to geometrical (shape) changes in the brain or head. For other situations where the internal detail is indistinct or significant intensity changes are induced for other reasons (such as BOLD changes) it is often more appropriate to use linear transformations or low-order warps, which are less affected by these changes as compared to the global shape and structures. However, the final choice of transformation must be made according to the specific experiment and hypothesis to be tested, where other issues may also be important.

15.3.2 Interpolation

All images are acquired and stored as a collection of discrete points set on a spatial grid. However, in order to carry out the image transformations specified by the transformation parameters described above, the intensity at positions between grid points needs to be calculated. This process is called interpolation.

To illustrate what interpolation does, consider interpolating a one-dimensional signal using linear interpolation. The aim is to calculate the intensity at any location between the sample points. (One reason why we might want to do this would be to effect a sub-voxel—i.e. very small—translation.) To do this, the two nearest samples are chosen, and a hypothetical line is constructed between the intensities at these points so that the intensity at any point in between can be found. This is illustrated in Fig. 15.8.

There are several different methods of interpolation that can be used and these each produce slightly differ-

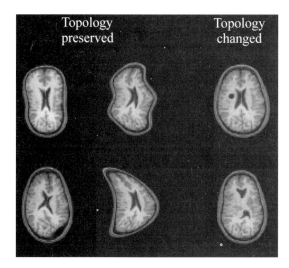

Fig. 15.7 Examples of topology preserving (*left*) and non-preserving (*right*) warps applied to the original image shown in Fig. 15.6. In particular, note that the topology is changed because of the extra hole introduced near the ventricle (*top image*) and the splitting of the ventricles (*bottom image*).

ent resulting intensities. Some of the most common methods in three dimensions are: nearest neighbour (take the value of the nearest original neighbour), tri-linear (the three-dimensional extension of the one-dimensional linear interpolation example given above), sinc (an interpolation function commonly applied in image processing) and spline approximations to sinc. Sinc interpolation uses information from local intensities in the original image which are further away from the point of interpolation than just the eight nearest neighbours, taking into account the fact that a single raw data point (in *k*-space) affects the intensity across a wider portion of the image than just the nearest neighbours. However, sinc interpolation is usually quite a lot slower than other methods and potentially more sensitive to noise and artefacts in the image.

When the precise value of the intensity at a point in the image is important, as it is in motion correction of fMRI volumes, the choice of interpolation can be significant. However, for many registration applications it is sufficient that the interpolated intensity be similar to surrounding tissue, allowing for some small interpolation inaccuracies. Therefore, the choice of interpolation method is usually not critical, although in general, nearest neighbour interpolation should be

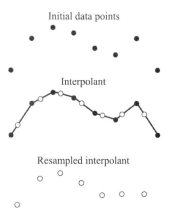

Fig. 15.8 A one-dimensional linear interpolation. The top figure shows the original discrete samples. In the middle figure the original samples are connected with lines (hence linear interpolation) forming the interpolant. This interpolant is then resampled at the new points (*open circles*), effectively performing a sub-voxel translation.

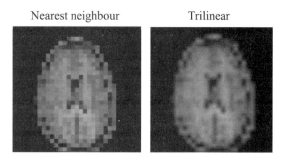

Fig. 15.9 An example showing the (block-like) artificially sharp boundaries created by nearest neighbour interpolation. The images shown here (for illustration purposes only) were produced by increasing the resolution (upsampling) from a voxel size of $8 \times 8 \times 8$ mm to a voxel size of $1 \times 1 \times 1$ mm, using the two different interpolation methods, thus enhancing the effect in order to make it visually obvious.

avoided as it produces artificially non-smooth boundaries, as shown in Figs 15.9 and 15.10.

15.3.3 Manual registration

The goal of registration is to align two images. One way to do this is to identify unique landmarks (points, lines, curves or surfaces) in each image, and then use corresponding pairs of landmarks to align the images. Manual registration requires a user to select several

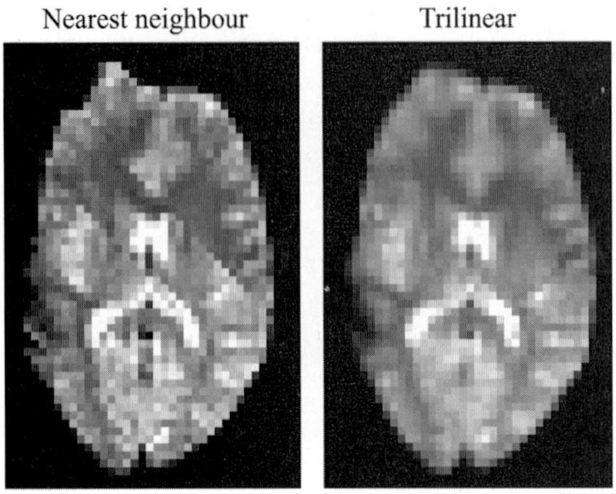

Nearest neighbour   Trilinear

Fig. 15.10 An example showing the 'artefacts' (diagonal discontinuities) generated by nearest neighbour interpolation when a rotation is applied to the original image before resampling, compared with the smoother result when trilinear interpolation is used.

anatomically unique structures (for example, the inter-hemispheric plane, corpus callosum, lateral sulcus, anterior commissure, etc.) via suitable interactive software. After the selection is done, the software uses these points to calculate the transformation that best aligns the selected landmarks.

There are several benefits in doing manual registration. First, the calculation of the transformation is very simple and fast. Therefore, it is relatively easy to write software that performs such manual registration. Consequently, it was the first form of registration available and is still easy to adapt for new modalities or variations of the basic registration problem. Second, there is no need to perform brain extraction or bias field correction prior to registration, as the presence of non-brain structures and moderate bias field will not adversely affect the manual selection of landmarks. Third, as the landmarks are selected by an expert user, the alignment of the images is guaranteed to be close around these structures. That is, manual registration will not give obviously erroneous registrations (such as a 180° rotation) which can occur when using automatic methods.

Manual registration also has some disadvantages. First, the selection of landmarks requires some expert knowledge and training. Second, even for an expert, the selection process can be quite time consuming, especially when there are many different images to

register. Third, the results are quite subjective as experts often do not agree on the precise locations of some structures in images. This can lead to quite large differences (of the order of 10 mm) between the registration results; this has been observed in studies on registration accuracy, e.g. (West *et al.* 1997). As well as the subjectivity involved, a manual method, whilst giving potentially good fit at the landmarks themselves, is not able to optimize the fit over the rest of the image, so there may be many areas where the fit is not as good as with an automatic method.

Identifying landmarks

Mathematically, the simplest and best landmarks to identify are unique points in the image. However, it is often the case that small, point-like anatomical landmarks, such as the anterior or posterior commissure, are very difficult to identify in images due to the lack of resolution or contrast. This is particularly true in typical fMRI images which are tuned for speed and BOLD contrast, not for finding anatomical structures. By comparison, larger anatomical landmarks such as the inter-hemispheric plane or the lateral sulcus are easier to identify but provide fewer constraints for the registration, as will be discussed below.

In some cases, where extra accuracy is needed or the anatomy is too indistinct, it is possible to provide additional physical markers, such as a stereotactic frame, fitted to the head, with six or more markers attached. These markers contain substances that are visible in the images and show up as small, easily identifiable points external to the head. In certain situations, such as neurosurgery, it is also possible to use more invasive markers such as screws which can be placed in strategic positions on or in the head. However, such markers are only useful if the frame is placed in exactly the same position with respect to the head for each image.

Calculating the transformation

Once the landmarks have been identified it is then possible to calculate the transformation. As is normally the case, the type of transformation being used must be specified beforehand. Moreover, the number of landmarks required depends on the number of DOF of the transformation. Specifically, each corresponding pair of landmarks will provide one or more constraints and there must be at least as many independent constraints as there are DOF in the transformation to be found.

The actual calculation of the transformation is done by solving a set of equations, where each constraint corresponds to one equation. The solution to these equations is the parameters that specify the transformation (one parameter for each DOF). For example, a rigid body transformation can be specified by six parameters consisting of three rotation angles and three translation offsets. However, it is often the case that there are more equations than parameters, in which case the system is mathematically over-determined and usually no single, exact solution exists. In this case the problem is converted into one of finding the best 'average' solution. This is very similar to finding a line of best fit by linear regression since in that case there are only two parameters (slope and intercept) but many points to fit. Therefore, in the same way, a least squares (or similar) fit is found so that the average error in aligning the landmark pairs is minimized.

15.3.4 Automatic registration

As manual registration requires considerable amounts of the user's time and gives somewhat subjective, less repeatable results, there has been considerable interest in automatic registration methods. However, the problem is much harder to solve for the fully automatic case and usually requires significantly more computation. Therefore a trade-off is usually required between, on the one hand, expected registration accuracy and repeatability, and on the other, time required for the computation.

One approach to automatic registration is to automate the process of finding landmarks in the images. This has the advantage that it is easy to validate by eye how accurate the landmark choices are and easily allows for some manual correction or intervention. However, it is very difficult to specify in a mathematical way how to find good landmarks. In addition, like manual registration, only a relatively small number of landmarks can be found and so only transformations with relatively few DOF can be used.

A far more popular approach is to define, for a given transformation, some global measure of similarity between the images, that is, a function which will quantify how similar the images are *after* some hypothesized transformation has been applied. This is done by defining a *similarity function* where better-aligned images give larger values. (Alternatively, a *cost function* can be used, where better aligned images give smaller values.)

Given a similarity function, the registration problem is solved by systematically trying different transformations in turn, to find the one which gives the maximum similarity value. It is this searching through a range of different possible transformations that increases the computation time.

Measuring similarity

One of the greatest challenges for automatic registration is the definition of a sensitive but robust similarity function. The first consideration when choosing a similarity function is whether registration is between two images of the same type (intra-modal) or different types (inter-modal). With intra-modal registration, one can normally assume that the two images will look fairly similar after correct registration—maybe just a change in overall brightness and contrast is necessary. However, in the latter case, one cannot assume that a given tissue type will have the same image intensity in each image. For instance, consider registering a T1-weighted MR image with a T2-weighted image. In the T1-weighted image the CSF has a lower intensity than the white matter, whereas in the T2-weighted image its intensity is higher. The unknown intensity transformation then becomes a confounding factor to be dealt with by the similarity function.

Intra-modal

For intra-modal image pairs, a given tissue should map to the same (or similar) intensity in each image. Therefore, the similarity can be measured by looking at the difference of intensities at corresponding voxels. Consequently, cost functions such as the mean absolute difference or mean squared difference can be used (see Appendix, Section 15.7.1). Note that since both positive and negative differences represent non-similar intensities, the absolute value or squared value of the difference is used. Figure 15.11 shows an image pair in several alignments together with the difference images.

| Image 1 | Image 2 | Difference image |

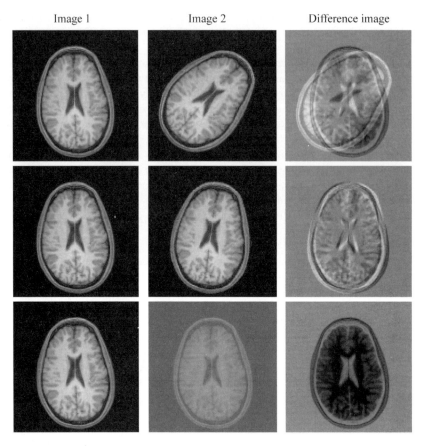

Fig. 15.11　An example showing the difference image formed by several image pairs. Each row contains an image pair (Image 1 and Image 2) together with the corresponding difference image (Image 2–Image 1), where light and dark areas in the difference image represent positive and negative values, respectively. The top two rows show the effect of a large and small rotation while the bottom row show the effect of a change in intensity brightness and contrast. Of these, the difference image with the least deviation from zero (either positive or negative) is in the middle row.

One problem with using the difference between images as a similarity measure is that the overall intensity level and contrast can vary (see Fig. 15.11) if, for instance, changes in scanner calibration occur. This means that there will be an overall bias in the difference image which can result in a poor registration being found. A way of overcoming this problem is to use a similarity function which is normalized so that global changes in brightness and contrast (global offset and scaling of intensity) do not change the similarity value. An example of this type of similarity function is normalized correlation. This is equal to the usual statistical covariance measure $(E\{I_1 I_2\} - E\{I_1\}E\{I_2\})$ divided by the standard deviation of the intensities in each individual image. It is the division by the two standard deviations that compensates for global scaling while the correlation itself is unchanged by global offsets.

Inter-modal

For inter-modal image pairs, the intensities associated with the various tissue types can be completely different from one image to another. However, within an area that contains a single tissue type the intensity should be nearly constant. This is true for each image, although the mean intensity of this area in each image is likely to be very different. For example, consider some tissue, say grey matter. The intensity in one image might be 100 ± 10, so that any intensity near 100 in the first image would be most likely to correspond to grey matter, whilst in the other image it might be 40 ± 5, a very different intensity, but again the intensity of all the grey matter within this image is nearly constant.

This observation is the basis of two related inter-modal similarity functions: the Woods function (as used in the AIR package (Woods *et al.* 1993)) and the Correlation Ratio (Roche *et al.* 1998) (as used in the FLIRT package (Jenkinson and Smith 2001)). These functions initially perform a segmentation of one image into areas of similar intensity. This segmentation is done by binning the intensity values as would be done to create a histogram. A bin number is then assigned to each location (voxel), so that all locations with the same bin number should correspond to the same tissue type. For example, choosing a bin size of 5 would assign all locations with an intensity value between 1 and 5 to bin 1, between 6 and 10 to bin 2, between 11 and 15 to bin 3, and so on. We will use the word *areas* to denote the set of locations with the same bin number (see Fig. 15.12). These areas represent spatial regions.

Then, each area is mapped onto the second image, and the intensities in each area examined. These intensities in the second image should be approximately constant if the image is aligned well, as each area should contain a single tissue type. However, if the images are poorly aligned there are likely to be several tissue types in any single area. Therefore, the similarity function is based on how much the intensity of the second image varies within each of the areas. Note that although the first image may be over-segmented (that is, a given tissue type may be split into more than one area) this does not matter since, if the alignment is good, the corresponding intensities in the other image will still be approximately constant, while if the alignment is poor, they will fluctuate greatly since the areas will be mapped across tissue boundaries.

More precisely, it is the variance of the intensities for each area in the second image that is of interest. In the Woods cost function (a cost function—see Appendix Section 15.7) the square root of the variance is taken for each area (giving the standard deviation) and then this is divided by the mean value in that area. After this the values are weighted by the size of each area and summed together to give a total (weighted) score. This total score represents the Woods function

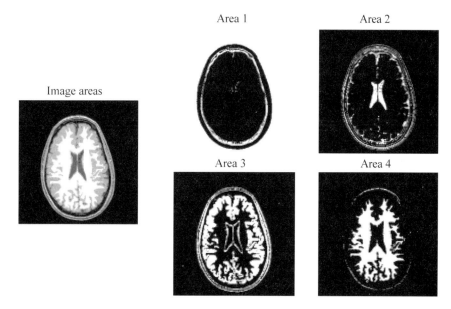

Fig. 15.12 An illustration of the spatial areas formed by binning the intensity values. On the left all the bins are shown in the one image, represented by different shades of grey, while on the right each area is shown, as white, in a separate image. For this example only four bins were used, but in practice often hundreds of bins are used.

and is unaffected by global intensity changes because of the normalization by the mean in each area.

For the Correlation Ratio (a similarity function—see Appendix, Section 15.7) the variance in each area is first weighted by the size of each area and summed together to give a total (weighted) variance score. This variance is then normalized by dividing it by the total variance of the second image, treated as a single area, and then subtracted from one. Once again this normalization ensures that the score is unaffected by global intensity changes.

Another commonly used inter-modal similarity function is Mutual Information (Maes *et al.* 1997; Viola and Wells 1997) (as used in the MRITOTAL (Collins *et al.* 1994) and UMDS (Studholme *et al.* 1996) packages) which is based on measuring the *joint entropy* of the intensities. Entropy, a quantity used in physics and communication engineering, is a measure of disorder; a substance with high entropy is one that is very disordered. Therefore, low entropy represents an ordered situation, and it is the relation between the corresponding intensities across the two images which should be orderly when the alignment is good.

In practice, the entropy is measured from the joint histogram of the two images. This histogram is formed by assigning a bin number to each voxel, in both images, based on the intensity at that voxel. Then a two-dimensional array of bins is formed with the bin numbers for the first image along the vertical axis, and those for the second image along the horizontal axis. This array is the (unfilled) joint histogram and to fill it requires looking at a each voxel position in turn, finding the bin numbers from each image at this position, then adding one to the cell corresponding to the pair of bin numbers found.

For example, consider a voxel position of (10, 3, 7). If the bin number is 4 at this position in the first image, and is 6 at this position in the second image, then the cell (4, 6) in the joint histogram has one added to it. So, by starting with zero in all cells, the joint histogram is built by examining each voxel location in turn (for both images together) and adding one to the appropriate bin. Figure 15.13 shows some joint histograms formed from an inter-modal pair of images in various alignments. Note how the dispersion of the histogram entries decreases as the images become well aligned.

Given the joint histogram, the entropy quantifies how orderly the entries are. This is defined mathematically

with both joint and marginal (individual) entropies, which are combined to form the mutual information. Section 15.7 (Appendix) contains the mathematical definitions of this and the other similarity/cost functions discussed above.

Finding the transformation

Once the similarity function has been chosen, the transformation that maximizes this similarity must be found. Due to the complexity of the similarity functions there is usually no analytical (that is, directly calculable) solution available, as opposed to the landmark method, and so the solution must be found by searching. The problem of searching for the parameter values which give the best function value (global maximum) is a standard problem in mathematics, called the optimization problem. Consequently, there are many different algorithms available for solving the optimization problem.

A difficulty with optimization in the context of registration is that only the global maximum is of interest, not local maxima, but many optimization algorithms only aim to find local maxima. The difference between local maxima and the global maximum is shown in Fig. 15.14. As can be seen, there is only one global maximum for a function (the single biggest value), which may be hidden in amongst many local maxima. In practice, some registration methods simply find the nearest local maximum, and so rely on starting close enough to the global maximum, but this can lead to non-robust registration. To solve this problem in general requires more sophisticated optimization algorithms.

Optimization

Searching for the transformation that gives the best similarity value (the global maximum) is the task of the optimization algorithm. Conceptually, the problem seems simple, as it is easy to spot the global maximum in a graph like that shown in Fig. 15.14. However, there is one main factor which makes the task difficult—the fact that only the values at particular transformations can be found with no other values or general trends known in advance.

To illustrate this problem consider an old sailing ship in coastal waters that wants to find the deepest

Image 1   Image 2   Joint histogram

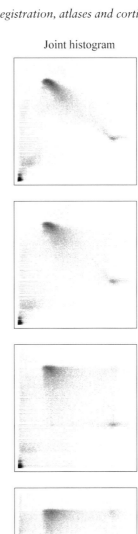

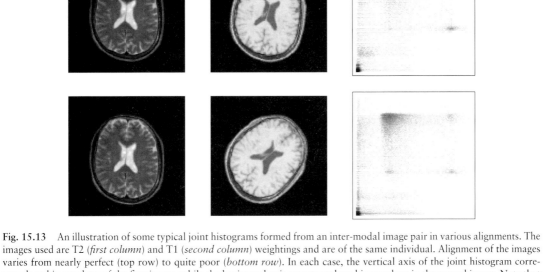

Fig. 15.13 An illustration of some typical joint histograms formed from an inter-modal image pair in various alignments. The images used are T2 (*first column*) and T1 (*second column*) weightings and are of the same individual. Alignment of the images varies from nearly perfect (top row) to quite poor (*bottom row*). In each case, the vertical axis of the joint histogram corresponds to bin numbers of the first image, while the horizontal axis corresponds to bin numbers in the second image. Note that as the alignment gets worse the dispersion increases, but even for the nearly perfect alignment there is some dispersion. In this case the dispersion is due to the fact that the relationship between tissue type and intensity is not perfect but only approximate.

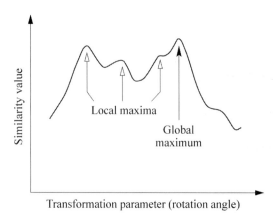

Fig. 15.14 An illustration, using similarity function values calculated for a real image pair, showing both local maxima and the global maximum.

point within some region. At any particular position that the ship is in, it can measure the depth by letting out a chain and measuring how far it has to go before hitting the seabed. Initially, the depth is unknown at all positions, and the depth can only be measured at particular positions. Thus it is necessary to start somewhere and then progressively try new positions until the captain is satisfied that the deepest point has been found. What makes this search difficult is that it is largely blind. Given a handful of depth measurements, the difficult part is deciding where to look next, and when to stop and assume that the deepest point has been found. Unfortunately, there is no general guarantee at any stage that the deepest point has indeed been found.

In this analogy the process of letting out the chain is simply equivalent to the calculation of the similarity function. The position of the ship is equivalent, not to a position in the image, but to a particular choice of the transformation parameters (for instance, rotation angles, and translation values). That is, the ship attempts to find the position where the depth is greatest, but the optimization algorithm needs to find the transformation parameters that give the greatest similarity. This makes the problem much harder because for the ship analogy there were only two dimensions to search, but for transformations there are many dimensions (equal to the DOF) which makes the general scope of the search much, much larger.

For automatic registration, choosing an appropriate optimization algorithm is crucial for two reasons. First, this is the most time-consuming part of the registration process, and second, if the optimization gives bad results then the overall registration will be bad, regardless of what similarity function is chosen. Therefore, the algorithm used should ideally be both efficient (quick) and robust (unlikely to give bad results such as finding local maxima).

Although there are many mathematical local optimization algorithms available (like gradient ascent, Powell's method, etc.—see Press *et al.* 1995 for more) there are few global optimization algorithms. Of these, Simulated Annealing (also see Press *et al.* (1995)) is the most well known, and does provide a statistical guarantee of finding the global maximum, but has the disadvantage that it requires many, many evaluations of the similarity function (which takes a long time) before finding the desired solution. In many cases there is no standard optimization algorithm that is suitable, and so a custom-made algorithm is often designed to satisfy both efficiency and robustness requirements, given the particular similarity function that is chosen.

For warps, the problem is even more difficult as there are potentially millions of parameters to find, and any form of search in such a high dimensional parameter space is prohibitively slow. Therefore, most optimization algorithms for warping registrations start by finding the best initial affine transformation and then assume that this is 'close' to the desired solution so that all other parameter values will be small and can be found using quick, local optimization algorithms. In addition, they usually rely on using multi-scale analysis techniques to speed the search; this is discussed next.

Multi-scale analysis

When looking at brain images it is normally easy for a person to identify a rough alignment based on the gross features in the image, such as the outline of the skull or brain. Mathematically, a similar thing can be achieved by using a multi-scale approach. The basic idea is to initially blur the images so that the fine detail is lost; then only the gross features are used to get an initial alignment. This is usually repeated at several different scales (amounts of blurring) so as to refine the fit using progressively finer and finer details.

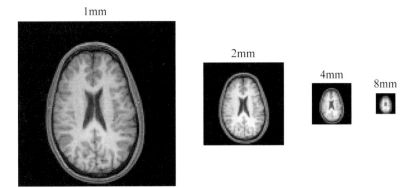

Fig. 15.15 Example showing an image with $1 \times 1 \times 1$ mm voxels, and three subsamplings of this image with $2 \times 2 \times 2$ mm, $4 \times 4 \times 4$ mm and $8 \times 8 \times 8$ mm voxels.

There are two main advantages to using such a multi-scale approach. One is to improve the robustness of the optimization, by ensuring that the initial fit is 'close' to the desired solution (the global maximum), and the other is to speed up the optimization process. This speed-up is possible because the blurred image can be resampled at a coarser resolution (larger voxel size) without loss of detail. Consequently, there are fewer voxels in the subsampled image which allows the similarity function to be evaluated more quickly. For example, subsampling an image from $1 \times 1 \times 1$ mm voxels to $4 \times 4 \times 4$ mm voxels decreases the number of voxels in the image by a factor of 64, allowing the optimization at this scale to be 64 times faster. Figure 15.15 shows an illustration of this subsampling scheme, with an initial image (1 mm cubed voxels) and three typical subsamplings (2 mm, 4 mm, and 8 mm cubed voxels respectively). Note that in order to ensure robustness the images must be blurred by an appropriate amount prior to subsampling.

Summary

Generally, automatic registration requires: (1) a similarity function and (2) an optimization algorithm. Many different approaches have been proposed (see (Maintz and Viergever 1998) for a review of manual and automatic registration methods). Of the similarity functions used, some are only suitable for intra-modal registration, while others are suitable for inter-modal registration as well. (Note that any inter-modal similarity function should also be capable of working for intra-modal image pairs, but it may not give as good results as using an intra-modal similarity function.) However, the optimization algorithm is equally important, and is what principally determines the speed and robustness of the method.

The implementation of any registration method (as a software package) is not simple and many small, but important, details which have not been discussed here need to be worked out. Therefore it is advisable to rely on an existing, tested package. Some of the (freely available) packages currently available are: AIR (Woods *et al.* 1993) (using the Woods function); FLIRT (Jenkinson and Smith, 2001) (using the Correlation Ratio); MRITOTAL (Collins *et al.* 1994) (using Mutual Information); SPM (Friston *et al.* 1995) (using a set of modality-specific templates and Mean Square Difference); UMDS (Studholme *et al.* 1996) (using Mutual Information).

With any automatic registration method there is always the possibility that the results will be erroneous. This is usually due to finding a local maximum of similarity rather than the global maximum. Therefore, it is always advisable to check the results visually.

15.4 Atlases

Just as road maps are useful for navigating around towns, brain atlases are useful for navigating around brain images. In particular, there are two basic tasks for which an atlas is helpful. These are:

- to specify the location of a place in a common reference framework (like using the grid references on a road map); and
- to find other information, like histological or functional data, about some location of interest (which is similar to looking for tourist attractions, hotels, etc. on a road map).

Atlases can be used for both tasks; however, for the first task it is also possible to use a template rather than a full atlas. A template is a subclass of atlas; one where there is no extra information about the significance of locations beyond assigning them a standard (grid reference) coordinate system.

Atlases (and templates) are only useful after the image being examined is registered to the atlas. In some cases, affine registration is sufficient, but for many high resolution atlases, full warping registrations are necessary to take advantage of the detail provided. However, the choice of transformation also depends, as stated before, on the type of images available, and for images like fMRI EPI, there is only minimal anatomical detail. This makes full warping registration difficult and potentially inaccurate for these cases compared to registrations using linear transformations.

15.4.1 Templates

When only a standard coordinate system is required (say for comparing the locations of activations or lesions between two groups) then a template is sufficient. This template may either be based on the image of a single subject, or derived from a group of subjects. Normally a template lies in a standard coordinate frame.

When a template is generated as an 'average' of a group of subjects, various registration and averaging steps are required. First an initial target for registrations is created—this may either be one of the individual images or an existing template, or may be derived from one or more of the subjects' images on the basis of manual landmark determination. Next, all images are registered to this target. Finally the mean of the resulting registered images is found, producing a blurred average image. Most template creation procedures are somewhat similar to this outline. Variations on this method include iterating the main steps to give

a more representative average image, and using non-linear registration, in order to give a less blurred average.

15.4.2 Example: Atlas of Talairach and Tournoux

A commonly used atlas is the one developed by Talairach and Tournoux (Talairach and Tournoux 1988). This atlas was constructed from a detailed examination of a single post-mortem brain. In addition, 3D coordinates were assigned relative to a system based on eight landmark points. These landmarks are: the Anterior Commissure (AC); the Posterior Commissure (PC); the most anterior (A) and posterior (P) points on the brain surface along the AC-PC line; the most superior (S) and inferior (I) points on the brain surface along a line passing through AC, perpendicular to the AC-PC line and within the inter-hemispheric plane; the most extreme right (R) and left (L) points on the brain surface along a line passing through AC and perpendicular to the inter-hemispheric plane. Figure 15.16 shows an example of these selected points. Consequently, by identifying these points in another brain image the image can be manually registered (with a piece-wise affine transformation) to the standard space of Talairach and Tournoux.

15.4.3 Probabilistic atlases

An atlas can contain any sort of information, such as histological or anatomical data. Usually this information is associated with fixed reference points (or areas) in the atlas. However, there is significant variability in normal brain anatomy and such variability can also be incorporated into the atlas by making it a probabilistic atlas.

Consider a tissue-type atlas. When registering a group of images to an atlas, the normal variation in anatomy means that the tissue type at any particular location will not be consistent across all individuals. There will often be two or more tissue types at each location, each with a probability of occurrence, which reflects how likely a voxel at this location is to contain a particular tissue type. For example, a point in the atlas may state that there is a 30 per cent probability of it being grey matter and a 70 per cent probability of it being white matter. This reflects the fact that, for the

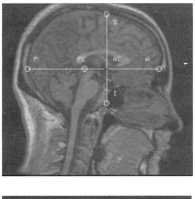

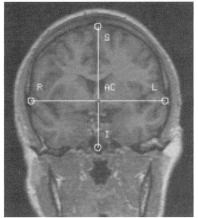

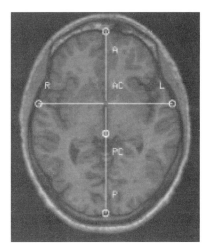

Fig. 15.16   An example showing the points used to specify Talairach coordinates.

group that was used to make the atlas, the point corresponded to white matter in only 70 per cent of cases. Such points are common, given, for instance, the variation of sulci and gyri in the cortical surface.

One of the useful features of a probabilistic atlas is that it allows probabilities to be assigned to measurements. For instance, the probability of an activation having occurred in a given Brodmann's area can be quantified given a probabilistic atlas. Furthermore, for warping transformations a probabilistic atlas can be constructed which records the relative movement of individual points in the warps. This warp information shows how likely different structures are to change shape and in what ways (see (Toga and Thompson 1999) for more details). Such atlases allow quite sophisticated questions about structure, shape or functional localization between groups to be answered. Often this will require that an atlas be built for the particular groups being studied; however, as such atlases become more widely available, it will become increasingly possible to compare a group to the 'normal' population by using an atlas that represents this population.

15.5 Cortical flattening

The surface of the human cortex, comprising a relatively thin layer of grey matter, is very convoluted; it is folded into a pattern of sulci and gyri that whilst broadly similar for all humans also shows individual variation. Furthermore, when analysing the functional response of the brain, it is the spatial relationships between different parts of the cortical surface that are of interest. Therefore, an understanding and analysis of these spatial relationships is critical for the understanding of cognitive function.

Analysing the spatial relations in three dimensions, however, is complicated. It is more natural to express the relations in a two-dimensional representation, since the cortical grey matter is in effect a folded two-dimensional surface. Cortical flattening provides a way of creating such a two-dimensional map from the three-dimensional images of the brain. Therefore, it allows the cortical surface (either whole or part) and its connections to be visualized more easily as a single entity. Furthermore, in the flattened map all parts are visible at once, which is not possible in three dimensions due to its convoluted, self-occluding structure.

The process of cortical flattening involves three major stages: extraction of the cortical surface (including necessary cuts); inflation in three dimensions; and flattening of the inflated surface. This process can be automated; however, some manual intervention is usually necessary to take account of the differences in the anatomy, especially for the extraction and placement of cuts.

15.5.1 Extraction and cuts

In the first stage of processing, the cortex must be extracted from the image. This usually involves removing non-brain structures initially (see Section 15.2.2) and then segmenting the grey and white matter. Once a satisfactory segmentation has been performed (either manually or automatically), only the outer or inner (or in some cases internal) surface of the grey matter is retained (resembling a thin shell); this represents the cortical surface.

The next step is to identify natural boundaries in the cortical surface such as the inter-hemispheric plane and the lateral sulcus. These boundaries are marked as cuts, meaning that the spatial relations between points on either side of the boundary will not be preserved in the flattening process. As it is quite common to only be interested in a certain cortical area (visual cortex for example), any additional relevant boundaries on the cortex also become cuts.

Cuts are necessary; without them, either extreme within-surface distortions arise during flattening, or it may even be impossible to flatten the cortical surface. For instance, consider the familiar flattened maps of the world. Typically, a cut is taken down the Pacific Ocean, so that the American continent is on the far left and the Asian continent is on the far right. This effec-

tively separates areas of the Pacific which, although near each other on the globe, are on opposite sides of the flattened map. In a similar way points on either side of the inter-hemispheric plane will be separated in the flattened map, which is sensible since they are not directly connected across the cortex, but internally, via the corpus callosum.

15.5.2 Inflation

Once the cortical surface has been found, and the cuts marked, an optional intermediate stage is to expand this cortex so that it becomes smooth. This step is known as inflation and is similar to inflating a wrinkled balloon. The expansion is done by simulating the effect of two forces: one which pushes all points away from the centre of the brain (the inflationary force) and one which attempts to hold neighbouring points together (like surface tension). Note that the second force is not applied to points either side of a cut as these are allowed (indeed encouraged) to separate. This inflation of the surface results in a new surface which is both larger and smoother, making it easier to flatten, but still retains all the spatial connectivity of the original surface.

15.5.3 Flattening

The final stage in cortical flattening is to take the inflated surface, which is still three-dimensional, and warp it into a two-dimensional map. However, for most curved surfaces (cylinders being a notable exception) this warping into two dimensions involves some distortions. For example, in most 2D maps of the world, Greenland appears to have a much greater area relative to other countries than it does on a globe. The objective for this process, therefore, is to reduce the amount of distortion.

One measure of distortion is the difference in distance between two corresponding points in the flattened map compared to the original, non-inflated surface. It is then possible to find the warp (that is, the coordinate transformation) which generates the least distortion. This then becomes equivalent to the registration problem where the distortion measure is used as a cost function, and the optimization algorithm finds the transformation that has minimal cost.

When the best transformation has been found this can be applied to the original images, including activation maps, so that they can be viewed in this flattened, two-dimensional map. It is common to also show the locations of the sulci/gyri on the flattened map so that it is easier to visualize where the original locations were. These flattened maps then allow many types of functional connectivities to be analysed and the structure of the functional organisation to be mapped. Such maps are commonly used to study the visual cortex, and have allowed various retinotopic mappings to be found, leading to an understanding of the early stages of visual processing.

Example images showing the stages of flattening in one particular approach (see (Dale *et al.* 1999; Fischl *et al.* 1999)) are shown in Fig. 15.17.

15.6 *Example applications*

This section looks at three typical applications of structural analysis in fMRI. Although this is only a small sample from the range of possible applications, it should give a sense of how the theory, explained in previous sections, is applied in the course of an fMRI experiment.

15.6.1 Localising activations

The most common application of structural analysis in fMRI is the registration of activation images to a template in order to assign standard coordinates. Typically a two-stage registration process is used to register a functional image with a template. This involves several steps:

(1) Pre-process the original functional image, correcting for distortion, removing bias field and/or non-brain structures.
(2) Pre-process a structural image (of the same subject) to remove non-brain structures.
(3) Register the functional image with the structural image.
(4) Register the structural image with the template.
(5) Combine the two transforms and apply to original functional/statistical images.

The reason for using a two-step registration, with the structural image as the intermediary, rather than a one-step registration of functional image directly to the template, is that the functional images typically have poor anatomical detail, as the sequence is tuned to be fast and give good BOLD contrast. This, together with the fact that the functional images are usually low resolution, means that registrations with the template are often not very accurate, especially when large DOF transformations are used. However, when registering with the structural image of the same subject, a low DOF transformation is sufficient (usually between 6 and 12 DOF), as the anatomy should be exactly the same (provided geometric scanning distortions are minimized). The structural image, which has higher resolution and better anatomical contrast, can then be registered to the template with a high DOF transformation (12 DOF or more). This allows a good match to be found despite the difference in anatomy between the individual and the template, since there is sufficient detail in the structural images for the registration to utilize.

To perform these registrations requires three images: a functional image from the fMRI experimental time-series; a structural image of the same subject; and a template. Therefore, when running the experiment it is necessary to acquire a structural image in addition to the usual fMRI time-series. For the structural image, any imaging modality that highlights anatomy is useful, although it may be helpful to use the same modality as the template in order to assist the second stage registration. The functional image, however, requires no extra acquisition as any arbitrary image from the time-series (excluding the first few which show saturation effects) is suitable.

Finally, the reason that the two transforms are combined in the last step into a single transform (which takes functional data into template space), rather than applying two separate transforms, is that any errors due to interpolation then occur only once rather than twice. This transformation is applied to statistical activation maps (which are originally in the same coordinate system as the functional image) so that they can be combined with structural information in standard (template) space. This allows the locations of activation sites to be reported in this standard space.

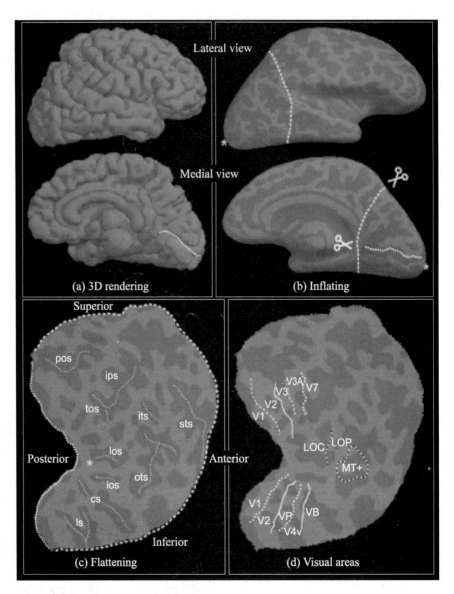

Fig. 15.17 Example images showing the different stages of flattening in one particular approach (Dale *et al.* 1999; Fischl *et al.* 1999), courtesy of R. Tootell and N. Hadjikhani. Inflation removes the main folds of the sulci and gyri, and flattening produces a planar surface, on which different functional areas are shown.

15.6.2 Correlating functional and anatomical information

Another use of registration for activation images is to determine not only standard coordinates, but the anatomical area of an activation. In the simplest case this involves registering a subject's structural and functional images. This is the first stage registration outlined in the previous example, and the same preprocessing steps apply. Then, by examining the structural image in detail (which has better contrast and resolution than the functional image), the location of an activation can be determined with respect to that subject's anatomy. For example, such a registration can be used to determine whether an activation occurred in the hippocampus.

In some cases, however, the subject's structural image lacks sufficient detail or contrast to enable structures of interest to be isolated accurately. This can occur because the imaging sequence did not have sufficient contrast in the region of interest, or subject motion caused motion artefact in the scan, or because the resolution had to be reduced in order to keep the scanning time down to an acceptable length. It is in these situations that it is best to use a probabilistic atlas instead.

The difficulty in using an atlas to relate functional and anatomical information is that the difference in individual anatomy becomes an unwanted confound. Therefore it is better to attempt a two-stage registration as described in the previous example, since this constrains the initial functional to structural registration while allowing a more general structural to atlas registration. However, the situation here is made harder by the fact that the structural image lacks detail in the region of interest. Consequently, the registration in this region is likely to be less accurate. But, by using a probabilistic atlas some statistical inferences about the location can be made, since the confound of differing anatomies is taken into account by the atlas. So the final result is no longer a simple yes or no as to whether it is in some area (the hippocampus for example), but instead it is a probability which expresses the likelihood of it being in this area.

Fig. 15.18 An example of 'flattened activation' courtesy of R. Tootell and N. Hadjikhani. The different parts of the visual cortex are identified using phase-encoded visual stimulation. (See also colour plate section.)

15.6.3 Mapping functional activations in visual cortex

One goal of fMRI experimentation is to map out and explain the functional organisation of the human brain. Cortical flattening is a valuable tool in this endeavour as it allows the activations to be visualized in a two-dimensional map. Consequently it can show the flow of activations across the cortex, and this is particularly evident in the visual cortex.

Consider an experiment to demonstrate the functional architecture of the visual cortex. This must involve some paradigm which allows the activation to be tracked through different locations in order to fully explore the functional connectivities. To do this for the visual cortex is simple, as the organisation is retinotopic for the first few areas (V1, V2, etc.) and so a stimulus that moves across the retina is sufficient to create a moving activation in the cortex. For instance, an expanding set of concentric rings will cause a wave of activation to pass over the primary visual areas.

The experiment must be planned so that results that are time-locked to the stimulus can be found with an appropriate analysis of the time-series. Then, after this analysis has been done, a series of time-locked activa-

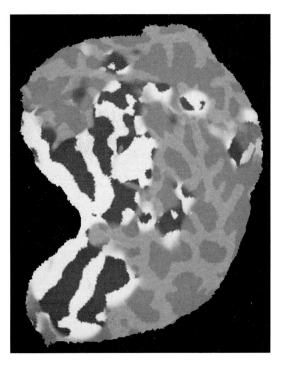

tion maps are available, but in the original three-dimensional space. To convert these into a series of two-dimensional activation maps requires cortical flattening.

In order to perform cortical flattening, a single anatomical scan is initially required. The cortex is then extracted from this scan by removing non-brain structures and placing cuts along the boundaries of the visual cortex. Once this is done, the cortex is inflated and then flattened as described in Sections 15.5.2 and 15.5.3. This produces a warping transformation that can be applied to each of the activation maps (after they are registered with the anatomical scan), producing a series of two-dimensional activation maps which allow the cascade of activations to be tracked across the visual cortex from one area to another. An example of this kind of 'flattened activation' is shown in Fig. 15.18.

15.7 Appendix—mathematical definitions

This appendix contains mathematical definitions of some commonly used similarity/cost functions for both intra-modal and inter-modal registration.

Let the two images be I_A and I_B with the voxel intensity at a location j (in I_A) denoted by I_{Aj}. Furthermore, let N be the total number of voxels in an image.

15.7.1 Intra-modal

$$\text{Mean Absolute Difference} = \frac{1}{N} \sum_j |I_{Aj} - I_{Bj}|$$

$$\text{Mean Square Difference} =$$

$$\frac{1}{N} \sum_j (I_{Aj} - I_{Bj})^2$$

$$\text{Normalized Correlation} =$$

$$\frac{(1/N) \sum_j (I_{Aj} - \overline{I_A})(I_{Bj} - \overline{I_B})}{\sqrt{(1/N) \sum_j (I_{Aj} - \overline{I_{Aj}})^2} \sqrt{(1/N) \sum_j (I_{Bj} - \overline{I_{Bj}})^2}}$$

where

$$\overline{I_A} = \frac{1}{N} \sum_j I_{Aj} \quad \text{and} \quad \overline{I_B} = \frac{1}{N} \sum_j I_{Bj}.$$

Note that the MAD and MSD are cost functions, NC is a similarity function.

15.7.2 Inter-modal

$$\text{Woods Function} = \sum_k \frac{n_k}{N} \frac{\sigma_k}{\mu_k}$$

$$\text{Correlation Ratio} = 1 - \sum_k \frac{n_k}{N} \frac{\sigma_k^2}{\sigma^2}$$

$$\text{Mutual Information} = H(I_A) + H(I_B) - H(I_A, I_B)$$

where σ_k^2 is the variance, μ_k is the mean value, and n_k is the number of voxels in area k; and σ^2 is the total variance across the whole image. Joint entropy is given by

$$H(I_A, I_B) = - \sum_{ij} \frac{n_{ij}}{N} \log\left(\frac{n_{ij}}{N}\right)$$

where n_{ij} is the number of voxels that were assigned to bin (i, j). The marginal entropies, $H(I_A)$ and $H(I_B)$, are defined similarly, but using the individual image histograms rather than the joint histogram. Note that the Woods function is a cost function, and CR and MI are similarity functions.

References

Collins, D., Neelin, P., Peters, T., and Evans, A. (1994). Automatic 3D intersubject registration of MR volumetric data in standardized Talairach space. *Journal of Computer Assisted Tomography*, 18(2), 192–205.

Dale, A., Fischl, B., and Sereno, M. (1999). Cortical surface-based analysis I: Segmentation and surface reconstruction. *NeuroImage*, 9, 179–94.

Fischl, B., Sereno, M., and Dale, A. (1999). Cortical surface-based analysis II: Inflation, flattening, and a surface-based coordinate system. *NeuroImage*, 9, 195–207.

Friston, K., Ashburner, J., Frith, C., Poline, J.-B., Heather, J., and Frackowiak, R. (1995). Spatial registration and normalization of images. *Human Brain Mapping*, 2, 165–89.

Jenkinson, M. and Smith, S. (2001). A global optimisation method for robust affine registration of brain images *Medical Image Analysis*, 5(2), 143–156..

Jezzard, P. and Balaban, R. (1995). Correction for geometric distortion in echo planar images from B_0 field variations. *Magnetic Resonance in Medicine*, 34, 65–73.

Maes, F., Collignon, A., Vandermeulen, D., Marchal, G., and Suetens, P. (1997). Multimodality image registration by maximisation of mutual information. *IEEE Transactions on Medical Imaging*, **16**(2), 187–98.

Maintz, J. and Viergever, M. (1998). A survey of medical image registration. *Medical Image Analysis*, **2**(1), 1–36.

Press, W., Teukolsky, S., Vetterling, W., and Flannery, B. (1995). *Numerical Recipies in C*, 2nd edn. Cambridge University Press, Cambridge, UK.

Roche, A., Malandain, G., Pennec, X., and Ayache, N. (1998). The correlation ratio as a new similarity measure for multi-modal image registration. MICCAI '98. Lecture Notes in Computer Science, LNCS, Vol. 1496, 1115–1124, Editors: W. Wells, A. Colchester, S. Delp.

Sled, J., Zijdenbos, A., and Evans, A. (1998). A nonparametric method for automatic correction of intensity nonuniformity in MRI data. *IEEE Transactions on Medical Imaging*, 17, 87–97.

Smith, S. (2000). *Robust automated brain extraction*, p.625. *Sixth International Conference on Functional Mapping of the Human Brain*, San Antonio, Texas, USA.

Studholme, C., Hill, D., and Hawkes, D. (1996). Automated 3D registration of MR and CT images of the head. *Medical Image Analysis*, **1**(2), 163–75.

Talairach, J. and Tournoux, P. (1988). *Co-planar stereotaxic atlas of the human brain*. Thieme Medical Publisher Inc., New York.

Toga, A. and Thompson, P. (1999). *Brain Warping*, Ch. 1. Academic Press, San Diego.

Viola, P. and Wells, W. (1997). Alignment by maximization of mutual information. *International Journal of Computer Vision*, **24**(2), 137–54.

West *et al.*, J. (1997). Comparison and evaluation of retrospective intermodality brain image registration techniques. *Journal of Computer Assisted Tomography*, **21**(4), 554–66.

Woods, R., Mazziotta, J., and Cherry, S. (1993). MRI–PET registration with automated algorithm. *Journal of Computer Assisted Tomography*, **17**(4), 536–46.

Zhang, Y., Brady, M., and Smith, S. (2001). Segmentation of brain MR images through a hidden Markov random field model and the expectation maximization algorithm. *IEEE Transactions on Medical Imaging*, **20**(1), 45–57.

16 | *Extracting brain connectivity*

Christian Büchel and Karl Friston

16.1 Introduction

In the late nineteenth century the early investigations of brain function were dominated by the concept of functional segregation. This approach was driven largely by the data available to scientists of that era. Patients with circumscribed lesions were found who were impaired in one particular ability while other abilities remained largely intact. Indeed, descriptions of patients with different kinds of aphasia (an impairment of the ability to use or comprehend words), made at this time, have left a permanent legacy in the contrast between Broca's and Wernicke's aphasia. These syndromes were thought to result from damage to anterior or posterior regions of the left hemisphere respectively. In the first part of the twentieth century the idea of functional segregation fell into disrepute and the doctrine of 'mass action' held sway, proposing that higher abilities depended on the function of the brain 'as a whole' (Lashley, 1929). This doctrine was always going to be unsatisfying. However, with the resources available at the time it was simply not possible to make any progress studying the function of the 'brain as a whole'. By the end of the twentieth century the concept of functional segregation returned to domination.

The doctrine is now particularly associated with cognitive neuropsychology and is enshrined in the concept of double dissociation (see Shallice 1988, Chapter 10). A double dissociation is demonstrated when neurological patients can be found with 'mirror' abnormalities. For example, many patients have been described who have severe impairments of long-term memory while their short-term memory is intact. In 1969 Warrington and Shallice, described the first of a series of patients who had severe impairments of phonological short-term memory, but no impairments of long-term memory. This is a particularly striking example of double dissociation. It demonstrates that different brain regions are involved in short and long-term memory. Furthermore, it shows that these regions can function in a largely independent fashion. This observation caused major problems for theories of memory, extant at the time, which supposed that inputs to long-term memory emanated from short-term memory systems (e.g. Atkinson and Shiffrin 1968).

Functional brain imaging avoids many of the problems of lesion studies, but here too, the field has been dominated by the doctrine of functional segregation. Nevertheless, it is implicit in the subtraction method that brain regions communicate with each other. If we want to distinguish between brain regions associated with certain central processes for example, then we will design an experiment in which the sensory input and motor output is the same across all conditions. In this way activity associated with sensory input and motor output will cancel out. The early studies of reading by Posner and his colleagues are still among the best examples of this approach (Posner *et al.* 1988; Petersen *et al.* 1990). The design of these studies was based on the assumption that reading goes through a single series of discrete and independent stages; visual shapes are analysed to form letters, letters are put together to form words, the visual word form is translated into sound, the sound form is translated into articulation, and so on. By comparison of suitable tasks (e.g. letters vs. false font, words vs. letters, etc.), each stage can be isolated and the associated brain region identified. Although subsequent studies have shown that this characterization of the brain activity associated with reading is a considerable oversimplification, the original report still captures the essence of most functional imaging studies; a number of discrete cognitive stages are mapped onto discrete brain areas. Nothing is revealed about how the cognitive processes interact, or how the brain regions communicate with each other. If word recognition really did depend on the passage of information through a single series of discrete stages, we would at least like to know the temporal order in which the associated brain regions were engaged. Some evidence comes from EEG and MEG studies. In fact, we know that word recognition depends upon at least two parallel routes; one via meaning, and the other via phonology (Marshall and Newcombe 1973). Given this model we would like to be able to specify the brain regions associated with each route and have some measure of the strengths of the connections between these different regions.

In this chapter we will show that new methods for measuring effective connectivity allow us to characterize the interactions between brain regions that underlie the complex interactions among different processing stages of functional architectures.

16.2 Definitions

In the analysis of neuroimaging time-series (i.e. signal-changes in a set of voxels, expressed as a function of time), functional connectivity is defined as the *temporal correlations between spatially remote neurophysiological events* (Friston *et al.* 1993*b*). This definition provides a simple characterization of functional interactions. The alternative is effective connectivity (i.e. *the influence one neuronal system exerts over another*) (Friston *et al.* 1993*a*). These concepts originated in the analysis of separable spike trains obtained from multiunit electrode recordings (Gerstein and Perkel 1969; Aertsen and Preissl 1991). Functional connectivity is simply a statement about the observed correlations; it does not comment on how these correlations are mediated. For example, at the level of multiunit micro-electrode recordings, correlations can result from *stimulus-locked transients,* evoked by a common afferent input (that is, signal input into the neural system as a result of external stimulation), or reflect *stimulus-induced oscillations;* phasic coupling of neural assemblies, mediated by synaptic connections (Gerstein *et al.* 1989). Effective connectivity is closer to the notion of a connection, either at a synaptic (cf. synaptic efficacy) or cortical level. Although functional and effective connectivity can be invoked at a conceptual level in both neuroimaging and electrophysiology they differ fundamentally at a practical level. This is because the time-scales and nature of neurophysiological measurements are very different (seconds vs. milliseconds and hemodynamic vs. spike trains). In electrophysiology it is often necessary to remove the

confounding effects of stimulus-locked transients (that introduce correlations *not* causally mediated by direct neural interactions) in order to reveal an underlying connectivity. The confounding effect of stimulus-evoked transients is less problematic in neuroimaging because propagation of signals from primary sensory areas onwards is mediated by neuronal connections (usually reciprocal and interconnecting). However it should be remembered that functional connectivity is not necessarily due to effective connectivity (e.g. common neuromodulatory input from ascending aminergic neurotransmitter systems or thalamo-cortical afferents) and, where it is, effective influences may be indirect (e.g. polysynaptic relays through multiple areas). In this chapter we will only focus on effective connectivity. More details about functional connectivity can be found in (Friston *et al.* 1993*b*).

16.3 Effective connectivity

16.3.1 A simple model

Effective connectivity depends on two models: a mathematical model, describing 'how' areas are connected and a neuroanatomical model describing 'which' areas are connected. We shall consider linear and non-linear models. Perhaps the simplest model of effective connectivity expresses the hemodynamic change at one voxel as a weighted sum of changes elsewhere. This can be regarded as a multiple linear regression, where the effective connectivity reflects the amount of rCBF (regional cerebral blood flow) variability, at the target region, attributable to rCBF changes at a source region. As an example, consider the influence of other areas M on area $V1$. This can be framed in a simple equation:

$$V1 = Mc + e \qquad (16.1)$$

where $V1$ is a $n \times 1$ column vector with n scans, M is a $n \times m$ matrix with m regions and n observations (scans), c is a $m \times 1$ column vector with a parameter estimate for each region. e is a vector of error terms.

Implicit in this interpretation is a mediation of the influence among brain regions by neuronal connections with an effective strength equal to the (regression) coefficients c. This highlights the fact that the linear model assumes that the connectivity is constant over the whole range of activation and does not depend on input from other sources.

Experience suggests that the linear model can give fairly robust results. One explanation is that the dimensionality (the number of things that are going on) of the physiological changes can be small by experimental design. In other words the brain responds to simple and well organized experiments in a simple and well organised way. Generally however neurophysiological interactions are non-linear and the adequacy of linear models must be questioned (or at least qualified). Consequently we will focus on a non-linear model of effective connectivity (Friston *et al.* 1995).

Reversible cooling experiments in monkey visual cortex, during visual stimulation, have demonstrated that neuronal activity in V2 depends on forward inputs from V1. Conversely neuronal activity in V1 is *modulated* by backward or re-entrant connections from V2 to V1 (Schiller and Malpeli 1977; Sandell and Schiller 1982; Girard and Bullier 1988). Retinotopically corresponding regions of V1 and V2 are reciprocally connected in the monkey. V1 provides a crucial input to V2, in the sense that visual activation of V2 cells depends on input from V1. This dependency has been demonstrated by deactivating (reversibly cooling) V1, while recording from V2 during visual stimulation. In contrast, cooling V2 has a more *modulatory* effect on V1 activity. The cells in V1 that were most affected by V2 deactivation were in the infragranular layers, suggesting V2 may use this pathway to modulate the output from V1 (Sandell and Schiller, 1982). Because, in the absence of V1 input, these re-entrant connections do not constitute an efficient drive to V2 cells, their role is most likely 'to modulate the information relayed through area 17'.

To examine the interactions between V1 and V2, using fMRI in humans, it is possible to use a non-linear model of effective connectivity, extended to include a modulatory interaction (cf. eqn (16.1)):

$$V1 = M.c_o + \text{diag}(V1)\, Mc_M + e \qquad (16.2)$$

where diag(V1) refers to a diagonal matrix with elements in the vector V1; this premultiplies the (scan × region) matrix M so that each region's contribution to the model is affected by the activity in V1.

This model has two terms that allow for the activity in area V1 to be influenced by the activity in other areas M (our hypothesis being that V2 is prominent amongst those areas). The first represents an effect that depends only on afferent input from other areas M. This is the activity in M scaled by c_o. The coefficients in c_o are referred to as *obligatory* or driving connection strengths, in the sense that a change in areas M results in an *obligatory* response in area V1. This is similar to c in the simple linear model above. Conversely the second term reflects a *modulatory* influence of areas M on area V1. The coefficient determining the size of this effect (c_M) is referred to as a *modulatory* connection strength, because the overall effect depends on both the afferent input ($M.c_M$) and intrinsic activity in V1. This effect can be considered as a greater responsiveness of V1 to inputs with higher intrinsic activation of V1.

This intrinsic activity-dependent effect, determined by the value of c_M, provides an intuitive sense of how to estimate c_M. Imagine one were able to 'fix' the activity in V1 at a *low* level and measure the connectivity between the regions in M and V1 assuming a simple linear relationship (eqn (16.1)): A value for the sensitivity of V1 to changes elsewhere could be obtained, say c_1. Now, if the procedure were repeated with V1 activity fixed at a *high* level, a second (linear) estimate would be obtained, say c_2. In the presence of a substantial modulatory interaction between regions in M and V1 the second estimate (c_2) will be higher than the first (c_1). This is because the activity intrinsic to V1 is higher and V1 should be more sensitive to inputs. In short $c_2 - c_1$ provides an estimate of the modulatory influence on V1 (similarly $c_1 + c_2$ is related to c_o). By analogy to reversible cooling which allows one to remove the effects of isolated cortical regions, we 'fix' activity *post hoc* by simply selecting a subset of data in which the V1 activity is confined to some small range (*high* or *low* activity).

A relevant example analysis is now described. The data used in this analysis were a time-series of 64 gradient-echo EPI 5 mm coronal slices through the calcarine sulcus and extrastriate areas. Images were obtained every 3 s from a normal male subject using a 4T whole body system. Photic stimulation (at 16 Hz) was provided by goggles fitted with light emitting diodes. The stimulation was off for the first 30 s, on for the second 30 s, off for the third, and so on. The first four scans were removed to eliminate saturation effects and the remainder were realigned.

A reference voxel was chosen in right *V1* and the effective connection strengths c_M were estimated allowing a map of c_M (and c_o) to be constructed. This map provides a direct test of the hypothesis concerning the topography and regional specificity of modulatory influences on *V1*. The lower row in Fig. 16.1 shows maps of c_O and c_M (neurological convention—right *V1* is marked); these reflect the degree to which the area exerts an obligatory (left) or modulatory (right) effect on *V1* activity. These maps have been thresholded at 1.64 after normalization to a standard deviation of unity. This corresponds to an uncorrected threshold of $p < 0.05$.

The obligatory connections to the reference voxel derive mainly from *V1* itself, both ipsilaterally and contralaterally with a small contribution from contiguous portions of *V2*. The effective connectivity from contralateral *V1* should not be over-interpreted given that (i) the source of many afferents to *V1* (the lateral geniculate nuclei) were not included in the field of view and that (ii) this finding can be more parsimoniously explained by 'common input'. As predicted, and with remarkable regional specificity, the modulatory connections were most marked from ipsilateral *V2*, dorsal and ventral to the calcarine fissure (note that 'common input' cannot explain interactions between *V1* and *V2* because the geniculate inputs are largely restricted to *V1*).

To address functional asymmetry[1] in terms of forward and backward modulatory influences the modulatory connection strengths between two extended regions (two 5×5 voxel squares) in ipsilateral *V1* and *V2* were examined. The estimates of effective connection strengths were based on hemodynamic

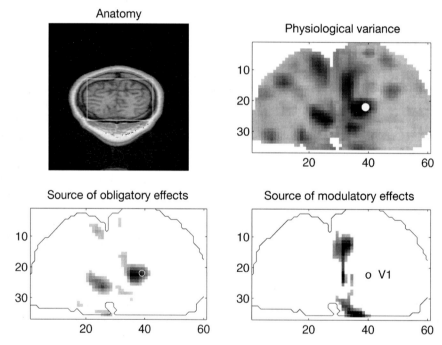

Fig. 16.1 Maps of the estimates of obligatory and modulatory connection strengths to right *V1*. *Top left*: Anatomical features of the coronal data used. This image is a high resolution anatomical MRI scan of the subject that corresponds to the fMRI slices. The box defines the position of a sub-partition of the fMRI time-series selected for analysis. *Top right*: The location of the reference voxel designated as right *V1* (white dot). This location is shown on a statistical parametric map of physiological variance (calculated for each voxel from the time-series of 60 scans). *Lower left and lower right*: Maps of c_O and c_M. The images have been scaled to unit variance and thresholded at p = 0.05 (assuming, under the null hypothesis of no effective connectivity, the estimates have a Gaussian distribution). The reference voxel in *V1* is depicted by a circle. The key thing to note is that *V1* is subject to modulatory influences from ipsilateral and extensive regions of *V2*.

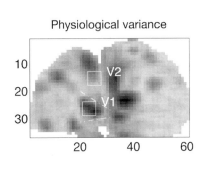
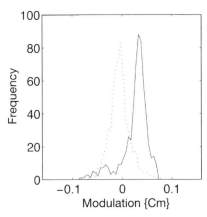

Fig. 16.2 Graphical presentation of a direct test of the hypothesis concerning the asymmetry between forward and backward *V1–V2* interactions. Left: a map of physiological variance showing the positions of two boxes defining regions in left *V1* and *V2*. The broken lines correspond (roughly) to the position of the *V1/V2* border according to the atlas of (Talairach and Tournoux 1988). The value of c_M was computed for all voxels in each box and normalized to unity over the image. The frequency distribution of c_M connecting the two regions is presented on the right. The modulatory backward connections (*V2* to *V1*—solid line) are clearly higher than the modulatory forward connections (*V1* to *V2*—broken line).

changes in all areas and the subset of connections between the two regions were selected to compare the distributions of forward and backward modulatory influences. Fig. 16.2 shows the location of the two regions (this time on the left) and the frequency distribution (i.e. histogram) of the estimates for connections from the voxels in the *V1* box to the *V2* box (broken line) and the corresponding estimates for connections from voxels in the *V2* box to *V1* (solid line). There is a remarkable dissociation, with backward modulatory effects (*V2* to *V1*) being much greater than forward effects (*V1* to *V2*). This can be considered a confirmation of the functional asymmetry hypothesis.

16.3.2 Structural equation modelling

The simple model above was sufficient to analyse effective connectivity to one region at a time (e.g. *V1* or *V2*). We will now introduce structural equation modelling as a tool allowing for more complicated models comprising many regions of interest and demonstrate how non-linear interactions are dealt with in this context. The basic idea behind structural equation modelling

(SEM) differs from the usual statistical approach of modelling individual observations. In multiple regression or AnCova models the regression coefficients derive from the minimisation of the sum of squared differences of the predicted and observed dependent variables (i.e. activity in the target region). Structural equation modelling approaches the data from a different perspective; instead of considering variables individually, the emphasis lies on the variance-covariance structure.[2] Thus models are solved in structural equation modelling by minimising the difference between the observed variance-covariance structure and the one implied by a structural or path model. In the past few years structural equation modelling has been applied to functional brain imaging. For example (McIntosh *et al.* 1994), demonstrated the dissociation between ventral and dorsal visual pathways for object and spatial vision using structural equation modelling of PET data in the human. In this section we will focus on the theoretical background of structural equation modelling and demonstrate this technique using fMRI.

In terms of neuronal systems a measure of covariance represents the degree to which the activities of

---

[1] Here we are referring to asymmetry in connections, not asymmetry between hemispheres.

[2] The variance–covariance structure describes in detail the dependencies between the different variables (in this case, the measured regional responses to stimulation).

two or more regions are related (i.e. functional connectivity). The study of variance–covariance structures here is much simpler than in many other fields; the interconnection of the dependent variables (regional activity of brain areas) is anatomically determined and the activation of each region can be directly measured with functional brain imaging. This represents a major difference to 'classical' structural equation modelling in the behavioural sciences, where models are often hypothetical and include latent variables denoting rather abstract concepts like intelligence.

As mentioned above, structural equation modelling minimizes the difference between the observed or measured covariance matrix and the one that is implied by the structure of the model. The free parameters (path coefficients or connection strengths c above) are adjusted to minimize the difference[3] between the measured and modelled covariance matrix (see Büchel and Friston (1997) for details).

An important issue in structural equation modelling is the determination of the participating regions and the underlying anatomical model. Several approaches to this issue can be adopted. These include categorical comparisons between different conditions, statistical images highlighting structures of functional connectivity and non-human electrophysiological and anatomical studies (McIntosh and Gonzalez-Lima 1994).

With respect to anatomical connectivity in humans, the advent of new MR techniques promises a better characterization of neuronal connectivity in humans. Diffusion tensor imaging (DTI) measures the anisotropy of diffusion in the brain. The main anisotropy exists in the white matter because the orientation of neuronal fibres (axons) allows molecules to diffuse easier along the fibre than in other directions. Therefore the main direction of the diffusion tensor reflects the underlying orientation of white matter tracts. Through tracing algorithms it is now possible to infer the connectivity of individual regions (e.g. activations derived from an fMRI study) in an individual brain.

A model is always a simplification of reality; exhaustively correct models either do not exist, or would be too complicated to understand. In the context of effec-tive connectivity one has to find a compromise between complexity, anatomical accuracy and interpretability. There are also mathematical constraints on the model; if the number of free parameters exceeds the number of observed covariances the system is underdetermined and no single solution exists.

Each estimated model can be analysed to give an overall goodness of fit measure, for use when comparing different models with each other. A 'nested model' approach can be used to compare different models (e.g. data from different groups or conditions) in the context of structural equation modelling. A so-called 'null-model' is constructed where the estimates of the free parameters are constrained to be the same for both groups. The alternative model allows free parameters to differ between groups. The significance of the differences between the models is expressed by the difference of the goodness of fit statistic. Consider the following hypothetical example. Subjects are scanned under two different conditions, e.g. 'attention' and 'no attention'. The hypothesis might be that within a system of regions A, B, C and D, the connectivity between A and B is different under the two attentional conditions. To determine whether the difference in connectivity is statistically significant, we estimate the goodness of fit measure for two models: Model 1 allows the connectivity between A and B to take different values for both conditions. Model 2 constrains the path coefficient between A and B to be equal for 'attention' and 'no attention'. If the change of connectivity between 'attention' and 'no attention' for the connection of A and B is negligible, the constrained model (Model 2) should fit the data equally well compared to the free model (Model 1). We can now infer whether the difference of the two goodness of fit measures is significant. Non-linear models can also be accommodated in the framework of SEM by introducing additional variables containing a non-linear function (e.g. $f(x) = x^2$) of the original variables (Kenny and Judd 1984). Interactions of variables can be incorporated in a similar fashion, wherein a new variable, containing the product of the two interacting variables, is introduced as an additional influence. This is similar to the approach used in the previous section, where the interaction was expressed by the influence of

---

[3] The free parameters are estimated by minimizing a function of the observed and implied covariance matrix. To date the most widely used objective function in structural equation modelling is the maximum likelihood (ML) function.

the product of *V1* and *V2* on *V1*. We will now demonstrate these ideas using an example. More details of structural equation modelling, including the operational equations can be found in Büchel and Friston (1997).

Example—learning

In this first example we were interested in changes in effective connectivity over time as expected during paired associates learning (Büchel *et al.* 1999). In the case of object-location memory, several functional studies have demonstrated activation of ventral occipital and temporal regions during the retrieval of object identity and, conversely, increased responses in dorsal parietal areas during the retrieval of spatial location (Milner *et al.* 1997). These results suggest domain-specific representations in posterior neocortical structures, closely related to those involved in perception, a finding that accords with the segregation of ventral and dorsal pathways in processing categorical or spatial stimulus features, respectively. Another phenomenon observed in some learning studies is a decrease of neural responses (i.e. adaptation) to repeated stimulus presentations. This repetition suppression has been replicated consistently in primate electrophysiological and human functional imaging studies (Desimone 1996). For object-location learning, it is intuitively likely that two specialized systems need to interact to establish an association. Domain-specific representations or repetition suppression are not sufficient to account for this associative component. In other words, functional segregation and localized response properties cannot account for associative learning alone.

In our fMRI experiment, decreases in activation during learning, indicative of repetition suppression, were observed in several cortical regions in the ventral and dorsal visual pathway. Within the framework of repetition suppression it has been hypothesized that decreases in neural responses are a secondary result of enhanced response selectivity (Wiggs and Martin 1998). By analogy to the development and plasticity of cortical architectures, this refined selectivity is likely to be due to changes in effective connectivity within the system at a synaptic level. We explicitly addressed this notion by characterizing time-dependent changes in effective connectivity during learning.

The experiment was performed on a 2T MRI system equipped with a head volume coil. fMRI images were obtained every 4.1 s with echo planar imaging (48 slices in each volume). Six subjects had to learn, and recall, the association between 10 simple line drawings of real world objects and 10 locations on a screen during fMRI. Each learning trial consisted of four conditions, 'encoding', 'control', 'retrieval' and 'control' (Fig. 16.3(a)). The behavioural data acquired during 'Retrieval' demonstrated that all six subjects were able to learn the association between object identity and spatial location, for all 10 objects, within eight learning blocks, as indicated by the ensuing asymptotic learning curves (Fig. 16.3(b)).

The structural model used in the analysis embodies connections within and across ventral and dorsal visual pathways and was based on anatomical studies in primates (Figure 16.3(c)). Primary visual cortex was modelled as the origin of both pathways. In addition to 'interstream' connections between dorsal extrastriate cortex (DE) and the fusiform region (ITp) and between the posterior parietal cortex (PP) and ITp, we included direct connections based on a hierarchical cortical organization. Given our hypothesis relating to changes in effective connectivity between dorsal and ventral pathways, the path analysis focused on the connection between posterior parietal cortex (PP, dorsal stream) and posterior inferotemporal cortex (ITp, ventral stream). We divided each learning session into EARLY (first part) and LATE observations (second part) and estimated separate path coefficients for each partition.

The path coefficient between PP and ITp increased significantly during learning in the group (p < 0.05) and was confirmed by an analysis of individual subjects showing an increase in effective connectivity between PP and ITp of 0.27. In contrast to the connections between streams, connections within the dorsal pathway decreased over time.

The estimated change in connectivity from PP to ITp clearly depended on the cut-off point between EARLY and LATE. To unequivocally establish a relationship between neurophysiologically mediated changes in connectivity and behavioural learning, we examined the relationship between the temporal pattern of effective connectivity changes and learning speed for all sessions and subjects. We estimated the differences in effective connectivity for seven EARLY and LATE partitions, by successively shifting the cut-off. The cut-

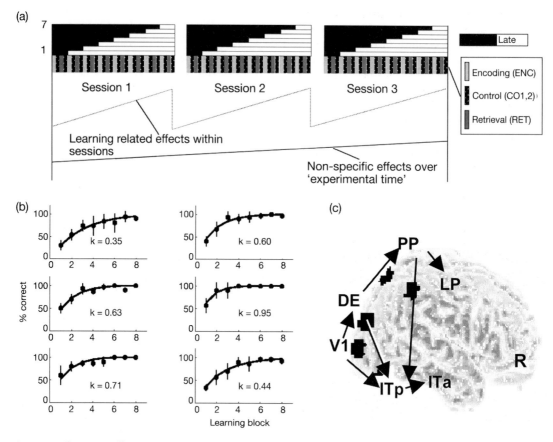

Fig. 16.3 Changes in effective connectivity over time in paired associates learning. (a) the design of the study. Blocks of 'encoding' and 'retrieval' were alternated by control conditions. Subjects had to perform three individual learning sessions, to avoid the confounding effect of time. (b) the behavioural performance data for each of the six subjects averaged across all three learning sessions. (c) the anatomical model. Processing of object identity is mainly a property of the ventral visual pathway, whereas object location is a property of the dorsal stream. We focussed on the interstream connections (mainly PP to ITp) based on the hypothesis that learning the association of object identity and spatial location will lead to an increase in effective connectivity between the ventral and the dorsal stream.

off time at which the connectivity change peaked was used as a temporal index of changes in effective connectivity (i.e. plasticity). The significant regression of k, a measure of learning speed,[4] on this plasticity index indicated that for sessions showing fast learning (i.e. high k) the maximum difference in path coefficients between PP and ITp was achieved earlier in the session (i.e. EARLY comprises less scans relative to LATE) (Fig. 16.4). In other words, the temporal

pattern of changes in effective connectivity strongly predicted learning or acquisition.

Example—attention

Electrophysiological and neuroimaging studies have shown that attention to visual motion can increase the responsiveness of the motion-selective cortical area V5 (O'Craven and Savoy 1995; Treue and Maunsell

---

[4] All individual behavioural learning curves were well approximated by the function $1 - e^{-kx}$ where $0 < k < 1$ indexes learning speed. Small values of k indicate slower learning.

1996) and the posterior parietal cortex (PP) (Assad and Maunsell 1995). Increased or decreased activation in a cortical area is often attributed to attentional modulation of the cortical projections to that area. This leads to the notion that attention is associated with changes in connectivity.

Here we present fMRI data from an individual subject, scanned under identical visual motion stimulus conditions, while changing only the attentional component of the tasks employed. First, we identify regions that show differential activations in relation to attentional set. In the second stage, changes in effective connectivity to these areas are assessed using structural equation modelling. Finally, we show how these attention-dependent changes in effective connectivity can be explained by the modulatory influence of parietal areas using a non-linear extension of structural equation modelling. The specific hypothesis we addressed was that parietal cortex could modulate the inputs from $V1$ to $V5$.

The experiment was performed on a 2T MRI system equipped with a head volume coil. fMRI images were obtained every 3.2 s with echo-planar imaging (32 slices in each volume). The subject was scanned during four different conditions: 'fixation', attention', 'no attention' and 'stationary'. Each condition lasted 32 s giving 10 volumes per condition. We acquired a total of 360 images. During all conditions the subjects looked at a fixation point in the middle of a screen. In this section we are only interested in the two conditions with visual motion ('attention' and 'no attention'), where 250 small white dots moved radially from the fixation point, in random directions, towards the border of the screen, at a constant speed of $4.7°$ per second. The difference between 'attention' and 'no attention' lay in the explicit command given to the subject shortly before the condition: 'just look' indicated 'no attention' and 'detect changes' the 'attention' condition. Both visual motion conditions were interleaved with 'fixation'. No response was required.

Regions of interest were defined by categorical comparisons using an output statistical image ('SPMZ'), comparing 'attention' and 'no attention', and 'no attention' and 'fixation'. As predicted, given a stimulus consisting of radially moving dots, we found activation of the lateral geniculate nucleus (LGN), primary visual cortex ($V1$), motion sensitive area $V5$ and the posterior parietal complex (PP). For the subsequent analysis of

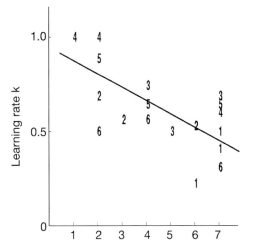

Length of EARLY (in learning blocks) that maximised the EARLY vs. LATE difference in connectivity between PP and ITp

Fig. 16.4 Changes in effective connectivity predict learning. This graph shows the correlation between the temporal index of change in effective connectivity and learning. The temporal index is defined as the time of a maximum increase in effective connectivity between PP and ITp. For example, a temporal index of three indicates that the maximum increase in effective connectivity occurred between the third and fourth blocks. The numbers denote the subject from which this temporal index of effective connectivity was obtained. Each subject was scanned during three independent learning sessions, therefore each number appears three times. A negative slope means that the maximum increase in effective connectivity occurs earlier in fast learning.

effective connectivity, we defined regions of interest (ROI) with a diameter of 8 mm, centred around the most significant voxel as revealed by the categorical comparison. A single time-series, representative of this region, was defined by the first eigenvector of all the voxels in the ROI (Büchel and Friston, 1997).

Our model of the dorsal visual stream included the LGN, primary visual cortex ($V1$), $V5$ and the posterior parietal complex (PP). Although connections between regions are generally reciprocal, for simplicity we only modelled unidirectional paths.

To assess effective connectivity in a condition-specific fashion, we used time-series that comprised observations during the condition in question. Path coefficients for both conditions ('attention' and 'no attention') were estimated using a maximum likeli-

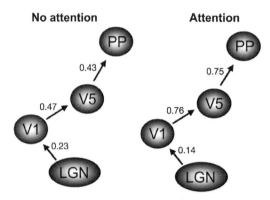

Fig. 16.5 Structural equation model of the dorsal visual pathway, comparing 'attention' and 'no attention'. Connectivity between right V1 and V5 is increased during 'attention' relative to 'no attention'. This is also shown for the connection between V5 and PP.

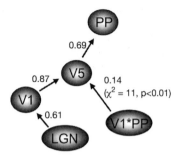

Fig. 16.6 Structural equation model of the dorsal visual pathway incorporating the interaction of right PP on the connection from right V1 to V5.

hood function. To test for the impact of changes in effective connectivity between 'attention' and 'no attention', we defined a free model (allowing different path coefficients between V1 and V5 for 'attention and no attention') and a constrained model (constraining the V1 → V5 coefficients to be equal). Figure 16.5 shows the free model and the estimated path coefficients. The connectivity between V1 and V5 increases significantly during attention. Note that there is also a significant difference in connectivity between V5 and PP.

The linear path model comparing 'attention' and 'no attention' revealed increased effective connectivity in the dorsal visual pathway in relation to attention. The question that arises is: Which part of the brain is capable of modulating this pathway? Based on lesion studies (Lawler and Cowey 1987) and on the system for directed attention as described in (Mesulam 1990), the posterior parietal cortex is hypothesized to play such a modulatory role.

We extended our model accordingly to allow for non-linear interactions, testing the hypothesis that the PP acts as a moderator of the connectivity between V1 and V5. Assuming a non-linear modulation of this connection, we constructed a new variable 'V1PP' in our analysis. This variable, mediating the interaction, is simply the time-series from region V1 multiplied (element by element) by the time-series of the right posterior parietal region.

The influence of this new variable on V5 corresponds to the influence of the posterior parietal cortex on the connection between V1 and V5 (i.e. the influence of V1 on V5 is greater when activity in PP is high). The model is shown in Fig. 16.6. Because our non-linear model could accommodate changes in connectivity between 'attention' and 'no attention', the entire time-series was analysed (i.e. attention-specific changes are now explicitly modelled by the interaction term).

As in the linear model, we tested for the significance of the interaction effect by comparing a restricted and free model. In the restricted model the interaction term (i.e. path from V1PP to V5) was set to zero. Omitting the interaction term led to a significantly reduced model fit (p < 0.01), indicating the predictive value of the interaction term.

The presence of an interaction effect of the PP on the connection between V1 and V5 can also be illustrated by a simple regression analysis. If PP shows a positive modulatory influence on the path between V1 and V5, the influence of V1 on V5 should depend on the activity of PP. This can be tested, by splitting the observations into two sets, one containing observations in which PP activity is high and another one in which PP activity is low. It is now possible to perform separate regressions of V5 on V1 using both sets. If the hypothesis of positive modulation is true, the slope of the regression of V5 on V1 should be steeper under high values of PP. This approach is comparable to the one outlined in the first section, where we used high and low values to demonstrate a modulatory effect of activity intrinsic to V1 on the influence V2 has over V1.

16.3.3 Variable parameter regression

As demonstrated in previous sections, the basic linear model can be seen as a linear regression. The regression coefficient is then interpreted as a measure of the connectivity between areas. This interpretation of course implies that the influence is mediated by neural connections with an effective strength equal to the regression coefficient. Using this approach one immediately makes the assumption that the effective connectivity does not change over observations, because only a single regression coefficient for the whole time-series is estimated. This is unsuitable for the assessment of effective connectivity in functional imaging, as the goal in some experiments is to demonstrate changes in effective connectivity, for instance as a function of different conditions (e.g. 'attention' and 'no attention') or simply time itself. In the framework of regression analysis there are three ways to solve this problem. First, one could split up the data in different groups according to the experimental condition (e.g. 'attention' and 'no attention'), and then test for the difference of the regression coefficients. However, we may not know a priori the time-course of the changes that allow us to split the data in this way. A second, more general solution, is to expand the explanatory variable in terms of a set of basis functions to account for changes in connectivity. Here, we will present another alternative, variable parameter regression (VPR), which allows one to characterize the variation of the regression coefficient using the framework of state-space models and the Kalman filter (Kalman 1960).

Mathematical background

Consider the classical regression model

$$y = x\beta + u \tag{16.3}$$

where y is the measured data vector, x is a vector of explanatory variables and β is the unknown parameter. Usually β is estimated as

$$\hat{\beta} = \text{pinv}(x)y \tag{16.4}$$

where $\text{pinv}(x)$ is normally the Moore–Penrose pseudo-inverse, an optimal way of inverting a non-square matrix within the context of least-squares fitting. However, β can also be estimated recursively with the

advantage that inversion of a smaller matrix is necessary. This approach is known as recursive least squares (Harvey 1993). This basic model is now extended to allow β to evolve over time. Variable parameter regression assumes T ordered scalar observations $(y_1, \dots y_T)$ generated by the model:

$$y_t = x_t\beta_t + u_t, \quad t = 1, \dots, \text{T}, \tag{16.5}$$

$$u_t \sim N(0, \sigma^2) \tag{16.6}$$

where x_t is an n-dimensional row vector of known regressors and β_t is an n-dimensional column vector of unknown coefficients that corresponds to estimates of effective connectivity. u_t is drawn from a Gaussian distribution. All observations are expressed as deviations from the mean.

A recursive algorithm known as the Kalman filter (Kalman 1960) can now be applied to estimate the state-variable (β) at each point in time and also allows one to estimate the log-likelihood function of the model. A numerical optimization algorithm is then employed to maximize the likelihood function with respect to P. As the Kalman filter is a recursive procedure, the estimation of β_t is based on all observations up to time t. Therefore the filtered estimates will be more accurate towards the end of the sample. This fact is corrected for by the Kalman smoothing algorithm which is employed *post hoc* and runs backwards in time, taking account of the information made available after time t. Details of the Kalman filter and smoothing recursions can be found in standard textbooks of time-series analysis and econometrics (e.g. Chow 1983; Harvey 1990).

Example—attention to visual motion

To illustrate VPR we use the single-subject data set from the attention-to-visual-motion study. We concentrate on the effect of attention on the connection between the motion sensitive area *V5* and the posterior parietal cortex (PP) in the right hemisphere. Using structural equation modelling, we have demonstrated that it is principally this connection, in the dorsal visual stream, that is modulated by attention (Büchel and Friston 1997). In the current analysis we were interested whether variable parameter regression was capable of reproducing these findings. We therefore

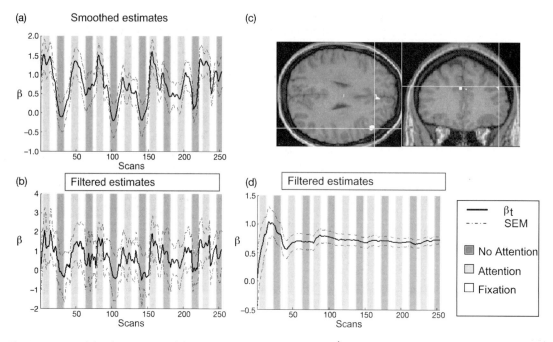

Fig. 16.7   (a) and (b) The trajectory of the smoothed and filtered estimates $\hat{\beta}_t(T)$ together with the associated standard errors for the variable parameter estimation of effective connectivity between V5 and PP. It is evident that $\hat{\beta}_t$ (the dynamic regression coefficient) is higher during the 'attention' conditions relative to the 'no attention' conditions. (c) Areas that significantly covaried with the time-dependent measure of effective connectivity between V5 and PP [i.e. $\hat{\beta}_t(T)$]. SPMZ thresholded at $p < 0.001$ (uncorrected) overlaid on coronal and axial slices of the subject's structural MRI. The maximum under the cross-hairs was at 45, 21, 39 mm, $Z = 4$. (d) The relationship between our technique and an ordinary regression analysis. In this analysis the variance term P was set to zero (i.e. fixed regression model). The trajectory of $\hat{\beta}_t$ now converges to β (= 0.73), the regression coefficient of the model $y = x\beta + u$.

assessed the effective connectivity β_t by regressing PP on V5. An alternate direction search, numerical optimization gave a chi-squared statistic of 56.4. We therefore had to reject the null-hypothesis of no variation at the 5 per cent level. P was estimated to be 0.074 and σ^2 was 0.23. The ordinary regression coefficient β for the model $y = x\beta + u$. was estimated at 0.73. Figure 16.7 (a and b) show the trajectories of the smoothed and filtered estimates $\hat{\beta}_t(T)$ together with the associated standard errors. It is clearly evident that $\hat{\beta}_t$ is higher during the 'attention' conditions relative to the 'no attention' conditions. Figure 16.7(d) relates our technique to an ordinary regression. In this analysis we constrained the variance term P to zero and re-estimated β_t. The trajectory of $\hat{\beta}_t$ now converges to β, the ordinary regression coefficient of the model $y = x\beta + u$. As expected the smoothed estimates are simply a constant (i.e. $\beta = 0.73$).

We interpret $\hat{\beta}_t$ as an index of effective connectivity between area V5 and the posterior parietal cortex. In our example, the connection between V5 and PP resembles the *site* of attention modulation. This leads to an interesting extension, where one might hypothesize that a third region is responsible for the observed variation in effective connectivity indicated by the trajectory of $\hat{\beta}_t(T)$. In other words after specifying the *site* and nature of attentional modulation we now want to know the location of the *source*. We addressed this by using $\hat{\beta}_t(T)$ as an explanatory variable in an ordinary regression analysis to identify voxels that covaried with this measure of effective connectivity. Figure 16.7(c) shows the result of this analysis. Among areas with statistically significant (p < 0.001, uncorrected) positive covariation was the dorsolateral prefrontal cortex and the anterior cingulate cortex. This result confirms the putative modulatory role of the dorsolateral prefrontal cortex in attention to visual motion, as suggested by previous analyses (Büchel and Friston 1997).

16.3.4 Effective connectivity versus categorical comparisons

One obvious advantage of the assessment of effective connectivity is that it allows one to test hypotheses about the integration of cortical areas. For example, in the presence of modulation, the categorical comparison between 'attention' and 'no attention' might reveal prestriate, parietal and frontal activations. However, the only statement possible is that these areas show higher cortical activity during the 'attention' condition as opposed to the 'no attention' condition. The analysis of effective connectivity revealed two additional results. First, attention affects the pathway from $V1$ to $V5$ and from $V5$ to PP. Second, the introduction of non-linear interaction terms allowed us to test a hypothesis about how these modulations are mediated. The latter analysis suggested that the posterior parietal cortex exerts a modulatory influence on area $V5$.

The measurements used in all examples in this chapter were *hemodynamic* in nature. This limits an interpretation at the level of *neuronal* interactions. However, the analogy between the form of the non-linear interactions described above and voltage-dependent (i.e. modulatory) connections is a strong one. It is possible that the modulatory impact of $V2$ on $V1$ (and of PP on $V5$) is mediated by predominantly voltage-dependent connections. The presence of horizontal voltage-dependent connections within $V1$ has been established in cat striate cortex (Hirsch and Gilbert 1991). We know of no direct electrophysiological evidence to suggest that extrinsic backward $V2$ to $V1$ connections are voltage-dependent; however, our results are consistent with this. An alternative explanation for modulatory effects, which does not necessarily involve voltage-dependent connections, can be found in the work of (Aertsen and Preissl 1991). These authors show that effective connectivity varies strongly with, or is modulated by, background neuronal activity. The mechanism relates to the efficacy of subthreshold EPSPs in establishing dynamic interactions. This efficacy is a function of post-synaptic depolarization, which in turn depends on the tonic background of activity.

16.4 Conclusions

This chapter has reviewed the basic concepts of effective connectivity in neuroimaging. We have introduced several methods to assess effective connectivity i.e. multiple linear regression, covariance structural equation modelling and variable parameter regression. The first example demonstrated that non-linear interactions can be characterized using simple extensions of linear models. In the second example structural equation modelling was introduced as a device that allows one to combine observed changes in cortical activity and anatomical models. The first example of this technique revealed changes in effective connectivity between the dorsal and the ventral stream over time in a paired-associates learning paradigm. The temporal pattern of these changes was highly correlated with individual learning performance and therefore changes in effective connectivity predicted learning speed. The second example of structural equation modelling focused on backwards modulatory influences of high order areas on connections among lower order areas. Both examples concentrated on changes in effective connectivity, and allowed us to characterize the interacting areas of the network at a functional level. Variable parameter regression was then introduced as a flexible regression technique, allowing the regression coefficient to smoothly vary over time. Again, we confirmed the backward modulatory effect of higher cortical areas on those areas situated lower in the cortical hierarchy. Although less than a mature field, the approach to neuroimaging data, and regional interactions, discussed above is an exciting endeavour that is starting to attract more and more attention.

References

Aertsen, A. and Preissl, H. (1991). Dynamics of activity and connectivity in physiological neuronal Networks. VCH publishers Inc., New York.

Assad, J.A. and Maunsell, J.H. (1995). Neuronal correlates of inferred motion in primate posterior parietal cortex. *Nature*, 373, 518–21.

Atkinson, R.C. and Shiffrin, R.M. (1968) Human memory: a proposed system and its control processes. In: *The psychology of learning and motivation: advances in research and theory*, Vol. 2, (ed. K.W. Spence and J.J. Spence). Academic Press, New York.

Büchel, C. and Friston, K.J. (1997) Modulation of connectivity in visual pathways by attention: Cortical interactions evaluated with structural equation modelling and fMRI. *Cerebral Cortex*, 7, 768–78.

Büchel, C., Coull, J.T., Friston, K.J. (1999) The predictive value of changes in effective connectivity for human learning. *Science*, 283, 1538–41.

Chow, G.C. (1983) *Econometrics*. McGraw Hill, New York.

Desimone, R. (1996) Neural mechanisms for visual memory and their role in attention. *PNAS*, 93, 13494–9.

Friston, K.J., Frith, C.D., and Frackowiak, R.S.J. (1993*a*) Time-dependent changes in effective connectivity measured with PET. *Human Brain Mapping*, 1, 69–80.

Friston, K.J., Frith, C.D., Liddle, P.F., and Frackowiak, R.S.J. (1993*b*). Funcational connectivity: The principal and component analysis of large (PET) data sets. *Journal of Cerebral Blood Flow in Metabolism*, 13, 5–14.

Friston, K.J., Ungerleider, L.G., Jezzard, P., and Turner, R. (1995) Characterizing modulatory interactions between $V1$ and $V2$ in human cortex with fMRI. *Human Brain Mapping*, 2, 211–24.

Gerstein, G.L., Bedenbaugh, P., and Aertsen, A. (1989) Neuronal assemblies. *IEEE Transactions on Biomedical Engineering*, 36, 4–14.

Gerstein, G.L., and Perkel, D.H. (1969) Simultaneously recorded trains of action potentials: analysis and functional interpretation. *Science*, 164, 828–30.

Girard, P. and Bullier, J. (1988) Visual activity in area $V2$ during reversible inactivation of area 17 in the macaque monkey. *Journal of Neurophysiology*, 62, 1287–1301.

Harvey, A.C. (1990) *Forecasting, structural time series models and the Kalman filter*, Cambridge University Press, Cambridge.

Harvey, A.C. (1993) *Time series models*. Harvester & Wheatsheaf, London.

Hirsch, J.A. and Gilbert, C.D. (1991). Synaptic physiology of horizontal connections in the cat's visual cortex. *Journal of Neuroscience*, 11, 1800–09.

Kalman, R.E. (1960) A new approach to linear filtering and prediction problems. *Transactions ASME Journal of Basic Engineering*, D82, 35–45.

Kenny, D.A. and Judd, C.M. (1984) Estimating nonlinear and interactive effects of latent variables. *Psychological Bulletin*, 96, 201–10.

Lashley, K.S. (1929). *Brain mechanisms and intelligence*. University of Chicago Press, Chicago.

Lawler, K.A. and Cowey, A. (1987) On the role of posterior parietal and prefrontal cortex in visuo-spatial perception and attention. *Experimental Brain Research*, 65, 695–8.

McIntosh, A.R. and Gonzalez-Lima, F. (1994). Structural equation modelling and its application to network analysis in functional brain imaging. *Human Brain Mapping*, 2, 2–22.

McIntosh, A.R., Grady, C.L., Ungerleider, L.G., Haxby, J.V., Rapoport, S.I., and Horwitz, B. (1994) Network analysis of cortical visual pathways mapped with PET. *Journal of Neuroscience*, 14, 655–66.

Marshall, J.C. and Newcombe, F. (1973) Patterns of paralexia: a neurolinguistic approach. *Journal of Psycholinguistic Research*, 2, 175–99.

Mesulam, M.M. (1990) Large-scale neurocognitive networks and distributed processing for attention, language, and memory. *Annals of Neurology*, 28, 597–613.

Milner, B., Johnsrude, I., and Crane, J. (1997) Right medial temporal-lobe contribution to object-location memory. *Philosophical Transactions of the Royal Society of London*, 352, 1469–74.

O'Craven, K.M. and Savoy, R.L. (1995) Voluntary attention can modulate fMRI activity in human MT/MST. *Investigative Ophthalmology and Visual Science*, (Suppl.) 36, S856.

Petersen, S.E., Fox, P.T., Snyder, A.Z., and Raichle, M.E. (1990). Activation of extrastriate and frontal cortical areas by words and word-like stimuli. *Science*, 249, 1041–4.

Posner, M.I., Petersen, S.E., Fox, P.T., and Raichle, M.E. (1988). Localization of cognitive operations in the human brain. *Science*, 240, 1627–31.

Sandell, J.H. and Schiller, P.H. (1982). Effect of cooling area 18 on striate cortex cells in the squirrel monkey. *Journal of Neurophysiology*, 48, 38–38.

Schiller, P.H. and Malpeli, J.G. (1977). The effect of striate cortex cooling on area 18 cells in the monkey. *Brain Research*, 126, 366–9.

Shallice, T. (1988). *From neuropsychology to mental structure*. Cambridge, Cambridge University Press.

Talairach, P. and Tournoux, J. (1988). *A stereotactic coplanar atlas of the human brain*. Thieme, Stuttgart.

Treue, S. and Maunsell, H.R. (1996). Attentional modulation of visual motion processing in cortical areas MT and MST. *Nature*, 382, 539–41.

Warrington, E.K. and Shallice, T. (1969). The selective impairment of auditory short term memory. *Brain*, 92, 885–96.

Wiggs, C.L. and Martin, A. (1998). Properties and mechanisms of perceptual priming. *Current Opinion in Neurobiology*, 8, 227–33.

V | *fMRI applications*

17 | *fMRI: applications to cognitive neuroscience*

Adrian M. Owen, Russell Epstein, and Ingrid S. Johnsrude

17.1 Introduction

Structural and functional imaging methods already have had an enormous impact on the way we assess human cognition *in vivo*. Detailed anatomical images, acquired through computerised tomography (CT) and magnetic resonance imaging (MRI), can now be combined with functional information from positron emission tomography (PET), functional magnetic resonance imaging (fMRI), quantitative electroencephalography (EEG), and magnetoencephalography (MEG) to produce a cohesive picture of normal and abnormal brain function. In less than a decade, the combination of high resolution structural MRI and fMRI in particular has become perhaps the single most powerful general pair of tools available to neuropsychologists, cognitive neuroscientists, and many others in the wider neuroscientific community with an interest in understanding the relationship between brain and behaviour.

This period has seen a rapid shift of emphasis in functional imaging away from PET 'activation studies' using H$_2$^{15}O methodology to fMRI. Not only is MRI more widely available than PET, but with no associated radiation burden, the new technology has quickly become an attractive alternative for large-scale cognitive studies in healthy volunteers. In addition, with the increased power afforded by fMRI, particularly at high field strengths, studies of brain activity in individual volunteers have become routine. Not only has this development largely negated the need for group 'averaging' within studies, but this also allows serial studies of responses in individual volunteers. One consequence is that many longer-term dynamic cognitive

processes, such as learning can be examined effectively (e.g. Karni *et al.* 1998). Undoubtedly however, it was the combined scientific promise of improved temporal and spatial resolution that most clearly established fMRI as a major tool for the study of human cognition.

In this chapter, there will be no attempt to provide an exhaustive review of fMRI studies of cognitive function or of the achievements of this field as a whole; while several reviews of this type have been attempted, they invariably occupy entire volumes and, in this rapidly evolving field, are long out-of-date even before they emerge from the publishing mill. Instead, we will focus paradigmatically on (i) areas where fMRI has *augmented* existing knowledge obtained using other techniques via the combination of its particular technical properties and their innovative application to the solution of diverse and novel problems in the field of human cognition and (ii) areas where fMRI has *superseded* alternative methodological approaches by providing more accurate, faster, safer or more cost effective information than was previously available.

As preceding chapters in this book have illustrated, MRI methods have matured rapidly and are continuing to evolve to allow better solutions to a broader variety of scientific questions. From within the cognitive neuroscience community, the impetus for much of this development has been the scientific questions themselves, with a clear emphasis on localization of function at the maximum possible spatial resolution. Broadly speaking, questions about functional localization of cognitive functions can be addressed using either subtractive methodology (PET or fMRI), correlational block designs (PET or fMRI) or event-related methods (fMRI only), and all of these procedures are described in detail elsewhere in this volume (see e.g. Chapter 9). In general terms, the increased effective power of high-field fMRI over PET activation studies means that such questions can be asked *within* an individual subject, allowing single-subject studies, group designs, or a mixture of the two to be implemented. Moreover, the superior temporal resolution of event-related fMRI designs over more traditional subtractive methods means that signal changes can be correlated with cognitive task performance on a trial-by-trial basis; in this way, differential time courses of activation within specific anatomical regions of interest may be examined and compared. Finally, fMRI can also be used to answer questions about functional connectivity (see Chapter 16); how activation in different cortical and sub-cortical regions covaries and how those relationships change with varying cognitive demands. In the sections that follow, we address each of these areas in turn, and evaluate their current relevance to, and future impact on, our understanding of normal cognitive function in humans.

17.2 Functional dissociation: an historical perspective

For many years, psychologists have sought to dissociate cognitive processes into multiple functional units or 'systems'. As an example, let us consider the field of human memory. Long-term versus short-term memory (or more recently, *working* memory), declarative (conscious or explicit) versus procedural (implicit) memory and semantic (knowledge) versus episodic (experiences) memory are popular dichotomies within the taxonomy of memory. Even within these groupings, further distinctions are often drawn; for example, between spatial working memory and non-spatial (e.g. verbal), working memory. Historically, a number of different methods have been employed in an attempt to map these putative functional models onto specific neural systems or anatomical regions, with varying degrees of success. For example, many contemporary cognitive models, including several of those relating to human memory, were derived from the study of the pattern of intellectual deficits that follows circumscribed cortical or sub-cortical excisions in patients. Unfortunately, however, in such patient studies it is often not possible to relate any particular cortical region to a given cognitive process with any degree of anatomical precision since the excisions are rarely confined to one, or even a few, cytoarchitectonic areas. In addition, structural and functional reorganisation of the cortex between the time of surgery and the subsequent neuropsychological test session may complicate matters still further. Electrophysiological studies in humans (EEG, ERP), have provided an alternative approach for investigating issues of functional localization and, when carried out in healthy individuals, can provide important information about 'normal' cognition with a high level of temporal resolution. Unfortunately, electrophysiological techniques suffer from poor spatial resolution, except in those exceptional circumstances where they can be used intraoperatively in patients.

The advent of high-resolution functional neuroimaging provided a possible solution to many of these problems, with PET activation studies rapidly becoming the early 'gold standard' for examining whether components of contemporary cognitive models are functionally localisable within the human brain. PET activation studies, by their very nature, required 'block' designs, usually of between 60 and 90 s duration, and throughout this period participants would perform a cognitive or sensory-motor task of interest. Comparisons between 'experimental scans' (involving the cognitive task of interest), and 'control scans' (usually involving a more basic visual/motor control task), yielded an indirect measure (regional cerebral blood flow), of the neural activity associated with the cognitive process under investigation. Critically, however, the PET activation method does not allow for the decomposition of this lengthy acquisition time into more psychologically meaningful temporal units. Thus, the derived estimates of local cortical blood flow represent the total accumulative effect of all of those cognitive, motor and perceptual processes taking place within the broad acquisition period. Therefore, since most cognitive processes occur over periods of milliseconds, rather than minutes, the temporal resolution of the technique has always been very poor. In spite of this clear limitation, many PET activation studies employed block designs to great effect and, as a consequence, this approach provided a natural starting point for many early fMRI studies.

17.3 fMRI and functional localization

Like PET activation studies, block design (or state-related; Friston *et al.* 1998) fMRI generally involves relatively lengthy 'epochs' of different conditions. Unlike PET activation studies, these conditions are often alternated with each other during the scanning session. For example, in one of the first experiments of this type (Kwong *et al.* 1992), 60 s 'blocks' of 8-Hz photic stimulation were alternated with 60 s 'blocks' of 'rest', in which no visual stimulation occurred. Comparison of the two conditions confirmed that the visual cortex was more active during visual stimulation than during rest. The basic theoretical assumption behind the design and analysis of this, and almost all subsequent fMRI experiments (both blocked and event-related) has been that of *cognitive subtraction*. If two conditions, A and B, are identical except that A requires a particular cognitive function *f* while B does not, then one can theoretically identify those cortical regions that are involved in *f* by subtracting the MR response during B from that during A. In general, the conditions, A and B, can differ in one of two ways. On the one hand, the stimuli presented during the two conditions may be identical, but the participants may be required to perform different tasks during each. On the other hand, the participants may be presented with different kinds of stimuli in each condition, but the task that they are required to perform may be identical. As one might expect, the latter method has been most widely used for studying the neural basis of perception, while most studies of non-perceptual processes have used the former approach.

In either case, however, the difficulty with cognitive subtraction is that the conditions employed frequently differ in several ways, some of which may not be interesting or obvious to the experimenter, but nevertheless elicit specific signal changes in the brain. This potential confound can be minimized in two ways; (i) one can systematically reduce the number of potential explanations for an observed effect by making the two conditions as similar as possible in all respects *except* for the dimension of interest. The problem with this approach, when used alone and/or early in an exploratory series of experiments is that two very similar

conditions may elicit no consistent difference in signal. (ii) in addition, however, converging evidence from comparisons between multiple conditions can be used to demonstrate that activation will be observed in a given target region whenever two conditions differ in one critical dimension, regardless of other non-specific differences between those two tasks. Unlike PET, fMRI is particularly well suited for this method of multiple comparisons, since experimental runs are not limited to only a few comparisons per session. Indeed, some fMRI experiments have used as many as eight different psychological conditions within a single session (e.g. Epstein and Kanwisher, 1998).

Using fMRI, it has become easier to use a systematic, hypothesis-driven approach to task design, employing the subtraction technique in a coarse-to-fine progression of comparisons between related conditions. Such studies usually begin by comparing two conditions that differ quite clearly along some dimension of interest, before focussing more precisely on what it is about the coarse comparison that drives the observed difference in MR activation. Face perception provides a paradigmatic example. Neuropsychological evidence from brain-damaged patients has long since suggested a role for the right occipital-temporal-lobe region in face recognition: patients suffering from prosopagnosia (the inability to recognize faces), frequently have damage to this region of cortex. Activation in what has often been referred to as 'the human face area' was also observed in many early PET studies that required participants to view face stimuli (e.g. Haxby *et al.* 1994), and, more recently, in a number of studies using fMRI. For example, Puce *et al.* (1995), reported that fMRI signal changes within a region of the right mid-fusiform gyrus were greater during blocked events in which subjects were required to view photographs of faces than during blocks in which they viewed equiluminant scrambled faces. In a follow-up study, Puce *et al.* (1996), compared signal changes between two different classes of meaningful visual stimuli, faces and letter-strings. The MR response during the face blocks was greater in some cortical regions (mid-fusiform gyrus, right occipitotemporal region, and middle temporal gyrus), while the MR response during letter-string blocks was greater in others (left occipital temporal sulcus and superior occipital sulcus). Although neither of these studies actually proves that the right fusiform gyrus is involved in face processing *per se* (for example, similar signal changes might well have been observed with any class of three-dimensional object), they did confirm that this region, among others, is more involved in the processing of meaningful objects than in the processing of nonsense visual patterns or letter-strings.

Kanwisher *et al.* (1997), extended these preliminary findings by identifying a cluster of voxels in the right middle fusiform gyrus that was consistently more active in 80 per cent of participants when they were viewing photographs of faces than when they were viewing photographs of common objects. Crucially, both sets of stimuli used were similar along many dimensions that are probably important for low- and mid-level vision, including that they both depicted interpretable, meaningful three-dimensional entities. The face > object comparison was then used to functionally define a putative 'fusiform face area' (FFA) in each of the participants and activity in this region was examined during additional tasks that involved different kinds of stimuli. For example, the hypothesis that the FFA might be involved in distinguishing between exemplars of a homogeneous object set was examined by comparing responses to faces with responses to houses. Despite the fact that both faces and houses are single basic-level object categories, the FFA response to faces was much greater. Similarly, the FFA response to pictures of faces was found to be significantly greater than response to pictures of hands, confirming that the FFA does not simply respond equally to any part of the body (see also Kanwisher *et al.* 1999). Thus, using only a systematic series of block design studies, Kanwisher *et al.* (1997; 1999), were able to conclude that the FFA was selectively involved in 'face perception', a result which clearly confirms a hypothesis that was originally, but inconclusively, derived from neuropsychological data in patients.

It is important to note that Kanwisher's results do not specify the precise role that the FFA plays in face perception. In general, a selective response to a specific stimulus category can result from at least two different kinds of cognitive process (Gauthier 2000). On the one hand, the brain region in question might be involved in processing a specific kind of perceptual information that is characteristic of that stimulus category. For example, one might argue that the FFA is specifically

involved in representing convex, rounded objects with protrusions in the right places (i.e. objects that look like faces), or some other low-level visual feature of faces (Ishai *et al.* 1999). On the other hand, this region might be involved in a specific kind of computation that is preferentially performed on that stimulus category. For example, Gauthier and colleagues have argued that the function of the FFA is not face perception *per se*, but subordinate level classification of objects for which the observer has expertise (Tarr and Gauthier 2000). According to that view, the large response in the FFA to faces simply reflects the fact that faces are almost always classified at the subordinate level rather than at the basic level (i.e. 'John's face' vs. 'a face'), and the fact that we are all face experts.

In short, one can either characterize the response of a given region in terms of the information processed by that region, or in terms of the cognitive operation performed on that information. A good deal of fMRI research involves attempts to reconcile these two competing kinds of hypotheses. As an example, many researchers have made claims about the relative functional contributions of the dorsolateral and ventrolateral regions of the frontal lobes to aspects of mnemonic processing (for review, see Owen 2000). These claims generally come in two flavours: either distinctions are drawn between the different kinds of information (e.g. spatial vs. non-spatial) processed by these particular regions (e.g. Goldman-Rakic 1994), or between the different kinds of specific (often polymodal) computations (e.g. retrieval vs. monitoring) performed by these regions (e.g. Petrides 1994; Owen 2000).

In a manner similar to that adopted by Kanwisher *et al.* (1997, 1999), above, the functional contributions of a number of other key cortical sites are being unravelled through a combination of existing neuropsychological data and more recent studies using fMRI. In this respect, it is those instances where the existing neuropsychology *would not* have predicted the fMRI results that perhaps yield the most interesting information. For example, for a number of years parahippocampal cortex has been implicated in topographical processing. This conclusion was based, originally, on the behaviour of a small number of patients who acquired difficulties with spatial navigation following damage to this region (Habib and Sirigu 1987; Aguirre and D'Esposito 1999; Barrash *et al.* 2000).

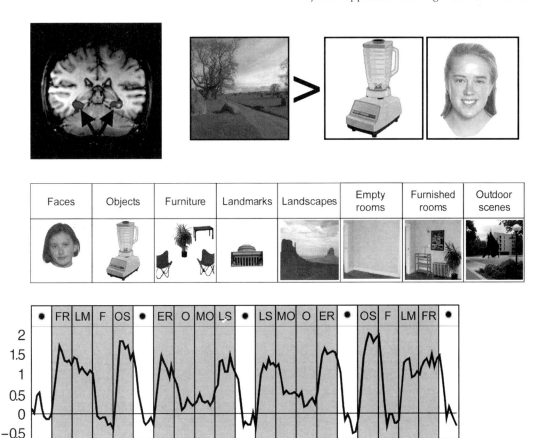

Fig. 17.1 Top panel: fMRI reveals a bilateral region in parahippocampal cortex that responds significantly more to scenes than to faces or objects. This region, the 'parahippocampal place area' (PPA), appears to overlap with voxels activated in spatial navigation tasks (e.g. Aguirre *et al.* 1996). What is the function of this region, and why does it respond so strongly to scenes? Several possible hypotheses present themselves. The PPA may respond more to the scenes because the scenes extend to the boundary of the stimulus, in contrast to the face and the object which both have bounding contours. Alternatively, the PPA may respond more to the scenes because the scenes contain a number of individual objects, while the other two stimuli depict only a single object. The middle panel illustrates stimuli used in a second experiment designed to address these hypotheses. The bottom panel illustrates the results of this experiment (i.e. mean time course within the PPA). The first hypothesis can now be eliminated, because the PPA responds strongly to landmarks, which like the object and the face has a bounding contour. The second hypothesis can also be eliminated because the PPA responds almost as strongly to empty rooms as it does to the same rooms filled with furniture and objects, and much more strongly to empty rooms than to arrays of furniture without spatial context. Thus, the PPA appears to respond strongly to any stimulus that gives information about the spatial structure of surrounding space. (Adapted from Epstein and Kanwisher 1998).

Three early neuroimaging studies (Aguirre *et al.* 1996; Maguire *et al.* 1996; Ghaem *et al.* 1997) confirmed this general result, demonstrating that this region responds more when participants perform a navigation task than when they perform a less navigationally-demanding control task. However, on the basis of these experiments alone, it was entirely unclear what *specific* role the parahippocampal region might play in such broadly-defined tasks. In a manner analogous to the systematic investigation of the FFA above, Epstein and Kanwisher (1998), extended these early findings to examine how this region might respond to different classes of visual stimuli, including faces, objects, buildings, and scenes (Fig. 17.1). Somewhat surprisingly, scenes appeared to activate parahippocampal cortex more than other stimulus classes in almost all subjects tested. Accordingly, in individual participants, the comparison scenes > (faces and other objects) provided a functional definition of the 'parahippocampal place area' (PPA) which was then used to define a region of interest for a further series of investigations (Epstein and Kanwisher 1998; Epstein *et al.* 1999). Using this approach, it was possible to establish that the PPA responded strongly to scenes even when they depicted empty rooms without any discrete objects (i.e. just bare walls) or abstract 'cityscapes' constructed from Lego blocks that were clearly not real places in the world. These findings led the authors to the conclusion that parahippocampal cortex is specifically involved in processing the geometric structure of spaces that one can imagine navigating through, or acting within. A patient study designed to test this new hypothesis established that parahippocampally-damaged patients were indeed *specifically* impaired at processing such geometric information (Epstein *et al.* in press).

The approach described above demonstrates how converging evidence from relatively simple block design studies can be used to draw rather specific and often unexpected conclusions about the cognitive processes subserved by different regions of the brain. Moreover, they demonstrate that, like all experimental paradigms, the conclusions that can be drawn from any neuroimaging study are only as good as the hypotheses that have been tested and rejected. For example, while some of the studies described above implicate the FFA in face perception, they do not clearly resolve whether this region is involved *only* in perception, or whether it is equally involved in recognition and/or memory encoding of face stimuli. (However, insofar as stimuli that recruit more perceptual resources are also more likely to be recognized and remembered, it is unclear whether neuroimaging will ever be able to distinguish conclusively between these possibilities.) Similarly, while this region does indeed appear to be specifically involved in face perception, it remains a possibility that faces simply represent a particular category of stimuli that we are extremely well practiced at perceiving and, in this sense, may not be represented neurally in any specific way at all (Tarr

and Gauthier 2000). Distinguishing between such possibilities will provide a significant challenge for future studies.

17.4 On the issue of 'greater activation'

In all of the experiments described above, which used block design, subtraction techniques, the conclusions were based on a simple principle: that is, that an increased MR response in a particular region corresponds to greater 'involvement' of that region in the task or process being investigated. In general terms, this assumption appears to be a valid one. For example, the fact that a greater MR signal is observed in area V1 of the occipital cortex when participants are visually stimulated than when they are not undoubtedly reflects the involvement of V1 in processing visual information. Unfortunately however, in most situations the relationship between the task in question and the observed MR signal is not so clear-cut. One problem is that the BOLD response may not be entirely linear and may saturate at relatively low stimulus presentation rates, for example (Robson *et al.* 1998; see Glover 1999). In addition, it is now well known that the MR signal can be strongly modulated by 'top-down' effects such as attention. Kastner *et al.* (1999), demonstrated that when subjects directed their attention to a quadrant of the visual field in anticipation of a visual stimulus, the MR signal change in the corresponding region of visual cortex was almost as high as when the stimulus actually appeared (see also, Kastner *et al.* 1998; Wojciulik *et al.* 1998; O'Craven *et al.* 1999). The size of these attentional effects clearly suggests that different conditions, within one experiment, should be designed to have equivalent attentional valence. One approach to avoiding such difficulties is to ensure that the putatively 'less-activating' condition requires at least as much attention as the 'more-activating' condition. For example, in the control condition of a perceptual experiment, subjects can be asked to perform a perceptually demanding 'one-back' repetition detection task that requires them to direct attention to all stimuli, including those that may be of less inherent interest.

A second problem with the general assumption that increased signal change equates to greater 'functional involvement' is that the overall MR signal reflects only the mass activity of a given region. It may not, therefore, reveal real differences in the neural firing *pattern* within an anatomical region, which do not translate into differences in the overall *level* of activity. For example, the fact that the FFA responds more during face perception than during object perception strongly *suggest*s that it is more involved in the processing of faces than in the processing of objects. Can it distinguish between different faces, however? Can it distinguish between different views of the same face? Whilst such processes are unlikely to affect overall activity of the region (the FFA is unlikely to respond more to Mary's face than John's face), they may well produce different neural firing patterns within this region.

17.5 Studies of adaptation, habituation and priming

Although fMRI cannot hope to measure firing patterns within individual neural ensembles, under certain circumstances it may be possible to observe such differences indirectly. Monkey neurophysiology studies have observed reduction of single-unit neural response with repeated presentation of the same stimulus (Miller *et al.* 1991; Li *et al.* 1993; Desimone 1996). This neural-level effect might be the basis of a similar adaptation effect found in several fMRI experiments, where a reduction in the overall MR signal was observed for repeated stimuli (Stern *et al.* 1996; Buckner *et al.* 1998; Schacter and Buckner, 1998; Henson *et al.* 2000). By recording the MR response to a new stimulus, it is possible to determine whether a given neural region, such as the FFA, considers this stimulus to be different to, or the same as, a previously stimulus to which it has already adapted (Grill-Spector *et al.* 1999; Kourtzi and Kanwisher 2000). Thus, if the region does not distinguish between the two stimuli, then the response to the second stimulus should be no greater than the response to the previously adapted stimulus. However, if the two stimuli differ along a dimension that is of importance to this region, then the MR response to the second should be greater than that to the first, because it contains novel information to which the region has not yet become adapted.

In one of the first studies to use this technique, Grill-Spector *et al.* (1999) examined signal changes in the lateral occipital complex, a region which had previously been implicated in object shape processing by virtue of its greater response to objects than to texture patterns (see also Malach *et al.* 1995). Adaptation in the lateral occipital complex was greater for repeated faces and for objects shown in different retinal locations or at different sizes, than for faces or objects shown from different viewpoints or under different illuminations. Indeed, there was very little adaptation at all in the latter conditions, suggesting that object representations in this region include viewpoint and illumination information, but are invariant with regard to retinal location and size.

17.6 Parametric studies

Correlational/parametric designs can also be used to answer questions about the relationship between MR signal response and the functional involvement of a given region, with a view to localising cognitive functions within the brain. More specifically, parametric studies are useful for determining whether neural responses to stimulation are linear, non-linear, whether they vary in different regions of the brain and whether they have any specific relevance to a particular cognitive function (Büchel *et al.* 1998). Correlational studies are based on the assumption that the magnitude of the haemodynamic response changes as a function of cognitive 'load': the more cognitive processing engaged by a task, the greater the haemodynamic response. Parametric designs can be used to examine the relationship between a stimulus parameter (such as word presentation rate) or a behavioural response (such as reaction time) and regional cerebral brain activity, as indexed by the BOLD response. This approach is elegant because it avoids many of the complexities of interpretation that are inherent in subtractive designs, including uncertainty about the assumption of additivity of cognitive processes (see Sidtis *et al.* 1999). In addition, concerns about the validity of 'rest conditions' or the physiological state of an individual during so-called 'baseline conditions' are neatly circumvented (see Binder *et al.* 1999). Like subtractive designs, correlational/parametric designs were first implemented in PET activation studies, but such designs generally require more data than a standard PET study can easily provide (unless sample sizes are very large). With fMRI many more measurements on the same subject can be obtained and statistical power increases dramatically, making it the method of choice in many cases.

As an example, several studies have used fMRI to examine the effect of word presentation rate on activation in auditory cortices in the human brain (Binder *et al.* 1994; Dhankhar *et al.* 1997; Rees *et al.* 1997; Büchel *et al.* 1998). The purpose of these studies was twofold: (i) to determine whether a parametric increase in auditory activation would be observed in response to increasing word presentation rate, and (ii) to determine whether anatomically differentiable auditory areas demonstrate different haemodynamic coupling to word rate (Dhankhar, *et al.* 1997; Büchel *et al.*1998). These studies generally demonstrate a positive relationship between presentation rate and activation in auditory areas, for word presentation rates between 0 and 50–90 wpm (Dhankar *et al.* 1997; Büchel *et al.* 1998), although signal saturation and even deactivation can occur at high stimulus rates (over 60–90 wpm). These results confirm that, for auditory areas at least, the underlying assumption of many parametric designs—that increasing regional neuronal activity is reflected in increasing haemodynamic response—is as valid for MRI as it is for PET (e.g. Price *et al.* 1992, Frith and Friston, 1996). Furthermore, although no evidence for differentiation in the nature of the coupling between processing load and haemodynamic response was obtained for auditory areas (Dhankhar, *et al.* 1997), Büchel *et al.* (1998) demonstrated that, whereas activation in auditory cortex increases monotonically (and generally linearly at low presentation rates) with presentation rate, frontal cortex shows a categorical response to the presence of words, irrespective of rate. This finding proves the principle that different areas can be distinguished functionally on the basis of the nature of the coupling between signal change and a parametric variable.

In several instances, correlational designs have been successfully employed in fMRI studies of 'higher-order' or 'executive' functions, to explore how activity within the frontal-lobes varies with parametrically increased task demands. This issue remains an important one, since it is often unclear whether the prefrontal changes observed during complex executive tasks (such as those involving working memory and planning) reflect the operation of general processes associated with task difficulty and mental effort, or processes specific to components of the executive tasks themselves, such as working memory. Unlike some of the more basic sensory-motor tasks described above, examination of these higher-level executive functions may be particularly difficult using the traditional subtractive approach. For example, many studies of working memory involve increasing the demand on processing resources in the experimental condition relative to the control condition (say, by increasing the number of items to be remembered). However, such a manipulation may cause volunteers to adopt novel strategies to solve the task, which while affecting frontal-lobe activity, may not be related to (or *reflect*) the increase in processing load *per se*. Again, parametric designs (particularly those using fMRI, since many thousands of data points can be obtained at each cognitive 'level'), neatly circumvent this problem, since an activity change related to a fundamental shift in task strategy will not generally manifest itself as a parametric change across multiple conditions or 'levels'. Braver *et al.* (1997) used this approach to explore frontal-lobe activity during performance of a sequential letter memory task in which working memory load was varied in a graded fashion. Volunteers observed a series of alphanumeric characters on a visual display and, in a number of different experimental conditions, were required to detect when a prespecified letter was observed (termed the '0-back' condition), when a letter was identical to the one presented in the previous trial (termed the '1-back' condition), or when a letter was identical to the one presented two or three trials earlier (termed the '2-back' and '3-back' conditions, respectively). Thus, working memory load was increased incrementally from the 0-back to the 3-back condition. Signal intensities in two prefrontal regions previously associated with working memory (the middle and inferior frontal gyri), showed a pattern of monotonic increase across the four load conditions and, on this basis, an average signal change per item of load was computed for these two regions. Thus, as the authors point out, although effects of this magnitude may be too small to detect reliably through individual comparisons (using a subtractive methodology, for example), the parametric design allowed them to demonstrate that the fMRI signal can track graded changes in cognitive load even in high-level executive tasks.

In summary, parametric designs may be thought of as providing something akin to a 'dose-response curve' for cognitive tasks in addition to allowing investigators to detect slight, but consistent, changes in the activity of specific cerebral regions in response to subtle task manipulations (Braver *et al.* 1997). In future, correlational designs will also be used to explore whether the coupling between processing load and haemodynamic response is dependent upon those task demands. For example, using PET, Frith and Friston (1996) observed a significant effect of attentional state on the correlation between rate of presentation of tones and blood flow in the thalamus, whereas attentional state did not effect this coupling in auditory cortex. In principle, such questions should be more easily addressed using fMRI since more data can be acquired on individual volunteers. More recently, several studies have used the principles of path analysis and structural equation modelling to explore similar questions of functional connectivity in greater detail using fMRI (see Chapter 16).

17.7 Event-related fMRI designs and their use in cognitive studies

While neuropsychological investigations of behavioural deficits in patients laid the foundations for much of what we now know about the functional neuroanatomy of human cognition, several key questions were largely impervious to these traditional techniques. One often quoted example is that of memory encoding; assessing the efficiency of memory encoding processes in patients is invariably confounded by the requirement to *retrieve* the previously encoded material during testing. Functional neuroimaging, on the other hand, does not suffer the same restrictions since data can be acquired separately during the encoding and retrieval operations. Many early PET studies and block design fMRI studies capitalised on this aspect of the technique and it was during this early period of functional neuroimaging that many significant advances were made in our understanding of human memory processes. Although block designs are a powerful and efficient method for investigating cognitive function, many important questions are trial (not block) specific. For example, within a given block of memory trials, a participant might perform correctly on some trials, but fail on others and a systematic comparison between the two types of trial is of obvious scientific interest. Accordingly, in recent years, sophisticated event-related procedures have been implemented within fMRI studies, stretching the temporal resolution of the technique close to, and sometimes well below, the haemodynamic response.

For example, two recent studies have used event-related designs to decompose memory encoding processes into even more fundamental components (Brewer *et al.* 1998; Wagner *et al.* 1998). Brewer and colleagues (1998) scanned subjects while making simple decisions about whether each of a series of novel pictures depicted an indoor scene or an outdoor scene. Thirty minutes after scanning the subjects were given an unexpected memory test for the pictures viewed in the scanner and their memory for each picture was judged as 'remembered', 'familiar, but not well remembered' or 'forgotten'. By comparing activity during the encoding of words that were subsequently remembered with that during the encoding of words that were subsequently forgotten, these researchers were able to demonstrate that the extent to which a stimulus was remembered well, correlated with activity in specific regions of the cortex. Similarly, Wagner *et al.* (1998) used the benefits of event-related fMRI to examine memory encoding while subject performed an *incidental* task. Volunteers were asked to judge whether each of a series of visually presented words was concrete (e.g. 'ticket'), or abstract (e.g. 'courage'). Twenty minutes after the scanning session, memory for the words was tested and, as in the study by Brewer *et al.* (1998), each word was classed as 'remembered (high confidence)', 'remembered (low confidence)', or 'forgotten'. Again, by comparing brain activity during the presentation of words that were remembered well with that during the presentation of words that were forgotten, the authors were able to define which cortical areas were associated with greater activation during 'successfully' remembered items. In short, these fMRI studies demonstrated, for the first time, that the degree of activation in specific cortical regions relates to how well a given stimulus will be encoded.

17.8 Embedded single-trial designs and their use in cognitive studies

Event-related analyses highlight the superior temporal resolution of fMRI over PET. Even though the haemodynamic response lags stimulus onset by several seconds, takes several seconds to develop fully and then decays, the shape of the curve is predictable enough that the effective temporal resolution of fMRI can be close to 1 s. This permits the examination of functional localization with a finer temporal grain than was possible with PET, and is perhaps the single characteristic which has most clearly identified fMRI as the gold-standard technique in a number of cognitive domains. For example, several investigators have used embedded single trial designs to maximized the effective temporal resolution of fMRI during cognitive tasks that are, by their very nature, presented too rapidly for examination using other techniques. Typically, trials are presented very quickly (say, one per second), although for the most part these trials are not *critical* to the question being addressed (i.e. do not involve the experimental parameter of interest), and essentially provide background neural activity against which signal changes are assessed (e.g. Dove *et al.* 2000; Pollman *et al.* 2000). Critical trials, involving the parameter of interest, occur at random intervals and are assumed to produce temporally correlated changes in fMRI signal which effectively 'rise above' the consistent background signal produced by the non-critical trials (Fig. 17.2). Such designs have proved to be particularly effective in studies of attention in which occasion shifts in cognitive set and/or response are required. Thus, occasional shift trials are embedded in a series of rapidly occurring non-shift trials, thereby allowing the signal changes associated with attentional shifting to be examined during tasks which can be presented and performed essentially exactly as they would be in any neuropsychological laboratory.

The temporal dynamics of the fMRI signal have also been used to answer specific questions about certain cognitive operations that are assumed to have reliable and identifiable temporal characteristics. For example, it may be reasonable to assume that neural ensembles that are involved in maintaining information within memory will produce prolonged and sustained fMRI signal changes during the maintenance phase of a memory task. On the other hand, those regions that are preferentially involved, say, in encoding operations might reasonably be expected to produce an initial signal change during the presentation of the stimulus to be remembered, which then decays away during the subsequent period of memory maintenance (e.g. see Courtney *et al.* 1997). Rowe *et al.* (2000) used a similar approach to determine whether regions of the frontal-lobe that have been implicated in working memory processes are involved in the maintenance of items in memory or in response selection using a novel spatial memory task (Fig. 17.3). As we discuss above, while the importance of the prefrontal cortex for 'higher-order' cognitive functions such as working memory is largely undisputed, no consensus has been reached regarding the fractionation of functions within this region. During working memory trials, the participants were shown three spatial locations and were then required to maintain those items throughout a variable delay. Response selection during this period was prevented by informing the participant which of the three remembered locations was the target only at the end of the delay period. The data were modelled such that transient neuronal activations in response to stimulus presentation, motor responses and selections from memory at the end of trials could be reliably distinguished from sustained activation during the memory delay. Selection, but not maintenance, was associated with activation of the dorsolateral frontal cortex, while maintenance preferentially recruited posterior frontal areas and intraparietal cortex. These results demonstrate the power of emerging methods in fMRI to delineate between the different psychological processes assumed to constitute working memory. Theoretically, however, they provide additional information about the role of the frontal-lobe in working memory *per se*: previous work in this area has suggested that the dorsolateral frontal cortex is essential for guidance of behaviour by internal representations in working memory (Goldman-Rakic, 1994), an operation typically described as 'holding stimuli on-line'. Rowe *et al.* (2000) demonstrate, however, that maintenance is not the critical operation at all and suggest instead that this region plays an essential role in the selection of representations *from* memory.

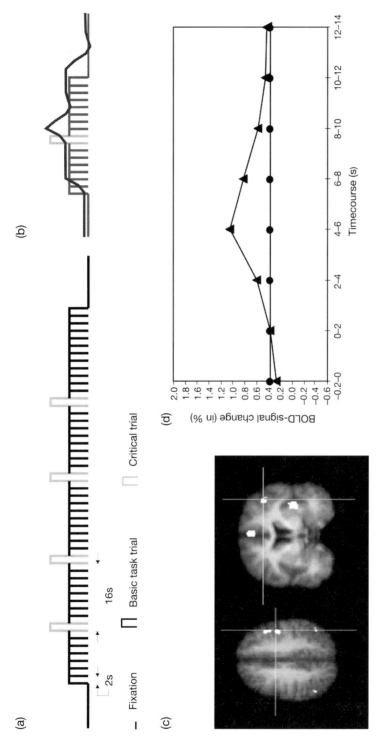

Fig. 17.2 An example of an embedded trial design. Procedure and selected results adapted from Pollmann *et al.* 2000. (a) Trials were presented very quickly (one every 2 s), although for the most part were not critical to the question being addressed. Critical trials, involving the parameter of interest, occur at random intervals and are assumed to produce temporally correlated changes in fMRI signal (b) which effectively 'rise above' the consistent background signal produced by the non-critical trials. (c) Summed activity at critical trials averaged across different participants revealed activity in various brain regions, including the prefrontal cortex. (d) Typical BOLD response measured at the banks of the inferior frontal sulcus. Circles = average responses during baseline trials, triangles = event-related responses during critical trials.

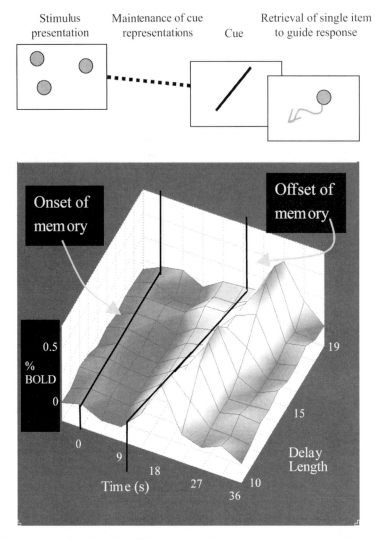

Stimulus presentation   Maintenance of cue representations   Cue   Retrieval of single item to guide response

Fig. 17.3 Procedure and selected results adapted from Rowe *et al.* (2000). Subjects were required to memorize the positions of three dots presented on a screen (*top row*) and hold this information in memory for several seconds (see text). At the end of the delay period a line presented on the screen indicated to the subjects which of the three locations was to be recalled (but did not reveal its exact location, which was somewhere on that line). Subjects were then presented with a single dot and were required to move it to the required location. The data were modelled such that transient neuronal activations in the prefrontal cortex in response to selections from memory (*shown in lower part of figure*), could be reliably distinguished from sustained activation during the memory delay (See also colour plate section.).

17.9 Studies of mental chronometry

The questions that Rowe *et al.* (2000), Courtney *et al.* (1997) and others were interested in were answered, essentially, by examining activation profiles across an individual time series, within a particular anatomical region. Indeed, it has been observed that, within subjects, the hemodynamic response is highly stable in shape, amplitude and timing within a particular brain area (Dale and Buckner 1997; Aguirre *et al.* 1998; Buckner 1998; Miezin *et al.* 2000). Several authors have concluded that event-related MR can be used to resolve timing differences of fractions of a second (Menon *et al.* 1998; Miezin *et al.* 2000), and this assumption has been empirically validated. Miezin and colleagues (2000) examined whether two events in motor cortex, happening about a second apart, could be differentiated. Their subjects viewed a flickering checkerboard and pressed a key with one hand at stimulus onset, and with the other hand at stimulus offset. They found that, within motor cortex, the hemodynamic response to the offset keypress lagged that to the onset keypress by about a second, which is about the same as the temporal difference between the two keypress events. Miezin *et al.* (2000) estimated from their data that timing offsets of as little as 100 ms were detectable, in theory. Thus, questions regarding the relative timing of events within an area can be answered with a high degree of temporal precision.

Activation timecourses demonstrate more variability when compared across regions (within an individual), and across subjects (within a region) (Aguirre *et al.* 1998, Miezin *et al.* 2000). In consequence, experimental questions requiring comparison across regions or across individuals cannot use information based on only the timecourse of the hemodynamic response. Instead, such questions must be posed in a way that relies on relative timing information, such as relative temporal offsets. For example, in the study by Miezin *et al.* (2000) described above, motor cortex was significantly influenced by the timing of responses (showing a lag when the response took longer, i.e. occurred at stimulus offset), whereas visual cortex was not. Thus, questions can be posed in the form of interactions across regions in the relative timing of brain activation under different conditions.

17.10 Studies of functional interaction between areas

The analysis methods that have been discussed so far are all designed to identify neural structures that participate in a cognitive process under study, but do not provide information about how these areas interact functionally. Several alternative analytic approaches aim to integrate over discrete activations, characterizing signal change in a system-wide, distributed fashion. This is usually accomplished using multi-variate tools (such as structural equation modelling) which model covariance in signal change among regions (McIntosh *et al.* 1994; Büchel and Friston 1997). FMRI is particularly well suited for examining functional relationships among activated areas because, through repeated scanning, it can provide many hundreds of data points in each of several conditions for an individual subject, allowing changes in interregional correlations to be evaluated as a function of time, level of performance, or task condition.

This kind of approach has been usefully employed to explore brain systems that underlie learning and has been used to demonstrate that brain systems are plastic: that is, that correlations in activity among areas change as a function of time and learned performance (e.g. Köhler *et al.* 1998; McIntosh *et al.* 1998; Büchel *et al.* 1999). For example, Büchel *et al.* (1999) required people to learn and recall the association between line drawings of real-world objects and locations on a screen during fMRI. Several blocks of trials in which subjects viewed objects in locations were administered, alternating with blocks of trials in which subjects were cued with the location and asked to recall the object associated with it. Over blocks, subjects became increasingly accurate at recalling which object 'went with' each location. At the same time, the correlation between a brain area in the dorsal visual ('where') pathway and one in the ventral visual ('what') pathway became stronger. The authors interpreted this finding as evidence of increased effective connectivity between cortical systems specialized for spatial and object processing, as a function of learning. Although this study focussed on data acquired during encoding blocks, other studies, most notably by McIntosh and colleagues (Köhler *et al.* 1998, McIntosh *et al.* 1998) have examined relationships among brain regions during retrieval, and, intriguingly, find similar learning-related changes in connectivity. These results indicate that the brain structures involved in retrieving items from memory are closely related, if not identical, to those that participate in the initial perceptual analysis and identification (Köhler *et al.* 1998).

17.11 Longitudinal studies

As we have noted above, a significant attraction of fMRI over more invasive functional neuroimaging methods such as PET is that multiple scans on individual volunteers are possible. Indeed, many of the more sophisticated analytical approaches described above, such as structural equation modelling, often rely crucially on there being many hundreds of data points within an individual subject. A more fundamental advantage of repeated scanning, however, is that many cognitive processes, such as learning, which were not easily accessible via existing functional neuroimaging techniques such as PET, can now be effectively examined. A number of investigators have used fMRI in this way, to map changing cortical representations during long-term practice, providing a means for examining the neurobiological correlates of skill learning over an extended time frame. For example, Karni *et al.* (1995, 1998), required volunteers to practice, for 10–20 min per day, a complex motor tasks (a rapid sequence of finger movements), over the course of several weeks of daily practice sessions. Six volunteers were scanned while performing the practised sequence, or a non-practised similar sequence, once per week for four to six weeks. Before training, a comparable extent of activation was observed in contralateral primary motor cortex (M1) during the two (unlearned) sequences. However, after four weeks of training, concurrent with asymptotic performance, the extent of motor cortex activated by the practised sequence enlarged compared with the unpractised sequence. The results suggest a slowly evolving, long-term, experience-dependent reorganisation of the primary motor cortex in adults, which may underlie the acquisition and retention of the motor skill.

In principle, studies such as this are possible with PET, although in practise, the associated radiation burden makes it unlikely that enough scanning sessions could have been conducted to achieve the same results. Moreover, since PET is theoretically limited to blocks of 60–90 s (the technique depends crucially on the decay of radioactive isotope), by definition, it is not possible to look at *continuous* (i.e. uninterrupted) learning. Such studies are entirely possible using fMRI, since the length of any one fMRI session is limited only be the technical limitations of the system being employed.

As well as being useful for examining certain specific types of 'slow changing' cognitive processes such as skill learning, it is clear that within-subject longitudinal fMRI designs are invaluable for investigating the ongoing effects of many different types of brain changes. Thus, through fMRI, monitoring the dynamics of disease progression, recovery of function after brain injury, normal and abnormal development and ageing and the effects of psychopharmacological intervention are all becoming scientifically tractable problems at the systems level.

17.12　Conclusion

Functional neuroimaging has revolutionised the way that cognitive neuroscientists investigate the relationship between brain and behaviour by providing a number of new tools for accessing, albeit indirectly, the neural basis of human cognition. fMRI is contributing to that revolution by providing a widely available, cost effective and non-invasive technique which combines high spatial resolution with critical information about the temporal dynamics of the cortical and sub-cortical signal changes observed.

That said, it *is* important to emphasize that, for the cognitive neuroscientist, fMRI remains only one of several possible approaches that may be recruited to investigate the relationship between brain and behaviour. As we have tried to illustrate here, the technique is suitable for accessing many aspects of human cognition. However, it is undoubtedly the case that many other questions may be more appropriately answered using alternative methods. In this respect, converging evidence from other disciplines within the cognitive neurosciences (including both other functional mapping techniques (see Chapter 19) and, of course, neuropsychological studies) remains essential. It has been said many times of the functional neuroimaging approach that these techniques can only provide *correlational* data; that is a map of those brain regions where activity co-occurs with a given cognitive function; unlike more traditional neuropsychological studies in patients, they can not provide evidence that a brain region is *essential* for that function. Integration of fMRI with a technique such as transcranial magnetic stimulation (TMS) that allows reversible interference with local brain functions may be critical for better establishing this.

Finally, what also continues to be clear is that the gulf between technological know how and depth of understanding has never been wider. Thus, the development of reliable, valid and efficient means for interpreting the information contained within a single functional image of the human brain still lags far behind our ability to acquire, measure and manipulate these images. While few would doubt that much has been achieved through the revolution in functional neuroimaging, the real cognitive neuroscientific promise provided by these new methods has yet to be fully realized.

References

Aguirre, G.K. and D'Esposito, M. (1999). Topographical disorientation: a synthesis and taxonomy. *Brain*, **122**(9), 1613–28.

Aguirre, G.K., Detre, J.A., Alsop, D.C. and D'Esposito, M. (1996). The parahippocampus subserves topographical learning in man. *Cerebral Cortex*, **6**, 823–29.

Aguirre, G.K., Zarahn, E. and D'Esposito, M. (1998). The variability of human, BOLD hemodynamic responses. *Neuroimage*, **8**, 360–69.

Barrash, J., Damasio, H., Adolphs, R. and Tranel, D. (2000). The neuroanatomical correlates of route learning impairment. *Neuropsychologia*, **38**(6), 820–36.

Binder, J.R., Rao, S.M., Hammereke, T.A., Frost, J.A. Bandettini, P.A., and Hyde, J.S. (1994). Effects of stimulus rate on signal response during functional magnetic resonance imaging of auditory cortex. *Cognitive Brain Research*, **2**, 31–38.

Binder, J.R., Frost, J.A., Hammeke, T.A., Bellgowan, P.S.F., Rao, S.M., and Cox, R.W. (1999). Conceptual processing during the conscious resting state: A functional MRI study. *Journal of Cognitive Neuroscience*, **11**(1), 80–93.

Braver, T.S., Cohen, J.D., Nystrom, L.E., Jonides, J., Smith, E.E., and Noll, D.C. (1997). A Parametric Study of Prefrontal Cortex Involvement in Human Working Memory. *Neuroimage*, **5**, 49–62.

Brewer, J.B., Zhao, Z., Desmond, J.E., Glover, G.H., and Gabrieli, J.D.E. (1998). Making memories: brain activity that predicts how well visual experience will be remembered. *Science*, **281**, 1185–87.

Büchel, C., and Friston, K.J. (1997). Modulation of connectivity in visual pathways by attention: cortical interactions evaluated with structural equation modelling and fMRI. *Cerebral Cortex*, **7**, 768–78.

Büchel, C., Holmes, A.P., Rees, G., and Friston, K.J. (1998). Characterizing stimulus-response function using non-linear regressors in parametric fMRI experiments. *Neuroimage*, **8**, 140–48.

Büchel, C., Coull, J.T., and Friston, K.J. (1999). The predictive value of changes in effective connectivity for human learning. *Science*, **283**, 1538–40.

Buckner, R.L. (1998). Event-related fMRI and the hemodynamic response. *Human Brain Mapping*, **6**, 373–77.

Buckner, R.L., Goodman, J., Burock, M., Rotte, M. Koutstaal, W., Schacter, D., Rosen, B., and Dale, A.M. (1998). Functional-anatomic correlates of object priming in humans revealed by rapid presentation event-related fMRI. *Neurone*, **20**, 285–96.

Courtney, S.M., Ungerleider, L.G., Keil, K., and Haxby, J.V. (1997). Transient and sustained activity in a distributed neural system for human working memory. *Nature*, **386**, 608–11.

Dale, A. M. and Buckner, R.L. (1997). Selective averaging of rapidly presented individual trials using fMRI. *Human Brain Mapping*, **5**, 329–40.

Desimone, R. (1996). Neural mechanisms for visual memory and their role in attention. *Proceedings of the National Academy of Sciences (USA)*, **93**, 13494–9.

Dhankhar, A., Wexler, B.E., Fulbright, R. K., Halwes, T., Blamire, A. M., and Shulman, R. G. (1997). Functional magnetic resonance imaging assessment of the human brain auditory cortex response to increasing word presentation rates. *Journal of Neurophysiology*, **77**, 476–83.

Dove, A., Pollmann, S., Schubert, T., Wiggins, C.J., and von Cramon, D.Y. (2000). Prefrontal cortex activation in task switching: An event-related fMRI study. *Cognitive Brain Research*, **9**, 103–9.

Epstein, R. and Kanwisher, N. (1998). A cortical representation of the local visual environment. *Nature*, **392**, 598–601.

Epstein, R., Harris, A., Stanley, D., and Kanwisher, N. (1999). The parahippocampal place area: Recognition, navigation, or encoding? *Neurone*, **23**, 115–25.

Epstein, R., DeYoe, E.A., Press, D.Z., Rosen, A.C. and Kanwisher, N. (in press). Neuropsychological evidence for a topographical learning mechanism in parahippocampal cortex. *Cognitive Neuropsychology*.

Friston, K.J., Fletcher P., Josephs, O., Holmes, A., Rugg, M.D., and Turner, R. (1998). Event-Related fMRI: Characterizing Differential Responses. *NeuroImage*, **7**, 30–40.

Frith, C.D. and Friston, K.J. (1996). The role of the thalamus in 'top down' modulation of attention to sound. *NeuroImage*, **4**, 210–15.

Gauthier, I. (2000). What constrains the organization of the ventral temporal cortex? *Trends in Cognitive Sciences*, **4**, 1–4.

Ghaem, O., Mellet, E., Crivello, F., Tzourio, N., Mazoyer, B., Berthoz, A., and Denis, M. (1997). Mental navigation along memorized routes activates the hippocampus, precuneus, and insula. *NeuroReport*, **8**, 739–44.

Glover, G.H. (1999). Deconvolution of impulse response in event-related BOLD fMRI. *NeuroImage*, **9**, 416–29.

Goldman-Rakic, P.S. (1994). The issue of memory in the study of prefrontal functions. In: *Motor and cognitive functions of the prefrontal cortex* (ed. A.M. Thierry, J. Glowinski, P.S. Goldman-Rakic, Y. Christen), Springer-Verlag, Berlin Heidelberg.

Grill-Spector, K., Kushnir, T., Edelman, S., Avidan, G. Itzchak, Y. and Malach, R. (1999). Differential processing of objects under various viewing conditions in the human lateral occipital complex. *Neurone*, **24**(1), 187–203.

Habib, M. and Sirigu, A. (1987). Pure topographical disorientation: a definition and anatomical basis. *Cortex*, **23**, 73–85.

Haxby, J.V., Horwitz, B., Ungerleider, L.G., Maisog, J.M., Pietrini, P., and Grady, C.L. (1994). A PET-fCBF study of selective attention to faces and locations. *Journal of Neuroscience*, **14**, 6336–53.

Henson R, Shallice T, and Dolan R. (2000). Neuroimaging evidence for dissociable forms of repetition priming. *Science*, **18** 287(5456), 1269–72.

Ishai, A, Ungerleider, L.G., Martin, A., Schouten, J.L., and Haxby, J.V. (1999). Distributed representation of objects in the human ventral visual pathway. *Proceedings of the National Academy of Sciences (USA)*, **96**, 9379–84.

Kanwisher, N., McDermott, J., Chun, M.M. (1997). The fusiform face area: a module in human extrastriate cortex specialized for face perception. *Journal of Neuroscience*, **17**, 4302–11.

Kanwisher, N., Stanley, D. and Harris, A. (1999). The fusiform face area is selective for faces not animals. *NeuroReport*, **19**, 183–7.

Karni, A., Meyer, G., Jezzard, P., Adams, M.M., Turner, R., and Ungerleider, L.G. (1995). Functional MRI evidence for adult motor cortex plasticity during motor skill learning. *Nature*, **14**, 377(6545), 155–8.

Karni, A., Meyer, G., Rey Hipolito, C., Jezzard, P., Adams, M.M., Turner, R., and Ungerleider, L.G. (1998). The acquisition of skilled motor performance: fast and slow experience-driven changes in primary motor cortex. *Proceedings of the National Academy of Sciences (USA)*, **95**(3), 861–8.

Kastner, S., De Weered, P., Desimone, R., and Ungerleider, L.G. (1998). Mechanisms of directed attention in the human extrastriate cortex as revealed by functional MRI. *Science*, **282**(5386), 108–11.

Kastner, S., Pinsk, M.A., DeWeerd, P., Desimone, R., and Ungerleider, L.G. (1999). Increased activity in human visual cortex during directed attention in the absence of visual stimulation. *Neurone*, **22**, 751–61.

Köhler, S., McIntosh, A.R., Moscovitch, M. Winocur, G. (1998). Functional interactions between the medical temporal lobes and posterior neocortex related to episodic memory retrieval. *Cerebral Cortex*, **8**, 451–61.

Kourtzi, Z. and Kanwisher, N. (2000). Cortical regions involved in perceiving object shape. *Journal of Neuroscience*, **20**(9), 3310–8.

Kwong, K.K., Belliveau, J.W. Chesler, D.A., Goldberg, I.E. Weisskoff, R.M., Poncelet, B.P., Kennedy, D.N., Hoppel, B.E., Cohen, M.S., Turner, R., Cheng, H., Brady, T.J., and Rosen, B.R. (1992). Dynamic magnetic resonance imaging of human brain activity during primary sensory stimulation. *Proceedings of the National Academy of Sciences (USA)*, **89**, 5675–9.

Li, L., Miller, E.K. and Desimone, R. (1993). The representation of stimulus familiarity in anterior inferior temporal cortex. *Journal of Neurophysiology*, **69**, 1918–29.

McIntosh, A.R. and Gonzalez-Lima, F. (1994). Structural equation modelling and its application to network analysis in functional brain imaging. *Human Brain Mapping*, **2**, 2–22.

McIntosh, A.R., Cabeza, R.E., and Lobaugh, N.J. (1998).

Analysis of neural interactions explains the activation of occipital cortex by an auditory stimulus. *Journal of Neurophysiology*, **80**, 2790–6.

Maguire, E.A., Frackowiak, R.S.J., and Frith, C.D. (1996). Learning to find your way: a role for the human hippocampal region. *Proceeds of the Royal Society of London B [Biological Sciences]*, **263**, 1745–50.

Malach, R., Reppas, J.B., Benson, R.R., Kwong, K.K. Jiang, H., Kennedy, W.A., Ledden, P.J., Brady, T.J., Rosen, B.R., and Tootell, R.B. (1995). Object-related activity revealed by functional magnetic resonance imaging in human occipital cortex., *Proceedings of the National Academy of Sciences (USA)*, **92**(18), 8135–9.

Menon, R.S., Luknowsky, D.C., and Gati, J.S. (1998). Mental chronometry using latency-resolved functional MRI. *Proceedings of the National Academy of Sciences (USA)*, **95**, 10902–7.

Miezin, F.M., Maccotta, L., Ollinger, J.M., Petersen, S.E., and Buckner, R.L. (2000). Characterizing the hemodynamic response: effects of presentation rate, sampling procedure, and the possibility of ordering brain activity based on relative timing. *Neuroimage*, **11**, 735–59.

Miller, E.K., Li, L., and Desimone, R. (1991). A neural mechanism for working and recognition memory in inferior temporal cortex. *Science*, **254**, 1377–9.

O'Craven, K.M., Downing, P.E., and Kanwisher, N. (1999). fMRI evidence for objects as the units of attentional selection. *Nature*, **401**(6753), 584–7.

Owen, A. M. (2000). The role of the lateral frontal cortex in mnemonic processing: the contribution of functional neuroimaging. *Experimental Brain Research*, **133**, 33–43.

Petrides, M. (1994). Frontal lobes and working memory: evidence from investigations of the effects of cortical excisions in nonhuman primates. In: *Handbook of Neuropsychology*, (eds F. Boller and J. Grafman) vol. 9, pp. 59–82. Elsevier, Amsterdam.

Pollmann, S., Dove, A., von Cramon, D.Y., and Wiggins, C.J. (2000). Event-related fMRI: Comparison of conditions with varying BOLD-overlap. *Human Brain Mapping*, **9**, 26–37.

Price, C., Wise, R., Ramsay, S., Friston, K., Howard, D., Patterson, K., and Frackowiak, R. (1992). Regional response differences within the human auditory cortex when listening to words. *Neuroscience Letters*, **146**, 2, 179–82.

Puce, A., Allison, T., Gore, J.C., and McCarthy, G. (1995). Face-sensitive regions in human extrastriate cortex studied by functional MRI. *Journal of Neurophysiology*, **74**(3), 1192–9.

Puce, A., Allison, T., Asgari, M., Gore, J.C., and McCarthy, G. (1996). Differential sensitivity of human visual cortex to faces, letterstrings, and textures: a functional magnetic resonance imaging study. *Journal of Neuroscience*, **16**(16), 5205–15.

Rees, G., Howseman, A., Josephs, O., Frith, C.D., Friston, K.J., Frackowiak, R.S., and Turner, R. (1997). Characterizing the relationship between BOLD contrast and regional cerebral blood flow measurements by varying the stimulus presentation rate. *Neuroimage*, **6**, 4, 270–8.

Robson, M.D., Dorosz, J.L., and Gore, J.C. (1998). Measurements of the Temporal fMRI Response of the Human

Auditory Cortex to Trains of Tones. *Neuroimage*, **7**, 185–98.

Rowe, J.B., Toni, I., Josephs, O., Frackowiak, R.S.J., and Passingham, R.E. (2000). The prefrontal cortex: response selection or maintenance within working memory? *Science*, **288**, 1656–60.

Schacter, D.L. and Buckner, R.L. (1998). Priming and the brain. *Neurone*, **20**, 185–95.

Sidtis, J.J., Strother, S.C., Anderson, J.R., and Rottenberg, D.A. (1999). Are brain functions really additive? *Neuroimage*, **9**, 5, 490–6.

Stern, C.E., Corkin, S., Gonzalez, R.G., Guimaraes, A.R., Baker, J.R., Jennings, P.J., Carr, C.A., Sugiura, R.M., Vedantham, V., and Rosen, B.R. (1996). The hippocampal formation particpates in novel picture encoding: evidence from functional magnetic resonance imaging. *Proceedings of the National Academy of Sciences (USA)*, **93**, 8660–5.

Tarr, M.J. and Gauthier, I. (2000). FFA: A flexible fusiform area for subordinate-level visual processing automatized by expertise. *Nature-Neuroscience*, **3**(8), 764–9.

Wagner, A.D., Schacter, D.L., Rotte, M., Koutstaal, W., Maril, A., Dales, A.M., Rosen, B.R., and Buckner, R.L. (1998). Building memories: remembering and forgetting of verbal experiences as predicted by brain activity. *Science*, **281**, 1188–91.

Wojciulik, E.H., Kanwisher, N. and Driver, J. (1998). Covert visual attention modulates face-specificity activity in the human fusiform gyrus: fMRI study. *Journal of Neurophysiology*, **79**(3), 1574–8.

18 | *Clinical applications of mapping neurocognitive processes in the human brain with functional MRI*

Keith R. Thulborn and Antonio Gisbert

18.1 Introduction

The diagnosis and treatment of sensory, motor and cognitive dysfunction is of central importance to medicine yet there are substantial limitations in our strategies for their diagnoses and monitoring. In current medical practice, diseases of the central nervous system (CNS) are broadly categorized into those that are neurological (when a biological basis for the illness is known) and those that are psychiatric (when a specific biological basis has not been determined). This rather arbitrary division is rooted in an emphasis on structural pathology. Functional testing has until recently been very limited. The neurological and psychiatric examinations of traditional medicine interrogate the CNS by testing if specific stimuli elicit expected responses. The assumption made from normal responses is that the CNS is normal. This 'black box' approach can now be questioned as the brain can produce apparently normal responses even in the face of severe insult (Thulborn *et al.* 1999*a*). Finally, while, much has been learned by integrating clinical experiences with pathology, such studies represent only single time point comparisons.

The dynamics of pathological changes must be inferred. With the advent of modern neuroimaging, and specifically magnetic resonance imaging (MRI), understanding of the pathological brain and disease and its dynamics has been greatly accelerated. This is true for neurology where the anatomic changes underlying the clinical signs and symptoms become readily apparent. Psychiatry and clinical psychology have benefited less from such approaches, as imaging has been used primarily to exclude any anatomic basis for impaired mental function. The introduction of functional MRI (fMRI) to medicine promises a major advance by providing functional discrepancies for the causes of neurological and psychiatric disease.

Besides the drive to use these methods to understand normal brain function, the momentum for the clinical development of fMRI has been generated by immediate opportunities for applications in presurgical planning. Such planning includes epilepsy, tumor resection and treatment of arteriovenous malformations. Neurosurgeons are already capitalizing on fMRI to map those areas of eloquent cortex to be avoided during resection of parts of the brain, shorten the length of surgical procedures and to minimize craniotomy size (Patel *et al.* 1999; Lee *et al.* 1999). Such work already has emphasized that the assumptions underpinning such functional mapping must be examined for each patient, as the consequences of errors are extreme for that individual. Unlike research studies of normal individuals in which generalized results are sought from a subject group, clinical studies especially focus on individual patients and the results are applied to their management. The robustness of individual results therefore must be assured. The presence of pathology immediately raises the issue of how the pathology may affect interpretation of the results of fMRI. Thus, clinical applications of fMRI pose challenges that must be addressed. This chapter presents strategies that serve to meet these challenges.

18.2 Quality assurance for clinical fMRI

Unlike research studies in which groups of subjects are studied in a highly controlled environment to reach a group result, clinical studies yield essentially single subject results to be used to manage that individual's medical problem. There are a number of immediate problems that such studies must confront. Patients may be ill and taking multiple medications. They can be from a wide range of educational and cultural backgrounds. The clinical challenge is to achieve a high fMRI success rate (> 90 per cent) within the typical 60 min MRI examination time such that all the clinically relevant information, both anatomic and functional, can be obtained. To ensure this level of success, several aspects of the fMRI examination must be considered. This topic of quality assurance has been reviewed in more detail elsewhere (Thulborn 1999*a*) and will be summarized here.

18.2.1 Personnel

Patients must show higher degrees of cooperation with fMRI studies than are required in more conventional MRI examinations. Such patient cooperation is dependent in part on the skills of MR technologists and nursing staff. The patient must be helped to feel comfortable and understand the nature of the examination. This process takes time and must be planned for in the daily schedule if stress on both the staff and patients is to be minimized. Establishing rapport with the patient by thoroughly demonstrating the nature of the paradigm and answering any questions is mandatory for achieving high success rates. The importance of the clinical staff to any success in this needs to be recognized by the physicians or surgeon asking for such investigative procedures.

18.2.2 Patient preparation

The anxious or ill patient must be reassured and trained to perform the paradigm with special care. This may require extra time and effort on the part of the MR technologist and nursing staff. Training can be done on a computer screen initially but ultimately the novelty of the scanner must be reduced. This can be achieved efficiently by use of a MRI system simulator (Rosenberg *et al.* 1997), one specially-designed to mimic the scanner environment (even to the point of having recorded gradient noise). Truly claustrophobic patients can be readily identified at this time and their studies can be abandoned without loss of scanner time. Initial training also provides behavioral feedback on the appropriateness of the paradigm for each patient.

For example, if response times are unduly long or accuracy low, the paradigm should be changed or modified to match the skill level of the patient.

Visual stimuli require patients to have appropriate visual acuity. Otherwise, contact lenses should be worn or MR-compatible eye corrective lenses should be supplied. Such glasses are available commercially. Although fMRI is noisy, auditory stimuli can be used even with the use of earplugs using currently available sound projection systems (Binder *et al.* 1994; Booth *et al.* 1999; Jancke *et al.* 1999).

18.2.3 Patient safety

Patient safety must be ensured. Although fMRI does not impose additional risks over conventional MRI, the use of more equipment around the patient should raise concern about introducing ferromagnetic objects into the scanner room. This issue is immediately resolved by leaving all fMRI equipment in the scan room and allowing only qualified personnel into the room with patients. Although researchers use bite bars to reduce subject head motion, such devices increase the risk of aspiration in some patients and decrease cooperation in others. The visor system containing a sighting system to provide visual feedback as to head position and a tight-fitting, yet comfortable, pillow have been successful in the hands of the author (Thulborn 1999*b*).

Noise from gradient switching can reach levels of 90–120 dB. Protection against such potentially damaging levels must be given using earplugs, headphones, or other passive blocks. It is hoped that future systems may have active noise cancellation.

Considerable electromagnetic radiation is generated in the scanner. Conduction loops can generate substantial heat and must be kept away from patients to avoid burns. Even pools of water, incontinence or a leaked saline infusion solution can prove hazardous.

18.2.4 Paradigms

Paradigms should be calibrated in healthy control subjects matched for age, gender and handedness prior to being used clinically. Depending on the paradigm, each of these parameters can have a significant effect. As there is a seemingly endless choice of paradigms being used in research settings, the selected use of well-characterized tasks that interrogate many areas of the brain simultaneously provides a working solution in the clinical setting. Matching patient skills to the degree of task difficulty is important to ensure that the task is performed throughout the entire fMRI study. Paradigms with a flexible means of adjusting the difficulty to match the skill set of different patients are exceedingly helpful and time efficient. By way of example, younger children have auditory skills that are more advanced than reading skills. Auditory stimuli then may be a better choice over visual stimuli for language comprehension paradigms using sentences and questions for the pediatric population (Booth *et al.* 1999).

As discussed elsewhere in this book, three basic experimental designs are available for fMRI: block or event-related designs and low-frequency correlations. Because of its simplicity of design and analyses, the block design is most commonly used and is the basis of the paradigms illustrated in this chapter. Each condition of the paradigm is maintained for a fixed time (usually in the order of 30–60 s) and the conditions are cycled until sufficient statistical power is reached to demonstrate the activation (usually in the order of 5–12 min or greater than 60–80 images per condition). During the stimulus block the maximum haemodynamic response is achieved by repeated stimulus presentation and then the MR signal intensity re-equilibrates during the rest condition prior to the next stimulus period. The active condition contains repeated stimuli of equivalent cognitive load, but assumes that task performance is maintained during the active condition and across cycles. The second approach of event-related fMRI uses short duration stimuli and image averaging as a function of time after stimulus. This design allows the behavioral response to each stimulus to be measured separately. Although an individual stimulus produces much less activation than the grouped stimuli of a block, signal change associated with similar behavioral responses can be averaged (Rosen *et al.* 1998; Richter 1999). Although it remains less well-characterized, a potentially very useful new approach is the use of low frequency correlations in MR signals across the brain even in the absence of any overt paradigm (Biswal *et al.* 1995). This approach would only require that the patient remain still for several minutes.

To illustrate the block design paradigm in greater detail, those paradigms illustrated in the clinical examples described later in this chapter are now explained and justified. The visually guided saccade (VGS) paradigm (Luna *et al.* 1998) is a simple reflexive eye movement to a bright target on a dark background. The details are described in the caption of Figs 18.1(a,b) which show a schematic of the paradigm and an example of the corresponding normal activation map. Because the eye movement control pathway is perhaps one of the best understood and intensively studied pathways in non-human primates and humans, it can provide a useful general strategy for interrogating human brain function in the setting of disease. An excellent review of the state-of-the-art for these paradigms has been provided elsewhere (Luna *et al.* 1999*a*). The VGS paradigm allows mapping of areas in the superior and lateral frontal lobes (frontal eye fields, FEF, along the precentral sulcus), medial frontal cortex (supplementary eye fields, SEF), parietal lobes (intraparietal sulcus, IPS), occipital lobes (primary visual cortex, V1), and temporal lobes (visual motion cortex, MT/V5). This paradigm is very robust and has been successful in children (Luna *et al.* 1999*b*), and in patients with Alzheimer's disease (Thulborn *et al.* 2000). Modifications of this paradigm to test cognitive functions such as working memory (memory-guided saccades) and impulse control (antisaccades) have been demonstrated (Sweeney *et al.* 1997; Berman *et al.* 1999; Luna *et al.* 1999*b*). With the introduction of commercially available MR-compatible eye trackers, behavioral monitoring of eye movement will be useful for correlated assessments of task performance.

Language is central to studies of human cognition. Regions of brain involved in processing and expressing language are vital to preserve when planning surgery in eloquent areas. This is particularly evident in temporal lobe epilepsy, which is sometimes treated with a partial temporal lobectomy. Given the involvement of the superior temporal gyrus and sulcus (Wernicke's area in the left temporal lobe and contralateral homologous area) and its connections to the inferior frontal lobe (Broca's area in the left frontal lobe and contralateral homologous area), functional mapping of these areas provides useful help in surgical planning. Language comprehension paradigms, first described elsewhere (Just *et al.* 1996), also can be robust in clinical applications. The paradigm that has been calibrated in adults and used routinely for patients is shown in Figs 18.2(a,b) The details of the parameters are given in the

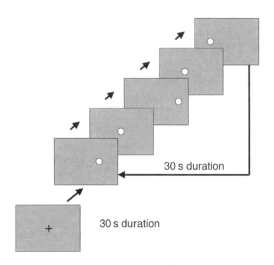

Fig. 18.1 (a) Schematic for the visually-guided saccade (VGS) paradigm which has up to 10 cycles in which condition 1 (central fixation of 30 s duration on a small crosshair) is compared to condition 2 (saccades to a spot of light appearing randomly at one of five locations along the horizontal meridian). (b) Group activation map of a group (*n* = 10) of adults performing the VGS paradigm analysed by a simple *t*-test (*t* threshold > 3.5) after excluding the 6 s transition periods. The supplementary eye fields (1), frontal eye fields (2) and intraparietal sulcus (3) are identified. (See also colour plate section for part (b).)

30 s duration

30 s duration

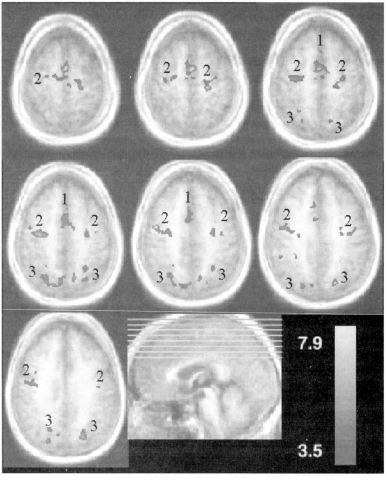

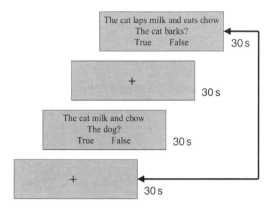

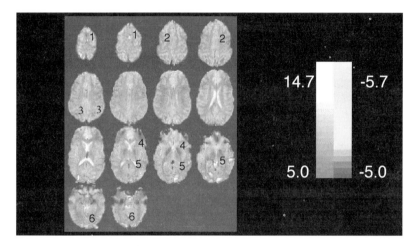

Fig. 18.2 (a) Schematic for the reading comprehension paradigm which has up to 10 cycles in which condition 1 (central fixation of 30s duration on a small crosshair) is compared to condition 2 (reading word lists made by deleting verbs from sentences) and condition 3 (reading a sentence followed by a question answered as TRUE or FALSE by depressing a finger switch). (b) Representative activation map of a normal adult performing the reading task paradigm analysed by a simple *t*-test (threshold > 5.0) after excluding the 6 second transition periods. In addition to the supplementary eye fields (1), frontal eye fields (2), and intraparietal sulcus (3), Broca's area (4) and Wernicke's area (5) and often the contralateral homologous areas are identified. Primary and association visual cortices (6) are identified. (See also colour plate section for part (b).)

caption. The paradigm compares central fixation (30 s) with periods (30 s) of reading either word strings or sentences, followed by a question to be answered as TRUE or FALSE by depressing one of two finger-switches held in each hand. As this paradigm also measures the behavioral responses (accuracy, latency) from each of the questions, task performance can be measured to ensure that the patient has understood the paradigm and cooperated throughout the duration of the study. For children, the task is presented as a listening rather than reading task to ensure age appropriateness (Booth *et al.* 1999).

Finally, the motor cortex is also an area that is critically important to preserve during surgery. Possible changes in its function or organization also may be important to understand stroke rehabilitation. Tasks need not be complex. Even simple finger tapping tasks

have been used for presurgical planning. Figs 18.3(a,b) show a schematic of a simple finger apposition paradigm and the activation map of a normal subject, respectively.

18.2.5 Scanner

The BOLD contrast effect is small (only 1–2 per cent at 1.5 Tesla) and dependent on the scanner applied magnetic field strength. Systems operating at less than 1.5T are not recommended and the use of 3T and higher has much to be recommended (Thulborn, 1999*c*). Higher field strengths (e.g. ≥ 3T) provides the signal-to-noise needed for practical use of smaller voxel dimensions, which allows better localization of activations with larger signal changes (Thulborn *et al.* 1997*a*). The MR scanner to be used for fMRI also

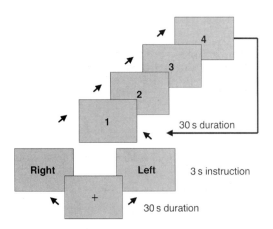

Fig. 18.3 (a) Schematic for the finger tapping (ft) paradigm which has up to 10 cycles in which condition 1 (central fixation of 30 s duration on a small crosshair without finger movement) is compared to condition 2 (central fixation of 30 s duration on a small crosshair with finger opposition at the rate shown by the rate of appearance of the counting numbers). Handedness of the finger tapping can be alternated or both hands can be used simultaneously depending on the clinical question to be answered. The visual fixation task is used to maintain head position with the visor. (b) Representative activation map of a normal adult performing the ft paradigm analysed by a simple t-test (threshold > 9.0) after excluding the 6 s transition periods. The supplementary motor area (1), primary motor area (2) and primary somatosensory cortex (3) are identified. (See also colour plate section for part (b).)

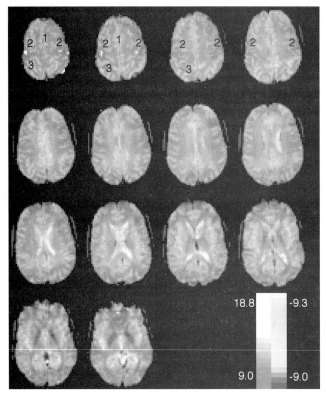

must meet some basic requirements that exceed performance criteria for conventional MRI. Some form of ultrafast imaging, such as echo-planar (EPI) or spiral imaging should be available (Cohen *et al.* 1991; Glover 1999).

As BOLD contrast is weak, image averaging is required. The typical clinically acceptable acquisition time for a cooperative patient is less than 10 min. Longer times may introduce extra variance from patient fatigue with loss of attention and increased head motion. Ultrafast imaging effectively removes the effect of head motion in single images but motion correction algorithms have limited success in removing scan-to-scan motion effects, particularly those through

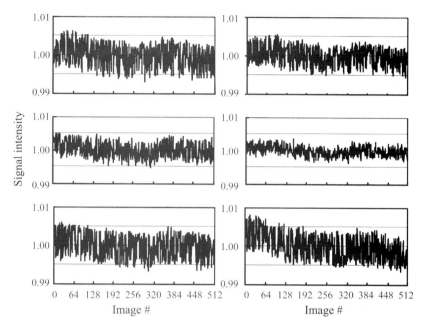

Fig. 18.4 Stability of signal intensity for the 3 T whole body scanner (Signa LX, Version 8.2.5.5, General Electric Medical Systems, Milwaukee, WI) is measured using the standard head radiofrequency coil and TLT spherical water phantom (without phantom loader) positioned at the magnet isocenter. The acquisition parameters using the gradient-echo EPI (psd epiRT) are: repetition time (TR) = 2000 ms; echo time (TE) = 25 ms; flip angle = 90°; field of view (FOV) = 20 × 20 cm²; acquisition matrix = 64 × 64, slice thickness = 3 mm; slice gap = 12.5 mm; number of slices = 10, and number of averages per slice (NEX) = 1. Autoshim, phase correction and two reference images for ghost correction are performed. A total of 512 images for each of 10 slices acquired over 17 min mimics the design of a typical fMRI study. A region of interest (ROI, 10 × 10 voxels) placed in the centre of the images of the central six slices produces the time courses of the normalized signal intensity shown in the figure. The signal intensity of each image is normalized against the mean signal intensity of the entire time course of that slice. The resultant analysis reveals signal stability to be well within 1 per cent (peak-to-peak) of the normalized signal at the centre of the phantom (0.7 per cent).

the imaging plane (see chapter by Brammer). In addition over time, signal intensity drifts from scanner instability may be as serious as patient head motion. Typically, scanner stability with ultrafast imaging has been reported to be less than 1 per cent peak-to-peak variation over 30 min (Thulborn 1999*a*). The signal to noise ratio must be maintained and monitored regularly on each fMRI scanner. Increasing noise may indicate that the radiofrequency shielding of the magnet room is no longer within specifications. Declining signal intensity may indicate problems with the radiofrequency coil, transceiver or preamplifier system. Such changes usually precede major scanner failures but can jeopardize fMRI sensitivity and robustness. As all equipment is subject to failure with time, daily quality assurance ensures that such loss of performance does not impact on patient studies. A representa-

tive stability test for daily quality assurance performed on a 3T whole body scanner (LX Signa, General Electric Medical Systems, Milwaukee, WI) is shown in Fig. 18.4. The test uses the commercial volume head radiofrequency coil and TLT spherical doped water phantom (without loader) with the acquisition parameters described in the figure caption. The multi-slice data are plotted as normalized signal intensity and typically has a peak-to-peak variation of less than 1 per cent over 17 min. This has been a satisfactory target performance as such variation on a human head is typically greater than this (> 5 per cent). Other quality assurance parameters should include signal-to-noise ratio, EPI ghosting levels, spike level, cryogen boil-off rate and magnetic field homogeneity. Quantitative performance criteria that have been demonstrated to be reproducible are important.

The scanner should have patient handling capabilities similar or identical to those typical on clinical scanners to allow rapid setup and for safety reasons. As patient comfort and cooperation decrease with time, fMRI examinations should be performed as efficiently as possible. Thus, fMRI should precede conventional MRI where possible in comprehensive imaging protocols (Thulborn 1999*a*; Thulborn *et al.* 1999*b*, 2000).

As on any high quality clinical service, all images should be reviewed by a qualified physician prior to releasing the patient. Some simple activation studies can be reviewed in real-time on some of the newer scanners. This is an important advantage to ensure that the data are adequate before the patient is discharged from the scanning suite. This avoids the inconvenience of repeating costly studies.

18.2.6 Control system

Given the many data streams to be synchronized in a routine clinical fMRI study (which ideally can be done by a single MR technologist) the synchronization control system is as important as the scanner. The presentation of a task to the patient has thus far usually been through visual or auditory means. The stimuli must be synchronized to the MR image acquisition and sometimes also with respect to physiological (cardiac cycle, respiratory cycle) responses. Information on behavioural response (accuracy, latency) can be important for ensuring quality control, and for data interpretation. Such a control system has been previously described (Thulborn *et al.* 1996) and several systems are now commercially available. Visual stimuli may be presented on rear-projection screens at the foot of the patient table or within the bore of the magnet. Goggles and LCD displays within the bore also are possible. One rear-projection screen incorporates a sighting system to control head movement in the cooperative subject (Thulborn, 1999*b*). Routine quality assurance of the accuracy in synchronization timing is mandatory. Constancy of the stability of the luminance of high quality visual stimuli and fidelity of auditory stimuli should be verified routinely.

18.2.7 Data analysis

As image averaging is necessary to detect the small signal changes associated with brain activation, numerous statistical methods have been used for isolating activation from background signal fluctuations (see Part IV). The image data can be examined for head motion subjectively by visual inspection in an animation loop or objectively with estimated displacement (translation, rotation) parameters based on the images (Eddy *et al.* 1996). Head motion should be less than 30 per cent of a voxel dimension to avoid the need for correction. If head motion has occurred, the data may be censored to remove images in which there has been too much motion or another acquisition is required. Different software packages are available for motion correction, all of which make assumptions that may be questionable in certain circumstances (see Chapter 13). Three-dimensional corrections such as by AIR (Woods *et al.* 1992) require a three dimensional data set whereas fMRI data are usually multi-planar. Other corrections, such as FIASCO (Eddy *et al.* 1996), are two-dimensional, being limited to in-plane motion whereas head motion is usually three-dimensional. A recently reported approach for correction of multi-planar data in three dimensions has been proposed (Kim *et al.* 1999). Clearly the best approach is to cultivate a cooperative patient and enhance the opportunity for a motionless state by using comfortable positioning, biofeedback (Thulborn, 1999*b*), and efficient fMRI studies.

Behavioral measures of paradigm performance should be examined for accuracy and latency. If the patient is not performing to the expected standard, the paradigm may be mismatched to the skills of the patient. Readjustment of the paradigm may be required so that the activation map can be interpreted in light of control data. In general, more difficult tasks can elicit more activation and results acquired over a range of task difficulty can provide a useful additional measure of brain response (Just *et al.* 1996; Carpenter *et al.* 1999*a,b*).

A caution in this work is that physiological responses may follow the paradigm time course but be unrelated to the paradigm task. Fluctuations in respiratory and cardiac rates have been reported to change MR signal intensities (Hu *et al.* 1995). Such changes may occur by altering venous drainage from the brain or by bulk magnetic susceptibility effects. Care therefore should be taken that the small signal changes that may be *attributed* to activation are not just physiological effects. Several approaches can be used, these include: prospective gating of image acquisition to physiological responses, retrospective corrections to signal intensity time course data based on physiological cycles, and examining activation under specified physiological conditions by sorting the image data into specified phases of these physiological cycles.

Once these preliminary inspections of the data indicate that a valid data set is available, the activation map can be calculated from the statistical comparison of the conditions examined in several ways (as outlined in Chapter 14). The use of the voxel-wise student t-test to compare signal intensities between different paradigm conditions is the simplest and most conservative approach. It assumes an unrealistic boxcar response defined by the duration of each condition of the paradigm. The boxcar response can be refined to omit the known haemodynamic response delay of 5–10 s for transitions between paradigm states. Correlations can use any shape of reference function and offer the next step in refining the shape of the haemodynamic response by retaining the time course information. Other approaches include fitting the response to model functions (Cohen 1997; Genovese, 1997; Buxton *et al.* 1998; Cohen and Dubois 1999). Statistical parametric mapping software, SPM, (Cohen 1997), developed initially for analyzing data from positron emission tomography (PET), has been used also for fMRI. Clustering methods such as fuzzy clustering (Baumgartner *et al.* 1997; Moser *et al.* 1997), principle components analysis and a multitude of other methods have been described (Strupp, 1996). The methods have been applied according to the quality of the data, nature of the paradigms and the requirements of individual research laboratories. A review of various software packages has been reported elsewhere (Gold *et al.* 1998). As such, there is no entirely unequivocal answer as to the best statistical test to be used in a particular setting. This is determined in part by local resources and expertise. We have used the most conservative t-test for analysis of clinical studies presented in this chapter.

18.2.8 Data presentation

The communication of the full richness of the fMRI data to the referring physician is a challenge for a clinical service. The use of a standard reference frame such as that of Talairach (Talairach and Tournoux,

1988) to provide coordinates from activation is of little use in clinical management of individual patients. In clinical applications, the best approach is to register the functional data to the surface topography of the individual brain, e.g. as a colour scale of statistical significance overlaid onto multi-planar high-resolution grey-scale structural images of the same patient. The multi-dimensional aspects of the data thus can be conveyed visually to the neurosurgeon. However, when low-resolution fMRI images are acquired with a gradient-echo sensitized echo-planar or spiral sequence and displayed over high-resolution conventional images, care must be taken to understand the magnitude of any differences in distortions that may exist between the different image types. Errors may be quite large (as large as 10 mm) in certain areas of the brain, such as the inferior frontal lobes or the orbitofrontal cortex because air-tissue interfaces can produce magnetic susceptibility distortions that decrease accuracy of spatial localization or led to signal dropout (Kurata *et al.* 1999).

Another aspect of display that is useful for presurgical planning is to allow three orthogonal planes to be viewed. This is particularly useful if this is done in conjunction with registration to an external coordinate frame as is done in image-guided stereotaxis surgery. However, although three-dimensional rendering can be visually impressive and useful, it is computationally and time intensive. Given the experience with planar displays of data traditionally used clinically, this familiar approach currently remains the best form of communicating fMRI data.

Software packages are available for presentation of fMRI results, some of which are well documented and maintained as public domain software. The data presented in this chapter uses the Analysis of Functional NeuroImages (AFNI) (Dr. R. Cox, Medical College of Wisconsin) (Cox, 1996). In addition to functional data, the clinician often requires other data, including anatomic imaging, perfusion or diffusion imaging, and often (depending on the patient) MR angiography. The integration of so much multi-dimensional data from a comprehensive MR protocol (Thulborn *et al.* 1996) has been a challenge recently met by another software package (Thulborn *et al.* 1997*b*).

18.3 Mechanism of BOLD fMRI and its assumptions in clinical applications

A description of the mechanism of blood oxygenation level dependent (BOLD) contrast has been presented elsewhere in this text. A brief review will be given here only to emphasize how its assumptions relate to clinical applications. The importance of increasing spatial resolution to increase the magnitude of the BOLD signal change is also explained.

18.3.1 Spatial resolution

The optimum voxel size may be comparable to, or even smaller than the size of the functional unit of the cortex. This would minimize any partial volume effect that would decrease the relative signal change that occurs when activation in one part of a voxel is averaged with other areas of the voxel that do not activate. However, minimum practical voxel dimensions are limited by the concomitantly smaller signal. Greater signal-to-noise at higher magnetic field strengths enhances the magnitude of any BOLD contrast signal by permitting smaller voxels in addition to the direct effects of field strength on the magnitude of the BOLD effect. Results reported at 3.0 Tesla (Thulborn *et al.* 1997*a*) show that, at voxel dimensions of 0.8 mm in-plane and with slice thickness of 3 mm, both spin-echo and gradient-echo echo planar images can produce BOLD signal changes of about 8–12 per cent for stronger stimuli. Larger voxels at 3 mm in-plane resolution have smaller signal changes of 3–6 per cent despite better intrinsic signal-to-noise. This suggests that higher strength magnets (3 T or higher) offer a more robust BOLD response that may be useful in clinical settings where individual results are to bear on the management of that patient.

Comparisons at 3 T of high- and low-resolution activation maps with high-resolution venograms (Reichenbach *et al.* 1997), and apparent diffusion coefficient maps (Thulborn *et al.* 1997*a*) show that activation is associated with vessels under 300 microns in diameter as shown in Fig. 18.5 and Table 18.1. The single region of activation at low resolution is resolved into two regions at high resolution and each region has a signal intensity on the venogram that is much lower than that of veins. Similarly the apparent diffusion

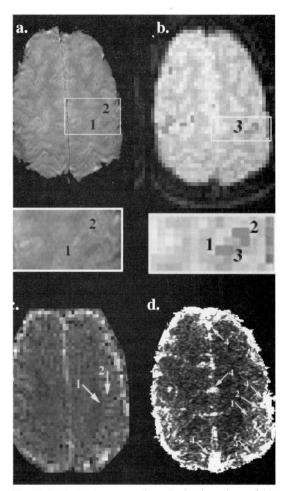

Fig. 18.5 Activation maps through the frontal eye fields from (a) high-resolution fMRI and (b) low-resolution using the VGS paradigm on the same subject. The gradient-echo echo planar imaging was performed with acquisition parameters: TR = 3000 ms, TE = 25 ms, with voxels dimensions of $0.8 \times 1.6 \times 3.0$ mm^3, and $3.1 \times 3.1 \times 3.0$ mm^3, respectively. Corresponding (c) apparent diffusion coefficient maps from diffusion weighted imaging and (d) high resolution venograms were obtained and used to localize tissue properties of the activation areas as shown in Table 18.1. The locations of the voxels with maximum t-value for the two clusters in the left frontal eye field on the high resolution map (1,2) are shown along with the voxel (3) at the center of the single equivalent cluster on low resolution image. These areas are projected onto the diffusion map and venogram. Areas (4) on the venogram represent veins. (See also colour plate section.)

Table 18.1 Parameters characterizing percent changes (%Δ) in signal intensities (SI) in areas 1 and 2 on high-resolution (HR) activation maps, areas 3 and 2 on low-resolution (LR) activation maps, signal intensities from veins on venogram, and apparent diffusion coefficient (ADC) in grey matter (GM), white matter (WM), and cerebrospinal fluid (CSF) on apparent diffusion coefficient (ADC) maps. The maps and regions are shown in Fig. 5. Area 1 on the HR map corresponds to area 3 on the LR map

	Area 1 (3)	Area 2	Veins	GM	WM	CSF
HR fMRI (%Δ SI)	2.0	3.3				
LR fMRI (%Δ SI)	1.1	−0.1				
Venogram (SI)	10	21	275	19	4.5	72
ADC (10^{-3} mm^2/s)	0.9	1.1	1.4	1.2	0.7	2.4

coefficients of the activation areas are consistent with grey matter, not white matter or cerebrospinal fluid. This may not be the case at 1.5 T (Krings *et al.* 1999). Very high-field MR imaging thus has advantages for accurate localization: allowing smaller voxel size, increasing the magnitude of the BOLD response, and increasing the contribution from brain relative to draining veins.

18.3.2 Haemodynamic coupling in disease

The second issue relevant to clinical applications is the assumption that the haemodynamic coupling of neuronal activity to the vascular response remains normal in the setting of pathology. If the normal coupling is disrupted, then the sensitivity of the BOLD response may be decreased or ablated completely, irrespective of any changes in the responsiveness of the underlying brain. Such a case has been reported for cortex adjacent to a glioblastoma multiforme (Holodry *et al.* 1999). Similarly, medications (including 'occult' drugs such as nicotine or caffeine) may also produce changes in the cerebrovascular circulation of a patient, thereby compromising the sensitivity of BOLD contrast. Interpretation of such clinical studies using a paradigm response calibrated in normal subjects (even when matched for age, gender, handedness, and skill set) may be misleading. One strategy for examining this issue has been to measure the adequacy of the baseline brain perfusion with diffusion weighted imaging

(DWI) and to measure the haemodynamic reserve by perfusion imaging before and after vasodilation.

As perfusion and diffusion imaging and the appropriate analyses are described elsewhere in this text, no further description will be given here. The use of these approaches will be demonstrated in the clinical examples below. The interpretation of BOLD contrast is limited to regions of normal diffusion and perfusion and adequate reserved perfusion capacity. No method currently exists for the interpretation of BOLD contrast in areas of abnormal perfusion in the clinical setting.

18.4 Clinical cases demonstrating fMRI applications

18.4.1 Presurgical planning

Arteriovenous malformations

An arteriovenous malformation in the brain is usually a congenital abnormality of vessels in which there is a direct connection of arteries to veins without an intervening capillary bed. Due to the absence of the normal precapillary control of blood flow, this abnormal anastomosis produces a high flow state that may become symptomatic at any age. Presentation in adults may be at the time of catastrophic haemorrhage or from development of neurological symptoms from encroachment of the blood supply of adjacent tissues. The treatment requires a reduction of the blood flow through these vessels. Such a result can be achieved by any combination of endovascular embolization to block the abnormal vessels, surgical resection or selective radiation therapy. Such lesions can be expected to show disturbances of tissue perfusion around the lesion. Thus, the issue of haemodynamic coupling arises in the very area in which functional information is required. The first case demonstrates an approach to this clinical setting.

Case 1 is a 30 year old right-handed man who presented with left-hand parathesia and poorly controlled hypertension. Extensive neuroimaging was performed as shown in Figs 18.6, 18.7, and 18.8 for anatomy, diffusion and perfusion imaging, respectively.

The conventional anatomic imaging shows the tangle of abnormal vessels in the right posterior frontal

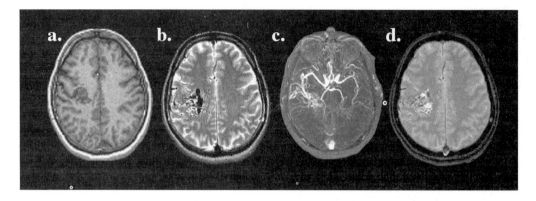

Fig. 18.6 Selected images from comprehensive anatomic imaging of Case 1 showing the arteriovenous malformation in the right posterior frontal lobe. (a) T1-weighted, gradient-echo, axial image, (b) T2-weighted, fast spin-echo image, (c) three-dimensional, time of flight, MR angiogram through the Circle of Willis and (d) susceptibility-sensitive, gradient-echo image demonstrate the AVM supplied from the enlarged right middle and anterior cerebral arteries, but without evidence of prior haemorrhage.

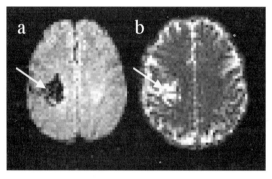

Fig. 18.7 Selected slices through the AVM (arrow) of Case 1. (a) Diffusion weighted image and (b) corresponding apparent diffusion coefficient trace map showing normal water diffusion up to the borders of the lesion.

lobe between the precentral and central sulci on both T1 and T2 weighted images (Figs 18.6(a) and 18.6(b)). The MRA (Fig. 18.6(c)) demonstrates arterial input is from enlarged right middle and anterior cerebral arteries while venous drainage is to the superior sagittal sinus. No previous haemorrhage is evident in terms of increased magnetic susceptibility signal loss on gradient-echo imaging (Fig. 18.6(d). Planning for the treatment of this lesion raised the question about the locations of motor, premotor and supplementary motor cortex which anatomically surround this lesion.

Given the symptoms, the surrounding cortex may have been ischaemic. This was tested with diffusion weighted imaging and the calculation of apparent diffusion coefficient maps (Thulborn *et al.* 1997*a*; Thulborn, 1999*c*) as shown in Fig. 18.7(a,b). As there is no restricted diffusion up to the edge of the AVM, it was concluded that substantial ischaemia was not present.

As the AVM has a high flow state, the surrounding cortex may not have sufficient haemodynamic reserve to show a BOLD response. This was tested by performing a perfusion study (Thulborn, 1999*c*; Thulborn *et al.* 1997*a*) based on susceptibility contrast bolus tracking before and after vasodilation with acetazolamide (1 g administered i.v. over 1 min and allowed 15 min for full effect). Pre- and post-vasodilation maps of tissue transit time (TTT) and relative cerebral blood volume (rCBV) are shown in Figs 18.8(a) and 18.8(b), respectively. Pre-vasodilation maps show normal values of TTT and rCBV up to the edge of the lesion. Post-vasodilation results in uniform lengthening of TTT and increased rCBV throughout the cerebral hemispheres up to the edge of the lesion. These data suggest that there is preserved haemodynamic reserve despite the AVM. Thus, according to this criterion, the interpretation of BOLD fMRI studies up to the edge of the AVM should not be compromised. Subsequently, fMRI studies were performed with the visually-guided saccade (Fig. 18.9) and finger tapping (Fig. 18.10) paradigms.

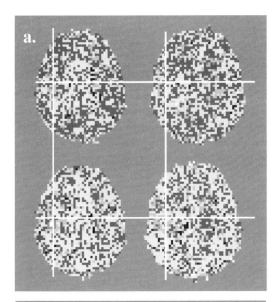

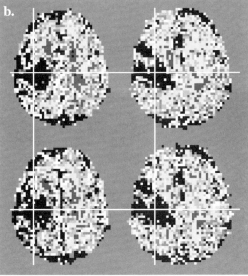

The VGS and finger tapping paradigm activated the frontal eye fields (FEF) in the precentral cortex clearly abutting the lesion. The more medial supplementary eye fields (SEF) and the supplementary motor area (SMA) were also activated. The motor cortex (M1) was anterior to the AVM whereas the activated somatosensory cortex (S1) was displaced posteriorly with the central sulcus. Given the close proximity of these functions to the lesion, the management of this AVM via the initially proposed endovascular and surgical approaches was changed to gamma knife irradiation.

Brain tumors

Treatment of brain tumors depends on their histological grade. The surgical resection of selected malignancies requires a wide margin to maximize the opportunity of complete removal. On the other hand, the proximity of eloquent cortex handicaps generous margins to avoid compromising patient function. The second case illustrates the role of functional mapping with the language paradigm, emphasizing its potential role even in paediatric applications. The bilaterality of language in most people (Thulborn *et al.* 1999*a*; Just *et al.* 1996) suggests that prognosis may be better than expected based on the anatomic location of the tumour.

Case 2 is a 14-year-old boy status post previous resection of an astrocytoma in the left parietal lobe but with recurrence of seizures. Anatomic neuroimaging was performed as shown in Fig. 18.11. The encephalomalacic change in the left parietal region from the previous resection is shown on both T1-, T2- and proton density weighted images (Figs 18.11a,b,c). No previous haemorrhage is evident in terms of increased magnetic susceptibility signal loss on gradient-echo imaging (Fig. 18.11d). The gadolinium contrast enhanced T1-weighted imaging in the axial and coronal planes shows a 5 mm enhancing nodule in the

Fig. 18.8 (a) Selected adjacent slices from the TTT perfusion parametric map through the AVM (centre marked by crosshairs) for the pre-vasodilation (*upper row*) and post-vasodilation (*lower row*). The color scale graded in seconds is: black, 0–5 s; blue, 5–10 s; green, 10–15 s; pink, 15–20 s; red, 20–25 s; and yellow, >25 s. The displacement of blue voxels by green voxels is clearly evident, indicating vasodilation with concomitant longer transition times in all areas including the AVM. Thus perfusion reserve appears to be maintained. (b)Selected adjacent slices from the rCBV perfusion parametric map through the AVM (centre marked by crosshairs) for the pre-vasodilation (upper row) and post-vasodilation (lower row). The color scale is a relative scale of: blue, 1–50; green, 50–100; pink, 100–150; red, 150–200; yellow, 200–250 s and black, >200. The trend from low blood volumes (blue and green colors) to higher blood volumes (pink, yellow and black colors) is evident up to the edge of the AVM, indicating a relative haemodynamic reserve in all areas despite the AVM. (See also colour plate section.)

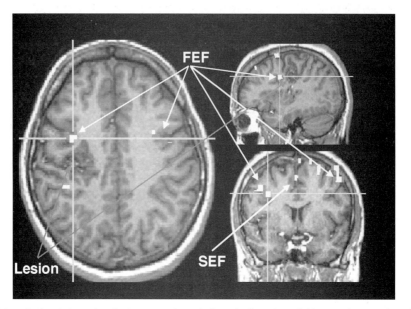

Fig. 18.9 Axial, sagittal and coronal activation maps through the right frontal eye field (FEF) showing the relative positions of the FEF and supplementary eye fields (SEF) to the AVM (lesion, red arrows) of Case 1. The t-statistic (threshold of 3.5) is displayed as a color scale: yellow > red > 3.5. The green lines show the relative location of each mapping plane. This presentation was derived from AFNI software. (See also colour plate section.)

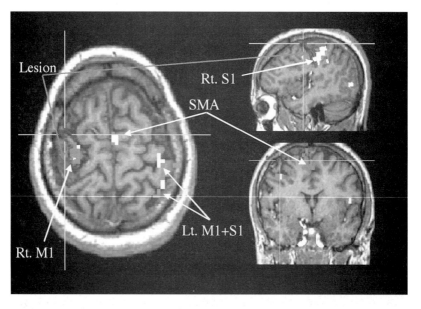

Fig. 18.10 Axial, sagittal and coronal activation maps through the right motor cortex (M1) showing the relative positions of M1 and supplementary motor area (SMA) to the AVM (lesion, red arrows) of Case 1. The t-threshold was set at 3.5 and is displayed as a color scale: yellow > red > 3.5. The green lines show the relative locations of each plane. The SMA is posterior to SEF shown in Fig. 18.9. M1 is posterior to FEF but anterior to the lesion. The left M1 and S1 were also strongly activated whereas this only weakly occurs in normal subjects. The right S1 (shown on the sagittal map) identified on a more inferior axial slice is posterior to the AVM.(See also colour plate section.)

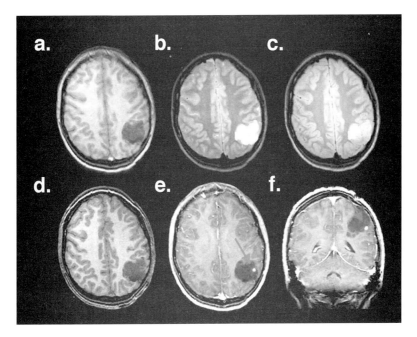

Fig. 18.11 Selected images from comprehensive anatomic imaging of Case 2 showing the encephalomalacic area in the left frontoparietal region. (a) T1-weighted, spin-echo axial image, (b) T2-weighted, fast spin-echo image, (c) proton density-weighted fast spin-echo image, (d) 3D gradient-echo image and post intravenous gadolinium contrast enhancement in the (e) axial and (f) coronal planes. The enhancing nodule is indicated by the arrow in (e) and (f).

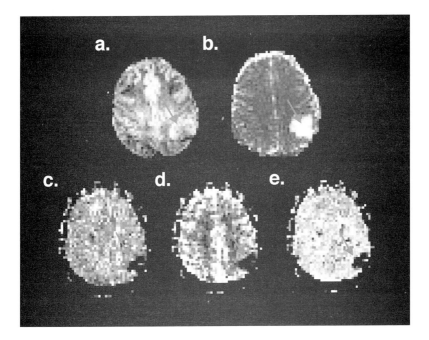

Fig. 18.12 Selected slices through the encephalomalacia (arrow) of Case 2. (a) Diffusion weighted image and (b) corresponding apparent diffusion coefficient trace map showing normal water diffusion up to the borders of the encephalomalacia. The equivalent slice from the perfusion parametric maps are shown as (c) tissue transit time (TTT) map, (d) relative cerebral blood volume (rCBV) map and (e) time of arrival (TA) map. These parameters are also normal up to the edge of the encephalomalacia. BOLD contrast studies should be interpretable up to these boundaries.

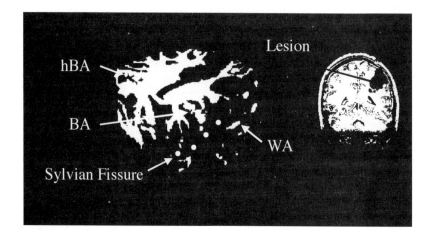

Fig. 18.13

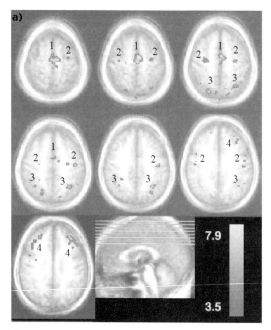
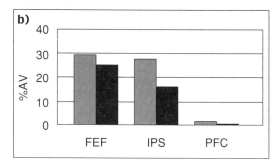
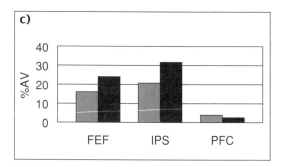

Fig. 18.14

inferior lateral aspect of the surgical bed (Figs 11e,f). Planning for the resection of this tumour recurrence raised the question about the proximity of Wernicke's area in the anatomically close superior gyrus of the temporal lobe. The surrounding cortex was examined for ischaemia with diffusion weighted imaging and the calculation of apparent diffusion coefficient maps (Baumgartner *et al.* 1997; Thulborn, 1999*c*,) as shown in Fig. 18.12a,b). As there is no restricted diffusion up to the edge of the nodule, ischaemia is not present. The encephalomalacic region shows ADC values comparable to cerebrospinal fluid (CSF) as would be expected. A simple perfusion study based on susceptibility contrast bolus tracking (Thulborn *et al.* 1997*a*; Thulborn 1999*c*,) was performed and maps of the tissue transit time (TTT), relative cerebral blood volume (rCBV) and arrival-time (TA) were normal up to the margin of the lesion (Fig. 18.12c,d,e). The fMRI studies were performed with both the language and motor (finger tapping) tasks. Only the language task is shown in Fig. 18.13. Wernicke's area was functionally defined to be more inferior and anterior to the nodule. The surgical approach was from anterior and superior to the nodule with uneventful resection. The patient is doing well without loss of language skills.

18.4.2 Diagnosis

Alzheimer's disease

Although fMRI requires cooperative subjects, this example demonstrates that even demented patients can be examined successfully with an appropriate paradigm. This example also demonstrates an approach to expressing fMRI data in terms of the distribution of activation. The laterality ratio (LR) reflects the distribution of activation between equivalent areas of the two cerebral hemispheres as: $LR = (L\text{-}R)/(L + R)$, where L and R are the volumes of activation for equivalent areas in the left and right hemispheres, respectively. This ratio is positive for left dominant processes, negative for right dominant processes and zero for co-dominant processes.

Young adult and elderly control subjects show a negative laterality ratio for the intraparietal sulcal (IPS) activation of the VGS paradigm (Thulborn *et al.* 2000). This area may be involved in visual spatial attention. In contrast, for patients with probable Alzheimer's disease, a positive LR(IPS) for the VGS paradigm has been found, consistent with pathologically dysfunction of the parietal lobe. Although these data are expressed as group maps for scientific reporting as shown in Fig. 18.14, results for clinical reports of individual patients also can be expressed as laterality ratios. Comparisons of activation volumes between left and right hemispheres for the normal and probable Alzheimer's disease groups (Fig. 18.15(b) and (c), respectively) show that the normally dominant right intraparietal sulcal activation is reduced below that of the left hemisphere by Alzheimer's disease.

18.4.3 Rehabilitation therapy

Stroke

Patients who survive the acute and subacute phases of stroke show variable recovery. The uncertain nature of this recovery process is now open to investigation with fMRI. Recently two cases of recovery from aphasia were examined with serial fMRI and the language

Fig. 18.13 *(Above left)* Three-dimensional (3D) rendering of the activation map for Case 2. The exposed axial, coronal and sagittal planes through the AVM (lesion, red arrows) show the lesion's relative position to Wernicke's area (WA, posterior left superior temporal gyrus), Broca's area (BA, left inferior frontal lobe) and homologous Broca's area (hBA, right frontal lobe) and the Sylvian fissure (green dots). The t-threshold was set at 3.5 and is displayed as a color scale: yellow > red > 3.5. The coronal contrast enhanced image to the right shows the gadolinium contrast-enhancing nodule medial and superior to WA. This 3D presentation is an alternative presentation to three planes of Figures 18.9 and 18.10 and is also derived from AFNI software. (See also colour plate section.)

Fig. 18.14 *(Below left)* (a) Group activation map for a group of patients with Alzheimer's disease in which the group averages of the activation and the structural studies are superimposed. Such a group analysis is readily performed with AFNI software. Bar graphs expressing the percentage activation volume (per cent AV) for the dorsal pathway activated by the VGS paradigm are shown for (b) normal elderly control subjects (n = 5) and (c) patients with Alzheimer's disease (n = 9). Three areas; frontal eye fields (FEF), intraparietal sulcus (IPS), and prefrontal cortex (PFC), of the right (gray) and left (black) cerebral hemispheres are plotted. The reversed sign of the LR is statistically significant (p < 0.1) for IPS with the diagnosis of probable Alzheimer's disease. The total activation is reduced in this disease also. (See also colour plate section.)

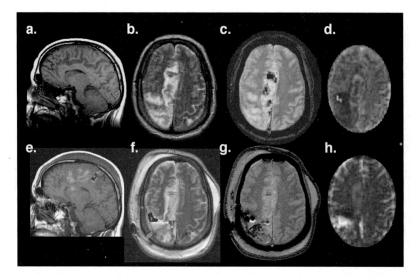

Fig. 18.15   Selected anatomic images from Case 3 through the large right hemispheric stroke involving territories of both the right anterior and middle cerebral arteries at two days post event: (a) sagittal T1-weighted spin-echo image, (b) axial T2-weighted fast spin-echo image, (c) axial gradient-echo image and (d) ADC map showing reduced ADC in the areas of signal abnormality on the anatomic images. Comparable images following strokectomy at four days post event are: (e) sagittal T1-weighted spin-echo image, (b) axial T2-weighted fast spin-echo image, (c) axial gradient-echo image and (d) ADC map showing reduced ADC at the periphery and high ADC centrally in the surgical site. The right motor cortex was resected in the emergent strokectomy required to halt brain herniation during an acute neurological decline.

paradigm (Thulborn *et al.* 1999*a*). The results indicated that recovery was not based on the survival of tissue in the damaged zone but rather due to the redistribution of cognitive workload over the existing large-scale neurocognitive network. The current case serves to emphasize this point.

Case 3 is a 30 year old right-handed man who presented with dense left hemiplegia at 6 hours showed a stroke in the posterior distribution of the right middle and anterior cerebral arteries. The conventional T1- and T2-weighted MR images showed abnormal signal along the right cingulate gyrus and over the right temporoparietal regions (Figs 18.15a,b). The gradient echo MR images showed haemorrhage within the stroke involving the anterior cerebral artery (Fig. 18.15c) (although the stroke was termed non-haemorrhagic based on an earlier computed tomographic examination). There was restricted diffusion and reduced ADC in the stroke region (Fig. 18.15d). The patient was maintained on heparin therapy. By day 4, the patient experienced a rapid neurological decline, consistent with cerebral herniation from brain swelling and underwent a strokectomy. This resection removed the region of stroke encompassing the right motor cortex.

The anatomic imaging showing the post-operative anatomy is shown in Figs 18.15e,f,g,h). Given the removal of the right motor cortex, poor recovery from the hemiplegia would typically be expected. However, by the time that the patient returned for a fMRI study four weeks later, he was able to walk with a cane. Although unable to perform left finger tapping and foot movement easily, he was able to move his wrist and rotate his foot sufficiently to allow fMRI to be used to define brain activation associated with movements of the left upper and lower extremities. Responses from the left side were compared with those from the normal right side for finger tapping and foot dorsi- and plantar-flexion. The results for the foot movement are shown in Fig. 18.16.

Recovery of the left-sided extremity function was associated with activation of the left hemisphere for both upper and lower extremities. This redistribution happened rapidly and without any apparent activation in the right cortex.

Not only do such cases demonstrate that fMRI can be performed in the setting of abnormal physiology but that fMRI has a role in monitoring the rehabilitation process. As experience is gained with this

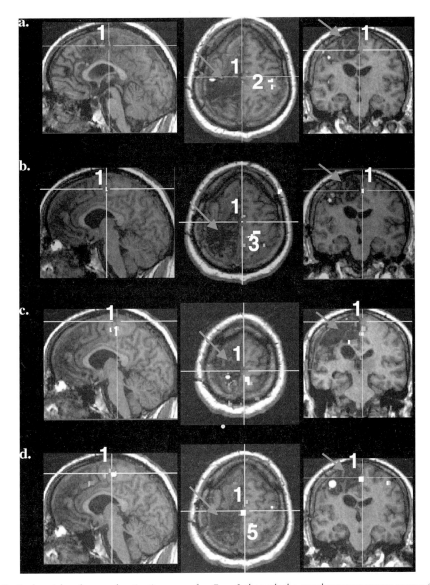

Fig. 18.16 Sagittal, axial and coronal activation maps for Case 3 through the supplementary motor cortex (1, SMA) and primary motor and somatosensory cortex of the left hemisphere in response to movement of the right upper (2), left upper (3), right lower (4) and left lower (5) extremities. The green lines show the relative locations of the three planes. This mapping shows robust activation elicited by movement of the left extremities in the left hemisphere adjacent to areas activated by the right extremities. The strokectomy (red arrows) clearly shows that the right motor cortex was resected. The patient was able to walk with a cane at 4 weeks following strokectomy suggesting that recovery was supported by redistribution of the cognitive workload to the left hemisphere. (See also colour plate section.)

devastating disease, fMRI may aid in the development of rehabilitation interventions to enhance these intrinsic compensation mechanisms.

18.5 Conclusion

As we consider using fMRI in the clinical arena, care must be taken to ensure high quality studies in the setting of single patient examinations in the presence of abnormal physiology. Mistakes have serious implications for the acceptance of this methodology as well as for the care of individual patients. Quality control of the imaging environment, patient preparation and selection, as well as appropriately calibrated paradigms are mandatory. With adequate attention to the points described in this chapter, fMRI becomes an exciting window onto brain function in many patient populations currently thought to be inappropriate for imaging.

Brain function appears to be distributed over large-scale neurocognitive networks with patterns based on workload and available resources. Such distributed processing seems to underlie the great plasticity of the human brain to buffer changes in cognitive function in at least some catastrophic acute and chronic diseases. Neuroimaging, especially fMRI, provides an opportunity to monitor these innate compensation mechanisms that cope with compromised performance due to disease. These compensation mechanisms offer potential for enhancing cognitive and behavioral function even in the presence of some types of diseases.

An interdisciplinary team of neuroradiologists, cognitive psychologists, MR physicists, statisticians, engineers, neurologists and psychiatrists will be required to ensure optimal clinical utilization of this emerging fMRI technology.

References

Baumgartner, R., Scarth, G., Teichtmeister, C., Somorjai, R., and Moser, E.. (1997). Fuzzy clustering of gradient-echo functional MRI in the human visual cortex. Part I: Reproducibility. *JMRI*, 7, 1094–01.

Berman, R.A., Colby, C.L., Genovese, C.R., Voyvodic, J.T., Luna, B., Thulborn, K.R., and Sweeney, J.A. (1999). Cortical-networks subserving pursuit and saccadic eye movements in humans: a fMRI study. *Human Brain Mapping*, 8, 209–25.

Binder, J.R., Rao, S.M., Hammeke, T.A., Yetkin, F.Z., Jesmanowicz, A., Bandettini, P.A., Wong, E.C., Estkowski, L.D., Goldstein, M.D., Haughton, V.M., and Hyde, J.S. (1994). Functional magnetic resonance imaging of human auditory cortex. *Annals of Neurology*, 35, 662–72.

Biswal, B., Yetkin, F.Z., Haughton, V.M., and Hyde, J.S. (1995). Functional connectivity in the motor cortex of resting human brain using echo-planar MRI *Magnetic Resonance in Medicine*, 34, 537–41.

Booth, J.R., MacWhinney, B., Thulborn, K.R., Sacco, K., Voyvodic, J., and Feldman, H.M. (1999). Functional organization of activation patterns in children: Whole brain fMRI imaging during three different cognitive tasks. Progress in *NeuroPsychopharmacology and Biological Psychiatry*, 23, 669–82.

Buxton, R.B., Wong, E.C., and Frank, L.R. (1998). Dynamics of blood flow and oxygenation changes during brain activation: the balloon model. *Magnetic Resonance in Medicine*, 39, 855–64.

Carpenter, P.A., Just, M.A., Keller, T.A., Eddy, W.F., Thulborn, K.R. (1999a). Time course of fMRI-activation in language and spatial networks during sentence comprehension. *NeuroImage*, 10, 216–24.

Carpenter, P.A., Just, M.A., Keller, T., Eddy, W., Thulborn, K.R. (1999b). Graded functional activation in the visuospatial system with the amount of task demand. *Journal of Cognitive Neuroscience*, 11, 9–24.

Cohen, M.S. (1997). A linear systems approach to the parametric analysis of fMRI time series. *Neuroimage*, 6:93–103.

Cohen, M.S. and DuBois, R.M. (1999). Stability, repeatability, and the expression of signal magnitude in functional magnetic resonance imaging. *Journal of Magnetic Resonance Imaging*, 10, 33–40.

Cohen, M.S. and Weisskoff, R.M. (1991). Ultra-fast imaging. *Magnetic Resonance Imaging*, 9, 1–37.

Cox, R.W. (1996). AFNI, software for analysis and visualization of functional magnetic resonance neuroimages. *Computers and Biomedical Research*, 29, 162–73.

Eddy, W.F., Fitzgerald, M., Genovese, C., Mockus, A., and Noll, D.C. (1996). In: *Functional imaging analysis software—computational olio*. Proceedings in Computational Statistics, pp.39–49. Physica-Verlagm, Heidelberg.

Friston, K.J., Frith, C.D., Liddle, P.F., and Frackowiak, R.S. (1991). Comparing functional (PET) images: the asessment of significant change. *Journal of Cerebral Blood Flow and Metabolism*, 11, 690–9.

Genovese, C.R. (1997). In: *A time-course model for fMRI data*, p.1669, ISMRM 5th Annual Meeting, Vancouver, B.C., Canada.

Glover, G.H. (1999). Simple analytic spiral *k*-space algorithm. *Magnetic Resonance in Medicine*, 42, 412–15.

Gold, S., Christian, B., Arndt, S., Zeien, G., Cizadlo, T., Johnson, D.L., Fiaum, M., and Andreasen, N.C. (1998). Functional MRI statistical software packages: a comparative analysis. *Human Brain Mapping*, 6, 73–84.

Holodny A.I., Schulder M., Lui W.C., Maldjian J.A., and Kalvin A.J. (1999). Decreased BOLD functional MR activation of the motor and sensory contices adjacent to a glioblastoma multiforme: implications for image - guided neurosurgery. *AJNR American Journal of Neuroradiology*, 20, 609–612.

Hu, X., Le, T.H., Parrish, T., and Erhard, P. (1995). Retrospective estimation and correction of physiological fluctuations in functional MRI. *Magnetic Resonance in Medicine*, **34**, 201–12.

Jancke, L., Buchanan, T., Lutz, K., Specht, K., Mirzazade, S., and Shah, N.J.S. (1999). The time course of the BOLD response in the human auditory cortex to acoustic stimuli of different duration. *Cognitive Brain Research*, **8**, 117–24.

Just, M.A., Carpenter, P.A., Keller, T.A., Eddy, W.F., and Thulborn, K.R. (1996). Brain activation modulated by sentence comprehension. *Science*, **274**, 114–16.

Kim, B., Boes, J.L., Bland, P.H., Chenevert, T.L., Meyer, C.R. (1999). Motion correction in fMRI via registration of individual slices into an anatomic volume. *Magnetic Resonance in Medicine*, **41**, 964–72.

Krings, T., Erberich, S.G., Roessler, F., Reul, J., and Thron, A. (1999). MR blood oxygenation level-dependent signal differences in parenchyma and large draining vessels: Implications for functional MR imaging. *AJNR American Journal of Neuroradiology*, **20**, 1907–14.

Kurata, J., Firestone, L.L., and Thulborn, K.R. (1999). In: *Accuracy of functional mapping with fMRI is limited by image distortions.* 25th Proceedings of Society for Neuroscience, Miami Beach, FL, 23–29 October 1999, #601.1.

Lee, C.C., Ward, H.A., Sharbrough, F.S., Meyer, F.B., March, W.R., Raffel, C., So, E.L, Cascino, G.D., Shin, C., Xu, Y., Riederer, S.J., and Jack, C.R. (1999). Assessment of functional MR imaging in neurosurgical planning. *AJNR American Journal of Neuroradiology*, **20**, 1511–19.

Luna, B., Thulborn, K.R., Strojwas, M.H., McCurtain, B.J., Berman, R.A., Genovese, C.R., and Sweeney, J.A. (1998). Dorsal cortical regions subserving visually-guided saccades in humans: a fMRI study. *Cerebral Cortex*, **8**, 40–7.

Luna, B. and Sweney, J.A. (1999a). Cognitive functional magnetic resonance imaging at very-high-field: eye movement control. *Topics in Magnetic Resonance Imaging*, **10**, 3–15.

Luna, B., Minshew, N.J., Keshavan, M.S., Merriam, E.P., Eddy, W.F., Thulborn, K.R., and Sweeney, J.A. (1999b). In: *Spatial working memory improves from late childhood to adulthood: eye movement and fMRI studies.* 25th Proceedings of Society for Neuroscience, Miami Beach, FL, 23–29 October 1999, #463.9.

Moser, E., Diemling, M., and Baumgartner, R. (1997). Fuzzy clustering of gradient-echo functional MRI in the human visual cortex. Part II: quantification. *JMRI*, **7**, 1102–08.

Patel, M.R., Blum, A., Pearlman, J.D., Naveed, Y., Ives, J.R., Saeteng, S., Schomer, D.L., and Edelman, R.R. (1999). Echo-planar functional MR imaging of epilepsy with concurrent EEG monitoring. *AJNR American Journal of Neuroradiology*, **20**, 1916–19.

Reichenbach, J.R., Venkatesan, R., Schillinger, D.J., Kido, D.K., Haacke, E.M. (1997). Small vessels in the human brain. MR venography with deoxyhemoglobin as an intrinsic contrast agent. *Radiology*, **7**, 266–79.

Richter, W. (1999). High temporal resolution functional magnetic resonance imaging at very-high-field. *Topics in Magnetic Resonance Imaging*, **10**, 51–62.

Rosen, B.R., Buckner, R.L., and Dale, A.M. (1998). Event-related functional MRI: Past present and future. *Proceedings of the National Academy of Sciences (USA)*, **95**, 773–80.

Rosenberg, D.R., Sweeney, J.A., Gillen, J.S., Chang, S.Y., Varanelli, M.J., O'Hearn, K., Erb, P.A., Davis, D., and Thulborn, K.R. (1997). Magnetic resonance imaging of children without sedation: preparation with simulation. *Journal of the American Academy of Child and Adolescent Psychiatry*, **36**, 853–9.

Strupp, J.P. (1996). Stimulate: a GUI based fMRI analysis software package. *NeuroImage*, **3**, 607.

Sweeney, J.A., Luna, B., Strojwas, M., Berman, R.A., McCurtain, B.J., Genovese, C.R., and Thulborn, K.R.(1997). *Functional MRI studies of eye movement control: a paradigm for clinical applications*, p.451, Proceedings Fifth Scientific Meeting International Society of Magnetic Resonance in Medicine, April 1997 Vancouver, Canada.

Talairach, J. and Tournoux, P. (1988). *Co-planar stereotaxic atlas of the human brain: 3D proportional system: an approach to cerebral imaging.* Georg Thieme Verlag, New York, NY.

Thulborn, K.R. (1999a). Quality assurance in clinical and research echo-planar functional MRI. In: *Medical radiology—diagnostic imaging and radiation oncology. Functional MRI* (ed. C. Moonen, P. Bandettini), chapter 28, pp.337–46. Springer-Verlag, Berlin.

Thulborn, K.R. (1999b). Visual feedback to stabilize head position for fMRI. *Magnetic Resonance in Medicine*, **41**, 1039–43.

Thulborn, K.R. (1999c). Clinical rationale for very high field (3.0 Tesla) functional MR imaging. *Topics in Magnetic Resonance Imaging*, **10**, 37–50.

Thulborn, K.R., Davis, D., Erb, P., Strojwas, M., and Sweeney, J.A. (1996). Clinical fMRI: implementation and experience. *NeuroImage*, **4**, S101-S107.

Thulborn, K.R., Chang, S.Y., Shen, G.X., and Voyvodic, J.T. (1997a) High resolution echo-planar fMRI of human visual cortex at 3.0 Tesla. *NMR in Biomedicine*, **10**, 183–90.

Thulborn, K.R., Uttecht, S., Betancourt, C., Talagala, S.L., Boada, F.E., and Shen, G.X. (1997b) A functional, physiological and metabolic toolbox for clinical magnetic resonance imaging: integration of acquisition and analysis strategies. *International Journal of Imaging Systems Technology*, **8**, 572–81.

Thulborn, K.R., Carpenter, P.A., and Just, M.A. (1999a). Plasticity of language-related brain function during recovery from stroke. *Stroke*, **30**, 749–54.

Thulborn, K.R., Gindin, T.S., Davis, D., and Erb, P. (1999b). Comprehensive MRI protocol for stroke management: tissue sodium concentration as a measure of tissue viability in a non-human primate model and clinical studies. *Radiology*, **139**, 26–34.

Thulborn, K.R., Martin, C., and Voyvodic, J. (2000). Functional MR imaging using a visually guided saccade paradigm for comparing activation patterns in patients with probable Alzheimer's disease and in cognitively able elderly volunteers. *American Journal of Neuroradiology*, **21**(3), 524–31.

Woods, R.P., Cherry, S.R., and Mazziotta, J.C. (1992). Rapid automated algorithm for aligning and reslicing PET images. *Journal of Computer Assisted Tomography*, **16**, 620–33.

VI | *Integrating technologies*

19 | Dynamic functional neuroimaging integrating multiple modalities

John S. George, David M. Schmidt, David M. Rector and Chris Wood

19.1 Introduction

The past few decades have witnessed extraordinary progress in the development of techniques for non-invasive structural and functional imaging of the human brain. However, despite this progress, no existing medical imaging modality provides all of the information required for best clinical practice or cutting edge research. MRI is the premier technique for characterizing the soft tissue anatomy of the human brain, but it has significant limitations for defining the geometry of the skull. Functional MRI provides detailed pictures of spatial patterns of neural activation based on associated haemodynamic changes, but does not capture the characteristic temporal dynamics of electrophysiological activation. MEG and EEG provide excellent temporal resolution of neural population dynamics but are limited in spatial resolution by the ambiguity and ill-posed nature of the source reconstruction problem. Electrical and magnetic stimulation offer capability for direct intervention in central or peripheral neural pathways, but depend on knowledge of anatomical and functional organization drawn from other sources. Other methods (including electrophysiology and microanatomy, optical and magnetic resonance spectroscopy, impedance tomography, PET, SPECT, endoscopy, neurosurgical intervention, behavioural and lesion studies), each provide important and unique, though more limited insight into neural function and functional organization. Although the mix and relative importance of imaging technologies will evolve, the need to integrate information from multiple methods will remain.

19.1.1 Anatomical MRI

The exquisite soft tissue images provided by magnetic resonance serve as the anatomical underpinning for functional neuroimaging of the human brain. An expanding array of methods depends on computational geometries derived from MRI to properly model the physical processes on which the measurements are based. 3D volume imaging allows researchers to define the anatomical substrate of functional activation. MRI allows documentation of the detailed anatomy of every subject in functional brain mapping studies. Emerging techniques will allow rigorous quantitative comparisons of anatomy and functional architecture across large numbers of normal individuals as well as populations with particular psychological or neurological abnormalities. A variety of brain warping or cortical unfolding strategies allow the individual anatomy to be mapped into a canonical brain coordinate system. Such capabilities have inspired initial efforts to develop statistical, probabilistic atlases of human brain structure (see Chapter 15). As atlases are extended to include functional data, they will become important sources of prior knowledge for MEG and EEG, and other forms of functional neuroimaging.

19.1.2 Functional MRI

The development of MRI-based techniques for mapping of the haemodynamic responses to neural activation has had profound effects on human neuroscience. fMRI provides spatial resolution unprecedented for noninvasive imaging. The underlying technology is widely accessible, and the methods are suitable for a wide range of paradigms. FMRI also has useful temporal resolution (see Chapter 7). As described in Chapters

17 and 18, responses to sensory stimuli or activation associated with cognitive or motor tasks separated by several seconds are readily resolved, so that the method allows tracking of many forms of problem solving or goal directed behaviour. The consistent lags associated with haemodynamic responses allow inference of physiological activation shifts of less than a second, particularly within a functional area. This allows tagging of stimuli and responses by time, a strategy exploited to map retinotopic organization and thereby identify early visual areas (Sereno *et al.* 1995).

Initial demonstrations of fMRI in humans (Belliveau *et al.* 1991) involved the injection of a paramagnetic contrast agent and required echo planar imaging capability (EPI) (Stehling *et al.* 1991) to resolve the initial passage of the injected bolus through the cerebral circulation. By measuring the local reduction in image intensity due to magnetic susceptibility, it was possible to calculate blood volume, which changes as a function of neural activation. As described throughout this book, current work exploits the paramagnetic nature of deoxyhaemoglobin to monitor changes in blood volume or venous blood oxygen content (Kwong *et al.* 1992; Ogawa *et al.* 1992). Because BOLD fMRI does not require administration of radioactivity or contrast agents, it is compatible with continuous recording, complex experimental paradigms and repeated experiments within individuals. As a practical matter, the relatively benign nature of the methodology helps insure a ready supply of volunteers. However, in spite of the phenomenal success of existing fMRI methods, there remain significant limitations. One of the most important is that the haemodynamic response is too slow to define brain activity adequately.

Many functions of the networks of the brain depend on the temporal interplay between spatially distinct spatial networks, interleaved through a particular cortical area, or spread across much of the cortical surface. Although the dynamics of some responses (e.g. action potentials) are sub-millisecond, the dominant time-scales for network interactions appear to be milliseconds and tens of milliseconds. MEG and EEG can record activities (averaged across populations of neurones) on these timescales. Unlike BOLD fMRI, these methods measure signals that are the direct physical consequences of electrophysiological activity.

19.1.3 MEG and EEG

With the advent of whole head sensor arrays and improved analytical strategies, neural electromagnetic (NEM) techniques (MEG, EEG, and related methods) are becoming increasingly important tools for human brain mapping, with particular advantages for tracking the temporal dynamics of brain activity (for review, see Hamalainen *et al.* 1993). Because these techniques provide no direct information about brain anatomy, they are typically used in conjunction with MRI to allow correlation of function with anatomical structure (George *et al.* 1989; Ranken and George 1993; Aine *et al.* 1996).

There now are several classes of computational techniques that allow the integration of data from MEG and MRI to improve the accuracy and reliability of functional neuroimaging by MEG (George *et al.* 1995*a,b*). In all of these MRI is used to build more realistic geometric models of primary compartments within the head volume conductor. This allows more accurate calculation of magnetic fields or potential distributions produced by primary currents within the head, which can improve the accuracy of source localization. MRI-derived models of the detailed geometry of cerebral cortex are used to constrain tomographic current reconstruction procedures. This strategy significantly reduces the number of parameters required to describe a general source model and thereby can enhance the performance of algorithms to solve the inverse problem. Functional MRI is used to constrain the inverse problem, allowing estimation of the timecourse of regions of activation identified through fMRI. This allows the integrated application of two powerful paradigms for functional neuroimaging, exploiting the strengths and minimizing the weaknesses of each.

19.2 Multi-modality imaging

The complementary strengths and weaknesses of available functional neuroimaging techniques have driven efforts by a number of investigators to combine multiple imaging modalities. However, this ambition poses a number of challenges—both fundamental and technical—that must be addressed.

19.2.1 Co-registration

One of the most basic requirements for multimodality imaging is that we are able to define the spatial relationships between the measures. Although the principles and some of the computational issues have been outlined in Chapter 15, there are technical and practical details that require careful attention for successful multi-modality investigations. Since MRI is used to define the anatomy, the general strategy is to define the coordinate system of other measurements relative to the implicit coordinate system of the MR volume imaging. Positions of the sensors used for MEG or EEG are typically measured in a head-centred reference frame defined by external anatomical references such as the bridge of the nose and the preauricular points adjacent to the external ear canals. The first step in multi-modality co-registration is to define the location of the sensor array relative to these anatomical landmarks.

A variety of systems have been used for this purpose, including calipers, mechanical arm digitizers, optical digitizers, and sonic probes. Perhaps the most widely used systems are magnetic 3D-space tracking and digitizing systems (e.g. as marketed by Polheimus Navigation Systems). The Polheimus systems employ magnetic field transmitter and pickup subsystems, each consisting of a set of three orthogonal coils. The transmitter is positioned at a fixed location and pickup coils embedded in a stylus or a discrete sensor are used to localize the pickup coils relative to the transmitter. Such systems can be used to digitize the location of each electrode of an EEG system, as well as the anatomical landmarks that define the coordinate system. Some MEG systems incorporate an active probe (or transmitter assemblies that are attached to the head) and use the MEG sensor array as the receiver for probe localization.

Once the spatial relationships between anatomical landmarks and the sensor array are established, it remains to define their spatial relationship to the MRI volume dataset. In early experiments MRI-visible fiducial markers (such as oil-filled capsules) were sometimes attached to the head surface. However, once full 3D volume imaging became routinely available, it became clear that there are significant advantages to locating the anatomical landmarks precisely on a head-surface defined from the MRI data itself.

With MEG data, the sensor array is fixed, so that it is only necessary to define the spatial relationship between the instrument and the head. With EEG, the relative locations of sensors can vary depending on the head shape and application techniques. Most EEG labs interested in precise source localization measure the position of each electrode, either with a 3D probe, or by video imaging.

Fitting procedures that employ anatomical landmarks in addition to defined electrode locations bring more data to bear on the coordinate reconciliation problem, and allow estimates of the localization variance based on different physical principles. In this regard, we note that the warping of images due to MRI gradient field inhomogeneities can introduce errors in the co-registration process, as can magnetic susceptibility effects, especially since external anatomical features often fall into the more troublesome regions of the acquisition volume. This sort of problem can be corrected with adequate instrument calibration and post-processing, but such corrections often are not made routinely.

Integrated visualization based on multiple co-registered data sets is a useful application of multimodality imaging, allowing neuroscientists to appreciate the relationship between neuroanatomy and functional architecture. The same capabilities are essential for most other applications of integrated computational modeling. The technical requirements are relatively straightforward, once the appropriate coordinate transforms are established.

19.2.2 Physical models

MEG and EEG (as well as other developing imaging methodologies) require nested computational models, to encapsulate measurement physics and to build plausible models of functional activation that account for experimental observations. Analytical head models consisting of one or more concentric spherical shells have been the mainstay of NEM source localization techniques to date (e.g. Sarvas, 1987), but a number of studies have shown that models incorporating a more realistic geometry of the principal conductivity boundaries can significantly improve source localization accuracy under some circumstances. A number of lines of evidence suggest that the dominant sources of NEM signals are postsynaptic currents in the cell bodies and dendrites of cortical grey matter (e.g. Mitzdorf, 1985). By assuming that sources lie within and normal to the thin layer of tissue comprising neocortex, it is possible to derive models that reduce the ambiguity and strengthen the power of reliable inference.

Building models of the gross anatomy of the head and the 3-D structure of neocortex remains a challenge, although the past decade has produced a number of advances. In present practice, *anatomical segmentation* is often undertaken on the basis of isotropic (or at least densely sampled) MR image volumes. After a certain measure of processing to remove inhomogeneities and artefacts in the images, semiautomatic voxel classification or region growing techniques can do an adequate job of identifying relevant classes of tissue. For many purposes a segmented volume or list of voxels is all that is required. However, many high performance rendering and volume modeling techniques require the additional step of tesselation: arbitrary boundary surfaces are divided into a series of contiguous triangles, or the volume is divided into a collection of tetrahedra. This strategy has the advantage that complex surfaces or volumes can be modelled with a minimum number of elements, leading to more efficient computations with acceptable accuracy.

19.2.3 Experimental strategy

Most multi-modality functional neuroimaging studies to date have employed experimental designs that could be utilized in separate trials with good reproducibility. This requirement is not a serious constraint. Most functional imaging techniques used in isolation require signal averaging over multiple trials in order to obtain reliable responses; it is a relatively small step to design experiments with repeated trials that can be staged as separate experiments with different functional mapping techniques. More than one experimentalist has argued that separate, modality-specific studies are the most practical strategy for multi-modality imaging.

Nevertheless, simultaneous measurements also have advantages. Experiments that collect more data can be more efficient, and can avoid the potential of confounding variables. For many applications, simultaneous measurements are essential for some experimental objectives. Studies of learning and memory, for example, are often influenced by the experience and state of the subject, including changes elicited by the experimental paradigm itself. It may not be possible to fully control for such effects with separate experiments. There also are special situations in which data from one modality determines the nature of that from a second. For example, fMRI studies of sleep need EEG to allow definition of the changing stages, and studies of epilepsy need simultaneous EEG to allow identification of interictal or mild seizure events. These signals allow relevant responses to be pulled out of ongoing fMRI data, or can be used to trigger acquisition of a series of images spanning the haemodynamic response.

In spite of the potential advantages, there are a number of technical and practical challenges for simultaneous EEG and fMRI. The magnetic resonance imaging system is an inhospitable environment for ultrasensitive, passive electromagnetic measurements. High magnetic fields set up interference in both the MR and EEG measurements. Susceptibility effects associated with electrodes can produce artefacts in MRI imaging. Imaging gradients induce currents in electrode leads or pickup coils adding a source of noise and creating a potential safety issue. The motion of conductive and paramagnetic materials (such as blood) within a strong magnetic field can produce strong noise components in the EEG signal, such as the ballistocardiogram. Even sequential experiments may be subject to interference between modalities. For example, MEG studies can be made difficult or impossible due to magnetization of metallic implants, fillings, etc., during a previous MRI session. Although there are analytical strategies or experimental strategies that can be used to address any of these problems, taken together they constitute a significant barrier.

19.2.4 Experimental design issues

Another challenge posed by multimodality experimental methods is the difficulty of simultaneously optimising the experiment for different modalities. Most fMRI studies to date have used blocked, steady-state sensory stimulation or behavioural paradigms in order to produce clearly detectable haemodynamic activation. Comparable steady-state stimulation paradigms can be used with MEG or EEG (Regan 1989), and clever methods have been developed to exploit the high bandwidth of NEM methods for 'frequency tagging' of stimuli—e.g. to identify the origin of responses to lateralized stimuli that may converge on the same cortical areas. However, steady-state methods also introduce problems. For example, phase ambiguity can obscure the details of timing between functional areas. EEG and MEG are easiest to analyse with event-related response paradigms, typically implemented through time-locked averaging of isolated stimulus presentations. Such methods allow randomization of interstimulus intervals to help avoid habituation, and to facilitate manipulation or control of attention, cognitive, or behavioural states. Pseudo-random stimulus sequences can be used to encode particular stimulus types within a rapidly presented train, and correlation techniques can be used to extract the response across time associated with each stimulus in spite of a high degree of temporal overlap.

19.2.5 Event-related fMRI

Recent work has established that even single, transient sensory stimuli elicit an incremental haemodynamic impulse response and that these responses sum approximately linearly, within limits of response saturation (see Chapter 9). Thus by adopting stimulus-locked averaging and overlap correction strategies similar to those used for NEM evoked responses (Woldorf 1993), it is possible to map responses to transient stimulation. This facilitates experimental designs that control for many of the potential confounds associated with studies of sensory processing, but requires more sophisticated synchronization, experimental control and record-keeping. This technique allows the same paradigms to be used for fMRI and NEM studies—an important consideration for comparative or integrated analysis.

Achieving the required stability across a sequence of images is the major challenge in functional MR imaging. This places demands on instruments and on experimental methods and designs. Motion is a principal source of artefact: gross movements (or sub-voxel shifts) can give rise to artefactual subtraction signals in areas of image intensity gradients, that may be confounded with regions of neuronal activation. Physiological motion (e.g. cardio-respiratory changes) also can give rise to apparent signals—or generate noise that reduces signal intensities (see Chapter 12). Fluctuations in blood oxygenation due to the cardiac and respiratory cycles are significant compared to

activity-correlated signals. In a slow steady-state experiment, such fluctuations can substantially average out, but, in an evoked response experiment, unfortunate correlations are more likely and more insidious. However, it is possible to correct for these effects by modeling the unwanted 'noise' by monitoring the physiological processes and removing correlated signals (Hu *et al.* 1995). With adequate models, it may be possible to make adequate corrections without extra measurements. Such considerations will probably drive a shift away from blind signal averaging techniques toward signal decomposition techniques applied on a trial by trial basis.

19.3 NEM source localization

Model-based analyses allow source localization based on MEG and EEG, but it is a demanding computational and theoretical problem. Source reconstruction is an ill-posed, ambiguous problem, and the calculation is often underdetermined for the general source models used for tomographic reconstruction. In general, NEM source localization requires nested models. The first is a head model that allows *forward calculations* of external magnetic fields and potential distributions at the head surface based on a given current source within the head volume conductor. The second component is a source model, describing the spatial distribution of driving currents. The source model is optimized by an *inverse procedure* that optimizes the parameters of the source model according to some criteria.

19.3.1 NEM forward problem

The electromagnetic forward problem employs a physical model of the electrical properties of the head to compute the magnetic fields or potential distribution observed at the surface, given a source current element (or distribution of elements) at a known location and orientation within the head. This scheme is illustrated in Fig. 19.1. A source current element is a distinct neuronal aggregate displaying coherent activity correlated with the task. This calculation may be complex but it is solvable. The computation may incorporate more or less detail, depending on available computational resources and our knowledge of the medium. For some

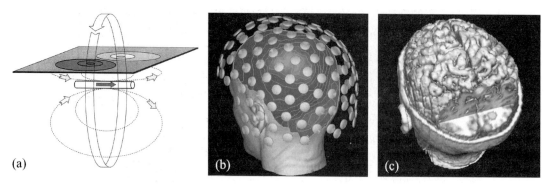

Fig. 19.1   Neural electromagnetic source localization. (a) Neuronal transmembrane currents give rise to longitudinal intracellular currents and extracellular volume return currents. A detectable magnetic field is associated with the intracellular current; extracellular currents tend to cancel in a spherical conducting volume. The extrema of the observed magnetic field distribution straddle and are orthogonal to the source current element. Extrema in the potential distribution are aligned with the current. (b) An array of electrodes or SQUID-based magnetic field detectors are positioned on or over the surface of the head. Potential and field distributions consistent with one or more simple dipole-like sources are often observed. (c) A source model based on a time-varying set of equivalent current dipoles is fit to the observed field distribution. In this figure, the uncertainty of source localization due to noise was estimated using Monte Carlo techniques and a 3D histogram of ECD location was constructed. (See also colour plate section.)

purposes (especially MEG) it may be adequate to assume a homogeneous spherical volume conductor, leading to an analytical solution. Piecewise homogeneous spherical shells may capture enough geometric detail to be adequate for EEG parametric model fitting. Alternatively, it is possible to use detailed anatomical geometry estimated from MRI to define the boundaries of the major conductivity compartments of the head for a boundary element calculation (e.g. Schlitt *et al.* 1995). Full 3D finite element or finite difference calculations can be performed at spatial resolution comparable to that of anatomical MRI. Such measures may be justified if data is available to further discriminate conductivity within compartments, or if fine anatomical details (such as the skull penetrations of the optic nerves and auditory canals) are likely to influence source localization.

19.3.2   Forward modeling in realistic geometries

Given tools for extracting anatomy of the skull and scalp from MRI data and building a computational mesh, it is possible to compute field or potential maps associated with a given current distribution using the boundary element method (BEM). Figure 19.2 shows the sort of information that can be extracted from a 3D

MRI data set. The meshes capture the geometry of the principal conductivity boundaries in a realistic geometry with minimal elements. However, solutions require a large matrix inversion, and may encounter numerical problems for sources locations close to the mesh. Although such problems can be addressed by local or global refinement of the computational mesh, it is unlikely that such an approach will prove practical for general use in a typical linear estimation problem or an iterative, non-linear optimization procedure. Huang and Mosher have developed a method based on *multiple spherical shells* approximating the local anatomy (Huang *et al.* 1998). After setup, this method has computational efficiency approaching that of analytical methods while retaining much of the improved accuracy of the BEM technique. This method, coupled with efficient forward calculations based on truncated Legendre polynomials may provide an adequate basis for EEG source localization. Note that it is not clear whether the computational overhead of full 3D forward calculations is justified, given our limited knowledge of tissue conductivities.

19.3.3   Conductivity estimation via MRI

Advanced MRI imaging strategies, e.g. diffusion tensor MRI (Pierpaoli *et al.* 1996) may provide empirical esti-

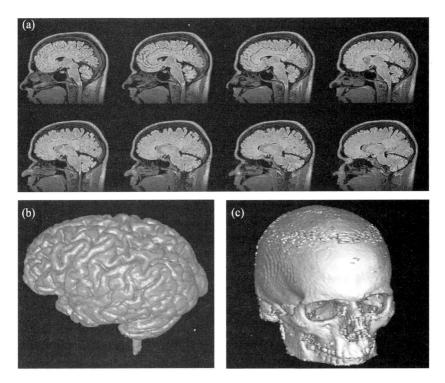

Fig. 19.2 Computational tools for interactive and semi-automatic segmentation of cortical anatomy allow extraction of computational geometries. (a) Region growing algorithms with adaptive criteria perform segmentation of white matter, and identification of grey matter by dilation. (b) 3D rendering of the cortical surface identified by an automatic algorithm. (c) Rendering of the skull segmented by region growing techniques from 3D MRI data. (See also colour plate section.)

mates of conductivity throughout the head for individual subjects. Diffusion tensor imaging discloses striking differences between white matter fibre tracts and grey matter, consistent with anticipated differences in the anisotropy of tissue conductivity. Analysis by Tuch suggests that these measures have a well-defined and predictable relationship to values of tissue conductivity (Tuch *et al.* 1999). Diffusion and conductivity tensors share the same eigenvectors due to the common geometry. The relationship between the eigenvalues for diffusion and conductivity can be derived by employing an 'effective medium' approximation. Making reasonable assumptions regarding the diffusivity, volume fraction and electrical properties of the membrane and intra- and extra-cellular space, this analysis concludes that the conductivity and diffusion are strongly and linearly related.

Whether or not this result is strictly true, diffusion tensor MRI clearly provides information regarding conductivity anisotropy. The consequences of conductivity anisotropy for source localization are not clear. Studies examining the effects of conductivity anisotropy on the EEG forward calculation suggest that white matter anisotropy can profoundly influence the magnitude of observed potential distributions at the head surface, but may not have significant effects on the observed spatial distribution. It is not clear whether this conclusion will apply generally to sources throughout the brain. Consideration of anisotropy may be one key to rationalizing the results of comparable MEG and EEG trials: EEG is strongly influenced by head volume conductivity, while the effects of this on MEG are minimal. The diffusion tensor method will be of only limited utility for estimating the conductivity of the skull, because of its limited water content. Unfortunately, the skull is the most important conductivity value for analysis of EEG data. These limitations underscore the need for more powerful methods to estimate the conductivity of structures within the head.

Wen and Balaban have coupled MRI with ultrasound to characterize conductivity boundaries within tissue (Wen *et al.* 1998). This method exploits the *Hall effect*: conductive bodies moving within a magnetic field accumulate charge at conductivity boundaries. The precise relationship between the signal and tissue conductivity is not clear, nor are the relative merits of the technique. *Current density MRI* measures perturbations of image data produced by passing current through electrodes at the head surface. Although these latter techniques are still under development, they can provide a direct measure of internal currents, which can be used to infer tissue conductivity. Ilmoniemi has described advantages of weak magnetic field detection based on MEG for impedance tomography. It might be feasible to employ MRI for volumetric characterization of the patterns of flow of applied current.

Geometrical constraints derived from head anatomy defined by MRI may play a critical role for conductivity estimation based on electrical impedance tomography (EIT). Techniques for impedance tomography

(passing currents and measuring resulting potentials at surface electrodes) hold unrealized promise for non-invasive measurements of tissue conductivity. MRI-derived anatomical geometry is expected to improve the accuracy of inverse procedures required to reconstruct tissue conductivity from such measures. EIT is a particularly useful strategy for conductivity estimations for EEG source modeling. The measurement can use an existing EEG electrode array with relatively minor modifications to the data system electronics to produce estimates of the most important conductances, in the context of the same head model that will be used for subsequent source localization.

19.3.4 Finite difference calculation

Although boundary element methods can capture the major features of the head geometry, they do have significant limitations. For example, most algorithms are limited to simple topologies, such as a set of non-intersecting shells, and conductivity asymmetries other than the simplest radial or tangential directions cannot be specified. 3D models solved using finite element and

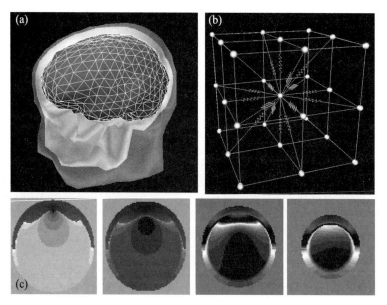

Fig. 19.3 NEM forward modeling in realistic geometries. (a) Boundary Element mesh based on simplified skull and scalp geometry derived from MRI volume imaging. (b) The regular computational mesh employed for finite difference computations in anisotropic media: The nodes for potential computation are at the corners of the spatial volume elements. (c) Several slices through a multi-layer system of spherical shells, used for validation of the finite difference code. A single current dipole source was positioned radially, just below the surface of the 'skull' layer.

finite difference methods can address these concerns, at the expense of computational complexity and time.

As typically employed, finite element methods achieve greater geometric accuracy in a more efficient representation, by constructing a specialized computational geometry. Finite difference methods generally employ a regular computational mesh, well suited to tagged volumetric data; however, new techniques involving embedded domains (such as subdivisions of voxels) promise to deliver improved geometrical fidelity. The essence of finite difference methods typically applied to bioelectric modeling is a simple solution of Poisson's Equation performed through successive over relaxation (SOR), a common linear equation solution method. The finite difference calculation is performed on a regular rectangular grid (Fig. 19.3) corresponding to the resolution of the MRI data used to drive the calculation. The computation of potential at any node is influenced by the 18 nearest neighbours: i.e. the peripheral elements on a $3 \times 3 \times 3$ grid without the eight corner elements (Salaheen and Ng 1997). This scheme can accommodate anisotropic conductivities, such as those estimated by diffusion tensor MRI.

One problem with traditional finite difference solutions is that the consequences of any localized perturbation propagate very slowly away from the site of introduction, since only the immediate neighbour nodes are influenced in any iteration. Thus, considerable computational time is spent waiting for the calculation to spread and settle. Multi-grid geometries can be used to address this problem. By solving the system on both coarse and fine scales and reconciling the results, it is possible to achieve substantial speedups in convergence. Parallel processing strategies and careful attention to updating schemes also can dramatically enhance performance. Multi-grid strategies may also prove useful when dealing with the geometry of fine structures below the resolution of the basic grid.

19.3.5 The neural electromagnetic inverse problem

The process of reconstruction of neural currents from surface MEG or EEG data is called the inverse problem. This problem can have no unique solution, but it is possible to build source models that account for the data. Required elements of a solution include a structure to describe the source model, and a scheme to select and optimize the source model. The accuracy of the solution depends on the validity and applicability of the assumptions that go into the model and the optimization procedure.

The conventional strategy for NEM source localization is to use sources consisting of one or more point current elements or dipoles. Each equivalent current dipole (ECD) is specified with 6–7 parameters, defining the location, orientation and current strength. Because the forward calculation is non-linear with respect to the location parameters, non-linear optimization techniques based on gradient descent strategies typically are used to fit the model. Optimization of dipole orientation and strength is often treated as a separate linear problem, for a given collection of sources. The success of this class of model depends on the selection of an appropriate model order—i.e. the number of dipole-like sources to be fit. As with any non-linear search procedure, there are potential problems with local minima in the error space of the model. The general strategy used to address this problem is to vary the starting parameters used for model optimization in order to identify consistent, robust patterns of convergence. This can be performed by the analyst, or by automatic computational procedures such as the multi-start algorithm described by Huang and Aine and their colleagues (Huang *et al.* 1998; Aine *et al.* 2000). Procedures such as simulated annealing or genetic algorithms incorporate procedural steps to help ensure that the algorithm finds global minima within a given class of models.

A second general strategy is to treat the inverse problem as an exercise in tomographic reconstruction. The reconstruction space is defined by a regular grid, a collection of voxels, or by vertices from a computational mesh. One to three current elements are associated with each possible source location. The objective of the reconstruction procedure is to assign a value to current in each model element. Most strategies for tomographic reconstruction employ large-scale linear methods based on the Moore–Penrose pseudo-inverse. This procedure, based on singular value decomposition, estimates a source distribution with minimum power over the collection of driving currents (Kullmann *et al.* 1989; Hamalainen and Ilmoniemi, 1994). A number of variants on this *minimum norm* procedure have been described, mostly based on different strategies for weighting the lead field basis matrix in order to select a solution with desired properties. Anatomical constraints based on cortical geometry can improve accuracy and efficiency (Wang *et al.* 1992). However, even with substantial reductions of the source space based on anatomy, the inverse is a highly underdetermined problem; there are many more source model parameters to estimate than the number of independent measures available from MEG or EEG.

The major problem with minimum norm procedures is that there is no guarantee that the solution of minimum Euclidean norm (i.e. the sum of squared currents) will be representative of the true solution. Because of the strong dependence of measured magnetic field on distance from the source, the basic minimum norm procedure tends to produce diffuse, superficial current reconstructions, even when the reconstruction space is constrained to the cortical surface (George *et al.* 1991). Currents closer to the sensor array can account for more power in the field map with less current and are therefore favoured by the method. However, more current elements are required to account for the shape of a field distribution that may actually arise from a more focal but deeper source.

In order to combat this tendency to favour solutions with more superficial generators, it is possible to scale the field distributions (or alternatively, the strength of the unit currents) in order to normalize the field power associated with each elemental source. Pseudoinverse procedures based on a normalized basis matrix offer some improvement in the fidelity of reconstructions. A similar idea motivates the magnetic field tomography (MFT) procedure described by Ionnides and colleagues (1990). Explicit or implicit basis matrix weighting procedures have proven to be a useful general strategy for modifying the properties of reconstruction algorithms. The FOCUSS algorithm described by Gorodnitsky *et al.* (1995) employs an iterative re-weighting procedure to derive sparse reconstructions based on focal activated patches. The LORETA algorithm described by Pascual-Marqui (1994), uses an alternative weighting scheme to find current reconstructions that are maximally smooth. As we shall see, weighting procedures can also be used to inject information from fMRI or PET into source localization procedures based on EEG or MEG.

For complex field or potential distributions, many different models might account for any particular observed field distribution. This is often true (to some extent) even for low-order parametric models based on multiple dipoles, although consistent results can often be obtained with proper model order and suitable optimization strategies. For tomographic reconstruction procedures the problem is exacerbated: an infinite number of models can account for the data, and the solution selected will depend critically on the explicit and implicit criteria employed for parameter estimation. Some criteria are based on numerical convenience, but others are driven by our assumptions regarding the nature of typical neural electric sources. For example, dipole models used to fit field or potential maps at a single instance in time are typically much less robust than strategies such as BESA (Scherg and Von Cramen 1986; Mosher *et al.* 1992; Mosher and Leahy 1999) that attempt to fit a temporal sequence of field maps with a minimum set of sources that each have an associated timecourse. For distributed source models it is useful to build models that assume a tendency toward temporal continuity, and source correlation across time and space.

19.4 Combined fMRI and MEG/EEG

Because of the ambiguity associated with the neural electromagnetic inverse problem, a number of investigators have pursued the strategy of using fMRI to define the locations of activation while using MEG or EEG to estimate time-courses.

A growing body of evidence suggests that there is a good (if imperfect) correspondence between neural electrical activation and the fMRI BOLD response, and that convergent information can be used to improve the reliability of macroscopic electrophysiological techniques (e.g. George *et al.* 1995*a*,*b*; Sanders *et al.* 1996). This approach has its pitfalls. In general, there is no guarantee that activation seen in one modality will be apparent in the other. For example, MEG or EEG typically require well-synchronized neuronal activity, consistent across many trials in order to produce a strong signal while fMRI requires a net response averaged over the observation time. The relationship between the precise area of electrophysiological activation and increased blood flow also is not certain. Clearly, at least in some circumstances, fMRI is more sensitive to changes in draining veins than in brain tissue (Frahm *et al.* 1994). It is not obvious in what brain regions or under what conditions the correspondence between NEM and fMRI may be compromised.

19.4.1 Extensions to conventional analytical methods

As described above, conventional source localization procedures for MEG and EEG involve non-linear optimization of a multiple source model based on equivalent current dipoles. The trick in such methods is to generate an initial guess of the structure of the model and its parameters that is close enough so that optimization procedures operating locally can find an adequate model.

If we assume that anatomical MRI constrains the location and orientations of possible source currents and that fMRI provides an estimate of the identity and relative strengths of active voxels, it is possible to define a field distribution associated with an extended source of arbitrary shape and size (George *et al.* 1999).

Figure 19.4 shows the results of such an analysis. These distributions can be used as spatial basis vectors to estimate the time courses of each source, although unless the basis vectors are orthogonal, a unique decomposition is not guaranteed. Alternatively, this putative source field distribution can be used to estimate an equivalent current dipole to be used for subsequent modeling procedures. Many investigators have located an ECD at the centre of mass of a cluster of activated voxels identified through fMRI. However, if the activated cluster has significant extent, the best fitting ECD may be located outside the region of activation (and perhaps outside of cortex). Depending on the distribution of source currents throughout the activated cluster (e.g. mostly parallel vs. antiparallel) the best ECD may be deeper or shallower than the activation extent apparent by fMRI. For these reasons, fMRI is best employed as a method to *seed* dipole source estimates, which then can be optimized using standard non-linear procedures (Ahlfors *et al.* 1999). This strategy provides a measure of flexibility to account for mismatches between assumptions and source model.

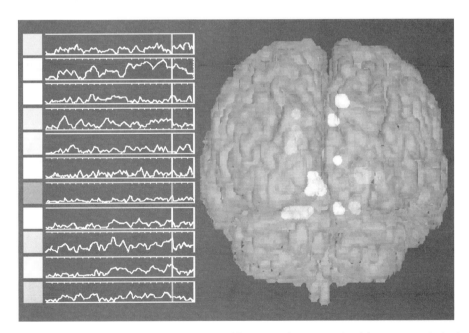

Fig. 19.4   Time courses of fMRI equivalent sources estimated from MEG data. FMRI visual data were acquired using blocked steady state stimulation, using the same video display as in a previous MEG experiment. Currents were assumed to vary within the source according to the distribution of FMRI activation. Currents were constrained to lie normal to cortex as indicated by anatomical MRI. Topographies were derived for each of the assumed sources, and used as basis functions for a linear decomposition of the time-varying field maps. Estimated time courses for 11 areas are coded in colour (See also colour plate section.).

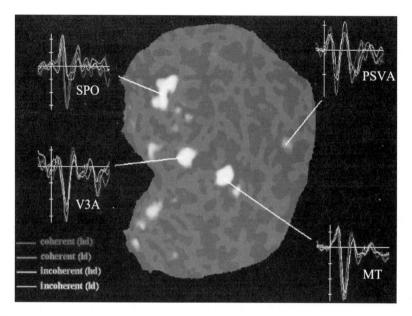

Fig. 19.5 MEG timecourses of fMRI sources using a weighted minimum norm procedure. Areas of activation from a visual fMRI experiment (involving visual motion) are shown on an unfolded cortex. A 0.9:0.1 weighted pseudoinverse procedure was applied to field maps at each time point. Estimated timecourses for activation in four identified visual areas are illustrated. Differences as a function of stimulus type are coded in color. (Data courtesy of Anders Dale and colleagues, Massachusetts General Hospital NMR Centre, Boston). (See also colour plate section.)

Given problems with local minima in non-linear optimization, it may be desirable to seed multiple optimization runs with ECDs based on a source probability distribution estimated from fMRI, or generated by stochastic perturbation of an estimated parameter set.

Dale and colleagues have championed an integrated tomographic inverse procedure based on a form of weighted minimum norm (Fig. 19.5). As in previous work, the inverse solution is constrained to lie within the cortical surface, and source current orientation may be constrained to lie normal to the local surface (Dale and Sereno 1993). Thresholded fMRI can be used as a hard constraint on the reconstruction; i.e. by weighting activated voxels as 1 and other voxels as 0, the solution can be forced to lie within the activated regions disclosed by fMRI. However, if fMRI analysis finds spurious activations (or worse, misses regions that contribute to field distributions observed with MEG or EEG) time course estimates will contain systematic errors. In simulated data, this problem is typically observed as 'crosstalk' between the estimated timecourses of component sources. Using crosstalk as a diagnostic metric, Liu and colleagues (1998) showed

that a 0.9:0.1 weighting scheme captured most of the advantages of fMRI constrained reconstruction while avoiding the most serious problems associated with sources not apparent in the fMRI data.

19.4.2 Bayesian inference

Given the fundamental ambiguity of the inverse problem and the complex error surface associated with the parameter space, there is no guarantee that the proper form of source model (e.g. the number of active sources) can be determined or that a single global minimum can be found, even by reference to fMRI data. The parameter values that are estimated depend critically on model assumptions and may vary widely as a function of small amounts of noise in the data. Methods for integrated analysis across modalities are mostly based on *ad hoc* strategies validated through simulations and tested on experimental data from well-studied systems.

Bayesian analysis techniques provide a formal method for integration of prior knowledge drawn from other imaging methods. In pure form, Bayesian techniques estimate a posterior probability distribution (a form of solution) based on the experimental data and prior knowledge expressed in the form of a probability distribution (Bernardo and Smith 1994; Gelman *et al.* 1997). In addition to providing a flexible mechanism for multimodality integration, these techniques allow rigorous assessment of the consequences of prior knowledge or assumptions about the nature of the preferred solution. Several investigators have explored traditional Bayesian methods, seeking a single 'best' solution that satisfies some criterion, such as a maximum likelihood, maximum a posteriori

(MAP), or maximum entropy solution (Baillet and Garnero 1997; Phillips *et al.* 1997). In this context, a weighted minimum norm solution can be shown to be a maximum likelihood solution with Gaussian priors. However, for reasons discussed previously, any given single solution is effectively guaranteed to be inaccurate, at least in its details. It may be very difficult to characterize the range of acceptable solutions or to quantify confidence intervals for a particular solution. Techniques such as Cramer–Rao bounds are model dependent and make assumptions that reduce reliability as general-purpose tools.

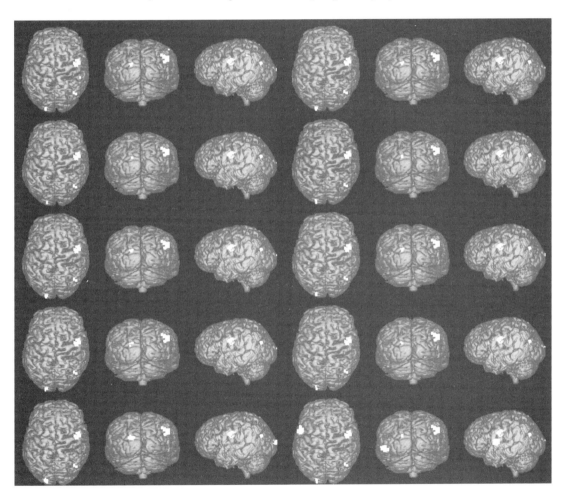

Fig. 19.6 A series of sample solutions from the posterior probability distribution. After 1000 iterations the Markov Chain Monte Carlo algorithm found the same set of three sources in almost every sample, although additional extraneous sources also appear in some solutions. These data were simulated and thus are known to contain three sources in the locations suggested by Bayesian inference.

Schmidt and colleagues (1999*a,b*) have described a technique for Bayesian inference that addresses this concern by explicitly sampling the posterior probability distribution. The strategy is essentially to conduct a series of numerical experiments and to see which stochastic solutions best account for the data. To make the method efficient enough to be practical, a Markov Chain Monte Carlo (MCMC) technique is employed. Figure 19.6 shows the results of a MCMC analysis using simulated data for validation. This is an importance sampling strategy; after the algorithm identifies regions of the source model parameter space that account for the data, by a stochastic process, the algorithm effectively concentrates its sampling in that region. Thus in the end, samples are distributed according to the posterior probability distribution—a probability distribution of solutions upon which all subsequent inferences are based. This method shares some conceptual linkage with the multi-start methods described by Huang and colleagues (Huang *et al.* 1998); however, the latter method is intended to avoid problems of local minima in parameter space, rather than to explore the topography. The Bayesian inference method does not employ optimization procedures and does not produce an estimate of the best fitting solution. Instead, it attempts to build a probability map of activation. This distribution provides a means of identifying and estimating probable current sources from surface measurements while explicitly emphasizing that multiple solutions can account for any set of surface EEG/MEG measurements.

The method for Bayesian inference uses a general neural activation model that can incorporate prior information on neural currents including location,

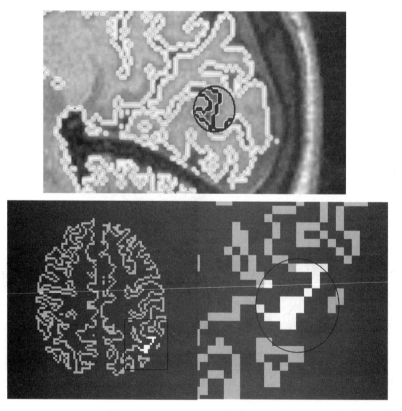

Fig. 19.7 Extended parametric source model used for Bayesian inference. A source defined by the intersection of cortex with a sphere centred on cortex. Note that adjacent sides of a sulcus or gyrus are often labeled together for extended sources. A source defined by a patch grown on the cortical surface. A location on cortex is seeded and adjacent bands of voxels are labeled in a series of dilation operations. (See also colour plate section.)

orientation, strength and spatial smoothness. The method uses an extended parametric model to define sources instead of equivalent current dipoles. An active region is assumed to consist of a set of voxels identified as part of cortex and located within a sphere centred on cortex, or a patch generated by a series of dilation operations about some point on cortex. Figure 19.7 shows examples of such source models There are no assumptions about the relative strength of currents across the source region—only that the active source currents are contained within the patch. Thus the approach incorporates the expectation of sparse and focal regions of neural activation exploited by dipole models without being nearly so restrictive. Studies with simulated data suggest that the extended parametric model may facilitate reliable estimation of the extent of electrical activation. The Bayesian inference technique is the first method for NEM source localization that offers encouragement in this regard.

In a typical analysis, 10 000 samples are drawn from the posterior distribution using a MCMC algorithm. Despite the variability among the samples, several sources common to (nearly) all are often apparent. Features such as these are associated with a high degree of probability, quantifiable because the MCMC samples are distributed according to the posterior probability distribution. By keeping track of the number of times each voxel is involved in an active

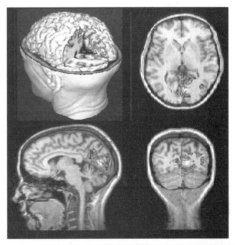

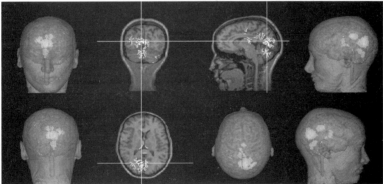

Fig. 19.8 Source probability maps estimated for visual evoked response data. Four views of a region found to contain activity at a 95 per cent probability level. This example is for left visual field stimulation. For right field stimulation, the most probable source is lateralized to the left hemisphere calcarine. Interactive visualization of spatial-temporal source probability maps co-registered with anatomical MRI for the same subject. The anatomical data set was used in the Bayesian inference procedure to constrain sources to lie in cortex. (see also colour plate section)

source over the set of samples, we effectively build a 3D histogram or probability map. By adjusting thresholds it is a simple process to derive confidence intervals. In addition to the information about the locations of probable sources, the Bayesian approach also estimates probabilistic information about the number and size of active regions (Fig. 19.8).

Because Bayesian methods explicitly employ prior knowledge to help solve the inverse problem, they provide a natural and formal method to integrate multiple forms of image data. The simplest strategy is to use fMRI data as a prior. This method can profitably employ the formalism introduced by Frank, and colleagues (1998) for analysis of fMRI data in which they quantify the probability of activation in any particular voxel on the basis of fMRI data. Bayesian methods will also benefit from the efforts to develop probabilistic databases of functional organization.

19.4.3 In-field EEG

Although integrated analysis poses the most serious conceptual challenges, it is only one piece of the puzzle. As previously discussed, it is not always feasible to design experiments that allow clean separation between the trials conducted with incompatible methodologies. Even when it is possible to use precisely the same experimental protocols, there can be confounds due to differences in the state or performance of the subject. A number of circumstances arise where simultaneous measurements are essential to achieve experimental objectives.

A number of laboratories have demonstrated the ability to collect interleaved EEG and fMRI data without endangering the subject or unduly compromising fMRI or EEG data (Lemieux *et al.* 1997). Experiments have employed standard gold plated EEG electrodes modified with a series resistor, or more recently, current-limiting JFET transistors surface mounted at the tip of the electrodes. These components serve as a safety measure to prevent inductive currents associated with time-varying magnetic fields of the MR measurement from being applied to the subject's scalp. In most present experiments the EEG electrodes are routed into a preamplifier box mounted near the MRI head coil. This device amplifies and filters the EEG signals, and encodes channels as a multiplexed analog optical signal that is fibre-optically coupled to the EEG data system

located outside the magnet room. In future systems, it may be useful to perform A/D conversion at the head stage, allowing transmission of digital data.

Several classes of experiments have been conducted to help validate these measurements: spontaneous EEG has been recorded interleaved with fMRI. Subjects were cued to open and close their eyes, modulating alpha activity (8–13 Hz). The anticipated differences in the power spectra were observed. Visual evoked potentials were elicited by photic stimulation, using a strobe flash or stimulation goggles. Responses were acquired interleaved with fMRI, and showed classical VEP waveform morphology, with well-resolved N1, P1, and N2 components (Bonmassar *et al.* 1999). Cognitive event-related potentials (e.g. visual P300) have been recorded during echo-planar imaging in a 3 Tesla magnet using 16 EEG leads. Ictal and interictal activity has been recorded in the magnet and used to trigger fMRI acquisition (Seeck *et al.* 1998; Krakow *et al.* 1999; Symms *et al.* 1999). Recent studies have demonstrated simultaneous acquisition of EEG and fMRI for continuous studies of epilepsy (Allen *et al.* 2000), as well as initial evoked response recordings.

In spite of these encouraging results, there area number of problems with the state of the art. Gradient and RF fields applied during MR imaging produce strong interference. There is no obvious strategy to eliminate this noise source. However, because the MRI acquisition sequences are repetitive and stereotypical, it is likely that the underlying physiological signal might be unmasked with appropriate signal processing strategies. In any case, the EEG recording system settles quickly, and it is possible to design echo planar acquisition sequences with quiescent interludes to allow interleaved EEG acquisition.

Metal electrodes with wire leads can introduce artefacts into the MR images. Induced currents in electrodes can produce heating or shock hazards. Current-limiting components help eliminate the problem of injection of induced currents while helping to insure safety of the imaging subject. A number of investigators (and companies) are examining electrode materials and geometries in an effort to reduce imaging artefacts due to susceptibility. The use of plastic or carbon fiber leads has shown promise for high quality EEG recording without MRI artefact, and soon will be commercially available.

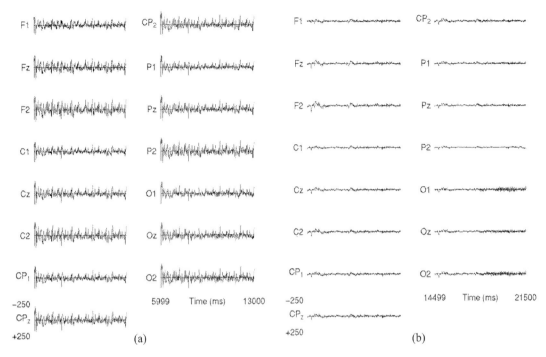

Fig. 19.9   Ballistocardiogram in EEG data. EEG data collected inside (a) and outside (b) the MRI B_0 field in the absence of imaging gradients or RF show the extra noise associated with blood flow (and other movements) within the magnetic field. Such noise can be reduced by spatial filtering, retrospective artefact removal, or by corrections based on references signals acquired during imaging. (Data courtesy of G. Bonmassar and colleagues.)

The human body introduces large noise sources due to mechanical or physiological motion within the ambient magnetic field. A noise component correlated with the respiratory cycle is rather low frequency and can be accommodated with conventional temporal filtering techniques. Another noise component associated with the cardiac cycle—the so-called *ballistocardiogram*—has temporal frequency components overlapping those in normal EEG (Fig. 19.9). Some investigators have employed a spatial Laplacian filter to reduce the ballistocardiogram contribution. Noise cancellation strategies based on monitoring of physiological reference signals such as ECG, blood pressure or perfusion also appear very promising.

19.5 *Impedance tomography*

Accurate forward solutions for both EEG and MEG require accurate specification of head geometry and head tissue conductivities. While it has become common to use structural MRI to provide geometric information, at present, most researchers take conductivity parameters from the literature, even though the large variability of the reported values suggests that these average values are likely to be unreliable. Electrical impedance tomography (EIT) is a method for measuring the head tissue conductivities *in vivo* by injecting small (1–10 µA) currents into the head and measuring the electric potential at the remaining electrodes of a dense EEG sensor array. Both modeling and experimental work suggest that it is possible to make EIT measurements at currents below the levels of 'leakage currents' allowable in FDA approved EEG equipment. Although EIT requires some modification of EEG equipment (e.g. to allow switching of electrodes between passing current and measuring potential) in general the issues for making EIT measurements compatible with MRI are the same as required for EEG.

19.5.1 Constrained parameter estimation

Although in principle, EIT allows 3D reconstruction (Gibson *et al.* 1999), in practice inverse procedures are highly model-dependent and ill-posed. While the actual conductivity of the human head is undoubtedly inhomogeneous and anisotropic, to a first approximation the major conductivity features are those of the brain, cerebrospinal fluid, skull and scalp. Several labs have described methods for estimating the average regional conductivity of each of these four major head tissue compartments (Glidewell and Ng, 1995; Ferree *et al.* 2000). The most obvious challenge to any impedance method in the human head is that, when current is injected into the scalp, the low skull conductivity causes much of the current to be shunted through the scalp. Yet while the skull conductivity is low, it is not zero. Computer simulations using a four-sphere model of the head have shown that scalp potentials so induced are sufficiently sensitive to all tissue conductivities to allow their accurate retrieval (Ferree *et al.* 2000). The method is directly extensible to head models of realistic geometry characterized by a small number of conductivity parameters. Such models are structurally identical to those required for EEG source reconstruction.

19.5.2 Functional EIT

EIT may prove to have substantial utility as a functional imaging technique in its own right. Recent work by Holder and colleagues (1996) has shown that EIT methods can be used to record functional responses. Studies with isolated nerves have recorded fast transient impedance responses (Holder 1992). Studies with whole head EIT measurements in humans have demonstrated evoked responses to sensory stimuli, although in this case, the measurements required long integration times (tens of seconds) that may have prevented resolution of the underlying responses. The mechanisms of such responses are not well understood. In principle, this sort of measurement might be made sensitive to the actual changes in neuronal membrane conduction that give rise to cellular electrical responses. The relative contributions of intracellular and extracellular conduction paths to currents injected at the scalp are not known, though conventional wisdom suggests that extracellular conductivity

will dominate such measurements. However, even extracellular currents might travel conductive paths modulated by neural activation. Several convergent lines of evidence suggest that significant swelling and shrinking of neurones (and thus changes in the extracellular space) accompany neural electrical excitation. These observations will be considered in more detail. Finally, changes in the volume and flow of blood during neural excitation also would be expected to produce detectable changes in impedance measurements from the head surface.

19.6 Optical methods

Optical methods have a number of important advantages for neurophysiological investigations. The technologies are sensitive, mature and cost effective. Detectors based on small high performance CCDs are cheap, yet offer high temporal resolution and information density. Importantly for our purposes, optical methods are compatible with (and complementary to) MRI. They provide a different and rather more specific measure of the haemodynamic processes that drive fMRI, including blood flow and blood oxygenation. Light scattering by tissue obscures the view of deeper processes; however, tomographic strategies based on temporally patterned illumination and time-resolved detection hold considerable promise for 3D measurements.

Optical measures may prove to be a particularly useful adjunct to functional MRI. They provide an alternative measure of haemodynamics; there are clear spectral signatures associated with the level of haemoglobin oxygenation in the visible bands as well as the near infrared. With appropriate techniques these measurements can be made quantitative, even for non-invasive measurements *in vivo*. Optical imaging studies have already provided important insights into the dynamics of haemodynamic regulation on a fine scale. It is likely that invasive optical studies will be one of the keys to unraveling the mechanisms of neurovascular coupling (Frostig *et al.* 1990). Similarly, non-invasive optical studies, probably employing dense fibre optic illumination and sensor arrays will prove useful for characterizing the timecourse of the various processes that taken together comprise the BOLD response.

19.6.1 Haemodynamic reference signals

Although regulation of the cerebral circulation is the basis of fMRI, cardiac and respiratory cycles are sources of periodic fluctuations that pose significant challenges for advanced functional imaging techniques. These cycles entail changes in blood volume and blood oxygenation—the same parameters that provide functional contrast for MRI. The movement of blood in a strong magnetic field gives rise to potentials at the head surface that constitute a large interfering signal. In fMRI paradigms employing blocked stimuli, most analyses integrate over many cycles in both trial and control blocks, so that the consequences of individual fluctuations are effectively suppressed. However, in single trial analyses or evoked response paradigms (where time-locked averages are constructed relative to a stimulus) there is greater potential for stochastic mischief. With limited numbers of trials, an unlucky conjunction of cycles can leave residue in an average response. This sort of problem may have a probability higher than chance, especially if the stimulus rate is fixed and near a harmonic of the frequency of the offending physiological cycle. Also, some subjects have a tendency to synchronize respiration with stimulus presentation, disrupting the phase dispersion that allows averaging to suppress signals not of interest.

Optical measurements can provide reference signals that track the cerebral circulation for the analysis and correction of dynamic interference seen in fMRI and EEG (Fig. 19.10). Using correlation techniques it is possible to characterize and correct for the periodic signals associated with respiration and the cardiac cycle (Allen *et al.* 1998). Although in principle it should be possible to gather the required data by monitoring ECG, respiration and perhaps blood pressure, optical measures can provide a direct measure of the relevant parameters collected at the most relevant site. Optical measures may be made particularly compatible with MRI. Emerging designs for dense optical sensor arrays typically employ optical fibres of plastic, glass or quartz to deliver light to the head surface and to detect light that has diffused through the head. Unlike the metallic leads and electrodes used for EEG and ECG, these materials do not perturb either transient or static magnetic fields. Thus fibre based optical sensors should not interfere with

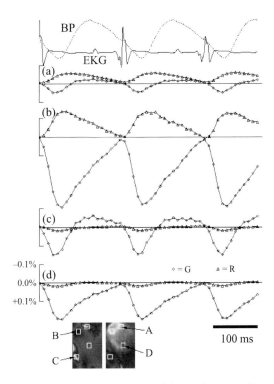

Fig. 19.10 Optical monitoring of haemodynamics, from fast video images collected over the dorsal medulla of rat (Rector *et al.* 1999). Averaged ECG and blood pressure traces are illustrated in upper traces. (a)–(d) illustrate correlated optical signals recorded from indicated regions of interest in the reference images below. Noninvasive optical monitoring may allow correction of cardiac and respiratory interference in event-related functional images.

magnetic resonance imaging, and imaging should not interfere with optical measurements.

19.6.2 Fast optical transient responses

Most functional optical measurements to date (including direct cortical imaging and noninvasive methods) depend on the same sorts of haemodynamic processes that are exploited by fMRI, i.e. changes in blood volume, perfusion and oxygenation. However, there are also a number of reports over the last thirty years or more, that describe fast optical signals that closely tract the dynamics of electrical activation in neural tissue. These fast intrinsic optical signals include changes in light scattering and birefringence. The physical basis of these signals has not been established, although a number of possible mechanisms have been proposed: conformational changes in membrane channels, release and dispersion of neurotransmitter packets, reorganization of cytoskeletal components, uptake of potassium by glial cells. Several lines of evidence suggest that the flow of ions in and out of neurones during electrical activation also may be associated with coincident flow of water to maintain osmotic balance. This suggests that neurones may swell and shrink on timescales comparable to postsynaptic responses or even action potentials. Indeed, there are direct physical measurements that support this interpretation (Watanabe, 1986; Tasaki and Byrne, 1992).

The early demonstrations of fast intrinsic optical signals employed isolated nerves and sensitive single channel detectors. The experiments are challenging because the signals are quite small—on the order of 1 part in 10^5. Given the signal-to-noise limitations of optical measurements, the prospects of imaging these fast signals appeared remote. In the face of these difficulties, efforts shifted toward the development of voltage sensitive and other indicator dyes, to enhance the signals available for fast optical measurements. In the meantime, Grinvald and colleagues demonstrated that intrinsic optical signals associated with local haemodynamic regulation in neural tissue could be imaged using high performance video technology. These signals are typically 1–2 orders of magnitude larger than the fast signals reported earlier. This method has disclosed remarkable features of the spatial organization of the information processing architecture of neural tissue. Although most experiments have involved exposing the tissue to be studied, acceptable images can be collected via endoscope, or even through the skull of small animals such as mice. The success of these optical imaging methods (like the success of BOLD fMRI) underscores the value of functional imaging methods based on intrinsic contrast mechanisms.

In spite of perceived obstacles, we have recently demonstrated that it is possible to image fast intrinsic optical changes in neural tissue *in vivo*.

19.6.3 Invasive dynamic microscopic imaging

We have conducted a series of experiments to characterize optical signals associated with ongoing physiological processes as well as those associated with responses to neural activation (Rector *et al.* 1999, submitted), as shown in Fig. 19.11. These experiments utilized a novel endoscopic imager and high performance CCD technology to record at fast acquisition rates and over a range of tissue depths. Back-scattered light images were continuously digitized (100 frames per second) together with blood pressure, ECG, tracheal pressure, and field potentials. To determine changes in light scattering across time after the stim-

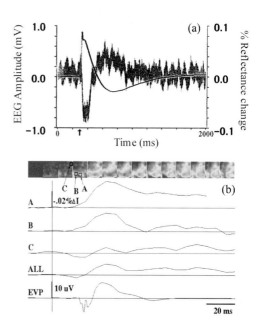

Fig. 19.11   Fast intrinsic optical signals measured *in vivo*. (a) Fast signal measured using a photodiode attached to a fiber optic probe placed on the hippocampus, during electrical stimulation of the corresponding site in the contralateral hippocampus. The noisy signal is optical; the electrical field potential recorded from the same site is illustrated for comparison. (Rector *et al.* 1997). (b) Video imaging of the fast intrinsic optical response from the dorsal medulla of rat, during stimulation of branches of the vagal bundle. A sequence of video frames (each 10 ms) is illustrated across the top. Timecourses of optical responses from identified regions of interest are displayed, along with the field potential measured with a microwire inserted under the focusing image probe. (Rector *et al.* 1999).

ulus, images from each sequence were averaged and divided by an average baseline image. Time averages aligned with the cardiac cycle show patterns that appear haemodynamic in origin. Image sequences using 780 nm illumination through several tissue depths show vessel perfusion. Vessel outlines are apparent in the surface images; images acquired at deeper levels are more diffuse and required a longer time-to-peak intensity, perhaps corresponding to capillary perfusion. Correlations between blood pressure and image intensity on a pixel-by-pixel basis reveal specific regions correlated with various phases of the blood pressure signal.

In these experiments we imaged the dorsal medulla of the rat, an area associated with cardiac and respiratory control. Nerve shocks to the vagal bundle elicited an electrical population spike 30 ms after the stimulus artefact and a population evoked potential with a peak 80 ms after the stimulus artefact. Image sequences showed a distinct spatial pattern of activation within the tissue, with four distinct temporal components: an early positive-going response at 30 ms (P30); an intermediate negative response (N80) which peaked 80 ms after the stimulus; a late and long-lasting negative response (N300); and a slow positive response lasting at least 800 ms (P800). Light-scattering images correlated with blood pressure at three different lag intervals showed various haemodynamic patterns, which differed significantly from the two early response patterns, and were similar to the two slower response patterns. Different stimulus related signals across depth were also observed. The time course and polarity of the slower components matched the haemodynamic mapping responses reported in earlier studies (Grinvald *et al.* 1988). The faster responses (P30, N80) were limited in their spatial distribution and appear to represent light scattering processes directly associated with neural activation (cf. Rector *et al.* 1997).

19.6.4 Non-invasive studies

In addition to these invasive optical imaging studies, a number of laboratories have undertaken the development of non-invasive macroscopic methods for optical tomography and spectroscopy (Fig. 19.12). These methods exploit the fact that light, particularly in the near infrared (NIR), is not strongly absorbed by tissue even though it is highly scattered. Light is differentially

absorbed as it diffuses through tissue; for example, oxy- and deoxyhaemoglobin have different absorption maxima in the NIR between 750 and 850 nm. The strategy for such measurements is to apply light to the scalp at one or many locations via optical fibres, and to collect light with other fibres, at varying distances from the source. Although light diffuses throughout the head, the amount of returning light drops off as a steep function of source-detector separation.

Spectral measurements can be made by applying light at a series of different wavelengths, or by illuminating with white light, dispersing the collected light with a prism or grating and measuring the spectrum in parallel with a detector array such as a CCD. Spectra cannot be analysed quantitatively if the effective path length of the measurement is unknown; the path may vary as a function of wavelength. By using pulsed or high frequency modulated illumination, and time-resolved detection, it is possible to estimate the effective path length for purposes of tomographic reconstruction or quantitative spectroscopy. Alternatively, differential spectroscopy as a function of time or experimental manipulation minimizes the problems with path length, since variations in absorbance are relatively small.

Measurements with continuous illumination and a white light spectrometer described by Mourant *et al.* (1996) detected clear changes in oxygenation of forearm muscle tissue as a function of respiratory manipulations (breath-holds and hyperventilation) and exercise (hand contractions). Changes in cerebral oxygenation were observed in response to respiratory manipulations. Small changes in perfusion and/or oxygenation over motor cortex were observed in response to a task requiring contraction of one hand or the other, consistent with haemodynamic changes in response to neural activation within the motor strip. These studies employed a cooled CCD camera to allow extended integration and high-resolution readout. However, the system did not provide frame rates adequate to resolve physiological fluctuations associated with the cardiac cycle and normal respiration.

19.6.5 Time of flight tomography and spectroscopy

Spectroscopy employing white light provides a wealth of information regarding the species involved in biochemical processes, but such methods are comparatively inefficient, since the light is dispersed among a number of detectors. Also, most white light sources do not provide capability for sub-nanosecond pulses or high frequency modulation. For these reasons, lasers, laser diodes or high output LEDs have typically been employed for time-resolved spectroscopy or optical tomography. Though generally of lower intensity, solid state devices provide a number of practical advantages. Small size facilitates the development of compact instrumentation. Also, power and cooling requirements are less demanding; and often individual devices can be devoted to each illumination channel, eliminating the need for multiplexing and allowing the identity of each source to be encoded in the modulation frequency or in the unique temporal sequence of activation.

Frequency domain techniques have been employed by a number of investigators for dynamic spectroscopy and even rudimentary tomography (Fig. 19.12). Such methods are particularly suitable for infants, given the small size of the heads and the relative transparency of the tissues, but spectrally resolved topographic maps of haemodynamic responses to neural activation can be reliably obtained in adults with suitable techniques (e.g. Benaron *et al.* 2000). 3D tomographic reconstructions are possible using time-resolved or frequency domain data; however, the computational challenges are similar to those confronted by MEG and EEG.

A forward calculation is required to predict the propagation of light through the highly scattering medium of biological tissue. For many purposes this process can be adequately treated as a diffusion process, allowing an analytical solution in simple geometries, and comparatively simple numerical solutions in realistic geometries. However, this approximation does not adequately treat the anisotropy of scattering by large structures such as cellular processes and is therefore least accurate for near-field measurements, which might otherwise provide the greatest spatial detail. While the effects of absorption or scattering centres are most apparent when the perturbation is located near the source or detector, time-resolved detection techniques can be used to selectively probe different volumes within a scattering medium. The path of any given photon can be described as a probability distribution in space. Finite difference procedures can be used to model the

processes of time-resolved (or steady-state) photon transport in considerable detail, given a reasonable model of the properties of the medium. There is little doubt that MRI data could be used to develop more accurate photon transport models and to serve as a spatial constraint on inverse procedures in ways that could substantially improve structural and functional imaging by optical techniques.

19.6.6 Fast noninvasive optical responses

Changes in light scattering by focal regions of neural tissue would be expected to alter the spatial and temporal distribution of light propagating from sources on the head surface. Since most of the probe light is lost through superficial reflection or scattering processes, it is important to design the measurement to maximize the sensitivity to light that penetrates the tissue deeply to interact with activated neural tissue, generally based on the separation between source and detector. Gratton and colleagues have described an apparent change in light scattering detected using non-invasive frequency domain techniques from the head surface (Gratton *et al.* 1997). These event-related optical signals (EROS) were detected as a phase shift in the modulated envelope of light returning to the head surface. These signals are fast, with components that correspond at least roughly to the major components of sensory activation observed with MEG or EEG, however, the signals are tiny. Detection depends on extensive averaging, (often across subjects) and corrections for physiological cycles. Signal topography across the head surface may be quite focal, so that dense sampling is required to resolve or even to reliably detect these signals, but the electronic investment required per channel for time-resolved or frequency domain measurements has limited the development of suitable systems. All of these problems have limited the ability of investigators in the field to extend or even reproduce these results, so that the claims have generated considerable controversy.

Recently, Villringer and colleagues have reported the detection of fast dynamic optic signals from the head surface, using simple continuous wave illumination and detection techniques (Steinbrink *et al.* 2000). Although presently described in a single report, these signals in many respects appear comparable to the images we have collected from the surface of neural

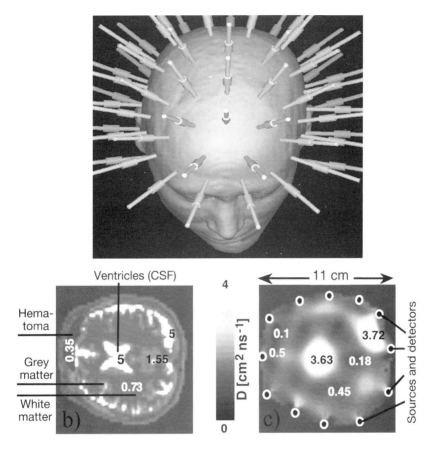

Fig. 19.12 Noninvasive dynamic optical imaging and time-resolved optical tomography. (a) Fiber optics in an array over the surface of the head are used as sources and detectors. Time resolved illumination and detection methods allow tomographic reconstruction or quantitative spectroscopy. Continuous wave methods (i.e. steady illumination and continuous detection) allow dynamic topographic imaging of haemodynamics and fast intrinsic neural signals. (b–c) Path length resolved optical techniques (time-resolved or frequency domain) can be employed for tomographic reconstruction. This reconstruction example used simulated data based on a MRI image (b) containing a haematoma as well as clear cerebral spinal fluid. The simulated optical data consisted of one source and eleven detectors for each of 12 source locations. Reconstructed data (c) captures the major features of the simulated medium although at low resolution. (See also colour plate section.)

tissue. The measurements employ much simpler technology and appear much more robust that the EROS signals reported by Gratton and colleagues. In particular, the technique should be adaptable to the construction of dense sensor arrays, based on low cost, solid state technologies. Figure 19.13 illustrates the type of response that can be obtained.

Such arrays can readily incorporate capabilities for simultaneous EEG and EIT and can be made compatible with MRI (Kleinschmidt *et al.* 1996). This array of complementary methodologies will no doubt enhance the accuracy and extend the range of applications of multi-modality functional imaging for basic neuroscience studies. A compact and low cost integrated sensor array would clearly have implications for the management of clinical conditions such as head trauma or stroke, allowing early and continuous monitoring of cerebral haemodynamics and neurological function while taking optimal advantage of more limited resources such as MR imager time.

19.7 Transcranial magnetic stimulation

The emergence of a range of technologies for non-invasive detection of neural activation has lead to a recent emphasis on the passive mapping of activity elicited by sensory stimulation or endogenous control processes. However, the history of functional brain mapping began with the analysis of functional and behavioural deficits produced by brain lesions associated with natural pathology or head trauma. The detailed mapping of cortical organization began with direct electrical stimulation of cortex, used by neurosurgeons to identify functionally important regions (e.g. for speech or motor control) that must be spared during cortical resection procedures.

Although electrical stimulation of cortex from the head surface is possible, the high resistance skull acts as an insulator to diffuse the focus of current and the scalp current densities required for cortical stimulation produce painful sensations. Magnetic fields are comparatively insensitive to the properties of the medium. A time-varying magnetic field can induce local currents that can stimulate neurones. This prospect has been a matter of concern as MRI has embraced stronger static fields, and strong, rapidly switched gradients. However, this phenomenon has been by exploited by instruments that employ strong transient fields for transcranial magnetic stimulation (TMS) of cortex.

19.7.1 TMS technology

TMS instruments typically employ capacitor discharge or other high current technologies to produce a transient magnetic field of 1 Tesla or more, lasting for a millisecond or less. Many designs employ shaped coils (for example, in a figure eight design) to maximize the intensity of field-induced currents and to sharpen the focus of the activated region. Stimulation coils, initially positioned by hand, are now precisely located with gantry systems or robotic arms (Paus and Wolford, 1998). Work is underway on arrays of coils that can be independently activated. By energizing multiple coils simultaneously, it may be possible to achieve a degree of focus in two dimensions. The physics of electromagnetism suggests that the maximum induced potential will always lie at conductivity

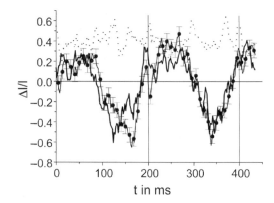

Fig. 19.13   Fast intrinsic optical signal recorded noninvasively using continuous wave technology. The experiment used source and detector fibers separated by 3 cm, positioned over the estimated location of somatosensory cortex. Electrical stimulation of the median nerve was delivered at intervals of 200 ms. A prominent response apparent at ~150 ms post-stimulation varied as a function of source and detector locations, and was not apparent in the control trial illustrated. (Steinbrink *et al.* 2000.)

boundaries with typical stimulation techniques, precluding true 3D focussing. However, by taking into account cortical microgeometry and the optimal current configuration for neuronal excitation, it may be possible to selectively stimulate neurones at other than the most superficial reaches of cortex.

The induction of currents within the brain by magnetic fields generated by external coils is a physics problem closely related to the modeling of MEG signals. In fact, the reciprocity principle suggests that precisely the same computations can be used for both. Thus high resolution electromagnetic models of the brain based on MRI will have utility for fine tuning the pattern of induced excitation. Already, the knowledge of anatomical structure and functional organization provided by MRI, coupled with simple analytical models of generated fields allow rather precise targeting of stimulation.

19.7.2 TMS applications

Existing TMS systems have been used for two principal applications: First, the system can be used to directly stimulate cortex. This effect can be detected through evoked motor responses, or by sensory percepts such as visual phosphenes. It is also possible to objectively measure the consequences of neural activation using EEG, fMRI or PET. Obviously any of these methods requires careful attention to safety as well as electronic interference issues (Virtanen *et al.* 1999). Second, by stimulating a selected region of neural tissue en masse, TMS can transiently interfere with the capacity of the tissue to process physiological input during the period of neuronal insensitivity following induced generation of an action potential. Thus, precisely timed TMS pulses can be used to disrupt neuronal processing, producing a 'transient lesion' that can be used to probe the location and timing of waystations in a processing stream of interest. For example, it is possible to block detection of visual stimuli (measured behaviourally) with a TMS pulse delivered 80–100 ms post-stimulus. This sort of effect might also explain anecdotal (and mostly discounted) reports of the efficacy of 'magnetic feedback' to suppress epileptic seizures. A TMS pulse delivered shortly after the onset of an ictal event might render the surrounding tissue refractory, limiting the spread and thus preventing the generation of a full blown seizure.

Previous work has demonstrated the feasibility of TMS measurements interleaved with functional imaging (Ilmoniemi *et al.* 1999; Bohning *et al.* 1997, 1999; Paus *et al.* 1997; Paus, 1999). Combination of TMS with PET (or even EEG) poses fewer technical problems than multi-modality studies with fMRI. Initial reported studies involved moving the TMS coil in and out of the vicinity of the head, in order to minimize possible electromagnetic interference as well as mechanical problems associated with the forces generated by strong magnetic fields. Some of the pioneers in this work suggest that the technical problems associated with fMRI/TMS might be addressed by engineered solutions, including integrated systems. For example, it could be possible to incorporate stimulation coil systems within the radiofrequency head coil assemblies used for MRI (O. Josephs, personal communication). The techniques required to minimize interactions between stimulating coil arrays and MR components are closely related to the engineering solutions required to minimize coupling between RF and gradient coils in high performance gradient inserts, and to accommodate RF transmission and receiving with the same tuned coils.

19.8 Advanced fMRI techniques

Initial fMRI techniques involved injection of paramagnetic contrast agents, and measurements of blood volume. Although these techniques are clearly more invasive they have advantages in SNR and are based on a well-established contrast mechanism. These methods have largely been supplanted by noninvasive contrast techniques such as arterial spin labeling (for perfusion) or BOLD, but they serve as a reminder that there are many physical correlates of neural activity that might be accessible to MRI measurement techniques.

19.8.1 Diffusion imaging

One method of interest is diffusion weighted MRI. This method, often used in conjunction with bolus tracking perfusion techniques, holds great promise for assessment of stroke. In such settings it sensitizes the image contrast to changes in the self-diffusion of water in tissue, which is found to change markedly following ischaemia. An interesting question that has been posed recently is: are there also reasons to think that there may be transient changes in the measured diffusion coefficient of water as a consequence of neural activation?

As described above, optical measures provide one line of evidence. Although some changes in scattered light may reflect haemodynamic changes, e.g. in the density of red blood cells or of haemoglobin, several investigators have provided evidence that some of the changes in neural tissue that give rise to changes in scattered light may depend on swelling and shrinking of cells. It is notable that optical changes can be observed in slice preparations, in the absence of circulation. Fast optical changes in isolated nerves were reported over thirty years ago. We have recently shown that fast intrinsic optical signals can be imaged from brain tissue *in vivo*. In addition to optical measures, evidence for such responses has been obtained with direct physical measurements of pressure and displacement (see Watanabe 1986 for reviews ; Cohen 1973).

Given the known physics of selective ion and water movements across neuronal cell membranes, it would be surprising if neuronal swelling and shrinking were not observed. It is not clear whether such responses would be more pronounced for the intra-cellular or extracellular spaces in diffusion-weighted MR measurements. Recent measurements (reported in abstract form by Le Bihan and colleagues) show changes in DW signals stimulated by neural activity. The experiments reported did not have the temporal resolution adequate to test predictions of fast signals, although the responses appear to be faster than the imaging rate. It is not clear that signal-to-noise will be sufficient for the technique to be useful. Still, the possibility of a diffusion weighted fMRI technique that might track neural activation dynamics is a very appealing prospect that deserves further investigation.

19.8.2 MRI measurements of neural magnetic fields

An even more appealing (though more challenging) prospect is the direct measurement of neural magnetic field transients *in situ* by MRI. This would deliver the advantages of MEG without the problems of source localization posed by the inverse problem: if we can map magnetic field throughout the volume, we can infer sources without the ambiguity of surface mapping techniques. The physics problem is closely related to current density MRI, except that current sources are located at unknown locations somewhere in the volume of the brain.

There are clearly serious technical challenges. The magnetic fields produced by neuronal activation are tiny—only tens to hundreds of femtoT (10^{-15} Tesla) at the head surface. These fields drop off rapidly with distance from the source; at the site of activation the local field perturbation is perhaps hundreds of picoT to 1 nanoT. Recent work involving computational simulation and experimental data from specialized phantoms has demonstrated the feasibility of detecting field perturbations of this magnitude in phase images acquired at 3 Tesla (recently published in abstract form by Bandettini and colleagues). However, given the small size of these perturbations there might be advantages to making measurements at lower field. Such a strategy might enhance contrast by increasing the ratio $\Delta B{:}B_0$, although it is likely to create problems in the signal-to-noise ratio, as the resonance peak would shift to a lower frequency. The limitations of thermal magnetization also become more apparent at lower field. The use of a pulsed B_0 field might allow

strong polarization while allowing spin preparation and signal acquisition to be accomplished at lower field strengths. Alternatively, optical pumping allows very high levels of polarization to be achieved at low fields. However, the delivery of adequate quantities of hyperpolarized gas through the circulation to the brain is an unresolved problem.

The prospect of fMRI imaging techniques capable of resolving the characteristic dynamics of neural activation poses new technical challenges as well as new opportunities. In the past, the MR image acquisition has been faster than the processes that give rise to functional contrast. If MRI is able to see processes that track the dynamics of the neural electrical response, the methods will require considerably faster imaging, with frame times of 5 ms or less. The most reasonable strategy to achieve this end is to reduce or eliminate the need for phase encoding. Several methods for faster imaging have been described in earlier work (e.g. Feinberg and Oshio 1992; Sodickson and Manning 1997; Sodickson 2000) and earlier chapters. Methods employing multiple receiver coils are at least superficially similar to MEG technology. As in MEG there are possible advantages in the use of cryogenic coils, superconducting detector circuitry, and measurements at lower ambient fields. Although such methods clearly involve significant technical challenges, the development path is reasonably clear, and the goal achievable given sufficient motivation. The prospect of tracking neural population dynamics using MRI-based techniques may provide such motivation.

19.9 *Summary*

No single imaging method provides all of the information desired by investigators exploring the principles of brain function, or by clinicians interested in diagnosing and intervening in cases of neurological pathology or mental health disorders. MRI is in many respects the leading methodology, in part because the same basic technology supports a wide range of techniques that can probe many different aspects of physiology and anatomy. Soft tissue geometry provided by MRI provides an organizational framework for all forms of functional data, and allows construction of the physical models required by many other functional measurement techniques. MRI can provide direct estimates of some of the physical parameters required by such models. FMRI can be used to develop source models that can be applied to data from EEG and MEG to estimate the timecourses of an ensemble of sources. Although such methods have pitfalls, emerging methods for integrated analysis can circumvent some of these problems. Bayesian techniques hold particular promise for providing dynamic spatio-temporal maps of activation in extended networks of the brain, complete with the information required to assess the confidence that should be placed in such results. Meanwhile, the continuing development of individual measurement technologies, as well as the methods to facilitate simultaneous measurements with rather incompatible technologies, will expand the arsenal of methods available to the neuroscientist or physician for understanding the architecture and dynamic function of the human brain.

Acknowledgement

Portions of the work described here were supported by MH 60993, a Human Brain Project/Neuroinformatics research project funded jointly by the National Center for Research Resources, National Institute of Mental Health, National Institute on Drug Abuse and the National Science Foundation.

References

Ahlfors, S.P., Simpson, G.V., Dale, A.M., Belliveau, J.W., Liu, A.K., Korvenoja, A., Virtanen, J., Huotilainen, M., Tootell, R.B., Aronen, H.J., and Ilmoniemi, R.J. (1999). Spatiotemporal activity of a cortical network for processing visual motion revealed by MEG and fMRI. *Journal of Neurophysiology*, **82**, 2545–55.

Aine, C.J., Supek, S., George, J.S., Ranken, D., Lewine, J., Sanders, J., Best, E., Tiee, W., Flynn, E.R., and Wood, C.C. (1996). Retinotopic organization of human visual cortex: Departures from the classical model. *Cerebral Cortex*, 6, 354–61.

Aine, C., Huang, M., Stephen, J., and Christner, R. (2000). Multi-start algorithms for MEG empirical data analysis reliable characterize locations and time-courses of multiple sources. *NeuroImage*, **12**, 159–72.

Allen, P.J., Polizzari, G., Krakow, K., Fish, D.R., and Lemieux, L. (1998). Identification of EEG events in the MR scanner: the problem of pulse artifact and a method for its subtraction. *NeuroImage*, 8(3), 229–39.

Allen, P.J., Josephs, O., and Turner, R. (2000). A method for removing imaging artifact from continuous EEG recorded during functional MRI. *NeuroImage*, **12**(2), 230–39.

Baillet, S. and Garnero, L. (1997). A Bayesian approach for introducing anatomical priors in the EEG/MEG inverse problem. *IEEE Transactions Biomedical Engineering*, 44(5), 374–85.

Bandettini, P.A., Wong, E.C., Hinks, R.S., Tikofsky, R.S., and Hyde, J.S. (1992). Time course EPI of human brain function during task activation. *Magnetic Resonance in Medicine*, 25, 390–97.

Belliveau, J.W., Kennedy, D.N., McKinstry, R.C., Buchbinder, B.R., Weisskoff, R.M., Cohen, M.S., Vevea, J.M., Brady, T.J., and Rosen, B.R. (1991). Functional mapping of the human visual cortex by magnetic resonance imaging. *Science*, **254**, 716–19.

Benaron, D.A., Hintz, S.R., Vilringer, A., Boas, D., Kleinschmidt, A., Frahm, J. *et.al.*, (2000). Noninvasive functional imaging of human brain using light. *Journal of Cerebral Blood Flow and Metabolism*, **20**(3), 469–77.

Bernardo J and Smith A (1994). *Bayesian Theory*. Wiley, New York.

Bohning, D.E., Shastri, A., Nahas, Z., Lorderbaum, J.P., Anderson, S.W., Dannels, W.R., Haxthausen, E.U., Vincent, D.J., and George, M.S. (1997). Echoplanar BOLD fMRI of brain activation induced by concurrent transcranial magnetic stimulation. *Investigative Radiology*, **33**(6), 336–40.

Bohning, D.E., Shastri, A., McConnell, K.A., Nahas, Z., Loderbaum, J.P., Roberts, D.R., Teneback, C., Vincent, D.J., and George, M.S. (1999). A combined TMS/fMRI study of intensity-dependent TMS over motor cortex. *Biological Psychiatry*, **45**(4), 385–94.

Bonmassar, G., Anami, K., Ives, J., and Belliveau, J.W. (1999). Visual evoked potential (VEP) measured by simultaneous 64-channel EEG and 3T fMRI. *NeuroReport*, **10**(9), 1893–97.

Cohen, L.B. (1973). Changes in neurone structure during action potential propagation and synaptic transmission. *Physiological Review*, **53**(2), 373–413.

Dale, A. and Sereno, M. (1993). Improved localization of cortical activity by combining EEG and MEG with MRI cortical surface reconstruction: A linear approach. *Journal of Cognitive Neuroscience*, **5**, 162–76.

Ferree, T.C., Eriksen, K.J., and Tucker, D.M. (2000). Regional head tissue conductivity estimation for improved EEG analysis. *IEEE Transactions of Biomedical Engineering*, 47(12), 1584–92.

Feinberg, P.A. and Oshio, K. (1991). GRASE (Gradient- and spin-echo imaging): a novel fast MRI technique. *Radiology*, **181**, 597–602.

Frahm, J., Merboldt, K.-D., Hanicke, W., Kleinschmidt, A., and Boecker, H. (1994). Brain or vein-oxygenation or flow? On signal physiology in functional MRI of human brain activation. *NMR in Biomedicine*, 7, 1–9.

Frank, L.R. Buxton, R.B., and Wong, E.C. (1998). Probabilistic analysis of functional magnetic resonance imaging data. *Magnetic Resonance in Medicine*, **39**, 132–48.

Frostig, R.D., Lieke, E.E., Ts'o, D.Y., and Grinvald, A. (1990). Cortical functional architecture and local coupling between neuronal activity and the microcirculation revealed by *in vivo* high-resolution imaging of intrinsic signals. *Proceedings of the National Academy of Sciences (USA)*, 87, 6082–6.

Gelman, A., Carlin, J.B., Stern, H.S., and Rubin, D.B. (1997). Bayesian Data Analysis. London. Chapman and Hall.

George, J.S., Jackson, P.S., Ranken, D.M., and Flynn, E.R. (1989). Three-dimensional volumetric reconstruction for neuromagnetic source localization. In: *Advances in Biomagnetism* (ed. S.J. Williamson, M. Hoke, G. Stroink and M. Kotani), pp.737–40, Plenum, New York.

George, J.S., Lewis, P.S., Ranken, D.M., Kaplan, L., and Wood, C.C. (1991). Anatomical constraints for neuromagnetic source models. *SPIE Medical Imaging V: Image Physics*, 1443, 37–51.

George, J.S., Sanders, J.S., Lewine, J.D., Caprihan, A., and Aine, C.J. (1995a). Comparative studies of brain activation with MEG and Functional MRI. In: *Biomagnetism: Fundamental Research and Clinical Applications* (ed. C. Baumgartner *et al.* pp. 60–5. Elsevier/ IOS, Amsterdam.

George, J.S., Aine, C.J., Mosher, J.C., Schmidt, D.M., Ranken, D.M., Schlitt, H.A., Wood, C., Lewine, J.D., Sanders, J.A., and Belliveau, J.W. (1995b). Mapping function in the human brain with MEG, anatomical MRI and functional MRI. *Journal of Clinical Neurophysiology*, 12(5), 406–31.

George, J.S., Schmidt, D.M., Mosher, J.C., Aine, C.J., Ranken, D.M., Wood, C.C., Lewine, J.D., Sanders, J.A., and Belliveau, J.W. (1999). In: *Dynamic neuroimaging by MEG, constrained by MRI and fMRI*, (ed. C.J. Aine, E.R. Flynn, Y. Okada, G. Stroink, S.J. Swithenby, and C.C. Wood), pp. 1134–37. *Biomag96: Proceedings of the Tenth International Conference on Biomagnetism vII*, Springer, New York.

Gibson, A., Bayford, R.H., and Holder, D.S. (1999). Development of a reconstruction algorithm for imaging impedance changes in the human head. *Annals New York Academy of Science*, 873, 482–92.

Glidewell, M.E. and Ng, K.T. (1995). Anatomically constrained electrical impedance tomography for anisotropic bodies via a two-step approach. *IEEE Transactions of Medical Imaging*, 14, 498–503.

Gorodnitsky, I., George, J.S., and Rao, B.D. (1995). Neuromagnetic source imaging with FOCUSS: A recursive weighted minimum norm algorithm. *Electroencephalography and Clinical Neurophysiology*, 95, 231–51.

Gratton, G., Fabiani, M., Corballis, P.M., and Gratton, E. (1997). Noninvasive detection of fast signals from the cortex using frequency-domain optical methods. *Annals New York Academy of Sciences*, 820, 286–98.

Grinvald, A., Frostig, R.D., Lieke, E., and Hildesheim, R. (1988). Optical imaging of neuronal activity. *Physiological Reviews*, 68(4), 1285–368.

Hamalainen, M.S. and Ilmoniemi, R.J. (1994). Interpreting magnetic fields of the brain: Minimum norm estimates. *Medical and Biological Engineering and Computing*, 32(1) 35–42.

Hamalainen, M.S., Hari, R., Ilmoniemi, R.J., Knuutila, J., and Lounasmaa, O.V. (1993). Magnetoencephalography— theory, instrumentation and applications to non-invasive studies of the working human brain. *Rev. Mod. Phys.*, 65(2), 413–97.

Holder, D.S. (1992) Impedance changes during the compound nerve action potential: implications for impedance imaging of neuronal depolarization in the brain. *Medical and Biological Engineering and Computing*, 30(2), 140–6.

Holder, D.S., Rao, A., and Hanquan, Y. (1996). Imaging of physiologically evoked responses by electrical impedance tomography with cortical electrodes in the anaesthetized rabbit. *Physiological Measurement*, 17(S4A), A179-A186.

Hu, X., Le, T.H., Parrish, T., and Erhard, P. (1995). Retrospective estimation and correction of physiological fluctuation in functional MRI. *Magnetic Resonance in Medicine*, 34, 201–12.

Huang, M., Aine, C.J., Supek, S., Best, E., Ranken, D.R., and Flynn, E.R. (1998). Multi-start downhill simplex method for spatio-temporal source localization in magnetoencephalography. *Electroencephalography and Clinical Neurophysiology*, 108, 32–44.

Ilmoniemi, R.J., Ruohonen, J., and Karhu, J. (1999). Transcranial magnetic stimulation: a new tool for functional imaging of the brain. *Critical Reviews in Biomedical Engineering*. 27, 241–84.

Ioannides, A.A., Bolton, J.P.R., and Clarke, C.J.S. (1990). Continuous probabilistic solutions to the biomagnetic inverse problem, *Inverse Problems*, 6, 523–42.

Kleinschmidt, A., Obrig, H., Requardt, M., Meboldt, K.D., Dirnagl, U., Villringer, A., and Frahm, J. (1996). Simultaneous recording of cerebral blood oxygenation changes during human brain activation by magnetic resonance imaging and near-infrared spectroscopy. *Journal of Cerebral Blood Flow and Metabolism*, 16(5), 817–26.

Krakow, K., Woermann, F.G., Symms, M.R., Allen, P.J., Lemieux, L., Barker, G.J., Duncan, J.S., and Fish, D.R. (1999). EEG-triggered functional MRI of interictal epileptiform activity in patients with partial seizures. *Brain*, 122, 1679–88.

Kullmann, W.H., Jandt, K.D., Rehm, K., Schlitt, H.A., Dallas, W.J., and Smith, W.E. (1989). A linear estimation approach to biomagnetic imaging. In: *Advances in Biomagnetism*. (ed. S.J. Williamson, M. Hoke, G. Stroink, and M. Kotani), pp.571–74, Plenum, New York.

Kwong, K.K., Belliveau, J.W., Chesler, D.A., Goldberg, I.E., Weisskoff, R.M., Pouncelet, B.P., Kennedy, D.N., Hoppel, B.E., Cohen, M.S., Turner, R., Cheung, H.-M., Brady, T.J., and Rosen, B.R. (1992). Dynamic magnetic resonance imaging of human brain activity during primary sensory stimulation. *Proceedings of the National Academy of Sciences (USA)*, 89, 5675–9.

Lemieux, L., Allen, P.J., Franconi, F., Symms, M.R., and Fish, D.R. (1997). Recording of EEG during fMRI experiments: Patient safety. *Magnetic Resonance in Medicine*, 38(6), 943–52.

Liu, A.K., Belliveau, J.W., and Dale, A.M. (1998). Spatiotemporal imaging of human brain activiy using functional MRI constrained magnetoencephalography data: Monte Carlo simulations. *Proceedings of the National Academy of Sciences (USA)*, 95(15), 8945–50.

Mitzdorf, U. (1985). Current source-density method and application in cat cerebral cortex: Investigation of evoked potentials and EEG phenomena. *Physiological Reviews*, **65**. 37–100.

Mosher, J.C. and Leahy, R.M. (1999). Source localization using recursively applied and projected (RAP) MUSIC. *IEEE Trans. on Sig. Proc.*, **47**(2), 332–40.

Mosher, J.C., Lewis, P.S., and Leahy, R. (1992). Multiple dipole modeling and localization from spatio-temporal MEG data. *IEEE Trans. Biomed. Eng.*, **39**, 541–57.

Mourant, J.R., Hielscher, A.H., Miller, H.D., and George, J.S. (1996). Broadband Monitoring of physiological changes with a continuous light tissue spectrometer. In: *OSA TOPS on Biomedical Spectroscopy and Diagnostics*. (ed. E.M. Sevick-Muraca and D.A. Benaron, **3**, 37–42, Optical Society of America.

Ogawa, S., Tank, D.W., Menon, R., Ellerman, J.M., Kim, S.-G., Merkle, H., and Ugurbil, K. (1992). Intrinsic signal changes accompanying sensory stimulation: functional brain mapping using MRI. *Proceedings of the National Academy of Sciences (USA)*, **89**, 5951–5.

Paus, T. (1999). Imaging the brain before, during and after transcranial magnetic stimulation. *Neuropsychologia*, **37**(2), 219–24.

Paus, T. and Wolforth, M. (1998). Transcranial magnetic stimulation during PET: reaching and verifying the target site. *Human Brain Mapping*, **6**, 399–402.

Paus, T., Jech, R., Thompson, C.J., Comeau, R., Peters, T., and Evans, A.C. (1997). Transcranial magnetic stimulation during positron emission tomography: a new method for studying connectivity of the human cerebral cortex. *Journal of Neuroscience*, **17**(9), 3178–84.

Pascual-Marqui, R.D., Michel, C.M., and Lehmann, D. (1994). Low Resolution Electromagnetic Tomography: a new method for localizing electrical activity in the brain. *International Journal of Psychophysiology*, **18**, 49–65.

Phillips, J.W., Leahy, R.M., Mosher, J.C. (1997). MEG-based imaging of focal neuronal current sources. *IEEE Trans. Med. Imag.*, **16**(3), 338–48.

Pierpaoli, C., Jezzard, P., Basser, P.J., Barnett, A., and Di Chiro, G. (1996). Diffusion tensor MR imaging of the human brain. *Radiology*, **201**(3), 637–48.

Ranken, D.M. and George, J.S. (1993). MRIVIEW: An interactive computational tool for investigation of brain structure and function. *Visualization {cq}93*, IEEE Computer Society.

Rector, D.M., Poe, G.R., Kristensen, M.P., and Harper, R.M. (1997). Light scattering changes follow evoked potentials from hippocampal schaffer collateral stimulation. *Journal of Neurophysiology*, **78**, 107–17.

Rector, D.M., Rogers, R.F., and George, J.S. (1999). A focusing image probe for assessing neural activity *in vivo*. *Journal of Neuroscience Methods*, **91**, 135–45.

Rector, D.M., Rogers, R.F., Schwaber, J.S., Harper, R.M., and George, J.S. (submitted). Rapid evoked optical responses imaged from the rat dorsal brainstem *in vivo*.

Regan, D. (1989). *Human brain electrophysiology: evoked potentials and evoked magnetic fields in science and medicine*, Elsevier, New York.

Salaheen, H. and Ng, K.T. (1997). New finite difference formulations for general inhomogeneous anisotropic bioelectric problems. *IEEE Transactions of Biomedical Engineering*, **44**(9), 800–09.

Sanders, J.A., Lewine, J.D., and Orrison, W.W. (1996). Comparison of primary motor cortex localization using functional magnetic resonance imaging and magnetoencephalography. *Human Brain Mapping*, **4**, 47–57.

Sarvas, J. (1987). Basic mathematical and electromagnetic concepts of the biomagnetic inverse problem. *Physics in Medicine and Biology*, **32**, 11–22.

Scherg, M. and Von Cramen, D. (1986). Evoked dipole source potentials of the human auditory cortex. *Electroencephalography and Clinical Neurophysiology*, **65**, 344–60.

Schmidt, D.M., George, J.S., and Wood, C.C. (1999*a*). Bayesian Inference applied to the electromagnetic inverse problem. *Human Brain Mapping*, **7**, 195–212.

Schmidt, D.M. and George, J.S. (1999*b*). A method for locating regions containing neural activation at a given confidence level from MEG data. In: *Biomag96: Proceedings of the Tenth International Conference on Biomagnetism v1*. (ed. C.J. Aine, E.R. Flynn, Y. Okada, G. Stroink, S.J. Swithenby and C.C. Wood), pp.334–37, Springer, New York.

Schlitt, H., Heller, L., Aaron, R., Best, E., and Ranken, D. (1995). Evaluation of boundary element methods for the EEG forward problem: effect of linear interpolation. *IEEE Transactions of Biomedical Engineering*, **42**(1), 52–8.

Seeck, M., Lazeyras, F., Michel, C.M., Blanke, O.I., Gericke, C.A., Ives, J., Delavelle, J., Golay, X., Haenggeli, C.A., de Tribolet, N., and Landis, T. (1998). Non-invasive epileptic focus localization using EEG-triggered functional MRI and electromagnetic tomography. *Electroencephalography and Clinical Neurophysiology*, **106**, 508–12.

Sereno, M.I., Dale, A.M., Reppas, J.B., Kwong, K.K., Belliveau, J.W., Brady, T.J., Rosen, B.R., and Tootell, R.B. (1995). Borders of multiple visual areas in humans revealed by functional magnetic resonance imaging. *Science*, **268**, 889–93.

Sodickson, D.K. (2000). Tailored SMASH image reconstructions for robust *in vivo* parallel MR imaging. *Magnetic Resonance in Medicine*, **44**(2), 243–51.

Sodickson, D.K. and Manning, W.J. (1997). Simultaneous acquisition of spatial harmonics (SMASH): fast imaging with radiofrequency coil arrays. *Magnetic Resonance in Medicine*, **38**(4), 591–603.

Stehling, M.K., Turner, R., and Mansfield, P. (1991). Echo-planar imaging: magnetic resonance imaging in a fraction of a second. *Science*, **254**, 43–50.

Steinbrink, J., Kohl, M., Obrig, H., Curio, G., Syre, F., Thomas, F., Wabntz, H., Rinneberg, H., and Villringer, A. (2000). Somatosensory evoked fast optical intensity changes detected non-invasively in the adult human head. *Neuroscience Letters*, **291**, 105–08.

Symms, M.R., Allen, P.J., Woermann, F.G., Polizzi, G., Krakow, K., Barker, G.J., Fish, D.R., and Duncan, J.S. (1999). Reproducible localization of interictal epileptiform discharges using EEG-triggered fMRI. *Physics in Medicine and Biology*, **44**(7), N161–68.

Tasaki, I. and Byrne, P.M. (1992). Rapid structural changes in nerve fibers evoked by electrical current pulses. *Biochemical and Biophysical Research Communications*, **188**(2), 559–64.

Tuch, D.S., Wedeen, V.J., Dale, A.M., George, J.S., and Belliveau, J.W. (1999). Conductivity mapping of biological tissue using diffusion MRI. *Annals New York Academy of Sciences*, **888**, 314–16.

Virtanen, J., Ruohonen, J., Naatanen, R., Ilmoniemi, R.J. (1999). Instrumentation for the measurement of electric brain responses to transcranial magnetic stimulation. *Medical and Biological Engineering and Computing*, **37**(3), 322–6.

Wang, J.-Z., Williamson, S.J., and Kaufman, L. (1992). Magnetic source images determined by a lead-field analysis: the unique minimum-norm least-squares estimation. *IEEE Transactions of Biomedical Engineering*, **39**, 665–75.

Watanabe, A. (1986). Mechanical, thermal and optical changes of the nerve membrane associated with excitation. *Japanese Journal of Physiology*, **36**, 625–43.

Wen, H., Shah, J., and Balaban, R.S. (1998). Hall Effect imaging. *IEEE Transactions of Biomedical Engineering*, **45**(1), 119–24.

Woldorf, M.G. (1993). Distortion of ERP averages due to overlap from temporally adjacent ERPs: Analysis and correction. *Psychophysiology*, **30**, 98–119.

Index